LOCAL ANESTHESIA
for the Dental Hygienist

Demetra Daskalos Logothetis, RDH, MS
Professor and Vice Chair, Department of Dental Medicine
Director, Division of Dental Hygiene
University of New Mexico
Albuquerque, New Mexico

ELSEVIER
MOSBY

ELSEVIER
MOSBY

3251 Riverport Lane
St. Louis, Missouri 63043

Vice President and Publisher: Linda Duncan
Acquisitions Editor: John Dolan
Managing Editor: Kristin Hebberd
Developmental Editor: Joslyn Dumas
Publishing Services Manager: Julie Eddy
Project Manager: Kelly Milford
Design Direction: Kim Denando

Printed in United States of America

Last digit is the print number: 9 8 7 6 5 4 3 2 1

To my husband Nick who means the world to me, without your constant love, support, and encouragement I would be lost.

To my children Stacey and Costa who have grown into wonderful, caring, and intelligent young adults, you both make me so proud.

And, in loving memory of my father-in-law, Costas Logothetis, his loving and kind spirit will remain with us always, may the memory of him be eternal.

REVIEWERS

CONTRIBUTORS

Diana M. Burnham, RDH, MS
Assistant Professor
University of New Mexico
Division of Dental Hygiene
Albuquerque, New Mexico

Margaret Fehrenbach, RDH, MS
Oral Biologist and Dental Hygienist
Adjunct Instructor, BASDH Degree
    Program
St. Petersburg College
St. Petersburg, FL
Educational Consultant and Dental
    Technical Writer
Seattle, WA

Christine N. Nathe, RDH, MS
Professor and Graduate Program
    Director
University of New Mexico
Division of Dental Hygiene
Albuquerque, New Mexico

Over the last 40 years, the delivery of local anesthetics has been added to the scope of dental hygiene practice in many states, and has been taught in most dental hygiene curriculums. Knowledge of local anesthetics is imperative to the successful administration of pain control agents. Although there are other local anesthetic textbooks available on the market for educating dental hygiene students to administer local anesthetics, none of them specifically relate to the practice of dental hygiene, until now! *Local Anesthesia for the Dental Hygienist* is a textbook that is directly related to the uses of local anesthesia in dental hygiene practice. It speaks directly to dental hygienist and offers examples of local anesthetic use during non-surgical periodontal therapy. *Local Anesthesia for the Dental Hygienist* is intended to help transform information into knowledge that is essential in both teaching and learning. This textbook will help transform the important information into a manageable knowledge base focusing on the significant information that is truly relevant to the practice of dental hygiene. *Local Anesthesia for the Dental Hygienist* offers comprehensive information on every aspect of the use of local anesthesia in dental hygiene practice. Irrelevant information important to specialty dental practices has been eliminated to focus on information important to the practice of dental hygiene.

INTENDED AUDIENCE

The intended audience of this textbook is the dental hygiene student, and the practicing dental hygienist who is taking the necessary coursework to become licensed in local anesthesia. In addition, practicing dental hygienists licensed to administer local anesthetics, and dentists may find this book useful for a quick reference or review during everyday practice. This textbook may also benefit the dental student as a classroom textbook or an additional resource.

ORGANIZATION

The material is divided into five sections to provide a clear and consistent organization of the content:

Section I: Introduction to Pain Control includes important general information on the history of local anesthetics, and pain control based on the human needs paradigm. Basic neurophysiology content is utilized for the dental hygienist to fully understand the generation and conduction of nerve impulses, and the mode of action of local anesthetics agents.

Section II: Local and Topical Anesthetic Agents includes pharmacology of local anesthetic and vasoconstrictor agents. This section provides detailed information on all local anesthetic agents, and offers color-coded local anesthetic tables to help in distinguishing among specific categories of agents and match the color codes of the American Dental Association (ADA). In addition, these tables offer helpful hints to local anesthetic selection. An entire chapter is devoted to topical anesthetics and their uses in dental hygiene practice. Local anesthetic and vasoconstrictor reference tables are included as an appendix for quick reference information.

Section III: Patient Assessment offers comprehensive information on the importance of preanesthetic patient assessment utilizing the patient's medical history. In addition, an entire chapter is devoted to determining individual patient drug doses with sample drug calculations, and several practice problems.

Section IV: Local Anesthetic Techniques for the Dental Hygienist includes a complete review of the anatomical considerations for the administration of local anesthetics. In addition, this section provides step-by-step instruction on how to set up the local anesthetic armamentarium, and technique/procedure boxes provide step-by-step instructions on how to perform specific injections for both the maxillary and mandibular arches with syringe stabilization examples for each injection. These technique/procedure boxes are a helpful tool for students to use during clinical practice section of their course, or for the practicing dental hygienist during everyday practice.

Section IV: Complications, Legal Considerations, Risk Management offers comprehensive material on how to prevent local and systemic anesthetic complications, and treatment of common local anesthetic emergencies. Legal considerations important to the administration of local anesthetics by dental hygienists are addressed. In addition, this section includes information on needle stick exposure prevention and post exposure management.

KEY FEATURES

Several key features are included in this book to assist the dental hygiene student studying and learning the fundamentals of local anesthesia:

- *Dental Hygiene Focus:* Although the focus of this textbook is on the administration of local anesthesia, the information is tailored to the specific role and needs of a dental hygienist administering local anesthetics.
- *Key Terminology:* Key terms are defined at the beginning of each chapter and bolded in blue throughout the chapter to help students learn new terminology. Local anesthesia terminology may be new to many dental hygiene students, and this will help draw attention to important key terms. These terms, along with other important concepts, are combined into a glossary at the end of the book.
- *Summary Tables and Boxes:* Throughout the text, important concepts are organized in summary tables and boxes

to assist visual learners, and are useful in studying and learning the material.

- *Procedure Tables and Boxes:* Procedure boxes for each injection are included that can be used as a guide in clinical situations. Tables are utilized for each injection to assist in the organization of information for each injection. Photos are placed in each relevant box for easy visualization of techniques and written material.
- *Consistent Presentation:* All injection techniques include detailed instructions and full-color photographs. All photos were taken by the author to maintain consistency and include examples of patient operator positioning.
- *Dental Hygiene Considerations:* At the end of each chapter, important dental hygiene considerations are presented summarizing the important concepts presented in the chapter and discussing its clinical relevance.

- *Case Studies:* Numerous case studies make it easier for students to apply knowledge to real-life situations and develop essential problem-solving skills.
- *Chapter Review Questions:* Twenty chapter review questions are presented at the end of each chapter to provide an opportunity for students to assess their knowledge.
- **A Companion Evolve Website:** Includes a timed mock board examination to assist students who will be taking the WREB, NERB, or other regional local anesthesia examination, technique exercises, glossary exercises, test-taking tips and strategies, competency skill sheets, and answers to the chapter review questions along with rationales and page-number references.

I hope that you will find the textbook and Evolve website to be the most comprehensive learning package available for local anesthesia.

Demetra Daskalos Logothetis

ACKNOWLEDGEMENTS

I would like to express my sincere gratitude to the many individuals who assisted in making this book a success. First, I would like to sincerely thank the contributors of this book, Diana Burnham, Christine Nathe, and Margaret Fehrenbach, for their hard work, perseverance, and attention to detail. Thank you to Christine Nathe, for her help with Departmental administrative work that allowed me the time to work on this project, and Vicki Gianopoulos who was always willing to help during the stressful moments of the book preparation. A special thank you to Cynthia Guillen who worked so hard to get me the images I needed for this book, and Gloria Lopez who spent hours in the dental chair allowing me to administer many local anesthetic injections to her for the photographs used in this book. I would like to thank my husband Nick who spent countless hours with me taking and retaking photographs to get them just right, and my children Stacey and Costa who supported and encouraged me throughout the work on this book. Thank you to my clinical anesthesia instructors, Sandy Bartee, and Kirstin Peterson, for assisting in the injection photographs, and for all their feedback. Thank you to my Graduate students Aleisha Barnaby and Lindsey Shay for their work in developing chapter review questions, and reviewing chapter content. In addition, I would like to thank all the reviewers for offering wonderful feedback and advice.

I would like to express my deepest gratitude to the Elsevier developmental team for their support and encouragement. This incredible team was so easy to work with that I cannot thank all of you enough for making this experience so enjoyable. A special thank you to Kristin Hebberd, Managing Editor of Health Professions, who is absolutely the sweetest person and so wonderful to work with, her continued support and advice throughout this project was deeply appreciated. Thank you to Joslyn Dumas, Developmental Editor for all her continuous help and encouragement, and to Kelly Milford, Project Manager for her assistance throughout the production phase.

In addition, I would like to thank the companies who provided their information and photographs as a contribution to this book. Thank you to Carestream Health, Inc., Dentsply Pharmaceuticals, Septodont USA, Milestone Scientific, Inc., and Onpharma Inc.

TABLE OF CONTENTS

PART I

Introduction to Pain Control

CHAPTER 1

Local Anesthesia in Dental Hygiene Practice: An Introduction

Christine N. Nathe RDH, MS

CHAPTER OUTLINE

LEARNING OBJECTIVES

1. Describe the history of pain control in health care.
2. Describe how local anesthesia is practiced by dental hygienists.
3. Describe the history of pain control provided by dental hygienists.
4. List state requirements for local anesthesia provided by dental hygienists.
5. Describe the human needs paradigm as it relates to pain control.
6. Describe patient perception of pain control.
7. Correctly complete the review questions and activities for this chapter.

KEY TERMS

Human needs paradigm Relationship between human need fulfillment and human behavior.
Local anesthesia Loss of sensation in a circumscribed area, creating a numbing feeling.
Pain An unpleasant sensory and emotional experience.
Pain control The mechanism to alleviate pain.
Pain perception Neurologic experience of pain that differs little between individuals.

Pain reaction Personal interpretation of and response to the pain message; highly variable between and among individuals.
Pain threshold The point at which a sensation starts to become painful and discomfort results.
Stress Physical and emotional response to a particular situation.
Visual analog scale An instrument used to measure pain.

INTRODUCTION

Pain is an unpleasant sensory and emotional experience, and can be thought of as one of the oldest of all dental problems. In fact, the control of pain during routine dental procedures is an important part of dental care delivery. Pain relievers routinely are referred to as analgesics. Specifically, the use of topical and local anesthetics provided by the dental hygienist is necessary for many dental hygiene appointments. Local anesthesia creates a numbing feeling which eliminates the feeling of sensation in a specific area, without loss of consciousness. Although pain is seemingly associated with dental care, dental providers have the ability to control and alleviate pain during and after procedures.

This chapter details the history of pain control and anesthetics in general, introduces the concept of anesthesia in dental hygiene practice, and discusses pain control in practice.

HISTORY OF PAIN CONTROL

Pain control is the mechanism that alleviates pain. Although some methods of pain control have probably always existed, historical evidence suggests that modern anesthetics can be traced to medieval times.[1] Early methods of pain reduction included religious techniques of scaring off demons and praying for the touch of God to stop the suffering.[2] Plants and herbs, including roots, berries, and seeds, became the prominent method for treating pain.[2]

The use of narcotics to reduce pain was a universally accepted practice and involved the use of cannabis, opium, and alcohol[3] (Box 1-1). However, these drugs used were not completely effective at altering pain, caused side effects, and were addictive. Opium was most useful for pain control. In fact, opium proved even more effective when converted into a more potent form, morphine, and injected into the bloodstream.[4]

Interestingly, chemists had also prepared acetylated salicylic acid, a plant compound used in headache powder, which often left the patient with severe gastric distress. A new compound, introduced as aspirin in 1899, was highly effective as an analgesic and antipyretic, and proved to be remarkably safe and well tolerated by patients.[2] However, for severe pain, more pain reducers and controllers were still in need.

The chemical to finally prove to be an effective surgical anesthetic was ether.[3] Several individuals were involved in the development of the concept of gas inhalation for anesthesia. In 1842, it was reported that William Clarke administered ether via a towel to a woman as one of her teeth was extracted by a dentist.[4] Horace Wells, a dentist, first tried nitrous oxide for dental pain control after attending several "laughing gas" parties. He practiced on himself by using nitrous oxide, which he considered safer than ether, and having a fellow dentist extract his tooth. He felt nothing during the extraction and discovered nitrous oxide to be an effective anesthetic. Halothane, a safe, stable chemical for inhalation anesthesia, was introduced in 1956. Short-acting anesthetics have also been introduced and are generally administered intravenously.[5]

In both Europe and the United States during the 1800's, there was an extended debate over the ethics of operating on an unconscious patient and whether the relief from pain might actually retard the health process. Furthermore, some found religious offense in the new practice. Evidently, some physicians felt that it violated God's law, whom they believe inflicted pain to strengthen faith.[2] Physicians used a calculus (measurement benchmark) to determine which patients were of the correct sensibility (exhibiting overall health) and need to benefit from the use of anesthesia.[2,6-7]

During World War II, Dr. Henry Beecher observed that seriously wounded soldiers reported much lower levels of pain than had his civilian patients. Based on his inference that clinical pain was a compound of the physical sensation *and* a cognitive and emotional reaction component he challenged laboratory studies in healthy volunteers and argued that pain could only be legitimately studied in the clinical situation. These observations formed the basis for real clinical research trials on pain control.[2,8-11] Eventually, in 1956, the gate control theory was published. The classic articles proposed a spinal cord mechanism that related the transmission of pain sensations between the periphery nervous system and the brain.[12]

HISTORY OF LOCAL ANESTHETICS

The first local anesthetic, cocaine, was isolated from coca leaves by Albert Niemann and Francesco Di Stefano in Germany in the 1860s.[13] Cocaine was first used as a local anesthetic in 1884 by Karl Koller, who demonstrated the use during painless ophthalmological surgery.[14,15] Although effective as an anesthetic, it was addictive, and many of those pioneer researchers who first studied cocaine's effects on themselves became addicted.[3]

In 1905, the ester procaine (Novacaine) was created in Germany and, when mixed with a proportion of epinephrine, was found to be effective and safe[1] (Box 1-2). Procaine took a long time to produce the desired anesthetic result, wore off quickly, and was not as potent as cocaine. Additionally, many patients were allergic to procaine because procaine is an ester and esters have a high potential for allergic reactions.

In the 1940s a new group of local anesthetic compounds, the amides, were introduced. The initial amide local anesthetic, lidocaine, was synthesized by Swedish chemist Nils Lofgren in 1943. Lidocaine revolutionized pain control in

---

BOX 1-1	Drugs Used in the Past to Reduce Pain

Alcohol
Cannabis
Hembane
Mandragora
Opium

BOX 1-2	History of Local Anesthetics

Cocaine: 1884
Procaine: 1904
Lidocaine: 1943
Bupivacaine: 1957
Mepivacaine: 1957
Prilocaine: 1959
Articaine: 1969; available in United States in 2000

dentistry worldwide, because it was both more potent and less allergenic than procaine. In the succeeding years, other amide local anesthetics (prilocaine in 1959, bupivacaine and mepivacaine in 1957) were introduced. These new amide local anesthetics provided the dental practitioner with an array of local anesthetics ranging in pulpal anesthesia for periods lasting from 20 minutes (mepivacaine) to 3 hours (bupivacaine with epinephrine). In 1969, Rusching and colleagues prepared a new drug, carticaine, which differed from the previous amide local anesthetics. Renamed *articaine* in 1984, the drug was derived from thiophene and thus contained a thiophene ring in its molecule instead of the usual benzene ring. Articaine became available in 2000 for marketing in the United States in a 4% 1 : 100,000 epinephrine formulation. Today, lidocaine remains the most popular anesthetic used in dentistry in the United States, but many patients do not understand the distinction between the agents and still ask for Novocain which is no longer available in dentistry.

ANESTHESIA IN DENTAL HYGIENE PRACTICE

Dental hygienists often treat patients with painful gingival and/or periodontal infections, which is why it is paramount for dental hygienists to be able to reduce and control pain while treating patients. Local anesthetics work by blocking the travel of the pain signal to the brain.[16] In addition to

pain control, local anesthetics can provide vasoconstriction if vasoconstricting drugs such as epinephrine or levonordefrin is added to the anesthetic. During the course of treatment, patients may have gingival inflammation and bleeding. Hemostasis is achieved via the vasoconstrictor in the anesthetic. By controlling the bleeding, proper visualization of the tissues and the working end of the instrument can be achieved.[17]

Many dental practices will hire a dental hygienist with certification in local anesthesia to provide local anesthesia for all dental and dental hygiene patients in the practice. Much like a nurse anesthetist or anesthesiologist focuses his or her nursing or medical specialization in the provision of anesthetics, so do many dental hygienists exclusively provide local anesthesia without providing any traditional dental hygiene services.

The delivery of local anesthetic has been added to the scope of dental hygiene practice over the past 40 years (Table 1-1 and Figure 1-1). Washington State added the provision of local anesthesia to state law in 1971, followed by New Mexico in 1972 and Missouri in 1973. Currently, 44 states allow dental hygienists to deliver local anesthetics. Maryland, New York, and South Carolina are states where dental hygienists may provide local infiltration but not block anesthesia.[18]

Proficiency is determined by coursework during the dental hygiene program or completion of appropriate training in an accredited continuing education setting. States

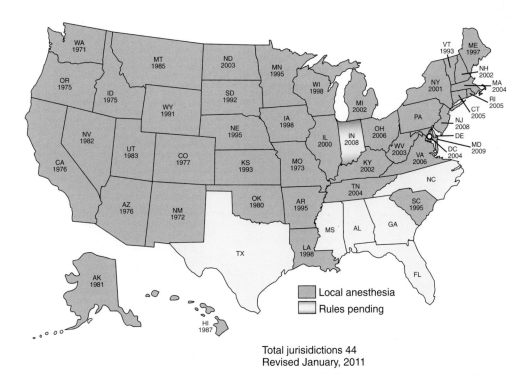

Total jurisidictions 44
Revised January, 2011

Figure 1-1 ■ States where dental hygienists may administer local anesthesia. (From American Dental Hygienists' Association: http://www.adha.org/governmental_affairs/downloads/localanesthesiamap.pdf. Accessed January 2011.).

TABLE 1-1	Local Anesthesia Administration By Dental Hygienists State Chart					
STATE & YEAR IMPLEMENTED	SUPERVISION REQUIRED	BLOCK AND/OR INFILTRATION	EDUCATION REQUIRED	EXAM REQUIRED	IMPLEMENT LANGUAGE IN STATUTE OR RULES	LEGAL REQUIREMENTS FOR LOCAL ANESTHESIA COURSES
AK 1981	General	Both	Specific	Yes—WREB and local anesthetic exam	Statute	16 didactic 8 clinical 8 lab
AZ 1976	Direct	Both	Approved	Yes—WREB and local anesthetic exam	Statute	36 hrs for local and N20
AR 1995	Direct	Both	Approved and Accredited	No	Statute	16 didactic 12 clinical
CA 1976	Direct	Both	Approved	Yes	Rules	No
CO 1977	General	Both	Accredited	No	Statute	12 didactic 12 clinical
CT 2005	Direct	Both	Accredited	No	Statute	20 didactic 8 clinical
DC 2004	Direct	Both	Board approved	Yes	Rules	32 hours total
HI 1987	Direct	Both	Accredited	Yes—Exam given by course	Statute	39 didactic and clinical
ID 1975	General	Both	Accredited	Yes—Clinical	Statute	No
IA 1998	Direct	Both	Accredited	No	Rules	Must be conducted by an accredited RDH or DDS school
IL 2000	Direct	Both	Accredited	No	Statute	24 didactic 8 clinical
IN 2008	Direct					
KS 1993	Direct	Both	Accredited	No	Statute	12 hrs total
KY 2002	Direct	Both	Specific	Yes—Written exam given by course	Statute	32 hour didactic 12 hours clinical
LA 1998	Direct	Both	Accredited	Yes	Rules	72 total hours
MA 2004	Direct	Both	Accredited	Yes	Statute	35 total; no less than 12 hours clinical
ME 1997	Direct	Both	Accredited	Yes	Rules	60 hours total
MD 2009	Direct	Infiltration	Accredited/Board approved	Yes	Rules	20 didactic 8 clinical
MN 1995	General	Both	Accredited	No	Rules	No
MO 1973	Direct	Both	Accredited/Board approved	Yes	Rules	No
MI 2002	Direct	Both	Accredited and Specific	Yes—State or regional board-administered written exam (NERB)	Statute	15 didactic 14 clinical
MT 1985	Direct	Both	Accredited	Yes—WREB local anesthetic exam or successful completion of clinical & written LA regional or state board exam	Statute	No
ND 2003	Direct	Both	Accredited	No	Rules	Course must include clinical and didactic components, but there are no specific hourly requirements.
NE 1995	Direct	Both	Accredited	No	Statute	12 didactic 12 clinical

STATE & YEAR IMPLEMENTED	SUPERVISION REQUIRED	BLOCK AND/OR INFILTRATION	EDUCATION REQUIRED	EXAM REQUIRED	IMPLEMENT LANGUAGE IN STATUTE OR RULES	LEGAL REQUIREMENTS FOR LOCAL ANESTHESIA COURSES
NH 2002	Direct	Both	Accredited	Yes—NERB local anesthesia exam	Statute	20 didactic 12 clinical
NV 1982	Direct/General	Both	Accredited	No	Rules	No
NM 1972	Direct	Both	Accredited	Yes—WREB local anesthesia exam	Statute	24 didactic 10 clinical
NJ 2008	Direct	Both	Accredited/Board approved	Yes—NERB local anesthesia	Rules	20 didactic 12 clinical Including a minimum of 20 hours monitored administration of local anesthesia
NY 2001	Direct	Infiltration	Accredited	No	Statute	30 didactic 15 clinical & lab
OH 2006	Direct	Both	Accredited	Yes—Written regional or state exam.	Statute	15 didactic 14 clinical
OK 1980	Direct	Both	Approved	No—Exam given by course	Rules	20½ hours
OR 1975	General	Both	Accredited	No	Rules	No
PA 2009	Direct	Both	Accredited/Approved	No	Rules	30 hours Didactic and Clinical Permit, must renew
RI 2005	Direct	Both	Accredited	Yes—NERB	Statute	20 didactic 12 clinical
SC 1995	Direct	Infiltration	Approved	Yes	Statute	Information not available
SD 1992	Direct	Both	Accredited/Approved	No	Statute	No
TN 2004	Direct	Both	Accredited/Approved	No	Rules	24 Didactic 8 Clinical
UT 1983	Direct	Both	Approved	Yes—WREB exam in anesthesiology (local)	Statute	No
VT 1993	Direct	Both	Accredited	Yes—Board administered	Statute	24 hours total
VA 2006	Direct	Both *Only on patients over age 18	Accredited	Yes—accredited program Board of another jurisdiction accepted	Statute	36 didactic-clinical
WA 1971	Direct	Both	Approved	No	Statute	No
WI 1998	Direct	Both	Accredited	No	Statute	10 didactic 11 clinical
WV 2003	Direct	Both	Pending	NERB local anesthesia exam or equivalent state or regional exam	Statute	12 didactic 15 clinical
WY 1991	Direct	Both	Approved	Yes = in state. No = out of state DH certified in local	Rules	No

Key: Accredited—Course must be provided within a CODA accredited HD program or an institution housing a CODA program.

Approved—Course must be approved by the state licensing agency.

Specific—Course is specified in law. Data compiled from 51 practice acts/rules.

Direct Supervision—means the dentist must be present.

General Supervision—means dentist need not be present.

vary in the amount of coursework, required minimal education, and necessity of examination before certification. Additionally, some states govern anesthetic practices by statute, some by rules.[17]

Twenty-eight states permit the administration of nitrous oxide by dental hygienists. The first state to enact this increase in the scope of practice for dental hygienists was Washington in 1971.[19] Some states may allow dental hygienists to monitor nitrous oxide, but not actually administer the drug. Simply, this means that the dental hygienist may not turn on the nitrous oxide but may change settings during the dental hygiene appointment as needed.

PATIENT PERCEPTION OF LOCAL ANESTHESIA

Patients often present to the dental office with pain. Specifically, pain is the sensation of discomfort and can range from mild to severe. It is well recognized that patients react differently to painful stimuli and many times the same patient will react differently to painful stimuli depending on a variety of environmental, social, emotional, or physical factors. The term *pain threshold* is often used when discussing pain. Pain threshold pertains to the point at which a sensation starts to be painful and discomfort results. This threshold varies among individuals and may be altered by some drugs such as local anesthesia. Pain perception is a neurologic experience of pain. Pain is perceived when painful stimuli are received and transmitted to the brain; pain perception differs little between individuals. Pain reaction is the personal interpretation and response to the pain message, and is highly variable among individuals.[20] Pain reaction threshold is the moment when pain crosses the threshold of tolerance, and at which point a reaction may occur. It may be influenced by the patient's emotional state, fatigue, age, culture, and fear and apprehension[20-21] (Table 1-2).

The fear of pain is not only associated with dental problems, but also with the administration of local anesthesia when patients present to the dental provider for relief from pain caused by the dental problems.[21] Basically, many patients fear the dental provider, because they are apprehensive about a "dental shot." Dental hygienists must be cognizant of the common fear associated with local anesthesia and communicate sincerely and empathetically to patients about the provision of pain control.

A tool used to help a person rate the intensity of certain sensations and feelings such as pain is the Visual Analog Scale (VAS). A VAS is a measurement instrument that attempts to measure pain that is believed to range across a continuum of values that cannot easily be directly measured. For example, the amount of pain that a patient feels ranges across a continuum from none to an extreme amount of pain. Operationally, a VAS is usually a horizontal line, 100 mm in length, anchored by word descriptors at each end as illustrated in Figure 1-2. The patient marks on the line the point that they feel represents their perception of

TABLE 1-2	Influences of Pain Reaction Threshold
INFLUENCE	**CLINICAL RELEVANCE**
Emotional state	Personal pain interpretation may vary within an individual based upon their emotional state at the time of dental treatment. Patients who are in a difficult emotional condition generally have a lower pain reaction threshold.
Fatigue and stress	Personal pain interpretation may vary within an individual based upon their level of fatigue and stress. Patients who are overly tired or stressed at the time of their appointment will generally have a lower pain reaction threshold.
Age	Older patients generally have higher pain reaction thresholds compared to younger patients, as they have accepted pain as part of life.
Cultural characteristics	Individuals from different cultures will react to pain differently as influenced by what is considered an appropriate reaction to convey within their culture.
Fear and apprehension	The more fear and apprehension the patient is regarding their dental appointment, the lower the pain reaction threshold. These are patients who frequently miss dental appointments.

From Human needs paradigm in relation to dental hygiene. In Darby ML, Walsh MM. *Dental hygiene theory and practice*, ed 2, St Louis, 2009, Saunders.

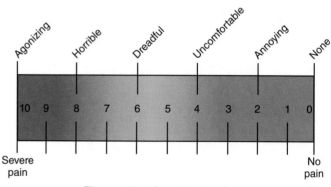

Figure 1-2 ■ Visual Analog Scale.

their current state. The VAS score is determined by measuring in millimeters from the left hand end of the line to the point that the patient marks. Pain scales are subjective but nonetheless will be useful for clinicians. The VAS scale will be used in Chapters 12 and 13 to describe the average level of pain associated with maxillary and mandibular injections.

HUMAN NEEDS PARADIGM

Dental hygiene care promotes health and prevents oral disease over the human life span through the provision of educational, preventive, and therapeutic services.[22] The human needs paradigm helps dental hygienists understand the relationship between human need fulfillment and human behavior. A human need is a tension within a person. This tension expresses itself in some goal-directed behavior that continues until the goal is reached.[23] The human needs theory explains that need fulfillment dominates human activity and that behavior is organized in relation to unsatisfied needs (Figure 1-3). Dental pain can be an unsatisfied need, because pain can be such an overwhelming force. Treating the cause of and alleviating dental pain using local anesthesia can be a welcome asset for the dental hygienist.

Interestingly, Darby discusses eight human needs related to dental hygiene that have many implications for pain control in dental hygiene[23] (Box 1-3). The human needs theory emphasizes the use of a patient-centered approach and relates to pain control and prevention, which may entail the provision of dental anesthesia.

Most of these needs relate directly to the need and use of local anesthesia for dental patients. Specifically, two of these needs relate to the provision of stress reduction principles and the use of local anesthesia. Freedom from fear and stress is the need to feel safe and to be free from emotional discomfort in the oral health care environment and

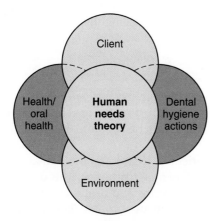

Figure 1-3 ■ Human needs paradigm in relation to dental hygiene. (From Darby ML, Walsh MM: *Dental hygiene: theory and practice*, ed 3, St Louis, 2010, Saunders.)

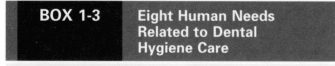

BOX 1-3	**Eight Human Needs Related to Dental Hygiene Care**

Protection from health risks
Freedom from fear and stress
Freedom from pain
Wholesome facial image
Skin and mucous membrane integrity of the head and neck
Biologically sound and functional dentition
Conceptualization and problem solving
Responsibility for oral health

From Darby ML, Walsh, MM: *Dental hygiene theory and practice*, ed 3, St Louis, 2010, Saunders.

to receive appreciation, attention, and respect from others. Freedom from pain is the need to be exempt from physical discomfort in the head and neck area. Once again, the use of local anesthesia by the dental hygienist can help attain these human needs.

MANAGEMENT OF FEARFUL PATIENTS

Fear prevents many patients from obtaining dental care, whether it is fear of dental treatment, local anesthesia or past experiences. Studies have revealed that from 50%–85% of patients who report dental anxiety had the onset of fear during their childhood or adolescence and the remainder became fearful of dental care during adulthood.[24] Patients who are anxious may have had unpleasant experiences in the past or may have a learned fear of dental care. Interestingly, the majority of studies confirmed a relationship between parental and child dental fear.[25] It is important to discuss this anxiousness with patients so that the dental hygienist can respond effectively to help alleviate fear.

Many patients do present to the dental provider when they are anxious and nervous. Although significant fear may be termed *dental phobia*, many patients are anxious about dental treatment, and all dental hygienists can expect to treat many anxious patients.[23] Patients with dental phobia may not be a regular (recall) dental consumer, based on the extreme fearfulness toward dental care in general.

The effects of fear on the body can physiologically evoke the stress response. Stress is a physical and emotional response to a particular situation. The response to stress is often termed *fight or flight* and occurs automatically. Studies suggest that patients who are fearful of dental treatment have elevated blood pressure, heart rate, and salivary cortisol levels immediately before dental checkups and treatment.[25,26] Dental hygienists must be cognizant of the important role patient fear plays in the provision of dental care.

STRESS REDUCTION PRINCIPLES

Prevention is the best method to manage an anxious patient. Basically, the dental hygienist should look for symptoms of stress immediately, so that stress reduction principles are enacted before stress levels elevate. Box 1-4 lists signs of moderate anxiety, including patient discussion with the receptionists or other patients in the waiting room about their fear, cold or sweaty palms, or unnaturally stiff posture. An astute practitioner looks for signs of anxiousness.

It is important for the dental hygienist to determine during the health and dental history review whether the patient is anxious. Some patients will express their apprehension and stress immediately, directly to the provider, whereas other patients may need questioning or persistent listening by the provider to find out about anxiousness. Ensuring a complete health history review at each appointment is important to recognize stressors and health conditions that may complicate procedures. Even a patient who is feeling fatigued or "under the weather" may be more

BOX 1-4 | **Clinical Signs of Moderate Anxiety**

RECEPTION AREA
Questions receptionist regarding injections or use of sedation
Nervous conversations with others in reception area
History of emergency dental care only
History of canceled appointments for nonemergency treatment
Cold, sweaty palms

DENTAL CHAIR
Unnaturally stiff posture
Nervous play with tissue
White-knuckle syndrome
Perspiration on forehead and hands
Overwillingness to cooperate with clinician
Quick answers

From Darby ML, Walsh, MM: *Dental hygiene theory and practice*, ed 3, St Louis, 2010, Saunders.

anxious and stressful during dental appointments. Obtaining the patient's vital signs is also important to understand a patient's total health history.

Considering shorter appointments, even though more appointments may be needed, may help some patients reduce stress levels, as can scheduling patients during specific time periods of the day. For example, some patients may do better in the morning, whereas others may do better in the afternoons. This is a completely personal preference as to whether an individual is better able to handle stressful situations at different periods during the day. Most patients are more rested and less fatigued in the mornings, and are better able to handle the stressful dental appointment if scheduled in the morning. Patients who are fearful of dental pain may be better served by appointments in the middle of the week, so they can be assured of seeing a provider the next day if needed. Telephone calls after treatment may be welcomed by some patients to ensure comfort and adequate care. The use of anesthesia as needed is an important key to prevention of fear associated with pain, which is discussed throughout this text.

SUMMARY

Dental hygienists have the unique responsibility and opportunity to alleviate pain for many patients. The history of pain control focuses on the use of different substances to help individuals endure pain. Anesthesia has been used in dentistry for more than a century and continues to improve. While treating infections that result in pain or while treating patients who perceive pain during regular procedures the dental hygienist may need to use anesthesia. Using the patient-centered approach to stress reduction and pain control in conjunction with the correct use of anesthesia can be advantageous to dental hygiene treatment.

DENTAL HYGIENE CONSIDERATIONS

Dental Hygiene Considerations
- Fear and anxiety during dental treatment is not uncommon, and affects approximately three-fourths of the population.
- Fear, anxiety, emotional distress, and fatigue lower the pain reaction threshold.
- Patients who are anxious or fear dental treatment are more likely to refuse local anesthesia for dental hygiene procedures. Explain that when local anesthetics are administered, the patient can relax during the treatment and will feel less pain.
- The attitude and demeanor of the dental hygienist will significantly influence the confidence and comfort of the patient and overall success of the administration of the local anesthetic.

- Although the patient may be fearful of receiving a local anesthetic injection, once the injection is administered the anesthesia will help attain the human need for comfort.
- Not all patients will inform the dental hygienist of their fear of dental treatment. The dental hygienist must recognize stress and health conditions that may complicate treatment through dialogue and a complete health history.
- Shorter, morning appointments in the middle of the week may better serve the apprehensive and fatigued patient.

CASE STUDY 1-1

Angel Loses Her Job
Angel is a single parent of two children ages 12 and 14. She has an appointment with the dental hygienist for her third quadrant of nonsurgical periodontal therapy with anesthesia. The dental hygienist is happy to see that Angel is on the schedule for today because she is a delightful person who is excited about the results she is seeing with her periodontal treatment. Her treatment has been progressing very nicely, and Angel is an ideal patient.

Angel is informed on the day of her dental visit that she will be laid off from her job in a month because of cutbacks in the company's budget. Angel is devastated

CASE STUDY 1-1

when she hears the news and considers rescheduling her dental appointment, but she is unsure how much longer she will have dental insurance provided to her by the company.

Angel decides to keep her dental appointment, and because she does not like to burden others with her problems, she decides not to tell the dental hygienist about her bad news.

Critical Thinking Questions

- How can Angel's bad news affect her pain reaction threshold?
- How can Angel's decision not to inform the dental hygienist of her emotional state affect the treatment scheduled for today?

CHAPTER REVIEW QUESTIONS

1. What potent drug used for pain control was derived from opium?
    A. Lidocaine
    B. Novocain
    C. Morphine
    D. Codeine
2. What drug did Horace Wells first introduce into dentistry for pain control?
    A. Nitrous oxide
    B. Local anesthetics
    C. Topical anesthetics
    D. Morphine
3. All of the following are reasons why procaine was not as desirable as cocaine for pain control EXCEPT:
    A. Difficult to produce the desired anesthetic result
    B. Its mechanism of action wore off too quickly
    C. It was not as potent
    D. All of the above
4. Injectable amides are recommended over esters because there is:
    A. Less risk of allergic reactions
    B. Increased potency
    C. Decreased mechanism of action
    D. Both A and B
5. What is the most popular local anesthetic used in the US today?
    A. Procaine
    B. Novocain
    C. Epinephrine
    D. Lidocaine
6. What is the definition of *pain threshold*?
    A. A neurologic experience of pain related to the process of receiving pain stimuli and transmission of this pain to the brain that differs little between individuals
    B. The point at which a sensation starts to be painful and discomfort results
    C. Personal interpretation and response to the pain message that is highly variable among individuals
    D. The sensation of discomfort that the patient feels, ranging from mild to severe

7. What is pain perception?
    A. A neurologic experience of pain related to the process of receiving pain stimuli and transmission of this pain to the brain that differs little between individuals
    B. The point at which a sensation starts to be painful and discomfort results
    C. Personal interpretation and responses to the pain message that is highly variable among individuals
    D. The sensation of discomfort that the patient feels, ranging from mild to severe
8. What is pain?
    A. A neurologic experience of pain related to the process of receiving pain stimuli and transmission of this pain to the brain that differs little between individuals
    B. The point at which a sensation starts to be painful and discomfort results
    C. Personal interpretation and responses to the pain message that is highly variable among individuals
    D. The sensation of discomfort that the patient feels, ranging from mild to severe
9. What is pain reaction?
    A. A neurologic experience of pain related to the process of receiving pain stimuli and transmission of this pain to the brain that differs little between individuals
    B. The point at which a sensation starts to be painful and discomfort results
    C. Personal interpretation and responses to the pain message that is highly variable among individuals
    D. The sensation of discomfort that the patient feels, ranging from mild to severe
10. Pain can be influenced by which of the following?
    A. Fear
    B. Fatigue
    C. Culture
    D. All of the above
11. What theory helps dental hygienists understand the relationship between human need fulfillment and human behavior?

CHAPTER REVIEW QUESTIONS

A. Pain threshold theory
B. Human needs theory
C. Human fulfillment theory
D. Behaviorism theory

12. What is the definition of stress?
    A. The sensation of discomfort that the patient feels, ranging from mild to severe
    B. A physical and emotional response to a particular situation
    C. Being anxious or nervous
    D. Having an unrealistic phobia

13. Which of the following may lower the pain reaction threshold?
    A. Fear
    B. Overeating
    C. Positive communication
    D. Explaining each procedure in advance

14. If a patient has a high pain threshold, he or she will experience more intense pain than a patient who has a low pain threshold.
    A. True
    B. False

15. Which of the following is the personal interpretation and response to the pain message, and is highly variable among individuals?
    A. Pain threshold
    B. Pain perception
    C. Pain reaction
    D. Pain reaction threshold

16. In what year was the first local anesthetic introduced?

A. 1884
B. 1904
C. 1943
D. 1957

17. It is best to schedule apprehensive patients for long appointments to complete as much work as possible, and it is best to schedule these appointments in the morning.
    A. Both statements are true
    B. Both statements are false
    C. First statement is true, second statement is false
    D. First statement is false, second statement is true

18. What percentage of patients have reported to have had onset of dental anxiety by adolescence?
    A. 5%–20%
    B. 20%–40%
    C. 40%–50%
    D. 50%–85%

19. Which of the following are signs of moderate anxiety?
    A. Slow to answer questions
    B. History of frequently missed appointments
    C. History of emergency appointments only
    D. B and C only
    E. All of the above

20. What is the best method of managing an anxious patient?
    A. Prevention
    B. Giving local anesthesia
    C. Giving general anesthesia
    D. Not telling the patient what is about to happen

REFERENCES

1. Goldie MP: The evolution of analgesia and anesthesia in oral health care, *RDH* 29(9):58-64, Sept 2009.
2. Meldrum ML: A capsule of history of pain management, *JAMA* 290(18): 2470-2475, 2003.
3. Gallucci JM: Who deserves the credit for discovering ether's use as a surgical anesthetic? *J Hist Dent* 56(1):38-43, 2008.
4. Keys TE: *The history of surgical anesthesia.* New York, 1963, Dover.
5. Fenster JM: *Ether day: the strange tale of American's greatest medical discovery and the haunted men who made it,* New York, 2001, HarperCollins.
6. Pernick MS: *A calculus of suffering: pain, professionalism and anesthesia in nineteenth-century America,* New York, 1985, Columbia University Press.
7. Rey R: *The history of pain,* Cambridge, MA, 1993, Harvard University Press.

8. Beecher HK: Pain in men wounded in battle, *Ann Surg* 123:96-105, 1946.
9. Beecher HK: *Measurement of subjective responses: quantitative effects of drugs,* New York, 1959, Oxford University Press.
10. Modell W, Houde RW: Factors influencing the clinical evaluation of drugs, with special reference to the double-blind technique, *JAMA* 167: 2190-2199, 1958.
11. Medlrum ML: Each patient his own control. James Hard and Henry Beecher on ten problems of pain measurement, *Am Pain Soca Bull* 9:3-5, 1999.
12. Melzack R, Wall PD: Pain mechanisms: a new theory, *Science* 150:971-979, 1965.
13. Gootenberg P: *Cocaine: global histories.* New York and London, 1999, Routledge.

14. Schulein TM: Significant events in the history of operative dentistry, *J Hist Dent* 53(2):69, 2005.
15. Dos RA: Sigmund Freud (1856-1939) and Karl Koller (1857-1944) and the discovery of local anesthesia, *Rev Bras Anestesiol* Mar-Apr 59(2):244-257, 2009.
16. Overman P: Controlling the pain, *Dimens Dent Hyg* 2(11):10, 12, 14, 2004.
17. Doniger SB: Delivering local anesthetic, *RDH* 25(4):68-73, 2005.
18. Local anesthesia by dental hygienists. Chicago, 2010, American Dental Hygienists' Association. http://www.adha.org/governmental_affairs/downloads/localanesthesia.pdf. Accessed August 4.
19. Nitrous oxide administration by dental hygienists. Chicago, 2010, American Dental Hygienists' Association.

http://www.adha.org/governmental_affairs/downloads/localanesthesia.pdf. Accessed August 4.

20. Wilkins EM: *Clinical practice of the dental hygienist*, ed 10, Philadelphia, 2009, Lippincott Williams and Wilkins.

21. Milgrom P, Coldwell SE, Getz T, et al. Four dimensions of fear of dental injections, *J Am Dent Assoc* 128:756-766, 1997.

22. American Dental Hygienists' Association. Dental hygiene: focus on advancing the profession, 2004-2005 (position paper). www.adha.org/downloads/ADHA_Focus_Report.pdf. Accessed August, 4 2010.

23. Darby ML, Walsh MM: *Dental hygiene theory and practice*, ed 3, St. Louis, 2010, Saunders.

24. Locker D, Liddell A, Depster L, Shapiro D: Age of onset of dental anxiety, *J Dent Res* 78:790, 1999.

25. Lahti S, Luoto A: Significant relationship between parental and child fear, *Evid Based Dent* 11(3):77, 2010.

26. Malamed SF: Sedation: a guide to patient management, ed 4, St. Louis, 2003, Mosby.

CHAPTER 2

Neurophysiology

Demetra Daskalos Logothetis RDH, MS

LEARNING OBJECTIVES

1. Describe the functional unit of a nerve system.
2. Explain the main function of the neuron.
3. Differentiate the role of the cell body in sensory and motor impulse transmission.
4. Describe the parts and functions of the neuron:
   - Neurilemma/axolemma
   - Neuroplasm/axoplasm
   - Endoneurium
   - Perineurium
   - Fascicle
5. Compare the ions in nerve transmission in regard to their functional element relative concentrations and location during the resting stage, depolarization, and repolarization.
6. Explain the stages of nerve conduction.
7. Describe the Na^+/K^+ pump and differentiate between active and passive energy requirements for the stages of nerve transmission.
8. Describe action potential and describe saltatory conduction.
9. Explain the anatomy of a sensory neuron.
10. Differentiate between type A, B, and C fibers in terms of their function, size, and relative speed of impulse transmission.
11. Discuss speed of impulse propagation with myelinated versus non-myelinated nerves.
12. Describe and recite the stages of nerve transmission in detail.
13. Describe the refractory periods.
14. Explain the role of neurotransmitters in nerve conduction.
15. Discuss the mode of action of local anesthetic agents on nerves.
16. Correctly complete the review questions and activities for this chapter.

KEY TERMS

Absolute refractory period The interval during which a second action potential absolutely cannot be initiated to restimulate the membrane, no matter how large a stimulus is applied.

Action potential Nerve impulse.

Afferent nerves Conduct signals from sensory neurons to the spinal cord or brain *(carry toward)*.

Autonomic nervous system (ANS) The part of the peripheral nervous system that acts as a control system and helps people adapt to changes in their environment. It adjusts or modifies some functions in response to stress.

Axon Cable-like structure of neuron.

Cell body Responsible for protein synthesis and provides metabolic support for the neuron.

Central fibers Nerve fibers that extend from the cell body toward the CNS.

Central nervous system (CNS) Structural and functional center of the nervous system includes the brain and the spinal cord.

Core bundles Fasciculi located in the core region (inner core).

Depolarization Action potential causes sodium channels to open allowing an influx of sodium ions changing the electrochemical gradient, which in turn produces a further rise in the membrane potential.

Efferent nerves Conduct signals away from the brain or spinal cord *(carry away)*.

Endoneurium Surrounds each axon by a layer of connective tissue.

Epineurium Connective tissue that wraps the entire nerve.

Faciculi Nerve fibers bundled together into groups.

Mantle bundles Fasciculi located in the mantle region (outer core).

Membrane potential Difference in voltage or electrical potential between the interior and exterior of a cell.

Myelinated nerve Lipoprotein sheath that almost completely insulates the axon from the outside.

Nerve Contains many bundles of peripheral axons.

Neuron Basic functional unit of the nervous system which manipulates information, and responds to either excitation or inhibition.

Neurotransmitters Endogenous chemicals that transmit signals from a neuron to a target cell across a synapse.

Nodes of Ranvier Uninsulated gaps formed between myelin sheaths covering axons allowing for the generating electrical activity.

Parasympathetic nervous system Coordinates the body's normal resting activities and is known as the "rest or digest" response.

Perineurium Connective tissue that wraps each fascicle.

Peripheral fibers Nerve fibers that extend from the cell body away from the CNS.

Peripheral nervous system (PNS) Nerve tissues that lie in the periphery.

Relative refractory period The interval immediately following the absolute refractory period and before complete reestablishment to the resting state, during which initiation of a second action potential is possible if a larger stimulus is achieved to produce successful firing.

Repolarization Occurs once the peak of the action potential is reached and the membrane potential begins to move back toward the resting potential (–70 mV). Results from efflux of K+ ions.

Resting state Non-stimulated neuron sitting with no impulse to carry or transmit, and its membrane is polarized.

Saltatory conduction The propagation of action potentials along myelinated axons from one node of Ranvier to the next node, increasing the conduction velocity of action potentials without needing to increase the diameter of an axon.

Somatic nervous system (SNS) Subdivision of the efferent division of the PNS and controls the body's voluntary and reflex activities through somatic sensory and somatic motor components.

Sympathetic nervous system Division of ANS that prepares the body to deal with an emergency situation and is involved with the "fight or flight" response.

▌INTRODUCTION

A local anesthetic is a drug that causes reversible local anesthesia and a loss of nociception (also called a pain receptor) as a result of the depression of excitation in nerve endings or the inhibition of the conduction process in peripheral nerves. Local anesthetic agents used in dental practice prevent both the generation and conduction of a nerve impulse. When it is used on specific nerve pathways (nerve block), effects such as analgesia (loss of pain sensation) can be achieved. Basically, local anesthetics provide a chemical roadblock between the source of the impulse and the brain. The impulse therefore is unable to reach the brain.[1,2]

Local anesthetics are known as membrane-stabilizing drugs, which work by decreasing the rate of depolarization when a membrane potential is initiated. Local anesthetic drugs work essentially by inhibiting sodium influx through stimulus-gated sodium ion channels in the neuronal cell membrane. When the local anesthetic binds to the sodium channels, the influx of sodium is interrupted, and the action potential cannot rise and signal conduction is inhibited. The receptor site is located at the cytoplasmic (axoplasmic, inner) portion of the sodium channel. When neurons are firing quickly, causing sodium channels to be in their activated state, the local anesthetic drugs bind easier to the sodium channels, increasing the onset of neuronal blockade. This phenomenon is called *state dependent blockade.*[2]

To fully understand how local anesthetics work, the dental hygienist must understand the inner working of the nervous system and its components.

ORGANIZATION OF THE NERVOUS SYSTEM

The nervous system is organized to detect changes (stimuli) from the environment, either internal or external, by processing and responding to the information received.

CENTRAL AND PERIPHERAL NERVOUS SYSTEMS

The central and peripheral nervous systems are divisions of the nervous system that are based upon location and direction of nerves (Figure 2-1).

The central nervous system (CNS) is the structural and functional center of the entire nervous system that includes the brain, contained within the skull, and the spinal cord, contained within the vertebral canal. The CNS is responsible for receiving sensory information, processing the information, and initiating an outgoing response.[3,4]

The peripheral nervous system (PNS) are nerve tissues that lie in the periphery, or "outer regions," of the nervous system, consisting of 31 pairs of spinal nerves arising from the spinal cord, and 12 pairs of cranial nerves arising from the brain.[3,4]

Nerve fibers that extend from the cell body toward the CNS are termed central fibers, and nerve fibers that extend from the cell body away from the CNS are termed peripheral fibers. Figure 2-2 illustrates the divisions and relationship of the CNS and PNS.

AFFERENT AND EFFERENT DIVISIONS

Afferent and efferent divisions of the CNS and PNS tissues are categorized according to the direction in which they carry information. The afferent division consists of all *incoming* information traveling along *sensory or afferent pathways.* The efferent division consists of all *outgoing* information along *motor or efferent pathways.* Figure 2-2 illustrates the afferent pathways in blue and the efferent pathways in red.

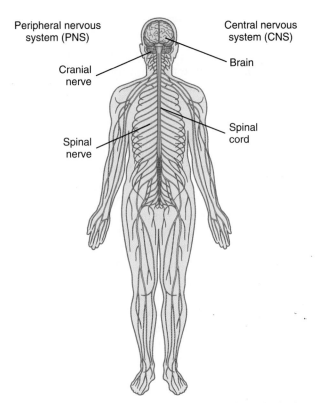

Figure 2-1 ■ The nervous system includes the brain and spinal cord (CNS) and the peripheral nerves and its branches (PNS). (From Drake RL, Vogl AW, Mitchell AWM: *Gray's anatomy for students*, ed 2, Philadelphia, 2010, Churchill Livingstone.)

SOMATIC AND AUTONOMIC NERVOUS SYSTEMS

Another way to organize the nervous system is based on function. The somatic nervous system is a subdivision of the efferent division of the PNS and controls the body's voluntary and reflex activities through somatic sensory and somatic motor components. External sense organs (including skin) are receptors. Somatic effectors are skeletal muscles and gland cells. The autonomic nervous system pathways carry information to the autonomic, or visceral, effectors that control involuntary (without conscious control) smooth muscle, cardiac muscle, or glandular tissue, and other involuntary tissue. The motor component controls smooth muscle contractions of viscera and blood vessels and the secretion of glands (eg: salivary glands). The autonomic nervous system is further divided into the *sympathetic* and the *parasympathetic* divisions. The sympathetic division prepares the body to deal with an emergency situation and is involved with the *"fight or flight"* response. The parasympathetic division coordinates the body's normal resting activities and is known as the *"rest or digest"* response.[3]

NEUROANATOMY

Nerve cells (neurons) are the basic functional unit of the nervous system which manipulate information and respond to either excitation or inhibition. Doing so involves changes

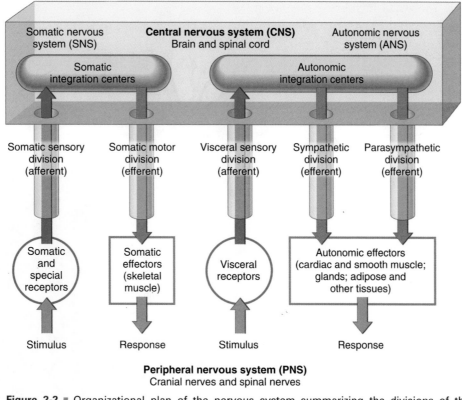

Figure 2-2 ■ Organizational plan of the nervous system summarizing the divisions of the nervous system. (From Patton K, Thibodeau G: *Anatomy and physiology*, ed 7, St Louis, 2010, Mosby.)

in the bioelectrical or biochemical properties of the cell, which require a vast expenditure of energy for each cell. The nervous system, compared with other organs, is the greatest consumer of oxygen and glucose. These energy requirements arise directly from the metabolic demand placed on cells, which have a large surface area and concentrate biomolecules and ions against an energy gradient. Along with maintaining its metabolism, each neuron receives information from the environment or from other nerve cells, processes information, and sends information to other neurons.[5-7]

For neurons to carry out the three tasks of receiving, processing, and sending information, they must have specialized structures that are designed to carry out each of these tasks. Basically, they conduct electrical impulses and communicate with other neurons through long cellular extensions (called *axons*) and synapses. The basic parts of a neuron are illustrated in Figure 2-3. Additionally, specialized mechanisms and structures exist for neurons to maintain a difference in the concentration of ions across their membranes. First, the mix of ions inside neurons is different from the mix of ions outside the cell. Maintaining this difference requires huge amounts of energy, because ions must be pumped against electrical and diffusion gradients. The large surface area of neurons compounds this problem. Second, those neurons that send information over long distances must have a way to supply these distant sites with macromolecules and energy. To fully understand the cell

biology of neurons, it is important to see the biochemical, anatomic, and physiologic properties of neurons as part of an integrated whole, the machinery that permits the neuron to do its specialized functions.[5-7]

THE STRUCTURE OF NEURONS

The neuron is an excitable cell that is the basic functional unit of the nervous system, specialized for sending impulses and making all nervous system functions possible. Basically, neurons are the functional unit for communication between the CNS and all parts of the body. A nerve contains many cable-like bundles of peripheral axons (the long, slender projections of neurons), which are encapsulated together. The nerve provides a pathway for the electrochemical nerve impulses to be transmitted along each of the axons. Nerves are found only in the PNS. In the CNS, the analogous structures are known as *tracts*.

Each nerve is a cordlike structure that contains many axons. These axons are often referred to as *nerve fibers*. Within a nerve, each axon is surrounded by a layer of connective tissue called the *endoneurium*. The nerve fibers are bundled together into groups called *fascicles*, and each fascicle is wrapped in a layer of connective tissue called the *perineurium*. Finally, the entire nerve is wrapped in a layer of connective tissue called the *epineurium* (Figure 2-4).

Fasciculi located in the mantle region are called *mantle bundles*, and fasciculi located in the core region are called *core bundles*. Mantle bundles are located near the outside

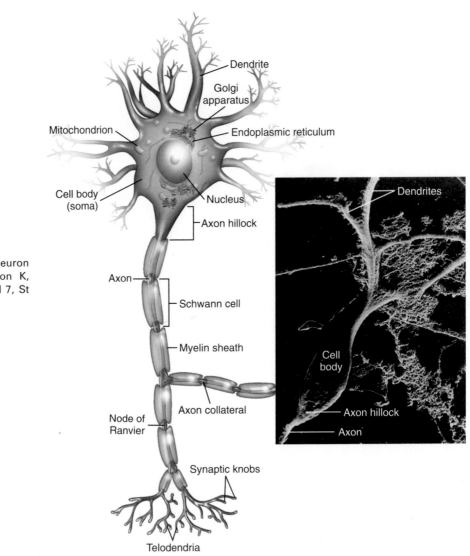

Figure 2-3 ■ Diagram of a typical sensory neuron innervating the oral mucosa. (From Patton K, Thibodeau G: *Anatomy and physiology*, ed 7, St Louis, 2010, Mosby.)

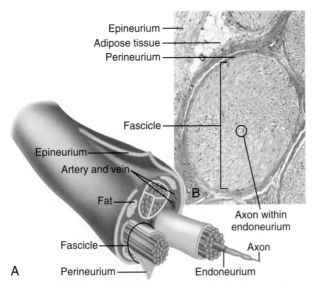

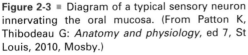

Figure 2-4 ■ The nerve. **A,** Each nerve contains axons bundled into fascicles. A connective tissue epineurium wraps the entire nerve. Perineurium surrounds each fascicle. **B,** A scanning electron micrograph of a cross section of a nerve. (From Patton K, Thibodeau G: *Anatomy and physiology*, ed 7, St Louis, 2010, Mosby.)

of the nerve, and core bundles are located on the inside of the nerve. The location of the bundles in larger nerves has an impact on which bundles are affected by the local anesthetic first. The local anesthetic, when administered diffuses through the nerve to the mantle bundles (outer core) at a higher concentration first and then to the core bundles (inner core) at a more diluted concentration due to some anesthetic being absorbed by capillaries and lymphatics. Because the mantle bundles are affected by the local anesthetic first, these bundles also lose anesthesia before the core bundles (Figure 2-5).[1,8]

CLASSIFICATION OF NEURONS

Nerves are categorized into three groups classified according to the direction that signals are conducted: Afferent nerves conduct signals from sensory neurons to the spinal cord or brain *(carry toward)*. Efferent nerves conduct signals away from the brain or spinal cord along motor neurons to their target muscles and glands *(carry away)*. *Mixed nerves* contain both afferent and efferent axons, and thus conduct both incoming sensory information and outgoing muscle

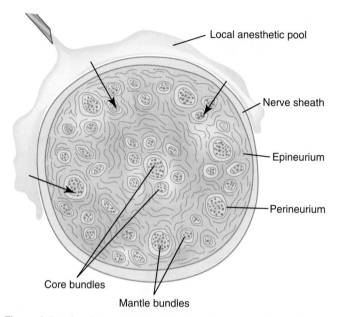

Figure 2-5 ■ A schematic cross section of a large peripheral nerve illustrating the composition of nerve fibers and bundles, and how the deposited local anesthetic solution near the nerve sheath must diffuse inward toward the core fibers, reaching the mantle fibers first. (Modified from de Jong RH: *Local anesthetics*. St Louis, 1994, Mosby.)

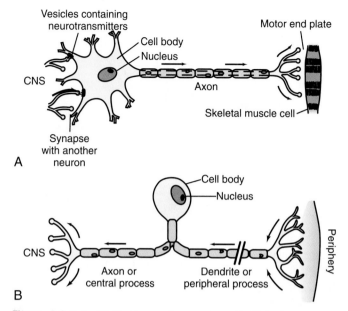

Figure 2-6 ■ **A,** Multipolar motor neuron. **B,** Unipolar sensory neuron. (From Liebgott B: *The anatomical basis of dentistry*, ed 3, St Louis, 2011, Mosby.)

commands in the same bundle. Although sensory and motor nerves are slightly different in structure, their main components of the neuron are the same, the cell body with a nucleus, axon, dendritic zone with free nerve endings (where stimulus is picked up) and terminal arborization (where the impulse is sent toward the CNS). The location of the cell body along the axon is the main difference between motor (efferent) neurons, and sensory (afferent) neurons. The cell body of the motor neuron participates in impulse conduction, and therefore is located at the terminal arborization. The cell bodies of sensory neurons do not participate in nerve conduction and therefore are located off the axon (Figure 2-6).

FUNCTIONAL REGIONS OF A SENSORY NEURON

There is a wide variation in the shape of sensory neurons, but they all have the same basic structures and functions (Figure 2-7).

Dendritic (Input) Zone

The dentritic zone is the most distal section of the neuron and is an arborization of nerve endings. These free nerve endings respond to stimulation (e.g., bradykinin, a "pain mediator" produced during cellular injury) produced in the tissues in which they lie, initiating nerve conduction. The dendrites of a neuron are cellular extensions with many branches, and metaphorically this overall shape and structure is referred to as a *dendritic tree*. This is where the majority of input to the neuron occurs.[3]

Cell Body (Soma)

The **cell body** is located at a distance from the axon in a sensory neuron, and is not involved in impulse transmission. The cell body is responsible for protein synthesis and provides metabolic support for the neuron (see Figure 2-6B).

Axon Hillock (Summation Zone)

The part of the axon where it emerges from the soma is called the *axon hillock*. The axon hillock decides whether to send the impulse farther down the axon. Besides being an anatomic structure, the axon hillock is also the part of the neuron that has the greatest density of voltage-dependent sodium channels. This makes it the most easily excited part of the neuron and the spike initiation zone for the axon: in neurologic terms it has the most negative action potential threshold. Whereas the axon and axon hillock are generally involved in information outflow, this region can also receive input from other neurons.[3]

Axon

If the axon hillock continues the impulse, it is then relayed from the periphery to the CNS by a thin, cable-like structure called the *axon*, which is made up of cytoplasm, or *axoplasm*, and is surrounded by a multilayer lipid membrane. Terminal branches of the axon distribute incoming signals to various CNS nuclei, which are responsible for their processing, similar to that seen in the dendritic zone, and form synapses. The axon is a finer, cable-like projection that can extend tens, hundreds, or even tens of thousands of times the diameter of the soma in length. The axon carries nerve signals away from the soma, and it carries some types of information back to it. Many neurons have only one axon,

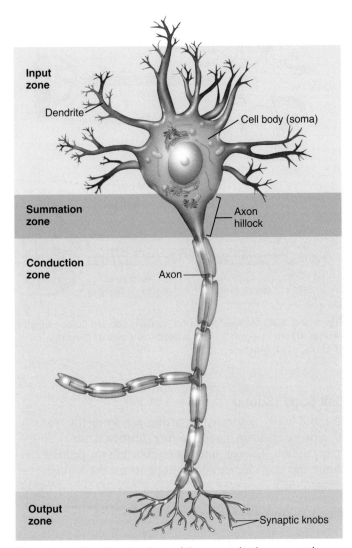

Figure 2-7 ■ Functional regions of the neuron's plasma membrane. The input zone receives input from other neurons or from sensory stimuli (stimulus-gated ion channels present). The summation zone serves as the site where the nerve impulses combine and possibly trigger an impulse that will be conducted along the axon, or conduction zone. Both the summation (trigger) zone and conduction zone have many voltage-gated Na$^+$ channels and K$^+$ channels imbedded in the plasma membrane. The output zone (distal end of axon) is where the nerve impulse triggers the release of neurotransmitters. The output zone includes many voltage-gated Ca^{++} channels in the membrane. (From Patton K, Thibodeau G: *Anatomy and physiology,* ed 7, St Louis, 2010, Mosby.)

but this axon may undergo extensive branching, enabling communication with many target cells. A single axon, with all its branches taken together, can innervate multiple parts of the brain and generate thousands of synaptic terminals.[3]

Output Zone (Synaptic Knobs)

The axon terminal contains synapses, specialized structures where neurotransmitter chemicals are released for possible reception by a nearby neuron. At a synapse, the membrane of the axon closely adjoins the membrane of the target cell,

---

BOX 2-1	Nodes of Ranvier and Myelin Sheath

Nodes of Ranvier are the gaps (approximately 1 μm in length) formed between the myelin sheaths generated by different cells. A myelin sheath is a many-layered coating, largely composed of a fatty substance called *myelin,* that wraps around the axon of a neuron and very efficiently insulates it. At nodes of Ranvier, the axonal membrane is uninsulated and therefore capable of generating electrical activity.

and special molecular structures transmit electrical or electrochemical signals across the gap.[3]

PERIPHERAL NERVE ANATOMY

The axon of a neuron is a single process and is the primary transmission lines of the nervous system, and as bundles they help make up nerves. Each individual axon is microscopic in diameter (typically about 1 μm across), and varies in both length and diameter. Some can be a meter long; others measure only a few millimeters long. In general, the larger the diameter of the axon, the faster the speed the impulse will travel across the nerve fiber. In vertebrates, the axons of many neurons are sheathed in myelin, which increases the speed of impulse conduction.

Myelinated Nerve

Myelin (lipoprotein sheath) is composed of about 75% lipid, about 20% protein, and about 5% carbohydrates. Myelin is made up primarily of a glycolipid called *galactocerebroside* and almost completely insulates the axon from the outside. Myelin is formed by either of two types of glial cells (which serve various roles in supporting the function of neurons): Schwann cells ensheathing peripheral neurons (Figure 2-8) and oligodendrocytes insulating those of the CNS (Figure 2-9). The myelin sheath of peripheral neurons is formed by many layers of thick Schwann cell membranes, which contain a fatty phospholipid myelin, called *myelinated fibers,* or white fibers (Figure 2-10). Along myelinated nerve fibers, gaps in the sheath, between adjacent Schwann cells, are called nodes of Ranvier (Box 2-1) and occur at evenly spaced intervals (see Figures 2-8 and 2-9). Only at the nodes of Ranvier, where the Schwann cells abut one another and the sheath is interrupted, does the myelinated axon have any direct contact with the extracellular space.

The myelination and its nodes of Ranvier enables an especially rapid mode of electrical impulse propagation called *saltatory conduction* (Box 2-2). Saltatory conduction (from the Latin *saltare,* to hop or leap) is the propagation of action potentials along myelinated axons from one node of Ranvier to the next node, increasing the conduction velocity of action potentials without needing to increase the diameter of an axon[1-3] (Figure 2-11).

Along *unmyelinated* fibers, impulses move continuously as waves and at a much slower rate compared to myelinated nerve fibers. When a peripheral fiber is severed, the myelin

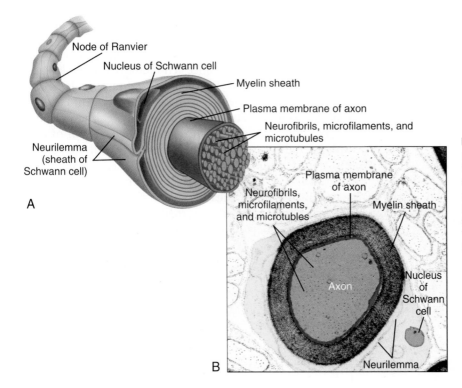

A

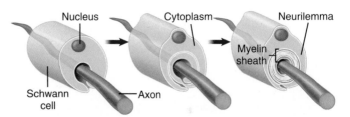

Figure 2-8 ■ Myelinated axon of the peripheral nervous system. **A,** Cross section of an axon and its coverings formed by a Schwann cell: the myelin sheath and neurilemma. **B,** Transmission electron micrograph showing how the densely wrapped layers of the Schwann cell's plasma membrane form the fatty myelin sheath. (From Patton K, Thibodeau G: *Anatomy and physiology,* ed 7, St Louis, 2010, Mosby.)

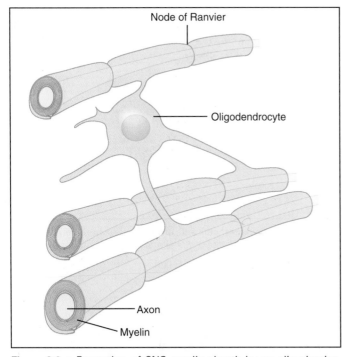

Figure 2-9 ■ Formation of CNS myelin sheath by an oligodendrocyte. (From Nolte J: *Elsevier's integrated neuroscience.* St Louis, 2007, Mosby.)

Figure 2-10 ■ Development of the myelin sheath. A Schwann cell (neurolemmocyte) migrates to a neuron and wraps around an axon. The Schwann cell's cytoplasm is pushed to the outer layer, leaving a dense multilayered covering of plasma membrane around the axon. Because the plasma membrane of the Schwann cell is mostly the phospholipid myelin, the dense wrapping around the axon is called a *myelin sheath.* The outer layer of cytoplasm is called the *neurilemma.* The extensions of oligodendrocytes also wrap around axons to form a myelin sheath. (From Patton K, Thibodeau G. *Anatomy and physiology,* ed 7, St Louis, 2010, Mosby.)

BOX 2-2   Saltatory Conduction

Because an axon can be unmyelinated or myelinated, the action potential has two methods to travel down the axon. These methods are referred to as *action potential conduction* for unmyelinated axons, and *saltatory conduction* for myelinated axons. Saltatory conduction is defined as an action potential moving in discrete jumps down a myelinated axon. This process is outlined as the charge passively spreading to the next node of Ranvier to depolarize it to threshold which will then trigger an action potential in this region which will then passively spread to the next node and so on. Saltatory conduction provides two advantages over conduction that occurs along an axon without myelin sheaths. First, it saves energy by decreasing the use of sodium-potassium pumps in the axonal membrane. Second, the increased speed afforded by this mode of conduction ensures faster interaction between neurons.

sheath provides a track along which regrowth can occur. Unmyelinated fibers and myelinated axons of the CNS do not regenerate. The demyelination of axons is what causes the multitude of neurologic symptoms seen in multiple sclerosis.[2,3]

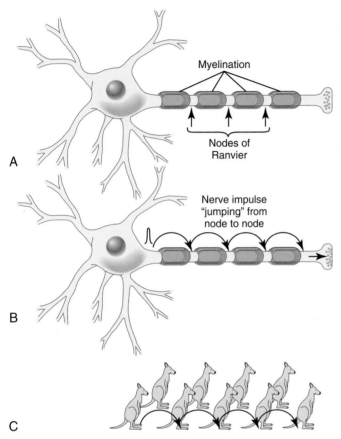

A

B

C

Figure 2-11 ■ Saltatory conduction. This series of diagrams shows the insulating nature of the myelin sheath prevents ion movement everywhere but at the nodes of Ranvier **(A). B,** The action potential at one node triggers current flow *(arrows)* across the myelin sheath to the next node, producing an action potential there. The action potential thus seems to "leap" rapidly from none to node resembling the jumping of a kangaroo **(C).** (From Herlihy B: *The human body in health and illness*, ed 4, St Louis, 2011, Saunders.)

Figure 2-13 ■ Impulse propagation along a myelinated axon compared to an unmyelinated axon. **A,** Myelinated axon allows a rapid propagation of the action potential by leaping from one node of Ranvier to the next node (saltatory conduction). **B,** Unmyelinated axon provides a much slower propagation of the action potential all along the nerve fiber.

Nonmyelinated Nerve

The nonmyelinated nerve fibers are long cylinder fibers with high-electrical resistance cell membranes that have no myelin sheath (Figure 2-12). These nonmyelinated nerve fibers are surrounded by low-resistance extracellular fluid. Ion diffusion occurs all along the nerve fiber through minute pores in nerve sheath. Therefore diffusion of electrolytes must occur all along the nerve cell membrane instead of jumping from node to node, causing these impulses to travel much slower than those traveling along a myelinated nerve sheath (Figure 2-13). Typically these are free nerve endings; the smallest nerve fibers are also known as C fibers. C fibers are the most numerous fiber type in the PNS.

CLASSIFICATION OF NERVE FIBERS

Peripheral nerve fibers differ substantially and can be classified based on axonal conduction velocity, frequency of firing, degree of myelination, and fiber diameter. For

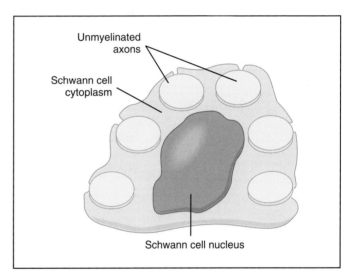

Figure 2-12 ■ Schwann cell and unmyelinated peripheral nervous system axons. (From Nolte J: *Elsevier's integrated neuroscience.* St Louis, 2007, Mosby.)

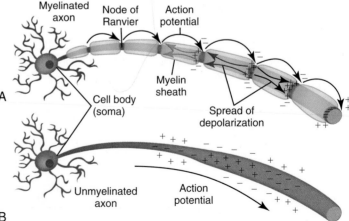

A

B

example, there are slow-conducting unmyelinated C fibers and faster-conducting myelinated Aδ fibers. All these factors influence the ability of the local anesthetic to block the nerve conduction.

Type A fibers are the largest fibers present in mammalian nerves, and with the rate of impulse transmission directly proportional to fiber diameter, this group comprises the most rapidly conducting axons. They are responsible for conducting pressure and motor sensations. Type A fibers are further divided into four groups, α through δ. Aδ fibers are distributed primarily in the skin and mucous membranes, and are responsible for the conduction of sharp, bright dental pain. Type B fibers are myelinated and moderate in size and are almost indistinguishable from Aδ fibers, but are not responsible for dental pain. Type C fibers are unmyelinated and the most numerous fibers in the PNS. They are responsible for carrying the sensations of dull or burning dental pain. As a result, in the lack of a myelin sheath, anesthetics block type C fibers more easily than they do type A fibers. Therefore patients who are adequately anesthetized still feel pressure and have mobility because of the unblocked type A fibers.[1,2,9,10]

Nerve fibers are classified as the following (Figure 2-14):

A Fibers: A fibers are the largest nerve fibers and can be either motor or sensory. In addition, these large fibers may require a stronger minimal stimulus compared to smaller C fibers. They are myelinated and have the fastest conduction velocity. A fibers, primarily delta fibers (Aδ) are responsible for sharp pain.

- *Alpha (α)*: Largest, fastest; responsible for muscle movement and light touch
- *Beta (β)*: Proprioception (awareness of position/ equilibrium)
- *Gamma (γ)*: Touch and pressure
- *Delta (δ)*: Pain, temperature

B Fibers: Fibers have medium diameters. They are lightly myelinated motor fibers.

C Fibers: Most numerous and smallest, usually unmyelinated and primarily responsible for dull, aching pain.

Both A and C fibers are found abundantly in the oral cavity, with C fibers in greater distribution.[1,2,9,10] Larger-diameter A fibers require more anesthetic volume than smaller C nerve fibers, to provide complete nerve blockade.

NEUROPHYSIOLOGY

All neurons are electrically excitable, maintaining voltage gradients across their resting membranes by sodium ion pumps, which combine with ion channels embedded in the membrane to generate intracellular-versus-extracellular concentration differences of ions such as sodium, potassium, chloride, and calcium. The relationship between the relative amounts of ions inside and outside the nerve membrane is known as the *concentration gradient* (Figure 2-15). Changes in the voltage across the nerve membrane can alter the function of the voltage-dependent ion channels. If the voltage changes by a large enough amount, an *all-or-none* (Box 2-3) electrochemical pulse called an action potential (nerve impulse) (Box 2-4) is generated, which travels rapidly along the cell's axon, and activates synaptic

Nerve fibers				
Fiber type	A	B	C*	
Diameter μm	2–20	<3	<1.5	
Conduction velocity (m/sec)	5–100	3–15	0.1–2.5	
Myelinated	Yes	Yes	No	
		Preganglionic, autonomic, vascular smooth muscle	Pain, temperature, postganglionic, autonomic	
Subtypes of A fibers	Aα	Aβ	Aγ	Aδ*
	Efferent, motor, somatic, reflex activity	Afferent, innervate muscle, touch sensation, pressure sensation	Efferent, muscle spindle tone	Afferent, pain, cold, temperature, tissue damage indication*

Figure 2-14 ■ Nerve fibers according to anatomic type. (From Wecker L, Crespo LM, Dunaway G, Faingold C, Watts S: *Brody's human pharmacology molecular to clinical*, ed 5, St Louis, 2010, Mosby.)

* Pain transmission fibers.

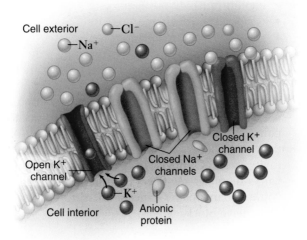

Figure 2-15 ▪ Role of ion channels in maintaining the resting membrane potential (RMP). Some K^+ channels are open in a "resting" membrane, allowing the K^+ to diffuse down its concentration gradient (out of the cell) and thus add to the excess of positive ions on the outer surface of the plasma membrane. Diffusion of Na^+ in the opposite direction would counteract this effect but is prevented from doing so by closed Na^+ channels. (From Patton K, Thibodeau G: *Anatomy and physiology*, ed 7, St Louis, 2010, Mosby.)

BOX 2-3   All-or-None Principle

Once a nerve is excited by the minimal threshold level (stimulus of sufficient magnitude to stimulate the nerve impulse), the impulse travels the full length of the fiber without additional stimulus. Impulse travels the same speed from any stimulus that exceeds minimum threshold level. The conduction of nerve impulses is an example of an all-or-none response. In other words, if a neuron responds at all, then it must respond completely and will be no longer dependent on the stimulus to continue. Conduction of an impulse is self-propagating energy. Greater intensity of stimulation does not produce a stronger signal but can produce *more* impulses per second.

BOX 2-4   Action Potential

An *action potential*, also known as a *nerve impulse*, is a spike of positive and negative ionic discharge that travels along the membrane of a cell. The creation and conduction of action potentials represents a fundamental means of communication in the nervous system. Action potentials represent rapid reversals in voltage across the plasma membrane of axons. These rapid reversals are mediated by voltage-gated ion channels found in the *plasma membrane*. The action potential travels from one location in the cell to another, but *ion flow* across the membrane occurs only at the nodes of Ranvier. As a result, the action potential signal jumps along the axon, from node to node, rather than propagating smoothly, as they do in axons that lack a myelin sheath. The clustering of voltage-gated sodium and potassium ion channels at the nodes permits this behavior.

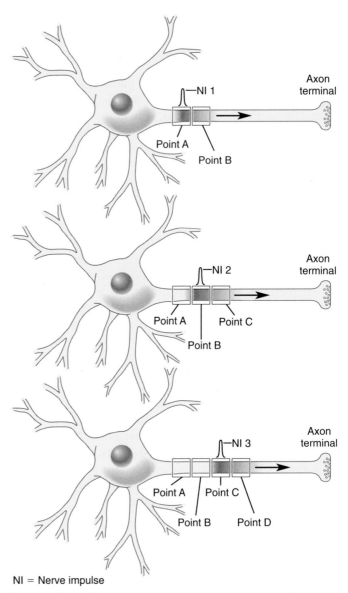

NI = Nerve impulse

Figure 2-16 ▪ All-or-none firing moves the nerve impulse at the same height as it depolarizes the next segment of the membrane without an addition stimulus. Nerve impulse #1 moves from axon hillock to point A; it depolarizes the next segment of the membrane point B, causing the nerve impulse #2 to form at the equal height and strength as impulse #1 (all-or-none firing). Impulse #2 then depolarizes the next segment, forming impulse #3, and so on. (From Herlihy B: *The human body in health and illness*, ed 4, St Louis, 2011, Saunders.)

connections with other cells when it arrives. The all-or-none firing means the height of each nerve impulse is the same as it depolarizes the next segment of the membrane, and so on. This ensures that the nerve impulse will travel the length of the nerve fiber at its initial strength and will not weaken (Figure 2-16).

A nerve conveys information, carried by neurons, in the form of electrochemical impulses (known as nerve impulses or action potentials). The impulses rapidly travel from one neuron to another by crossing a synapse; the message is converted from electrical to chemical and then back to

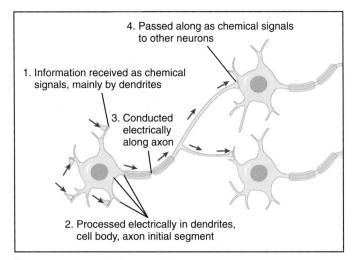

Figure 2-17 ■ Spread of electrical signals within a neuron and the use of chemical signals to transfer information from one neuron to another. (From Nolte J: *Elsevier's integrated neuroscience*. St Louis, 2007, Mosby).

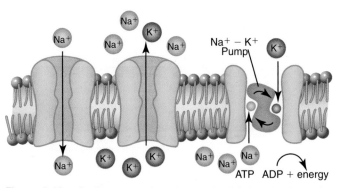

Figure 2-18 ■ Sodium-potassium pump. In this mechanism, the plasma membrane actively pumps sodium ions (Na+) out of the neuron and potassium ions (K+) into the neuron at an unequal (3:2) rate. Because very little sodium reenters the cell via diffusion, this maintains an imbalance in the distribution of ions and thus maintains the resting potential. (Modified from de Jong RH: *Local anesthetics*. St Louis, 1994, Mosby.)

electrical (see Figure 2-17). According to Tasaki[10] and Huxley,[12] the mechanism of nerve conduction occurs because the cytoplasm (axoplasm) of the axon is electrically conductive, and because the myelin inhibits charge leakage through the membrane (axolemma), depolarization at one node of Ranvier is sufficient to elevate the voltage at a neighboring node to the threshold for action potential initiation.[11-12] Thus action potentials in myelinated axons do not propagate as waves as in unmyelinated axons, but recur at successive nodes and in effect "hop" along the axon, by which process they travel faster than they would otherwise. The charge passively depolarizes the adjacent node of Ranvier to threshold, triggering an action potential in the neighboring node and subsequently depolarizing the next node, and so on.[10-12]

A stimulus—chemical, thermal, mechanical, or electrical—triggers nerve impulses that have a domino effect. Each neuron receives an impulse and must pass it through the synapses on to the next neuron to make sure the correct impulse continues on its path. Through a chain of chemical events, the dendrites pick up an impulse, shuttle it through the axon, and transmit it to the next neuron. The entire impulse passes through a neuron in about 7 milliseconds—faster than a bolt of lightning.[3,11-12]

GENERATION AND CONDUCTION OF NERVE IMPULSES

IONS IN NERVE TRANSMISSION AND RESTING MEMBRANE POTENTIALS

Polarization of the neuron's membrane: All living cells, which include neurons, maintain a difference in the ion concentration across their membranes. Sodium (Na+) ions are predominately in extracellular fluid, and potassium (K+) ions are predominately in the intracellular fluid. In addition to

the K+ ions intracellularly, negatively charged protein and nucleic acid molecules are synthesized within the cell and, because of their large size and solubility, do not diffuse across the resting membrane, causing the inside of the cell to be negatively charged in relation to the outside. This difference in the electrical charge on the outside of the cell versus the inside of the cell is called the membrane potential. Chloride (Cl−) ions assist in maintaining the membrane potential and are concentrated in the extracellular fluid with the sodium ions. When a neuron is not stimulated, it is sitting with no impulse to carry or transmit, and its membrane is polarized and in its *resting state*, also called the resting membrane potential (RMP). The electrical potential of nerve axoplasm in the resting state is approximately −70 mV with a range of −40 to −95 mV, and will remain this way until a stimulus comes along. Polarization (resting state) means that the electrical charge on the outside of the membrane is positive while the electrical charge on the inside of the membrane is negative. The outside of the cell contains excess sodium ions (Na+) at a ratio of 14:1; the inside of the cell contains excess potassium ions (K+). When a neuron is in its resting state, some of the K+ ion channels are open, but most of the Na+ channels are closed, allowing some intracellular K+ ions to diffuse out of the cell in an attempt to equalize the concentration gradient (Figure 2-15). The Na+/K+ pumps on the membrane, pump the Na+ back outside and the K+ back inside against resistance (Figure 2-18). The RMP is maintained by the cell with the operation of the sodium potassium pumps, and the cell's permeability characteristics remain stable. The use of adenosine triphosphate (ATP) energy is required for the pump to be fueled. The RMP is altered when either of these two mechanisms is altered.[3]

DEPOLARIZATION AND FIRING THRESHOLDS

Action potential: The action potential (see Box 2-4) is the membrane potential of an active nerve conducting an

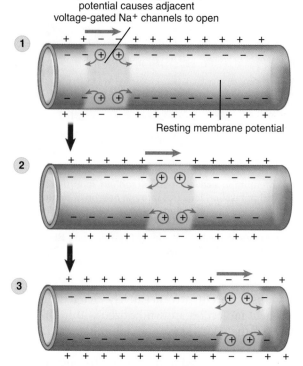

Figure 2-19 ■ Conduction of action potential. The reverse polarity characteristic of the peak of the action potential causes local current flow to adjacent regions of the membrane *(small arrows)*. This stimulates voltage-gated Na+ channels to open and thus create a new action potential. This cycle continues, producing wavelike conduction of the action potential from point to point along a nerve fiber. Adjacent regions of membrane behind the action potential do not depolarize again because they are still in their refractory period. (From Patton K, Thibodeau G: *Anatomy and physiology*, ed 7, St Louis, 2010, Mosby.)

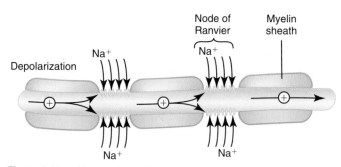

Figure 2-20 ■ Nerve conduction along a myelinated neuron moving between the uninsulated nodes of Ranvier, opening the stimulus gated channels, and allowing Na+ ions to rush into the cell, causing depolarization.

impulse. Excitation of a neuron occurs when a stimulus triggers the opening of a stimulus-gated channel, many of which are located in the membrane of the neuron's input zone (see Figure 2-7). Sodium ions move inside the membrane when a stimulus reaches a resting neuron, the gated Ca++ ion channels on the resting neuron's membrane release and open suddenly and allow the Na+ in the extracellular fluid to influx into the cell. As this happens, the resting neuron goes from being polarized to being depolarized. Figure 2-19 illustrates the conduction of the action potential.

Slow depolarization occurs until the axoplasm has depolarized approximately 15–20 mV, from −70 mV, which is the firing threshold. If the minimal threshold level is not achieved, the nerve slowly depolarizes and no impulses is generated, causing insufficient Na+ ion influx to depolarize the membrane.

Once the minimal firing threshold is achieved, more positive ions go charging inside the membrane, and the inside becomes positive as well; polarization is removed and the threshold is reached. Each neuron has a threshold

level—the point at which there is no holding back (*all-or-none principle;* see Box 2-3). After the stimulus goes above the threshold potential, more gated ion channels are stimulated to open and allow more Na+ inside the cell. This causes complete depolarization (rapid depolarization) of the neuron and an action potential is created. In this state, the neuron continues to open Na+ channels in response to voltage fluctuations all along the membrane. Complete depolarization occurs and the stimulus is transmitted along the neuron. When an impulse travels down an axon covered by a myelin sheath, the impulse must move between the uninsulated gaps called nodes of Ranvier that exist between each Schwann cell (Figure 2-20). To have the impulse cross the synapse to another cell requires the actions of either electrical synapses or chemical synapses. Electrical synapses occur where two cells are joined end-to-end by gap junctions (Figure 2-21A).[2,3] Action potentials can easily continue along the postsynaptic membrane because the plasma membrane and cytoplasm are functionally continuous in this type of junction.

Chemical synapses use chemical transmitters called neurotransmitters, which are packaged into synaptic vesicles that cluster beneath the membrane on the presynaptic side of a neuron. The neurotransmitters are discharged with the arrival of the action potential to send a signal from the presynaptic cell to the postsynaptic cell (see Figure 2-21B). These endogenous neurotransmitters transmit signals from a neuron to a target cell across the synapse. Neurotransmitters cause ion channels to open or close in the second cell, prompting changes in the excitability of that cell's membrane. Excitatory neurotransmitters such as acetylcholine and norepinephrine (in most organs) make it more likely that an action potential will be triggered in the second cell, causing depolarization (Figure 2-22). Inhibitory neurotransmitters such as dopamine and serotonin, cause K+ channels and/or Cl− channels to open. This causes K+ ions to rush outward and Cl− ions to rush inward. This response creates a more negative membrane than the resting potential, causing an action potential in the second cell less likely. Neurotransmitters are either destroyed by specific enzymes, diffuse away, or are reabsorbed by the neuron. Figure 2-23 summarizes the main events of chemical synaptic transmission.[2]

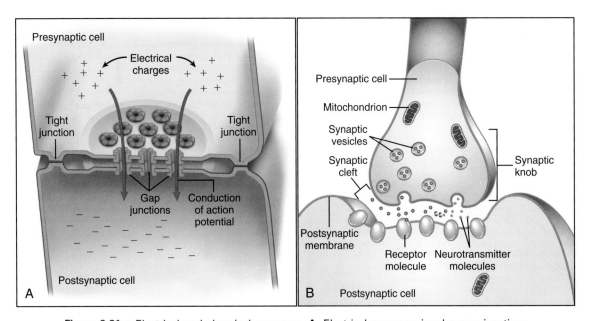

Figure 2-21 ■ Electrical and chemical synapses. **A,** Electrical synapses involve gap junctions that allow action potentials to move from cell to cell directly by allowing electrical current to flow between cells. **B,** Chemical synapses involve transmitter chemicals (neurotransmitters) that signal postsynaptic cells, possibly inducing an action potential. (From Patton K, Thibodeau G: *Anatomy and physiology*, ed 7, St Louis, 2010, Mosby.)

REPOLARIZATION

Repolarization occurs once the peak of the action potential is reached and the membrane potential begins to move back toward the resting potential (−70 mV). There is a change in membrane potential that returns the membrane potential back to this negative value. Repolarization results from the efflux of positively charged potassium ions out of the cell. After the inside of the cell becomes flooded with Na^+ ions and the nerve has reached a potential of approximately +40 mV, the gated ion channels on the inside of the membrane open to allow the reversal process to begin repolarization and restoring electrical balance.

The *refractory period* (Box 2-5) is when the Na^+ and K^+ ions are returned to their original sides: Na^+ on the outside and K^+ on the inside. While the neuron is busy returning everything to normal, it resists any additional incoming stimuli. The interval during which a second action potential absolutely cannot be initiated to restimulate the membrane, no matter how large a stimulus is applied, is known as the *absolute refractory period*, which coincides with nearly the entire duration of the action potential. In neurons, it is caused by the inactivation of the Na^+ channels that originally opened to depolarize the membrane. These channels remain inactivated until the membrane repolarizes, after which they close, reactivate, and regain their ability to open in response to stimulus. The *relative refractory period* is the interval immediately following the *absolute refractory period* and before complete

BOX 2-5	**Refractory Periods**

Absolute refractory period is the interval during which a second action potential absolutely cannot be initiated, no matter how large a stimulus is applied.

Relative refractory period is the interval immediately following the absolute refractory period, during which initiation of a second action potential is *inhibited* but not impossible if a larger stimulus is applied.

reestablishment to the resting state, during which initiation of a second action potential is *inhibited* but not impossible if a larger stimulus is achieved to produce successful firing. The return to the resting potential marks the end of the *relative refractory period*[3] (Figure 2-24).

RETURN TO RESTING STATE

After the Na^+/K^+ pumps return the ions to their rightful side of the neuron's cell membrane, the neuron is back to its normal polarized state of approximately −70 mV; the nerve is fully recovered and stays in the resting potential until another impulse comes along. Figure 2-25 illustrates the depolarization and repolarization mechanisms, and Table 2-1 describes the steps of the mechanism that produce an action potential. Nerve conduction requires only 1 msec to respond to a minimal threshold stimulus and recover (Figure 2-26).

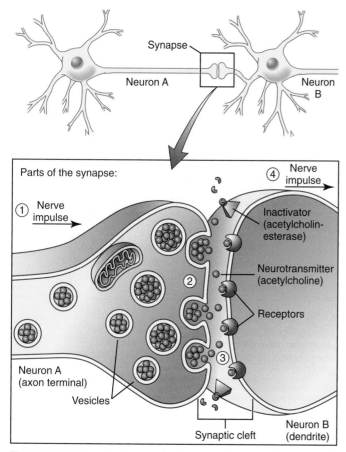

Figure 2-22 ■ Chemical synapse. Diagram shows detail of synaptic knob, or axon terminal, of presynaptic neuron, the plasma membrane of a postsynaptic neuron, and a synaptic cleft. On the arrival of an action potential at a synaptic knob, voltage-gated Ca^{++} channels open and allow extracellular Ca^{++} to diffuse into the presynaptic cell (step 1). In step 2, the Ca^{++} triggers the rapid exocytosis of neurotransmitter molecules from vesicles in the knob. In step 3, neurotransmitter diffuses into the synaptic cleft and binds to receptor molecules in the plasma membrane of the postsynaptic neuron. In step 4, the local potential may move toward the axon, where an action potential may begin. (From Herlihy B: *The human body in health and illness*, ed 4, St Louis, 2011, Saunders.)

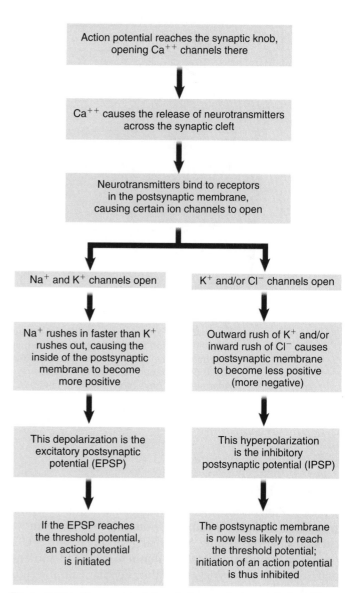

Figure 2-23 ■ Summary of chemical synaptic transmission. (From Patton K, Thibodeau G: *Anatomy and physiology*, ed 7, St Louis, 2010, Mosby.)

MODE OF ACTION OF LOCAL ANESTHETICS

Local anesthetic drugs act mainly by inhibiting sodium influx through sodium-specific ion channels in the neuronal cell membrane, in particular the so-called voltage-gated sodium channels. When the influx of sodium is interrupted, an action potential cannot arise and signal conduction is inhibited. The receptor site is thought to be located at the cytoplasmic (axoplasmic, inner) portion of the sodium channel. Local anesthetic drugs bind more readily to sodium channels in an activated state, thus onset of neuronal blockade is faster in neurons that are rapidly firing. This is referred to as *state dependent blockade* (Figure 2-27, and chapter 3).[2]

All nerve fibers are sensitive to local anesthetics, but generally, those with a smaller diameter tend to be more sensitive than larger fibers. Local anesthetics block conduction in the following order: small myelinated axons (e.g., those carrying nociceptive impulses), nonmyelinated axons, then large myelinated axons. Thus a differential block can be achieved (i.e., pain sensation is blocked more readily than other sensory modalities). In myelinated nerves, the local anesthetic blocks only at the nodes of Ranvier. Because of the excess current available in saltatory conduction (10 times more), at least two to three adjacent nodes must be blocked to ensure total block to the nerve. The larger the diameter of the nerve fiber, the greater the amount of local anesthetic needed to prevent depolarization (inferior alveolar (IA) and posterior superior alveolar (PSA) blocks require more anesthetic for successful nerve blockage than supraperiosteal injections).[2]

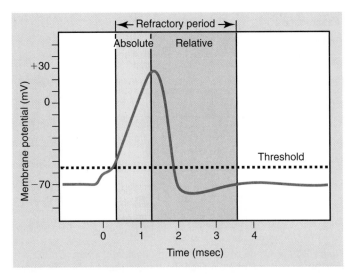

Figure 2-24 ▪ Refractory period. During the absolute refractory period, the membrane will not respond to any stimulus. During the relative refractory period, however, a very strong stimulus may elicit a response in the membrane. (From Patton K, Thibodeau G: *Anatomy and physiology*, ed 7, St Louis, 2010, Mosby.)

TABLE 2-1	Steps to the Mechanism that Produces an Action Potential

STEPS	DESCRIPTION
1	A stimulus triggers stimulus-gated Na⁺ channels in axonal membrane to open and allows inward Na⁺ diffusion. This causes the membrane to depolarize.
2	As the threshold potential is reached, voltage-gated Na⁺ channels open.
3	As more Na⁺ enters the cell through voltage-gated Na⁺ channels, the membrane depolarizes even further.
4	The magnitude of the action potential peaks (at +30 mV) when voltage-gated Na⁺ channels close).
5	Repolarization begins when voltage-gated K⁺ channels open, allowing outward diffusion of K⁺.
6	After a brief period of hyperpolarization, the resting potential is restored by the sodium-potassium pump and the return of ion channels to their resting state.

Modified from Patton K, Thibodeau G: *Anatomy and physiology*, ed 7, St Louis, 2010, Mosby.

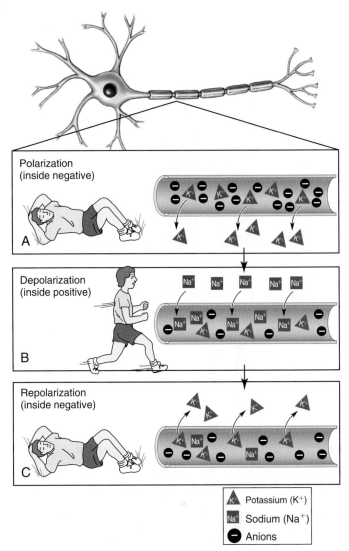

Figure 2-25 ▪ Depolarization and repolarization. **A,** Resting membrane potential results from an excess of positive ions on the outer surface of the plasma membrane. More Na⁺ ions are on the outside of the membrane than K⁺ ions are on the inside of the membrane. **B,** Depolarization of a membrane occurs when Na⁺ channels open, allowing the Na⁺ to move to an area of lower concentration (and more negative charge) inside the cell, reversing the polarity to an inside-positive state. **C,** Repolarization of a membrane occurs when K⁺ channels then open, allowing K⁺ to move to an area of lower concentration (and more negative charge) outside of the cell, reversing the polarity back to an inside-negative state. (From Herlihy B: *The human body in health and illness*, ed 4, St Louis, 2011, Saunders.)

DENTAL HYGIENE CONSIDERATIONS

Dental Hygiene Considerations
- Large nerve trunks (such as the IA and PSA nerves) are myelinated A fibers and require more local anesthetic volume to successfully block the core fibers.

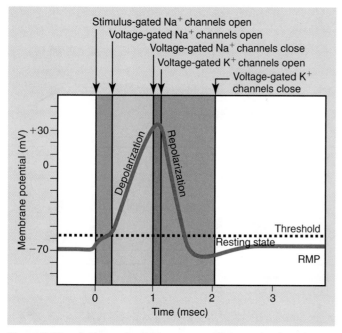

Figure 2-26 ■ Action potential in a neuron. Schematic of an electrophysiologic recording of an action potential showing the various phases that occur as the wave passes a point on the cell membrane. Each voltmeter records the changing membrane potential as a redline. (Modified from Patton K, Thibodeau G: *Anatomy and physiology*, ed 7, St Louis, 2010, Mosby.)

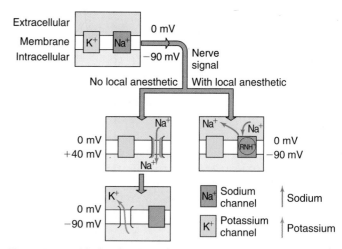

Figure 2-27 ■ Mode of action of local anesthetic agent. On the left is an open channel (the usual configuration after a sufficient stimulus has been applied), allowing sodium ion (Na^+) influx through the nerve membrane. The center channel remains closed to sodium ions, which is the usual configuration in the resting state. The right channel, although otherwise in the open configuration, has been closed by an anesthetic cation that is bound to the receptor site in the channel. (Modified rom Wecker L, Crespo LM, Dunaway G, Faingold C, Watts S: *Brody's human pharmacology molecular to clinical*, ed 5, St Louis, 2010, Mosby.)

CASE STUDY 2-1

Peter complains of inadequate anesthesia

Peter is in the office today for nonsurgical periodontal therapy of the mandibular right quadrant. The dental hygienist, Eliana, anesthetizes the mandibular right quadrant using an inferior alveolar nerve block and buccal injections, and she administers one cartridge of anesthetic. When Eliana begins scaling, Peter informs her that he feels numb in general, but not completely numb, especially on the anterior teeth and soft tissue.

Critical Thinking Questions

- What could be the reason why Peter is not completely numb?
- Why does Peter feel more sensitivity on the anterior teeth and soft tissues?
- How should Eliana respond to this situation?

CHAPTER REVIEW QUESTIONS

1. A stimulus is an electrical message from one part of the body to another, and an impulse is an environmental change in an excitable tissue.
   A. Both statements are true
   B. Both statements are false
   C. The first statement is true and the second is false
   D. The first statement is false and the second is true

2. Which fibers are the principle fibers in the transmission of sharp, bright dental pain?
   A. A δ fibers
   B. B fibers
   C. C fibers
   D. A β fibers
   E. A γ fibers

3. Local anesthetics work by:
   A. Penetrating the nerve to inhibit Cl^+ influx
   B. Penetrating the nerve to inhibit Na^+ influx
   C. Penetrating the nerve to inhibit K^- efflux
   D. Penetrating the nerve to inhibit Na^+ efflux
   E. Penetrating the nerve to inhibit K^- influx

4. Local anesthetics have their effect on myelinated nerves mostly in which way?
   A. All along the nerve membrane
   B. Mostly at the synapse
   C. Mostly at the cell bodies
   D. Mostly at the node of Ranvier

5. The minimal threshold stimulus required to excite a C fiber will also be sufficient to stimulate an A fiber.

CHAPTER REVIEW QUESTIONS

A. True
B. False

6. When energy for conduction is derived from the nerve cell membrane itself and is no longer dependent on the stimulus for continuance, the conduction is considered to be:
   A. Below the minimal threshold level
   B. Above the minimal threshold level
   C. Self-propagating
   D. In the absolute refractory period

7. The absolute refractory period occurs during the fraction of a millisecond when a nerve fiber can be excited only by a much stronger stimulus than the initial stimulus.
   A. True
   B. False

8. Saltatory conduction refers to:
   A. Rapid transmission of nerve impulses along a myelinated nerve fiber
   B. Diffusion of sodium chloride into the nerve cell during impulse conduction
   C. Conduction of an impulse along a nonmyelinated nerve at the nodes of Ranvier
   D. The movement of continuous waves along a nerve fiber

9. What is the type of glial cell located in the peripheral nervous system?
   A. Astrocytes
   B. Microglia
   C. Ependymal cells
   D. Oligodendrocytes
   E. Schwann cells

10. Myelin (lipoprotein sheath) is composed of :
    A. Approximately 75% lipid, 20% protein, and 5% carbohydrate
    B. Approximately 60% lipid and about 35% protein, and 5% carbohydrate
    C. Approximately 65% lipid and about 30% protein, and 5% carbohydrate
    D. 100% lipid

11. The sympathetic division is involved with the "rest or digest" response. The parasympathetic division is known as the "fight or flight" response.
    A. Both statements are true
    B. Both statements are false
    C. The first statement is true and the second is false
    D. The first statement is false and the second is true

12. The afferent division consists of all *incoming* information traveling along sensory or afferent pathways. The efferent division consists of all *outgoing* information along motor or efferent pathways.
    A. Both statements are true
    B. Both statements are false
    C. The first statement is true and the second is false
    D. The first statement is false and the second is true

13. The outer layer of the myelin sheath that wraps the entire nerve is called:
    A. Nucleus
    B. Schwann cell
    C. Epineurium
    D. Node of Ranvier

14. The axon hillock:
    A. Is where the majority of input to the neuron occurs
    B. Is not involved in impulse transmission
    C. Distributes incoming signals to various central nervous system nuclei
    D. Is where neurotransmitter chemicals are released for possible reception by a nearby neuron
    E. Decides whether to send the impulse farther down the axon

15. In a resting neuron, what positive ion is most abundant *outside* the plasma membrane?
    A. Potassium ions
    B. Sodium ions
    C. Calcium ions
    D. Chloride ions

16. In a resting neuron, what positive ion is most abundant *inside* the plasma membrane?
    A. Potassium ions
    B. Sodium ions
    C. Calcium ions
    D. Chloride ions

17. The electrical potential of nerve axoplasm in the resting state is approximately:
    A. −70 mV
    B. −30 mV
    C. Zero
    D. +30 mV
    E. +70 mV

18. Mantle bundles will be anesthetized first by a local anesthetic compared to core bundles.
    A. True
    B. False

19. Chemical synapses use chemical transmitters called:
    A. Neurotransmitters
    B. Chemical transmitters
    C. Synaptic transmitters
    D. Endogenous transmitters

20. The "all-or-none principle" occurs:
    A. With a spike of positive and negative ionic discharge
    B. In the interval during which a second action potential absolutely cannot be initiated
    C. Once a nerve is excited by the minimal threshold level
    D. Once a nerve is excited by a stimulus greater than the first stimulus

REFERENCES

1. Malamed S: *Handbook of local anesthesia*, ed 5, St Louis, 2004, Mosby.
2. de Jong RH: *Local anesthetics*, St Louis, 1994, Mosby.
3. Patton K, Thibodeau G: *Anatomy and physiology*, ed 7, St Louis, 2010, Mosby.
4. Liebgott B: *The anatomical basis of dentistry*, ed 3, St Louis, 2011, Mosby.
5. Nolte J: *Elsevier's integrated neuroscience*, St Louis, 2007, Mosby.
6. Castro A, Merchut MP, Neafsey E, Wurster R: *Neuroscience, an outline approach*, St Louis, 2002, Mosby.
7. Haines D: *Fundamental neuroscience for basic and clinical applications*, ed 3, St Louis, 2006, Churchill Livingstone.
8. Hargreaves K, Cohen S: *Cohen's pathways of the pulp*, ed 10, St Louis, 2011, Mosby.
9. Daniel S, Harfst S, Wilder R, Francis B, Mitchell S: *Dental hygiene concepts, cases and competencies*, ed 2, St Louis, 2008, Mosby.
10. Jastak T, Yagiela J, Donaldson D: *Local anesthesia of the oral cavity*, St Louis, 1995, Saunders.
11. Tasaki I: The electro-saltatory transmission of the nerve impulse and the effect of narcosis upon the nerve fiber, *Am J Physiol* 127:211-227, 1939.
12. Huxley AF, Stämpfli R: Evidence for saltatory conduction in peripheral myelinated nerve fibres, *J Physiol* 108:315-339, 1949.

ADDITIONAL RESOURCES

Becker D, Reed K: Essentials of local anesthetic pharmacology. American Dental Society of Anesthesiology, *Anesth Program* 53:98-109, 2006.

Paarmann C, Royer R: *Pain control for dental practitioners*, Baltimore, 2008, Lippincott Williams and Wilkins.

Haveles B: *Applied pharmacology for the dental hygienist*, ed 6, St Louis, 2011, Mosby.

Bahl R: Local anesthesia in dentistry, *Anesth Prog* 51:138-142, 2004.

PART II

Local and Topical Anesthetic Agents

CHAPTER 3

Pharmacology of Local Anesthetic Agents

Demetra Daskalos Logothetis RDH, MS

CHAPTER OUTLINE

LEARNING OBJECTIVES

1. Define local anesthetics.
2. Discuss the mechanism of actions of local anesthetics.
3. Describe the structure of local anesthetics.
4. Discuss the difference between esters and amides.
5. Discuss the properties and ionization factors of local anesthetics.
6. Describe the dissociation constant (pK_a), and its effects on the onset of action of local anesthetics.
7. Discuss how infection in the area of local anesthetic administration decreases its efficiency.
8. Describe the differences between the membrane expansion theory and the specific receptor theory.
9. Discuss the pharmacodynamics of local anesthetic drugs.
10. Discuss the pharmacokinetics of local anesthetics, including onset of action, duration, absorption, distribution, biotransformation, the difference between esters and amides, and differences within the same groups.
11. Discuss the systemic effects of local anesthetic drugs on the central nervous system and cardiovascular system.
12. Correctly complete the review questions and activities for this chapter.

KEY TERMS

Amide local anesthetic A local anesthetic agent made from a specific class of chemical compounds that are generally broken down by the liver and are more effective and longer-lasting than esters. This type of anesthetic rarely causes allergic reactions.

Anion Base form of the local anesthetic (lipid soluble and penetrates the nerve).

Cation Acid form of the local anesthetic (water soluble and active form of molecule).

Dissociation constant (pK$_a$) Represents the pH at which 50% of the molecules exist in the lipid-soluble tertiary form and 50% in the quaternary, water-soluble form.

Ester local anesthetic A short-acting local anesthetic agent made from a specific class of chemical compounds that are broken down by blood enzymes. They are less effective than amide anesthetics and more likely to cause allergic reactions.

Half-life of drug The period of time required to eliminate the amount of drug in the body by one-half of its strength.

Henderson-Hasselbach equation Calculates the pH of a buffer solution or the concentration of acid versus base molecules in an anesthetic solution.

Hydrophilic terminal amine Strong water-attracting properties that enable the diffusion of the agent through the water portions of the tissues to the nerves.

Intermediate hydrocarbon chain Determines if the local anesthetic is classified as an ester or an amide.

Ionized Cationic form of molecule.

Lipophilic aromatic ring Facilitates diffusion of local anesthetic through lipid rich membrane.

Pharmacodynamics The study of the physiological effects of drugs on the body and the mechanisms of drug action and its relationship between drug concentration and effect.

Pharmacokinetics The study of the action of drugs within the body.

Tachyphylaxis Increased tolerance to a drug that is administered repeatedly.

Unionized Anionic form of molecule.

INTRODUCTION

Local anesthetics are agents that block the sensation of pain by reversibly blocking nerve conduction when applied to a circumscribed area of the body. Local anesthetics interrupt neural conduction by interfering with the propagation of peripheral nerve impulses, thus inhibiting the influx of sodium ions during depolarization.

In most cases, this follows the anesthetic's diffusion through the neural membrane into the axoplasm, where they enter sodium channels and prevent them from assuming an active or "open" state. Local anesthetics block the conduction of a nerve impulse by preventing the nerve from reaching its firing potential. Local anesthetics bind to specific receptors in the nerve membrane to prevent the influx of sodium ions through the cell membrane. As long as the anesthetic remains bound to the receptor sites, the conduction of nerve impulses is prevented. If this process can be inhibited for just a few nodes of Ranvier along the axon, then nerve impulses generated farther down on the axon from the blocked nodes cannot propagate to the ganglion. In order to accomplish this process, the anesthetic molecules must enter through the cell membrane of the nerve and are dependent upon the potency, time of onset, and duration of the local anesthetic agent.

The use of reversible local anesthetic chemical agents is the most common method to secure pain control in dental practice. Box 3-1 describes the properties of ideal anesthetics. Not all local anesthetics that are available for use in

BOX 3-1	Properties of the Ideal Local Anesthetic

Potent local anesthesia
Reversible local anesthesia
Absence of local reactions
Absence of systemic reactions
Absence of allergic reactions
Rapid onset
Satisfactory duration
Adequate tissue penetration
Low cost
Stability in solution (long shelf life)
Ease of metabolism and excretion

Modified from Haveles B: *Applied pharmacology for the dental hygienist*, ed 6, St Louis, 2011, Mosby.

dentistry today meet all of these properties, although many are clinically acceptable.

CHEMISTRY

Local anesthetic agents are divided chemically into two major groups: the esters and the amides. The clinical significance of the two major groups is the potential for allergic reactions and the route of biotransformation. **Ester local anesthetics** have a high probability of producing an allergic reaction compared to amide local anesthetics. With ester local anesthetics, a patient who has an allergic reaction

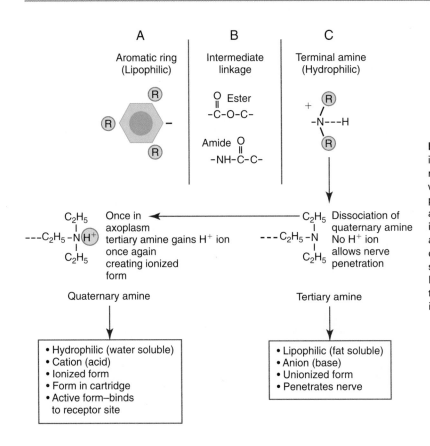

Figure 3-1 ■ Local anesthetic structure. All local anesthetics consist of three principal components. A, The aromatic ring is the lipophilic (base) portion of the molecule and is what penetrates the nerve, and determines the anesthetic potency. B, The intermediate chain determines if the local anesthetic is an ester or an amide. C, The terminal amine is the hydrophilic (acid) portion of the molecule; it is the active form in the cartridge and binds to the receptor sites on the nerve membrane. In order to bind to the receptor sites, it must first dissociate to a tertiary amine to become lipid soluble and penetrate the nerve. Upon nerve penetration it will regain a H^+ ion in the axoplasm, creating the ionized form necessary to bind to the receptor sites.

to one ester agent is likely to experience hypersensitivity to all ester anesthetics. This is less likely to occur within the amide local anesthetic group. Cross-hypersensitivity between esters and amides is unlikely. Due to the high degree of hypersensitivity to injectable esters, all injectable local anesthetics manufactured for dentistry today are in the amide group. Ester local anesthetics are hydrolized in the plasma by the enzyme pseudocholinesterase, and amide local anesthetics are biotransformed generally in the liver. Topical anesthetics are available in both the esters and amides. (See chapter 6.)

The local anesthetic molecule consists of three components: (1) the lipophilic aromatic ring, (2) intermediate hydrocarbon ester or amide chain, and (3) hydrophilic terminal amine (Figure 3-1). The lipophilic aromatic ring improves the lipid solubility of the molecule, which facilitates the penetration of the anesthetic through the lipid-rich membrane where the receptor sites are located. The greater the lipid solubility of the anesthetic molecule, the greater the potency of the drug. For example, the local anesthetic bupivacaine is more lipid-soluble than lidocaine, and it is therefore more potent because more of the anesthetic dose can enter the neurons. Because bupivacaine is more lipid-soluble and is more potent than lidocaine, it is prepared as a 0.5% concentration (5 mg/mL) rather than a 2% concentration of lidocaine (20 mg/mL).

The intermediate hydrocarbon chain determines if the molecule is an ester or amide, and this chain is important because it predetermines the course of biotransformation. Ester local anesthetics are hydrolyzed by appropriate ester-

ases, and amide local anesthetics generally require enzymatic breakdown by the liver.

The hydrophilic terminal amine (or acid cation form) may exist in a tertiary form (three bonds) that is uncharged and lipid-soluble (or base anion form) or as a quaternary form (four bonds) that is positively charged and renders the molecule water-soluble, which is how it is delivered from the dental hygienist's syringe into the patient's tissue. As explained earlier, the aromatic ring determines the actual degree of lipid solubility, but the terminal amine acts as an "on-off" switch allowing the local anesthetic to exist in either lipid-soluble or water-soluble configurations. Once the anesthetic is injected into the tissue, the quaternary amine dissociates into uncharged tertiary amine base and a hydrogen ion inorder to penetrate the lipid rich nerve membrane. The tertiary amine following penetration of the nerve will once again gain a hydrogen ion found within the axoplasm to successfully bind to the receptor sites. The tertiary and quaternary forms exhibit vital roles in the sequence of events leading to the conduction block[1] (discussed later, see Figure 3-1).

ROUTES OF DELIVERY

There are two major routes of delivery of local anesthetic drugs, topical and submucosal injection. Topical anesthetics are drugs applied to the surface of mucosal tissues that produce local insensibility to pain. Topical anesthetic agents are prepared in higher concentrations than injectable anesthetics to facilitate diffusion of the drug through the mucous

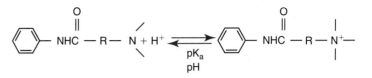

or written simply as

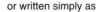

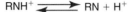

Figure 3-2 ■ Properties of base and salt forms of local anesthetics. (Modified from Haveles B: *Applied pharmacology for the dental hygienist*, ed 6, St Louis, 2011, Mosby.)

Salt	Free base
• Crystalline solids	• Viscid liquids or amorphous solids
• Water soluble (hydrophilic)	• Fat soluble (lipophilic)
• Stable	• Unstable
• Acidic	• Alkaline
• Charged, cation (ionized)	• Uncharged, nonionized
• Active form at site of action	• Penetrates nerve tissue
• Form present in dental cartridge (pH 4.5–6.0)	• Form present in tissue (pH 7.4)

membranes. Because of this, there is a risk for toxicity if large amounts of topical anesthetics are applied to limited areas. In contrast, submucosal injections of local anesthetics are more effective than topical routes of administration because the local anesthetic solution is injected and placed in close proximity to the nerve truck of the area to be anesthetized. This allows the solution to more effectively reach the nerve.

PHARMACODYNAMICS OF LOCAL ANESTHETIC DRUGS

Pharmacodynamics refers to the physiological effects of drugs on the body and the mechanisms of drug action and its relationship between drug concentration and effect. Synthetic local anesthetics are prepared as weak bases and during manufacturing precipitate as powdered unstable solids that are poorly soluble in water. They are combined with an acid to form a salt (hydrochloride salt) to render them water-soluble; these can be dissolved in sterile water or saline, creating a stable, injectable anesthetic solution. The molecules exist in a quaternary water-soluble state in the cartridge. In the cartridge, the solution contains an equilibrium of positively charged (ionized) molecules, the acid or cation $(RNH^+)^2$ and uncharged (unionized) molecules, the base or anion $(RN)^1$. The formula $RNH^+ \leftrightarrow RN + H^+$ represents the equilibrium between the two ions and H^+ as the hydrogen ion[2] (Figure 3-2). The equilibrium is dependent upon the pH of the solution and the pK_a (how easily the compound becomes charged). Discussed next, also see Box 3-2.

When the pK_a equals the pH there is an equal distribution of charged cations and uncharged base molecules. If there is a high presence of H^+ ions, the equilibrium shifts to the left and the anesthetic solution will have higher concentrations of the ionized (charged) cationic form (water-soluble) which is the active form of the molecule ($RNH^+ > RN + H^+$). In contrast, if the presence of H^+ ions is decreased, the equilibrium shifts to the right and the

anesthetic solution will have a higher concentration of unionized (uncharged) free base (fat-soluble), which is the form that penetrates the nerve membrane ($RNH^+ <$ $RN + H^+$).

The pH (the acid-base balance) of the solution is manipulated by the manufacturer to complement the specific molecular structure of each anesthetic. However, all local anesthetic solutions are acidic before injection. The lower the pH, the more acidic the solution, and the higher the pH, the more alkaline (basic) the solution. Local anesthetic solutions without vasoconstrictors range in pH from approximately 5 to more than 6; generally, preparations with vasoconstrictors are more acidic than plain formations because of the presence of the preservative (antioxidant) sodium bisulfite (see Chapter 4), and the pH ranges from approximately 3.3 to 5.5.[3] Once injected, the hydrophilic (ionized) cation component which is acidic facilitates diffusion through the extracellular fluid to the nerve. However, the cation form will not penetrate the nerve. Therefore the time of onset of the local anesthetic is based on the proportion of the molecule that converts to the tertiary, lipid-soluble (unionized) base structure when exposed to the normal physiologic pH (7.4) of the body. Once injected into the tissues (pH 7.4), the amount of local anesthetic in the free-base unionized form will increase to provide greater lipid penetration of the nerve. The increase in the base molecules is due to the dissociation of the H+ ion from the quaternary molecule, now rendering it a tertiary base molecule that can penetrate the nerve. The dissociation constant (pK_a) for the anesthetic predicts the proportion of molecules that exist in each of these states. By definition, the pK_a of a molecule represents the pH at which 50% of the molecules exist in the lipid-soluble tertiary anionic (uncharged base) form and 50% in the quaternary water-soluble cationic (charged acid) form[2] (see Box 3-2). As the pH of the tissues differs from the pK_a of the specific drug, more of the drug exists either in its charged or uncharged form. This is expressed in the Henderson-Hasselbalch equation: $pKa - pH = \log [RH+] / [R]$ where [R] is the concentration of unionized (uncharged) drug and [RH+] the concentration of ionized (charged) drug. This is important because the molecular form of the anesthetic that allows diffusion through the lipid rich nerve membrane is the free base (RN) (anionic) portion of the molecule. Once the free base of the molecule reaches the axoplasm inside the nerve membrane, the amine gains a hydrogen

ion and reverts back to the ionized quaternary (cationic) form (RNH^+), the active form of the molecule that binds to the receptor site preventing the influx of sodium (see Figures 3-1 and 3-3).

Because the pH of the body tissue is 7.4, the ideal pK_a of an anesthetic should be 7.4, indicating that 50% of the molecules are uncharged base and quick diffusion through the lipid membrane would occur. However, the pK_a of all local anesthetics have values greater than 7.5 except topical benzocaine which is 3.5, and have a pH of approximately 5 to 6 in plain solutions and lower with vasoconstrictors; therefore a greater proportion of the molecules exist in the quaternary water-soluble form when injected into tissue having normal pH of 7.4.[1] The higher the pK_a of the anesthetic, the lower the concentration of uncharged base molecules. This causes slower diffusion into the nerve cell and a slower onset of action of the local anesthetic. Table 3-1

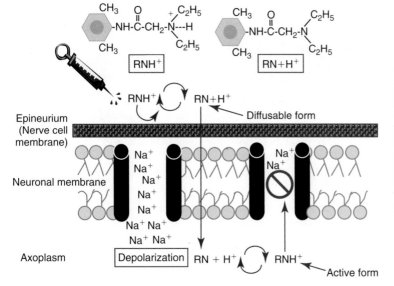

Figure 3-3 ■ Local anesthetic action. A local anesthetic exists in equilibrium as a quaternary salt (RNH^+) and tertiary base (RN). The proportion of each is determined by the pK_a of the anesthetic and the pH of the tissue. The lipid-soluble tertiary form (RN) is essential for penetration of both the epineurium and neuronal membrane. Once the molecule reaches the axoplasm of the neuron, the amine gains a hydrogen ion, and this ionized quaternary form (RNH^+) is responsible for the actual blockade of the sodium channel. Presumably, it binds within the sodium channel near the inner surface of the neuronal membrane.

TABLE 3-1	Characteristics Affecting Local Anesthetic Induction and Action	
CHARACTERISTICS	**ACTION AFFECTED**	**EXPLANATION**
Concentration of local anesthetic	Diffusion and onset	Higher concentration = more readily molecules diffuse through the nerve = rapid onset.
Dissociation constant (pK_a)	Onset	Determines the portion of administered dose in the lipid-soluble state (RN). Lower pK_a more rapid the onset of action. More RN molecules are present to diffuse through the nerve, decreasing the time of onset.
Lipid solubility	Potency	Greater lipid solubility enhances diffusion through the nerve, allowing a lower effective dose.
Protein binding	Duration	Increased protein binding allows more cations (RNH^+) to bind to the receptor sites within the sodium channels prolonging the presence of anesthetic at the site of action. Bupivacaine is a good example of this characteristic.
Perineurium thickness	Onset	Perineurium binds individual neurons together to form fasciculi. The thicker the perineurium, the slower the rate of diffusion and onset of action.
Nonnervous tissue diffusibility	Onset	Increased diffusibility = decreased time of onset.
Vasodilator activity	Anesthetic potency and duration	Greater vasodilator activity = increased blood flow to region = rapid removal of anesthetic molecules from injection site; thus decreased anesthetic potency and decreased duration.

TABLE 3-2	Dissociation Constants (pK$_a$) of Commonly Used Local Anesthetic Drugs		
AGENT	**PK$_A$**	**PERCENT BASE (RN) AT PH 7.4**	**APPROXIMATE ONSET OF ACTION (MIN)**
Lidocaine	7.7	29	2–4
Mepivacaine	7.7	33	2–4
Prilocaine	7.7	25	2
Articaine	7.8	29	2–4
Bupivacaine	8.1	17	5–8
Procaine	9.1	2	14–18
Topical benzocaine	3.5	100	1
Topical tetracaine	8.6	7	10–15

Source Malamed S: *Handbook of local anesthesia*, ed 5, St Louis, 2004, Mosby.

lists factors affecting local anesthetic induction time and action, and Table 3-2 lists dissociation constants (pK$_a$) of commonly used local anesthetic drugs. So, the proportion of cations and base molecules are determined by the pH of the anesthetic, pK$_a$ of the anesthetic, and the pH of the tissue. In addition, the uncharged tertiary amine base and the positively charged quaternary amine cation each have different important biophysical characteristics that influence the ability of the local anesthetic to block the nerve impulse.

INFECTION IN THE AREA OF INJECTION

Tissue acidity—a result of many dental diseases—can impede the development of local anesthesia. The normal pH of the tissue is 7.4, and the solution in the cartridge is predominately cationic (acidic). When the solution is injected into the tissue, the alkalinity of the tissue liberates the free base, allowing penetration of the local anesthetic molecule into the lipid rich nerve. The acidic environment associated with an active infection causes a much lower tissue pH in the vicinity of 5–6, which favors the quaternary water-soluble configuration and the amount of free base is reduced even further, leaving fewer base molecules to penetrate the nerve. This is one reason why it is difficult to achieve dental anesthesia when infection is present. Other factors for failure of anesthesia are edema and the increase in inflammation associated with infections. The selection of an anesthetic with a lower pK$_a$ such as mepivacaine (pK$_a$ 7.7), would most likely provide more effective anesthesia than bupivacaine (pK$_a$ 8.1) (Figure 3-4).

MECHANISM OF ACTION OF LOCAL ANESTHETIC AGENTS

As discussed in chapter 2, the primary effects of local anesthetics inhibit the depolarization of the nerve membrane by interfering with both sodium (Na$^+$) and potassium (K$^+$) currents. The action potential is not propagated because the

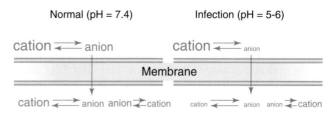

Figure 3-4 ▪ Effect of hydrogen ion concentration (pH) on local anesthetic drug action. In the normal extracellular environment (pH 7.4, left side of the diagram), the anion form of the local anesthetic drug exists in sufficient numbers to make anesthesia possible. In infection (pH 5.6, right side of diagram), the lower pH reduces the number of anesthetic anions available to penetrate the nerve membrane and the number of these base molecules needed for anesthesia may not be sufficient to be rendered effective. (Modified from Daniel S, Harfst S, Wilder R, Francis B, Mitchell S: *Dental hygiene concepts, cases and competencies*, ed 2, St Louis, 2008, Mosby.)

BOX 3-3	Mechanism of Action = Blockade of Voltage-Gated Sodium Channels

Membrane potential = –70 mV (range –90 to –60)
Excitatory impulse reaching minimal threshold
Na$^+$ channels open
Na$^+$ flown in (depolarizes membrane (+40 mV)
Na$^+$ channels close
K$^+$ channels open
K$^+$ flows out
K$^+$ channels close
Na$^+$/K$^+$ exchange (via Na$^+$/K$^+$ pump)
Repolarizes membrane (–70 mV)

Modified from Haveles B: *Applied pharmacology for the dental hygienist*, ed 6, St Louis, 2011, Mosby.

local anesthetic blocks the influx of sodium during the slow depolarization stage, and threshold level is never attained. Although the exact mechanism by which local anesthetics retard the influx of sodium ions into the cell is unknown, two theories have been proposed: the specific protein receptor theory which is more widely accepted, and membrane expansion theory (Box 3-3).

SPECIFIC PROTEIN RECEPTOR THEORY

Several theories concern the action of anesthetic on nerves. However, the specific receptor theory is the most widely accepted theory. One proven fact is that the anesthetic interferes with how the impulses travel down the length of the nerve. This is done by interfering with the influx of sodium ions across axonal membranes of peripheral nerves. The local anesthetic diffuses across the cell membrane and binds to a specific receptor at the opening of the voltage-gated sodium channel. The local anesthetic's affinity to the voltage-gated Na$^+$ channel increases significantly with the excitation rate of the neuron. Local anesthetics act during the depolarization phase of the nerve impulse generation by binding to the structural proteins known as *specific receptors* on the sodium channel.[3] The rate of depolarization is reduced and the nerve never reaches the firing potential.

Different anesthetics bind at different sites in the membrane. In myelinated nerves, local anesthetics have access to the nerve membrane only at the nodes of Ranvier where sodium channels are located. The anesthetic must permeate 8–10 mm of the nerve's length, approximately three to four nodes, to profoundly block the generation of the nerve impulse because an impulse can be strong enough to skip over one or two of the blocked nodes. The thickness of the nerve also has an effect on how much local anesthesia is needed to cover three to four nodes to achieve profound anesthesia. Therefore thicker nerve sheaths such as those found in the inferior alveolar nerve will require more anesthetic to achieve adequate nerve blockage (Figures 3-5 and 3-6).[4]

During the resting stage of nerve conduction, calcium ions (Ca^{++}) are bound to receptor sites within the ion channels of cell membranes. During depolarization, Ca^{++} ions are displaced and are thought to be the most significant factor responsible for the influx of sodium into the nerve. Local anesthetics work by competing with Ca^{++} ions to bind to these ion channels during slow depolarization and close (block off) these channels[3] (Figure 3-7).

THE MEMBRANE EXPANSION THEORY

The membrane expansion theory is not as readily accepted as the specific receptor theory and suggests that the local anesthetic agents that are highly lipid-soluble (e.g., benzocaine) insert themselves into the lipid bilayer of the cell membrane, causing three-dimensional changes in the configuration of the lipoprotein matrix by expanding the membrane. Local anesthetic agents that are highly lipid soluble are able to easily penetrate the lipid rich cell membrane. This leads to narrowing of the sodium channels, thus preventing depolarization by decreasing the diameter of the sodium channels[2] (see Figure 3-8). It has not been determined as to how much of the membrane expansion contributes to impulse blockade of excitable tissue. Therefore this theory remains speculative.

PHARMACOKINETICS OF LOCAL ANESTHETIC DRUGS

Pharmacokinetics is the study of the action of drugs within the body. These actions include mechanisms of drug absorption, distribution, metabolism, and excretion; onset of action; duration of effect; biotransformation; and effects and routes of excretion of the metabolites of the drug.

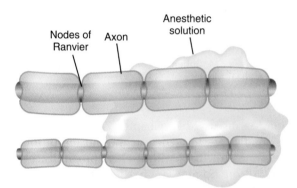

Figure 3-5 ■ Comparison of nodal interval nerve block between thin and thick axons. Two side-by-side axons—one thin, one thick—are bathed in a puddle of local anesthetic. The nodes of Ranvier interval of the thick fiber is twice that of the thin one. The local anesthetic solution covers four successive nodes of the thin axon (bottom) to ensure solid impulse block. At top, the impulses can easily skip one or even two inexcitable nodes, hence conduction along the thick axon continues uninterrupted and profound anesthesia is not achieved. (Modified from de Jong RH: *Local anesthetics*. St Louis, 1994, Mosby.)

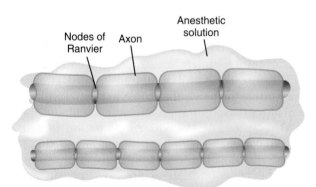

Figure 3-6 ■ Nodal interval nerve block between thin and thick axons when enough anesthetic is deposited. Both thick (top) and thin (bottom) axons have more than three nodes covered by local anesthetic solution. Conduction block will be complete in either group. (Modified from de Jong RH: *Local anesthetics*. St Louis, 1994, Mosby.)

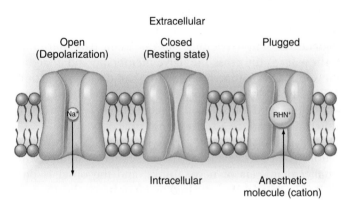

Figure 3-7 ■ Mode of action of local anesthetic agent. On the left is an open channel (the usual configuration after a sufficient stimulus has been applied), allowing sodium ion (Na^+) influx through the nerve membrane. The center channel remains closed to sodium ions, which is the usual configuration in the resting state. The right channel, although otherwise in the open configuration, has been closed by an anesthetic cation that is bound to the receptor site in the channel. (Modified from Malamed SF: *Handbook of local anesthesia*, ed 5, St Louis, 2004, Mosby.)

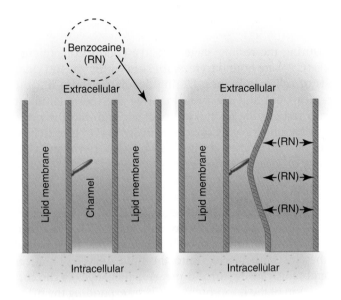

Figure 3-8 ■ Membrane expansion theory. (From Malamed SF: *Handbook of local anesthesia*, ed 5, St Louis, 2004, Mosby.)

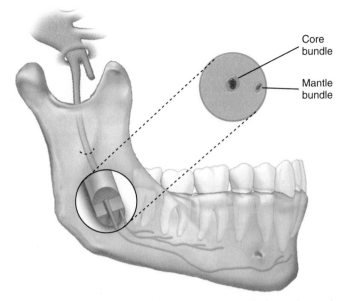

Figure 3-9 ■ The axons in the mantle bundle supply the molar teeth, and those in the core bundle supply the anterior teeth. The extraneural local anesthetic solution diffuse from the mantle to the core. (From Hargreaves KM, Cohen S: *Cohen's pathways of the pulp*, ed 10, St Louis, 2011, Mosby.)

ONSET OF ACTION

The onset of action of local anesthetics, the period from local anesthetic deposition near the nerve trunk to profound conduction block, is determined by several factors. The pK_a is the primary factor that determines the onset of action. The pK_a of a local anesthetic determines the amount of drug that exists in an ionized (acidic) form at any given pH. The lower pK_a levels increases tissue penetration and shortens onset of action due to more lipid-soluble unionized (base) particles. In contrast the higher pH level optimizes the dissociation of these base molecules and shortens the onset of action. This theory explains why local anesthetics often do not work in infected tissue. The infected tissue tends to be a more acidic environment and reduces the pH of the tissue, consequently reducing the number of unionized local anesthetic particles, causing a delay in the onset of action, or ineffective anesthesia. Anesthetics that have a high degree of lipid solubility and are in the base unionized form will readily cross the nerve membrane and attach to the sodium receptors, resulting in a rapid onset of action. Anesthetics that have a low degree of lipid solubility and are cationic and ionized will penetrate the nerve membrane slowly and produce a slower onset of action.

The administration site also influences the onset of action. The onset of a nerve block is faster in an area with smaller diameters of nerve trunks, and the onset is prolonged in areas with increased tissue or nerve sheath size.

INDUCTION OF LOCAL ANESTHETICS

The process by which the local anesthetic moves from its extraneural site of deposition toward the nerve is called *diffusion* and is governed by the initial concentration of the anesthetic. The higher the concentration of the administered local anesthetic, the more readily the diffusion of its molecules through the nerve, producing a more rapid onset

of action. As discussed in Chapter 2, the fasciculi in the mantle bundles are located near the outside of the nerve and innervate structures within close proximity, and fasciculi in the core bundles are located on the inside of the nerve and innervate structures at a distance. Using the inferior alveolar nerve as an example, the mantle bundles innervate the molar area, and the core bundles innervate anterior teeth at the end of the nerve fiber[4] (Figure 3-9). The location of the bundles in larger nerves has an impact on which bundles are affected by the local anesthetic first. Utilizing the example above, the local anesthetic when administered diffuses through the nerve to the mantle bundles (outer core) first providing concentrated anesthetic to the molar region, and then diffusing to the core bundles (inner core) providing a more diluted anesthetic solution to the anterior mandibular teeth, including the lip and chin.[2,5] Because the mantle bundles are affected by the local anesthetic first, they are exposed to higher concentrations of the local anesthetic, causing a complete, rapid, and easy blockage of these fibers. Because the core bundles are located at a further distance inside the nerve, they come in contact with a more diluted, lower concentration of local anesthetic[2] (Figure 3-10). The anesthetic loses its concentration from tissue fluids, capillaries and lymphatics at the site of administration, and anatomic barriers of the nerve. This results in a slower onset of action in these fibers, and complete blockage is most likely never achieved.[2,3] Although the presence of anesthetic symptoms expressed by the patient is a good indication that successful anesthesia has been achieved, it is not an adequate indication of profound anesthesia. Areas of inadequate anesthesia may be a result of the anesthetic molecules not reaching the most inner core bundles.

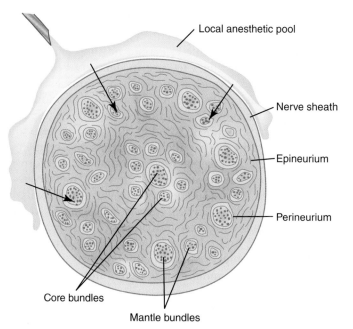

Core bundles

Mantle bundles

Figure 3-10 ■ The deposited local anesthetic solution near the nerve sheath must diffuse inward toward the core fibers, reaching the mantle fibers first. (Modified from de Jong RH: *Local anesthetics.* St Louis, 1994, Mosby.)

INDUCTION TIME

Induction time is defined as the time interval between the initial deposition of the anesthetic solution at the nerve site and complete conduction blockade. Factors that control induction time of an anesthetic and its clinical actions are listed in Table 3-1.

RECOVERY FROM LOCAL ANESTHETIC BLOCK

Fasciculi in mantle bundles lose anesthesia before the core bundles. Using the inferior alveolar nerve block as an example, anesthetic recovery begins in the molar teeth and ends with the anterior teeth, chin and lip. Anesthetic recovery is a slower process than induction because the anesthetic binds to the receptor site in the sodium channel releasing the anesthetic slowly into the systemic circulation. The degree of binding to the receptor site for each anesthetic determines the speed of recovery.

REINJECTION OF LOCAL ANESTHETIC

When the procedure lasts longer than the duration of the anesthetic, a second injection may be required to finish the procedure. If the patient has pain, the nerve has returned to function and it is usually more difficult to achieve profound anesthesia again. Because emergence of local anesthetics begins in the mantle fibers, it is important to reinject the anesthetic before the mantle fibers have fully recovered. Partially recovered mantle fibers can achieve rapid onset of action after a new high concentration of anesthetic is administered with a smaller volume than originally administered.[2] If the dental procedure lasts longer than the duration of the anesthetic and the mantle and core fibers have

fully recovered, the reinjection of local anesthetic will be ineffective. A term used to describe this phenomenon is tachyphylaxis which is described as an increased tolerance to a drug that is administered repeatedly.[2]

DURATION OF ANESTHESIA

The duration of local anesthetics is influenced by the following:
- *Protein binding:* longer acting local anesthetics such as bupivacaine are more firmly bound to the receptor sites than shorter acting local anesthetics such as lidocaine. Increased protein binding allows the cations (RNH^+) to bind/cling more firmly so duration is increased.
- *Vascularity of the injection site:* vascularity increases absorption of the anesthetic, allowing the drug to leave the injected area faster, decreasing potency as well as duration.
- *Presence or absence of a vasoconstrictor drug:* added vasoconstrictors to a local anesthetic decrease the vasodilatory properties of local anesthetics by constricting the surrounding blood vessels at the site of administration, increasing the duration of the anesthetic.

ABSORPTION OF LOCAL ANESTHETICS

The rate of systemic absorption of local anesthetics is dependent upon the total dose and concentration of the drug administered, the route of administration, the vascularity of the tissues at the administration site, and the presence or absence of a vasoconstrictor in the anesthetic solution.

All local anesthetics are vasodilators and produce a pharmacologic effect on blood vessels, varying slightly from type to type.[2] The importance of these vasodilating properties are the increase in the rate of absorption of local anesthetics and the decrease in the rate of action. Higher blood levels of the drug increase the chance of the patient developing an overdose. The local anesthetic molecules diffuse out of the sodium channels and are carried into the bloodstream. To reduce the rate of absorption, vasoconstrictors are added to local anesthetics to decrease the vasodilating properties of the local anesthetic by constricting the blood vessels and reducing the blood supply to the area of injection (see Chapter 4). The vasoconstrictor will reduce rapid systemic absorption, which reduces systemic toxicity and increases the duration of the anesthetic. Of equal importance is the site where the anesthetic is injected. If the anesthetic is inadvertently injected intravascularly, it will be absorbed into the bloodstream rapidly, significantly increasing the possibility of an overdose.

DISTRIBUTION OF LOCAL ANESTHETICS

After absorption of the local anesthetics into the bloodstream, they are distributed throughout the body to all tissues. High vascular organs such as the brain, heart, liver, kidneys, and lungs have higher concentrations of anesthetics.[2] Local anesthetics easily cross the blood-brain barrier, because nerves are predominantly susceptible to local anesthetics. The toxicity of local anesthetics is directly related to the amount of accumulation in the tissues.

METABOLISM (BIOTRANSFORMATION) OF LOCAL ANESTHETICS

The intermediate chain of the local anesthetic molecule determines the classification of the drug as either an ester or an amide. It also determines the pattern of biotransformation.

The elimination half-life of a local anesthetic is the period of time it takes for 50% of the drug to be metabolized/removed from the body. The first half-life removes 50% of the anesthetic from the bloodstream, the second half-life removes another 25%, the third half-life another 12%, the next half-life removes another 6%, and so on until the drug is completely removed from the body.[6] For example, lidocaine has a half-life of 90 minutes, by the time it gets through its last half-life, it takes approximately 10 hours for the drug to be completely removed from the body[6] (Table 3-3). The rate of absorption and the rate of elimination (half-life) of the local anesthetic from the blood and tissues influence the degree of toxicity. Also of important consideration are the drug-drug interactions with other medications that the patient may be taking that may compete with the metabolic process of the local anesthetic. This could increase the half-life of the local anesthetic and the possibility of an overdose. See Tables 3-3 and 3-4.

Ester Local Anesthetics

Esters, are hydrolyzed in the plasma by the enzyme pseudocholinesterase, and by liver esterases. Esters include

TABLE 3-3	Half-Life Example for Lidocaine	
MINUTES	**PERCENT LIDOCAINE REMOVED FROM BODY**
90	50
180	75
270	87
360	94
450	97
540	99
630	99.5

From Paarmann C, Royer R: *Pain control for dental practitioners.* Baltimore, MD, 2008, Lippincott Williams and Wilkins.

TABLE 3-4	Half-Life of Commonly Used Local Anesthetics
DRUG	**HALF-LIFE HOURS**
Lidocaine	1.6
Mepivacaine	1.9
Prilocaine	1.6
Articaine	.75
Bupivacaine	3.5

From Malamed S: *Handbook of local anesthesia,* ed 5, St Louis, 2004, Mosby.

benzocaine, tetracaine, and procaine. Benzocaine and tetracaine are commonly used in dentistry as topical anesthetics (see Chapter 6). Injectable esters are no longer manufactured in dental cartridges for use in dentistry because of their high potential for evoking allergic reactions. However, procaine is occasionally used in the medical profession and obtained in medical vials. Procaine is metabolized to para-aminobenzoic acid (PABA) and is the major metabolic by-product responsible for allergic reactions. Most patients are not allergic to the parent compound of ester drugs (e.g., procaine), but are allergic to the PABA metabolites. Approximately 1 in 2800 individuals have a hereditary condition known as *atypical pseudocholinesterase*, which causes the inability for these individuals to hydrolyze ester local anesthetics and other chemically related drugs. This condition causes higher anesthetic blood levels, increasing their risk for toxicity and therefore contrainidicating the use of esters.[2]

Amide Local Anesthetics

Amides are primarily metabolized in the liver, and the process is much more complex than for esters. Amides include lidocaine, mepivacaine, prilocaine, articaine, and bupivacine (see Chapter 5). Because the liver is the organ responsible for the entire metabolic process of most amides, the rate of biotransformation is slower in patients with significant liver dysfunction (e.g. cirrhosis) or patients with lower hepatic blood flow causing an increased risk of systemic toxicity. Biotransformation for lidocaine, mepivacaine, and bupivacaine occurs completely in the liver, while prilocaine is metabolized in the liver but some also occurs in the lungs. Because prilocaine is metabolized in the lungs and in the liver, it is more rapidly biotransformed and plasma levels decrease more quickly than with other anesthetics metabolized completely in the liver. Articaine is also an amide but contains a thiophene group/ester group. Only about 5 to 10% of articaine is biotransformed in the liver, with most of the drug being biotransformed by the enzyme plasma cholinesterase, the same route as esters. Amides that are primarily metabolized in the liver have a longer half-life that increases the risk for systemic toxicity. Because articaine is metabolized by plasma cholinesterese it has a very short half-life, approximately 45 minutes, that decreases the risk for systemic toxicity.

EXCRETION OF LOCAL ANESTHETICS

The kidneys are the primary excretory organ for the metabolites of all local anesthetic agents. A small percentage is excreted unchanged in the urine. Esters are almost completely hydrolyzed in the blood and only small amounts are excreted unchanged in the urine. Amides are relatively resistant to hydrolysis and therefore a greater percentage is excreted unchanged in the urine than that of an ester. With severe renal disease, such as end-stage renal disease, both the parent drug and the metabolites may accumulate in the kidneys, increasing the risk of systemic toxicity.

SYSTEMIC EFFECTS OF LOCAL ANESTHETICS

Unlike most medications that must be absorbed by the bloodstream to produce the desired effect, local anesthetics are chemical agents that are deposited in the area of nerve conduction to block the action potential before they are absorbed through the bloodstream. Once absorbed into the circulatory system and before biotransformation, local anesthetics will affect the central nervous system (CNS) and the cardiovascular system (CVS). The higher the blood plasma level, the greater the effects on these systems. Adverse reactions and toxicity to local anesthetics are directly related to the following:

- *Nature of the drug.* Amount of vasodilation of the anesthetic and the inherent toxicity of each agent are contributory factors to toxicity.
- *Concentration of the drug and dose administered.* Higher concentrations and doses administered produce higher blood levels of a drug.
- *Route of administration.* Intravascular injections rapidly produce high blood levels of a drug. Topical anesthetics are administered in high concentrations without vasoconstrictors and absorb quickly from the site of administration, increasing the possibility of toxicity.
- *Rate of injection.* Injections administered rapidly can increase the chance of toxicity because the tissues cannot accept the large, rapid volume of anesthetic.
- *Vascularity in the area of injection.* Vascularity in the area of the injection can be due to a dental infection, inflammation as a response to an infection, or vasodilation from a local anesthetic agent without a vasoconstrictor. Vascularity from any of these factors causes an increase in the risk of systemic toxicity by allowing the local anesthetic drug to be rapidly absorbed into the circulation.
- *Age of the patient.* Children and older patients are more susceptible to total dose administered and adverse reactions because in children their organs may not be fully developed to effectively metabolize the drug, and in contrast, the older patient's organs may not be functioning properly to effectively metabolize the drug.
- *Weight of patient.* Variations in patient weight affect blood levels of the drug. Maximum recommended doses must be calculated based on the patient's weight.
- *Patient health.* Patients with systemic conditions that affect the biotransformation of local anesthetics should be given reduced doses to prevent toxicity.
- *The route and rate of metabolism and excretion of the drug.* Patients with liver dysfunction may be unable to metabolize the anesthetic and amides may accumulate in the liver; amides and both amide and ester metabolites may accumulate in the kidneys from renal disease.[2,6]

Effect of Local Anesthetics on the Central Nervous System

Local anesthetics easily pass from the peripheral circulation into the CNS *which is especially sensitive to high blood* levels of local anesthetics (more than any other system) because local anesthetics readily cross the blood-brain barrier. In general, the concentrations of local anesthetics required to elicit CNS effects are inversely proportional to their anesthetic potencies. Although CNS effects from a local anesthetic are rare, at high blood levels, the local anesthetic overdose manifests as CNS depression. At low blood levels, they produce no significant effects on the CNS, but may have some anticonvulsant properties.[2,3,7,8] At much higher doses, the effects on the CNS are considered to be biphasic with phase I exhibiting initial excitatory signs (e.g., muscle twitching, tremors), progressing subsequently to phase II, depressive phase involving CNS depression, unconsciousness, convulsions, hypotension (because of the anesthetics, varying degrees of vasodilation), and eventually respiratory arrest.[1-3,5-7] Figure 3-11 demonstrates systemic influences of lidocaine, and Table 3-5 lists signs and symptoms of local anesthetic overdose on CNS.

Effect of Local Anesthetics on the Cardiovascular System

Local anesthetics can exert a variety of effects on the CVS. These effects are usually minimal. At mild overdose levels, the patient may exhibit a slight increase in blood pressure, heart rate, or respiration. Moderate overdose levels may occur with the administration of five cartridges of anesthetic. Similar to the CNS overdose symptoms, the CVS overdose symptoms are also biphasic in nature and change from stimulation to a depression phase at the higher end of the overdose level, demonstrating signs of depression. Reduced heart rate, blood pressure, and respiration rate would be observed. This decrease in myocardial contraction can lead to circulatory collapse and cardiac arrest[2,3,8] (Table 3-6).

The time lapse between the administration of the local anesthetic to the overdose reaction determines its severity. Symptoms that occur rapidly (within 5 minutes) are more likely to evolve into a more serious reaction. Delayed symptoms that occur after 5 minutes are usually easily resolved and do not develop into a serious reaction. In rare instances at extremely high levels, cardiac arrhythmia or hypotension and cardiovascular collapse occur (Table 3-7).

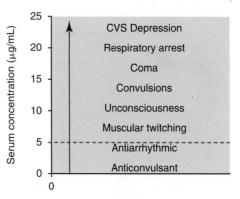

Figure 3-11 ■ Systemic influences of lidocaine.

TABLE 3-5	**Signs and Symptoms of a Local Anesthetic Overdose on the CNS**

SIGNS (OBSERVABLE-OBJECTIVE)	SYMPTOMS (SUBJECTIVELY FELT)
Low to moderate blood levels	Disorientation
• Excitatory-nervousness-talkativeness	Nervousness
• Slurred speech, general stutter	Flushed skin color
• Involuntary muscular twitching or shivering	Apprehension
• General light-headedness, dizziness	Twitching tremors
• Tremor or twitching in muscles of face and distal extremities	Shivering
• Confusion, apprehension	Dizziness
• Sweating	Light-headedness
• Vomiting	Visual disturbances
• Elevated respiration	Auditory disturbances
• Elevated heart rate	Headache
• Increased blood pressure	Tinnitus
Moderate to high blood levels	Metallic taste
• Convulsions generally tonic-clonic	
• Respiratory depression (at high blood levels of drug)	
• Depressed blood pressure and heart rate	
• CNS depression, coma, death	

TABLE 3-6	**Cardiovascular Effects of an Overdose***

LOW TO MODERATE OVERDOSE	MODERATE TO HIGH BLOOD LEVELS
Elevated blood pressure	Cardiovascular depression (decreased blood pressure)
Elevated heart rate	Decreased excitability (decreased heart rate)
	Cardiac arrest

*All injectable and most topical local anesthetics are absorbed and carried to the cardiovascular system.

TABLE 3-7	**Symptoms of Overdose on CVA**

• Headache
• Lethargy
• Increased slurring of speech
• Increased disorientation
• Possible loss of consciousness

DENTAL HYGIENE CONSIDERATIONS

• High degree of hypersensitivity to ester local anesthetic metabolites (PABA) has been documented; consequently, injectable esters are no longer available for use in dentistry.
• Bupivacaine has the greatest degree of lipid solubility and is therefore the most potent local anesthetic.
• The higher the pK_a of an anesthetic, the slower the onset of action. Bupivacaine has the highest pk_a and the slowest onset of action.
• Recovery of local anesthetic following an inferior alveolar-block begins in the molar teeth near the mantle bundles and ends with the anterior teeth near the core bundles.
• The degree of binding to the receptor site of each anesthetic determines the speed of recovery. Bupivacaine binds more firmly to the receptor site than shorter-acting local anesthetics.
• If more anesthetic is needed for a procedure, it is important to reinject the anesthetic before the mantle fibers have fully recovered. Partially recovered mantle fibers can achieve rapid onset of action with second dose at a smaller volume than initially administered.
• Tachyphylaxis is an increased tolerance to a drug that is administered repeatedly after the mantle and core bundles have fully recovered.
• Local anesthetics injected into tissue acidity, related to many dental infections, impedes the development of profound anesthesia.
• Local anesthetics are vasodilators and increase the absorption of the drug by the blood.
• Vasoconstrictors are added to local anesthetics to counteract the vasodilatory properties of the anesthetic, increasing the duration and decreasing the risk of systemic toxicity.
• The rate of systemic absorption of local anesthetics is dependent upon the total dose, concentration, route of administration, vascularity of tissues, and presence or absence of a vasoconstrictor.
• Intravascular injection significantly increased the possibility of an overdose.

DENTAL HYGIENE CONSIDERATIONS—cont'd

- Before biotransformation, local anesthetics affect the CNS and CVS.
- Local anesthetics easily cross the blood-brain barrier.
- The degree of local anesthetic toxicity is dependent upon the rate of absorption and elimination half-life. Articaine has a short half-life of 45 minutes and has the lowest risk of systemic toxicity of the amide anesthetics.

- Lidocaine, mepivacaine, and bupivacaine are biotransformed completely in the liver. Total dose for patients with liver dysfunction must be reduced.
- Pilocaine is biotransformed in the lungs and the liver. Total dose for patients with respiratory difficulties should be reduced.
- Articaine is biotransformed in the blood in the same manner as esters with only a slight amount (10%) metabolized in the liver.

CASE STUDY 3-1

Costa experiences difficulty with reanesthetization

Costa is in today for a 1-hour nonsurgical periodontal treatment of the mandibular left quadrant. The dental hygienist, Stefan, administers two cartridges of lidocaine 2% 1:100,000 epinephrine. Costa tells Stefan that he feels very numb. The procedure was much more difficult than Stefan expected, and the entire quadrant was not completed after the hour elapsed. Stefan's next patient canceled, and Stefan asked Costa if he would be able to stay longer to complete the procedure. Costa agreed. After approximately an hour and a half into the treatment,

Costa complains that he is feeling pain and asks for some more anesthetic. Stefan administers another cartridge of anesthetic, but Costa does not get numb.

Critical Thinking Questions

- Why did Costa not get numb the second time the anesthetic was administered?
- What could Stefan have done to prevent this from occurring?
- How should Stefan handle the situation?

CHAPTER REVIEW QUESTIONS

1. Infection and inflammation cause the following effects when administering a local anesthetic:
   A. Makes the local anesthetic more effective
   B. Increases tissue vascularity, which can inactivate the local anesthetic more rapidly
   C. Increases the duration of action of the local anesthetic
   D. Causes the inflamed tissue to have a high pH
2. Which of the following are desirable properties of local anesthetics?
   A. Reversible
   B. Rapid onset
   C. Stability in solution
   D. Potent
   E. All of the above
3. Which characteristic enhances the onset and effectiveness of local anesthetics?
   A. High lipid solubility
   B. High pK_a
   C. Low pH
   D. High concentration of cation molecules
4. Where is the action site for local anesthetics?
   A. The protein receptors
   B. The nerve membrane
   C. The central nervous system
   D. The calcium receptors

5. Which part of the chemical structure of a local anesthetic determines if the local anesthetic agent is classified as an ester or an amide?
   A. Intermediate chain
   B. Aromatic ring
   C. Terminal amine
   D. Quaternary amine
6. Local anesthetics have their effect on myelinated nerves mostly in which way?
   A. All along the nerve membrane
   B. Mostly at the synapse
   C. Mostly at the cell bodies
   D. Mostly at the node of Ranvier
7. The quaternary form of the local anesthetic molecule:
   A. Is the ionized form in the cartridge and is responsible for binding to the receptor site
   B. Is the unionized form in the cartridge and is responsible for binding to the receptor site
   C. Is the ionized form of the molecule that penetrates the nerve membrane
   D. Is the unionized form of the molecule that penetrates the nerve membrane
8. Ester type local anesthetics are no longer manufactured in injectable form for dentistry because:

CHAPTER REVIEW QUESTIONS

A. Of their difficulty penetrating the nerve
B. Of their high degree of hypersensitivity
C. They increase the potential for systemic overdose
D. They have significant vasodilatory properties

9. During manufacturing, local anesthetics are formulated as which of the following to render them water-soluble?
A. Muriatic acid
B. Sodium bisulfite
C. Hydrochloride salt
D. Sodium bicarbonate

10. Which of the following anesthetics will provide the most rapid onset based on its pK_a?
A. Mepivacaine
B. Lidocaine
C. Bupivacaine
D. Benzocaine

11. Which of the following local anesthetics is the most lipid-soluble?
A. Mepivacaine
B. Lidocaine
C. Bupivacaine
D. Prilocaine

12. The mantle bundles of the inferior alveolar nerve innervate which teeth?
A. The molar area
B. The anterior teeth
C. The lingual tissues
D. None of the above

13. When the local anesthetic is administered, the solution reaches the core bundles first.
A. True
B. False

14. What is tachyphylaxis?
A. A term used to describe the inability of the anesthetic to reach the nerve membrane because of anatomic barriers
B. Reinjection of anesthetic before the mantle fibers have fully recovered
C. Increased tolerance to a drug that is administered repeatedly
D. A term used to describe only partial anesthesia

15. Recovery of local anesthetics following the inferior alveolar block begins in the posterior teeth.
A. True
B. False

16. Which of the following are true regarding local anesthetics?
1. Are potent vasodilators
2. Exhibit anticonvulsant properties
3. Cause hemostasis
4. Cause hypotension
5. Have a pH of 7.5
A. 1, 4, 5
B. 1,2, 4
C. 2, 3, 5
D. 3, 4, 5

17. Which of the following is responsible for allergic reactions in ester anesthetics?
A. The parent compound
B. Para-amino benzoic acid
C. Pseudocholinesterase
D. Sodium bisulfite

18. Most amide local anesthetics are biotransformed in the:
A. Plasma
B. Lungs
C. Kidneys
D. Liver

19. Local anesthetic overdose has an effect on which system?
A. Central nervous system
B. Skeletal system
C. Lymphatic system
D. Respiratory system

20. Topical anesthetics are available in both esters and amides.
A. True
B. False

REFERENCES

1. Becker D, Reed K: Essentials of local anesthetic pharmacology, *Anesth Program* 53:98-109, 2006.
2. Malamed S: *Handbook of local anesthesia*, ed 5, St Louis, 2004, Mosby.
3. Jastak T, Yagiela J, Donaldson D: *Local anesthesia of the oral cavity*, St Louis, 1995, Saunders.
4. de Jong RH: *Local anesthetics*, St Louis, 1994, Mosby.
5. Paarmann C, Royer R: *Pain control for dental practitioners*, Baltimore, 2008, Lippincott Williams and Wilkins.
6. Bahl R: Local anesthesia in dentistry, *Anesth Prog* 51:138-142, 2004.
7. Finder RL, More PA: Adverse drug reactions to local anesthesia, *Dent Clin N Am* 46:447-457, 2002.
8. Patton K, Thibodeau G: *Anatomy and physiology*, ed 7, St Louis, 2010, Mosby.

ADDITIONAL RESOURCES

Liebgott B: *The anatomical basis of dentistry*, ed 3, St Louis, 2011, Mosby.

Nolte J: *Elsevier's integrated neuroscience*, St Louis, 2007, Mosby.

Castro A, Merchut MP, Neafsey E, Wurster R: *Neuroscience, an outline approach*, St Louis, 2002, Mosby.

Tetzlaff JE: *Clinical pharmacology of local anesthetics*. Woburn, 2000, Butterworth-Heinemann.

Haines D: *Fundamental neuroscience for basic and clinical applications*, ed 3, St Louis, 2006, Elsevier.

Haveles B: *Applied pharmacology for the dental hygienist*, ed 6, St Louis, 2011, Mosby.

Sisk A: Vasoconstrictors in local anesthesia for dentistry, *Anesth Prog* 39:187-193, 1992.

Rosenblatt MA, Abel M, Fischer GW, Itzkovich CJ, Eisenkraft JB: Successful use of a 20% lipid emulsion to resuscitate a patient after a presumed bupivacaine-related cardiac arrest, *Anesthesiology* 105:217-218, 2006.

CHAPTER 4

Pharmacology of Vasoconstrictors

Demetra Daskalos Logothetis RDH, MS

CHAPTER OUTLINE

LEARNING OBJECTIVES

1. Discuss the problems associated with the vasodilatory properties of local anesthetics.
2. Discuss the benefits and disadvantages of adding vasoconstrictors to local anesthetic solutions.
3. Discuss the effects and mechanism of action of vasoconstrictors.
4. Discuss the system effects of vasoconstrictors.
5. Discuss the possible adverse reactions to vasoconstrictors.
6. Describe how vasoconstrictors are inactivated.
7. Discuss the toxicity and contraindications of vasoconstrictors.
8. List the vasoconstrictors with their concentrations and effects on pain control, duration, and hemostasis.
9. Describe the maximum recommended dose for vasoconstrictors for healthy versus cardiovascularly compromised patients.
10. Correctly complete the review questions and activities for this chapter.

KEY TERMS

Absolute contraindication The offending drug should not be administered to the individual under any circumstances.
Adrenergic drugs Stimulate the adrenergic nerves directly by mimicking the action of epinephrine.
Catecholamine Sympathomimetic "fight or flight" hormones released by the adrenal glands in response to stress.

Endogenous Release from within.
Epinephrine Natural occurring catecholamine secreted by the adrenal medulla.
Exogenous Coming from outside the body.
Fight or flight response The body's primitive, automatic, inborn response that prepares the body to "fight" or "flee" from perceived attack, harm, or threat to survival.

continued next page

Levonordefrin A synthetic catecholamine manufactured in the United States as a 2% mepivacaine, 1:20,000 levonordefrin solution.

Maximum recommended dose Maximum dose of drug recommended for a patient depending on their physical health.

Norepinephrine Naturally occurring catecholamine affecting primarily α receptors.

Relative contraindication The administration of the offending drug may be used judiciously.

Sodium bisulfite Preservative providing a prolonged shelf life for the vasoconstrictor via anti-oxidant properties.

Sympathomimetic drugs Drugs that mimic the effects of the sympathetic nervous system.

Vasoconstrictors Adrenergic drugs, epinephrine and levonordefrin, that are added to local anesthetic cartridges to counteract the vasodilatory properties of local anesthetics, increasing the duration of action of local anesthetics, decreasing systemic toxicity, and providing hemostasis.

INTRODUCTION

Local anesthetics are vasodilators with the ester procaine having the most vasodilatory properties, compared to the amides mepivacaine and prilocaine having the least. No matter how readily the anesthetic can penetrate the nerve and bind to the receptor sites, the local blood vessels in the area of injection will immediately begin to absorb the anesthetic by causing vasodilation of the blood vessels, leading to increased blood flow to the site of injection *causing:*

- An increased rate of anesthetic absorption into the bloodstream by carrying the anesthetic away from the injection site.
- A decrease in the duration of the anesthetic's action by diffusing quickly from the site of administration.
- Higher bloodlevels of local anesthetics, increasing the risk of systemic toxicity.
- Increased bleeding in the area due to the increase in bloodflow.[1]

Vasoconstrictors are combined with local anesthetics to counteract the vasodilating properties of local anesthetics. Simply stated, vasoconstrictor drugs work by contracting the smooth muscle in blood vessels, which causes the vessels to constrict. Vasoconstrictors are important additives to the local anesthetic solution because of their ability to constrict blood vessels, thus providing the following beneficial effects:

- A decrease in the blood flow by constricting the blood vessels in the area of anesthetic administration, and reducing the amount of anesthetic needed to produce profound anesthesia.
- An increased duration of the anesthetic's effect by localizing the high concentration of the drug in the area of injection, within the nerve, improving the success rate and intensity of the nerve block. Using lidocaine 2% as an example, the duration of pulpal anesthesia in a plain solution (without a vasoconstrictor) is approximately 5-10 minutes, the duration of action dramatically increases approximately 6 times when a vasoconstrictor is added to 60 minutes of pulpal anesthesia.
- Slowing absorption of local anesthetic into the CVS, resulting in lower drug levels in the blood, reducing

the probability of systemic toxicity. Basically, the anesthetic metabolism is able to keep pace with drug absorption, providing hemostasis at the injection site, which is particularly useful in areas of heavy bleeding. Deep scaling procedures performed by the dental hygienist involve soft tissue manipulation resulting in hemorrhage, especially with severely inflamed tissues. These procedures generally require the patient to be anesthetized, and vasoconstrictors added to the anesthetic solution counteract unwanted bleeding caused by local anesthetic drugs.

CHEMISTRY

There are two vasoconstrictors that are added to local anesthetic drugs available in the United States, epinephrine and levonordefrin. Epinephrine is the most commonly used vasoconstrictor in dental local anesthetics, and is referred to as the benchmark. Vasoconstrictors used in dentistry are structurally identical with the natural, non-steroid mediators of the sympathetic nervous system (see Chapter 2), epinephrine and norepinephrine, which are secreted by the adrenal medulla (Figure 4-1). Because these drugs mimic similar effects as those caused by stimulation of the adrenergic nerves they are referred to as sympathomimetic or adrenergic drugs. The term catecholamine is also appropriate for these agents because they are naturally occurring

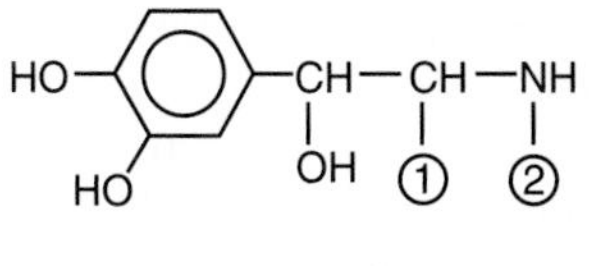

	①	②
Epinephrine	H	CH$_3$
Levonordefrin	CH$_3$	H
Norepinephrine	H	H

Figure 4-1 ■ Structural formulas of sympathomimetic amines commonly used as vasoconstrictors in local anesthesia for dentistry. (Redrawn from Jastak T, Yagiela J, Donaldson D: *Local anesthesia of the oral cavity.* St Louis, 1995, Saunders.)

catecholamines of the sympathetic nervous system and have a distinct structure of a benzene ring with two hydroxyl groups. Epinephrine and norepinephrine are naturally occurring catecholamines of the sympathetic nervous system, and levonordefrin is a synthetic catecholamine. They increase heart rate, contract blood vessels, dilate air passage, and participate in the "fight or flight" response of the sympathetic nervous system.

THE USE OF VASOCONSTRICTORS IN DENTISTRY

When a vasoconstrictor is not added to the local anesthetic solution, the drug is quickly removed from the injection site into the systemic circulation, increasing the possibility of systemic toxicity and decreasing the duration of action. As discussed previously, vasoconstrictors added to local anesthetic solutions have several potentially beneficial effects that counteract these undesirable properties of local anesthetics. However, epinephrine, which is the most widely used vasoconstrictor in dentistry, is not an ideal drug. Exogenous epinephrine is absorbed from the site of injection into the circulation just like local anesthetics, and measurable levels of epinephrine in the blood can affect the heart and blood vessels by causing the sympathomimetic "fight or flight" response of apprehension, increased heart rate, palpitations and sweating.[1] This has caused continued debate regarding the harmful influences of vasoconstrictors in some situations.[1,2] The benefits of vasoconstrictor use should be carefully weighed against the risks for patients who are medically compromised by severe cardiovascular disease, high blood pressure, or hyperthyroidism. However, completely avoiding the use of vasoconstrictors in these patients can cause a lack of profound anesthesia leading to pain during the dental procedure, and subsequently stimulating a significant release of endogenous epinephrine from the adrenal gland. This endogenous release of epinephrine in response to inadequate anesthesia during the dental appointment can be much greater than the amount which reaches the circulation from an injection of anesthetic with vasoconstrictor. Figure 4-2 illustrates the blood levels of endogenous epinephrine during rest and during mild-to-severe stress. Blood levels of endogenous epinephrine release are higher than the maximum recommended dose of epinephrine, 0.04 mg per appointment, for a cardiovascularly compromised patient. (See Chapter 8 for dosing calculations of epinephrine.)

Another important consideration is the endogenous release of epinephrine by the adrenal gland for healthy patients experiencing anxiety and stress before and during the dental appointment. As shown in Figure 4-2, endogenous release of epinephrine in minor to moderate stress is increased for particularly anxious patients. This can compound the adverse effects of exogenous administration of epinephrine via the anesthetic injection containing epinephrine (Figure 4-3). Fortunately, the undesirable systemic effects of epinephrine are short-lived. The rapid inactivation

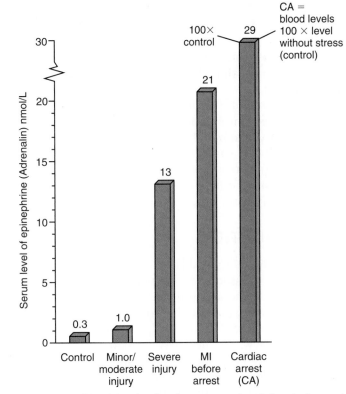

Figure 4-2 ▪ Blood levels of endogenous epinephrine during rest; with minor, moderate, or severe injury; myocardial infarction (MI; before arrest); and cardiac arrest (CA). (Modified from Haveles B: *Applied pharmacology for the dental hygienist*, ed 6, St Louis, 2011, Mosby.)

of epinephrine by the reuptake of adrenergic nerves quickly reduces the vasoconstrictor's harmful effects. According to Sisk, when epinephrine is administered intravenously, it has a half-life of 1 to 3 minutes.[4]

Patients with a recent myocardial infarction, coronary bypass surgery, or cerebrovascular accident within the past 6 months, and those with uncontrolled hypertension, angina, arrhythmias, or hyperthyroidism should not be given an anesthetic with a vasoconstrictor until their medical condition is controlled. Patients with a relative contraindication for vasoconstrictors can receive epinephrine-containing local anesthetic agents in the lowest possible dose, not to exceed the maximum recommended dose of 0.04 mg per appointment, using the best technique, which includes aspiration to reduce the risk of intravascular injection and injecting slowly to reduce the possibility of rapid systemic absorption. Depending upon the severity of the condition, the clinician must determine if a reduced amount of vasoconstrictor should be administered or if no vasoconstrictor should be administered at all. In general, there are only a few absolute contraindications to the use of a vasoconstrictor, and in most situations limiting the amount of vasoconstrictor a patient can receive produces the benefits of vasoconstrictor use in local anesthetics without compromising the patient. Absolute and relative contraindications to the use of vasoconstrictors are discussed in Chapter 7.

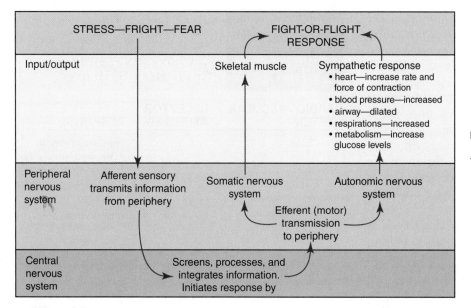

Figure 4-3 ■ Nervous system response during "fight or flight" or stress. (From McKenry L, Tessier E, Hogan M: *Mosby's pharmacology in nursing*, ed 22, St Louis, 2006, Mosby.)

TABLE 4-1	Epinephrine (Adrenalin) Concentrations and Uses in Dentistry

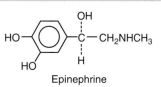

Epinephrine

CONCENTRATIONS	ANESTHETIC PREPARATIONS	USES
1:1000	Epinephrine alone	Emergency treatment of anaphylaxis and acute asthma attacks
1:50,000	2% Lidocaine	Most concentrated (least diluted) Provides greatest hemostasis Provides similar pain control as other anesthetic preparations containing epinephrine
1:100,000	2% Lidocaine 4% Articaine	Provides hemostasis but to a lesser degree than 1:50,000 Provides similar pain control as other anesthetic preparations Most commonly used concentration
1:200,000	4% Articaine 4% Prilocaine 0.5% Bupivacaine	Least concentrated (most diluted) Provides hemostasis but to a lesser degree than 1:100,000 and 1:50,000 Provides similar pain control as other anesthetic/vasoconstrictor preparations Good alternative for patients with significant cardiovascular disease Good alternative for elderly patients sensitive to epinephrine

EPINEPHRINE (ADRENALIN)

As previous discussed, epinephrine is a natural occurring catecholamine secreted by the adrenal medulla, consisting of approximately 80% of its secretions. It is also available as a synthetic catecholamine which is identical in structure with the natural hormone epinephrine. Epinephrine is the most widely used vasoconstrictor in dentistry, and the most potent. Epinephrine is the standard by which all other vasoconstrictors are measured (Table 4-1).[1]

MECHANISM OF ACTION

Epinephrine and norepinephrine cause vasoconstriction by activating adrenergic receptors located in most tissues. According to Ahlquist in 1948, these targeted receptor sites are divided into two major groups of adrenergic receptors, alpha (α) and beta (β), with several subtypes. Ahlquist recognized that α receptors have excitatory actions, and β receptors have inhibitory actions from catecholamines on smooth muscle. The excitatory action of α receptors by sympathomimetic drugs causes vasoconstriction of the smooth muscle in blood vessels. These α receptors have been further subcategorized into α_1 and α_2 depending upon differences in their location and function, α_1 receptors are excitatory–postsynaptic and α_2 receptors are inhibitory-postsynaptic.[1,2] The inhibitory action of β receptors by sympathomimetic drugs causes smooth muscle relaxation (vasodilation and bronchodilation), and cardiac stimulation. The β receptors have also been further subcategorized into β_1 found in the heart (causing cardiac stimulation) and small intestines (causing lipolysis), and β_2 found in the bronchi, vascular beds, and uterus causing bronchodilation and vasodilation.[1,3]

Norepinephrine activates predominately α receptors, and epinephrine activates both α and β receptors, causing vasoconstriction and vasodilation respectively. α Receptors are less sensitive to epinephrine.[3] However, once the α receptor is stimulated by high levels of epinephrine, this activation will override the vasodilation caused by β receptors and subsequently will cause vasoconstriction of the smooth muscle in peripheral arterioles and veins. This is the main reason sympathomimetic agents are added to local anesthetic solutions.

Stimulation of α receptors by adrenergic drugs such as epinephrine causes constriction of the smooth muscle in the blood vessels, also referred to as *vasoconstriction*. β_2 Receptor activation by epinephrine relaxes bronchial smooth muscles, causing the bronchi of the lungs to dilate. In addition, β_1 receptors have stimulatory effects that increase the rate and force of heart contractions. These stimulatory effects on β_1 receptors are undesirable side effects of incorporating sympathomimetic agents such as epinephrine into local anesthetic solutions. This is of particular concern in patients with preexisting cardiovascular and thyroid disease. The risks of adding the vasoconstrictor to the local anesthetic must be weighed against the benefits, and decreasing the amount of the drug administered should be considered (discussed next). Table 4-2 lists the major systemic effects of injected sympathomimetic agents involved in the cardiovascular and respiratory systems.[1,3]

EPINEPHRINE DILUTIONS

The concentration of vasoconstrictors in local anesthetic solutions is referred to as a ratio rather than a percentage as expressed by the local anesthetic drug. For example a concentration of 1:100,000 means there is 1 g (or 1000 mg) of drug contained (dissolved) in a 100,000 mL solution, or 0.01 mg/mL. The most common concentrations of epinephrine combined with local anesthetics are 1:50,000 (0.02 mg/mL), 1:100,000 (0.01 mg/mL), and 1:200,000 (0.005 mg/mL). The 1:50,000 concentration is manufactured in combination with 2% lidocaine, the 1:100,000 concentration is manufactured in combination with 2% lidocaine, and 4% articaine, and the 1:200,000 concentration is manufactured in combination with 4% prilocaine, 4% articaine, and 0.5% bupivacaine. Therefore, in a typical dental anesthetic cartridge containing both a local anesthetic drug and vasoconstrictor, the label will identify both drugs. Using lidocaine with epinephrine as an example, the cartridge may contain 2% lidocaine (referred to as a percentage) with 1:100,000 epinephrine (referred to as a ratio). Table 4-3 lists the vasoconstrictor concentrations combined with dental local anesthetics used in the United States and Canada.

The 1:50,000 dilution represents the highest concentration, and 1:200,000 dilution represents the lowest concentration and therefore produces fewer side effects.[1] Concentrations greater than 1:200,000 offer no advantage

TABLE 4-2	Systemic Effects of Adrenergic Amines on the Cardiovascular and Respiratory Systems

CARDIOVASCULAR SYSTEM	RECEPTOR AFFECTED	RESPONSE
Heart Rate	β_1, β_2	Increased (may be blocked or reversed by compensatory vagal reflex activity)
Contractile force	β_1, β_2	Increased
Coronary arterioles	$\alpha_1, \alpha_2, /\beta_2$	Constriction/dilation (local regulatory processes largely govern bloodflow)
Conduction velocity	β_1, β_2	Increased (may be blocked or reversed by compensatory vagal reflex activity)
Peripheral resistance	$\alpha_1, \alpha_2, /\beta_2$	Increased/decreased

RESPIRATORY SYSTEM	RECEPTOR AFFECTED	RESPONSE
Bronchial smooth muscle	β_2	Relaxation
Bronchial glands	$\alpha_1, /\beta_2$	Decreased/increased
Pulmonary arterioles	$\alpha_1, /\beta_2$	Constriction/dilation

Modified from Jastak, JT, Yagiela JA, Donaldson D: *Local anesthesia of the oral cavity.* St Louis, 1995, Saunders.

TABLE 4-3	Vasoconstrictors Used in Dental Local Anesthetic Solutions

GENERIC NAME	PROPRIETARY NAME	CONCENTRATIONS
Epinephrine	Adrenalin	1:50,000 1:100,000 1:200,000
Levonordefrin	Neo-Cobefrin	1:20,000

Modified from Darby M, Walsh M: *Dental hygiene theory and practice,* ed 3, St Louis, 2010, Sanders, Elsevier.

in prolonging the duration of anesthesia, reducing the plasma levels, or advancing pain control. Therefore, because a 1:50,000 offers no added benefits to most clinical situations, and can produce more profound undesired sympathomimetic actions (fight or flight), there is questionable rationale for using a 1:50,000 concentration of epinephrine for pain control. However, higher concentrations of epinephrine, specifically the 1:50,000 dilution are more effective for bleeding control (hemostasis). Local anesthetics with vasoconstrictors may be infiltrated for hemostasis even when pulpal anesthesia has been obtained. Therefore, using a 1:100,000 dilution of epinephrine for obtaining pulpal anesthesia may be used in combination with a relatively small infiltrated dose of 1:50,000 to decrease bleeding to less than half that recorded from a similar volume of 1:100,000. This is particularly important for bleeding control during periodontal surgeries, and for dental hygienists providing nonsurgical periodontal therapy.[5,6]

The selection of an appropriate vasoconstrictor concentration, if any, should be determined considering several factors such as the length of the dental procedure, medical status of the patient, and the need for hemostasis.[1] As discussed earlier, the addition of a vasoconstrictor to an anesthetic such as lidocaine can dramatically increase the pulpal anesthesia, and clinical effectiveness of lidocaine. The medical status of the patient must be reviewed and considered when selecting a vasoconstrictor. In general, patients with significant cardiovascular diseases ASA III and IV, patients with hyperthyroidism, sulfite allergies, and patients taking certain medications, the severity of each of these conditions must be evaluated to determine the appropriateness of a selected vasoconstrictor. The medical status of the patient in relationship to the use of vasoconstrictors will be covered thoroughly in Chapter 7. Finally, the need for hemostasis should be considered. Epinephrine is effective in decreasing blood flow during surgical procedures, and nonsurgical periodontal therapy. Because epinephrine possesses both α and β actions with α receptors being less sensitive to epinephrine than β receptors, higher doses of epinephrine are needed to produce the vasoconstriction action of α receptors. Although all epinephrine concentrations provide bleeding control, a 1:50,000 concentration (being double the concentration of 1:100,000, and four times the concentration of 1:200,000) provides the most rigorous bleeding control when compared to the 1:100,000 and 1:200,000 concentrations. However, an important consideration is that as the tissue level of epinephrine begins to decline, it produces a rebound vasodilatory effect when the β₂ action begins to predominate. This vasodilatory action can potentially lead to postoperative bleeding approximately 6 hours after the procedure.[1]

SODIUM BISULFITE PRESERVATIVE

Synthetic epinephrine is not very stable and must include the addition of an acidic preservative to stabilize the solution to prevent oxidation of epinephrine. Because a local anesthetic is manufactured as an acid salt, the drug is highly soluble in water and acidic pH 5–6. The addition of the preservative sodium bisulfite provides a shelf life of approximately 18 months because of its antioxidant properties.[1] However, there are disadvantages to the presence of the preservative sodium bisulfite. First, the preservative can further acidify the pH of the anesthetic solution to the range of 3.3 to 5.5, thus reducing the efficiency of the quaternary amine to dissociate (once injected) into the uncharged tertiary amine base necessary to penetrate the lipid rich membrane of the nerve, and slightly slowing the onset of action of the local anesthetic. This is of particular concern in the acidic environment associated with an active infection (see Chapter 3). Second, many individuals are allergic to the sodium bisulfite preservative associated with vasoconstrictors. Patients who have a true allergy to sodium bisulfite

should not receive an anesthetic/vasoconstrictor combination. Cartridges that do not contain a vasoconstrictor, such as 3% mepivacaine and 4% prilocaine, do not contain sodium bisulfite and are therefore safe to be administered to patients with sulfite allergies. Because mepivacaine and prilocaine produce only minor vasodilation compared with other available anesthetics, they can still produce adequate pulpal anesthesia for short dental appointments when administering nerve blocks. (See Chapter 5.)

ACTIONS OF EPINEPHRINE ON SPECIFIC SYSTEMS AND TISSUES

Mode of Action: Epinephrine exerts its action directly on the adrenergic receptors including both α and β receptors, affecting β receptors predominately.

Myocardium: The pharmacologic effect of epinephrine is essentially a result of its direct effect as agonist on specific α and β receptors (β₁ and β₂). Epinephrine increases heart rate, stroke volume, and cardiac output by stimulating β₁ receptors.

Pacemaker cells: Epinephrine stimulates β₁ receptors, increasing the incidence of dysrhythmias.

Coronary arteries: Epinephrine increases coronary artery flow by dilating coronary arteries.

Blood pressure: Small doses of epinephrine increase systolic pressure to a greater extent than the diastolic (diastolic pressure may decrease). Higher doses of epinephrine increase diastolic pressure.

Cardiovascular system: The β₁ effects of epinephrine have direct stimulation on the cardiovascular system, which leads to overall decrease in cardiac efficiency.

Vasculature: Epinephrine constricts the α receptors that are contained in the skin and mucous membranes. The effects of epinephrine on the blood vessels of the skeletal muscles, which contain both α and β₂ receptors, are dose dependent due to the predominance of β₂ receptors, which are more sensitive to epinephrine than α receptors. Therefore smaller doses are affected by β₂ actions and produce vasodilation, and larger doses are affected by α actions and produce vasoconstriction.

Metabolic system: Epinephrine inhibits insulin secretion, causing a rise in blood sugar and an increase in free fatty acids.

This is of particular concern in brittle diabetics taking large doses of insulin, especially if, in addition, these individuals have cardiovascular disease. Inconsistent blood sugar levels ranging from severe hypo- and hyperglycemia may result. Well-controlled diabetics may receive epinephrine without precautions.

Respiratory system: Epinephrine is a potent bronchial dilator due to the β₂ receptor effects. It is an invaluable drug for treating acute asthmatic attacks and anaphylactic reactions.

Central nervous system (CNS): In normal therapeutic doses, epinephrine does not stimulate the CNS. Overdose of epinephrine produces signs and symptoms of CNS stimulation, which may include anxiety, nausea, restlessness, weakness, tremor, headache, and hyperventilation.

Hemostasis: Epinephrine is added to local anesthetic solutions to provide hemostasis, and is frequently used during surgical procedures. High doses stimulate α receptors, causing vasoconstriction, followed by β₂ vasodilation after 6 hours.[1,6]

TERMINATION OF ACTION

The absorption of epinephrine is retarded because of the drug's vasoconstricting properties. It may take several hours for absorption to be completed. The effects of epinephrine following inadvertent intravascular injection becomes apparent within 1 minute and because of the body's efficiency at removing catecholamines the effects of epinephrine in the blood last only 5 to 10 minutes. Once absorbed, the action of epinephrine is terminated by the reuptake action of adrenergic nerves, any epinephrine that escapes the reuptake action is inactivated by enzymes catechol-O-methyltransferase (COMT), and monoamine oxidase (MAO) in the blood.[1,2] Only 1% of epinephrine, is excreted unchanged in urine. Figure 4-4 illustrates the distribution and fate of catecholamines injected into peripheral tissues.

MAXIMUM RECOMMENDED DOSE

The American Heart Association[7] and the New York Heart Association[8] indicate that the lowest possible effective

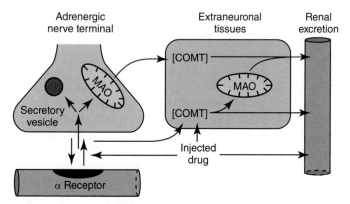

Figure 4-4 ■ The distribution and fate of catecholamines injected into peripheral tissues. *Dark arrows* indicate the predominant pathways for epinephrine and norepinephrine. (Redrawn from Jastak T, Yagiela J, Donaldson D: *Local anesthesia of the oral cavity.* St Louis, 1995, Saunders.)

dose should be used when administering local anesthetics with epinephrine to a healthy or medically compromised patients. Proper aspiration on several planes and slow injection should also be done when administering local anesthetics with epinephrine. The maximum recommended dose per visit of epinephrine for a healthy patient is 0.2 mg. The maximum recommended dose per visit of epinephrine for a cardiovascularly compromised patient is 0.04 mg. See Chapter 7 for medical history considerations when administering epinephrine. Maximum recommended doses for vasoconstrictors and local anesthetics, as well as calculation methods, are discussed in Chapter 8.

■ LEVONORDEFRIN (NEO-COBEFRIN)

Levonordefrin is a synthetic vasoconstrictor that is approximately one sixth (15%) as potent as epinephrine; it is manufactured in a higher concentration to achieve the same effects as epinephrine 1:100,000.[2] Levonordefrin is available in dentistry only with 2% mepivacaine, in a 1:20,000 concentration, which is 5 times greater than epinephrine in a concentration of 1:100,000, but because it is one sixth as potent as epinephrine, a 1:20,000 concentration of levonordefrin produces the same clinical effects as the epinephrine 1:100,000 concentration. Like epinephrine, levonordefrin contains the preservative sodium bisulfite to delay its deterioration (Table 4-4).

ACTIONS OF LEVONORDEFRIN ON SPECIFIC SYSTEMS AND TISSUES

Mode of Action: Levonordefrin is a selective α₂ agonist (75%) and produces vasoconstriction in low systemic concentrations; it has much less β activity (only 25%) compared with epinephrine that has 50% α and 50% β activity.[1]

Myocardium: The pharmacologic effect of levonordefrin on the myocardium is essentially the same as epinephrine by increasing cardiac output and heart rate, but to a lesser degree.

Pacemaker cells: Same as epinephrine by increasing dysrhythmias, but to a lesser degree.

Coronary arteries: Increases coronary artery flow by dilating coronary arteries similar to epinephrine, but to a lesser degree.

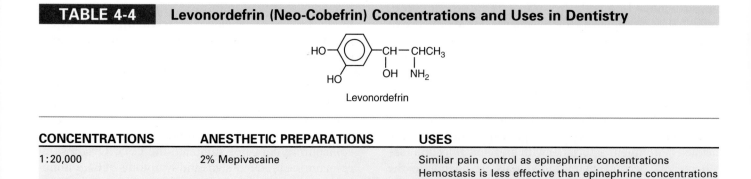

| **TABLE 4-4** | **Levonordefrin (Neo-Cobefrin) Concentrations and Uses in Dentistry** |

Levonordefrin

CONCENTRATIONS	ANESTHETIC PREPARATIONS	USES
1:20,000	2% Mepivacaine	Similar pain control as epinephrine concentrations Hemostasis is less effective than epinephrine concentrations

Blood pressure: Increases systolic pressure to a greater extent than the diastolic (diastolic pressure may decrease). Higher doses of levonordefrin increase diastolic pressure.

Cardiovascular system: Levonordefrin leads to a decrease in cardiac efficiency.

Vasculature: Effects on the vasculature are similar to epinephrine by providing α constriction of the skin and mucous membranes, but to a lesser degree.

Metabolic system: Levonordefrin inhibits insulin secretion, causing a rise in blood sugar and an increase in free fatty acids similar to epinephrine, but to a lesser degree.

Respiratory system: Levonordefin provides some bronchodilation but significantly less than epinephrine.

Central nervous system (CNS): In normal therapeutic doses, levonordefrin does not stimulate the CNS. In an overdose, it is not a potent stimulant when compared with epinephrine.

Hemostasis: Levonordefrin provides hemostasis, but significantly less effective than epinephrine.

TERMINATION OF ACTION

Levonordefrin is terminated by reuptake by adrenergic nerves and escaped levonordefrin is inactivated by COMT. Levonordefrin is not terminated by MAO.[2]

MAXIMUM RECOMMENDED DOSE

The maximum recommended dose per visit of levonordefin for a healthy patient is 1.0 mg. The maximum recommended dose per visit of levonordefrin for a cardiovascularly compromised patient is 0.2 mg. See Chapter 8 for maximum recommended dose and dosing methods.[7,8]

▋ OTHER VASOCONTRICTORS

NOREPINEPHRINE (LEVARTERENOL)

Norepinephrine is a naturally occurring catecholamine. Twenty percent of its production is from the adrenal medulla, but it is also available as a synthetic catecholamine. The usual concentration used in dentistry is 1:30,000. Norepinephrine has the same action as levonordefin on α receptors. It almost exclusively activates α receptors (90%) and minimally activates β receptors (10%).[1] Because of this, norepinephrine produces intense peripheral vasoconstriction with a possible dramatic increase in blood pressure. Therefore its use in dentistry is *not recommended.* The intense vasoconstriction/hemostasis caused by norepinephrine is likely to produce tissue necrosis, especially on the palate (Figure 4-5).

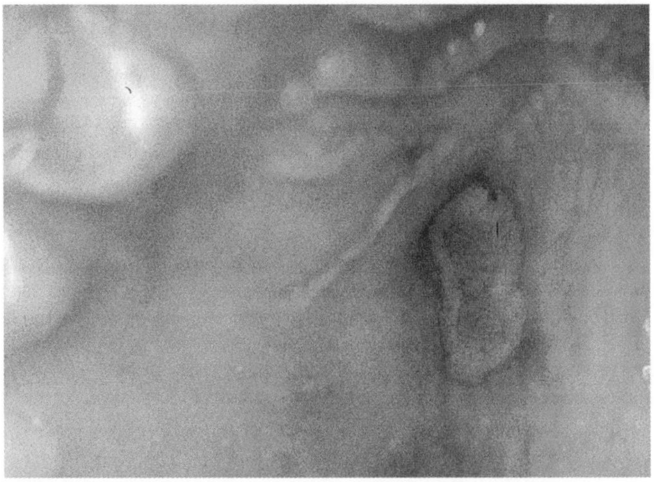

PHENYLEPHRINE (NEO-SYNEPHRINE)

Phenylephrine is a synthetic sympathomimetic amine that exerts its action predominately on α receptors (95%), with very little β effects on the heart. It is a very weak vasoconstrictor (only 5%) as potent as epinephrine and is formulated at much higher concentrations than epinephrine

Figure 4-5 ▪ Sterile abscess on the palate produced by excessive use of a vasoconstrictor (norepinephrine). (From Malamed S: *Handbook of local anesthesia,* ed 5, St Louis, 2004, Mosby.)

(1:2500 dilution). It is not used in dentistry, but is used in combination with local anesthetics for the management of hypotension and for nasal decongestants and ophthalmic solutions.

FELYPRESSIN

Felypressin is a synthetic hormone analogue of vasopressin.[1] It is a direct stimulator of vascular smooth muscles.[3] Felypressin causes few side effects because it has little or no direct effect on the myocardium or adrenergic nerve transmission. Therefore it may be safely administered to patients with uncontrolled hyperthyroidism, or patients taking tricyclic antidepressants or MAO inhibitors. Felypressin is available in Great Britain and other countries usually in combination with 3% prilocaine. It is favorably compared with epinephrine in anesthesia for restorative dentistry.[1,6]

▋ SIDE EFFECTS AND OVERDOSE OF VASOCONSTRICTORS

Overdose of vasoconstrictors from accidental intravenous injection or by administering more than the maximum recommended dose produces overstimulation of adrenergic receptors that can produce signs and symptoms normally observed from CNS stimulation. Table 4-5 lists the typical overdose responses to epinephrine.

With high plasma levels of epinephrine, dysrhythmias, ventricular fibrillation, dramatic increase in heart rate, and possible cardiac arrest are possible, more so in patients with increased susceptibility to the adverse cardiovascular effects of adrenergic drugs. Because the body is very efficient at removing vasoconstrictors, these adverse effects only last about 5 to 10 minutes. Even so, for patients with severe conditions such as unstable angina, recent myocardial infarction (within 6 months), recent coronary bypass surgery (within 6 months), uncontrolled hypertension,

TABLE 4-5	**Overdose Responses to Vasoconstrictors**
Tension	Increased heart rate
Anxiety	Increased blood pressure
Apprehension	Throbbing headache
Nervousness	Hyperventilation
Tremors	

Sources Malamed S: *Handbook of local anesthesia*, ed 5, St Louis, 2004, Mosby; Jastak T, Yagiela J, Donaldson D: *Local anesthesia of the oral cavity*. St Louis, 1995, Saunders.

uncontrolled hyperthyroidism, uncontrolled dysrhythmias, or congestive heart failure, the risk of using a vasoconstrictor may outweigh the benefits. The patient's physician should be consulted before using vasoconstrictors on these patients. These conditions, as well as drug interactions, are discussed in Chapter 7. For all patients, only the minimal effective dose should be administered, not to exceed the maximum recommended dose. (See Table 4-6 for recommended doses for vasoconstrictors).[1,6]

TABLE 4-6	**Recommended Maximum Dosages of Vasoconstrictors**			
CONCENTRATION	**MAXIMUM RECOMMENDED DOSE (MRD) PER APPOINTMENT HEALTHY PATIENT**	**NUMBER OF CARTRIDGES HEALTHY PATIENT (ASA I)**	**MAXIMUM RECOMMENDED DOSE (MRD) PER APPOINTMENT PATIENT WITH CARDIOVASCULAR DISEASE (ASA III OR IV)**	**NUMBER OF CARTRIDGES PATIENT WITH CARDIOVASCULAR DISEASE (ASA III OR IV**
1:50,000 Epinephrine	0.2 mg	5.5	0.04 mg	1.1
1:100,000 Epinephrine	0.2 mg	11.1	0.04 mg	2.2
1:200,000 Epinephrine	0.2 mg	22.2	0.04 mg	4.4
1:20,000 Levonordefrin	1.0 mg	11.1	0.2 mg	2.2

DENTAL HYGIENE CONSIDERATIONS

- Vasoconstrictors are added to local anesthetics to counteract the vasodilating properties of the local anesthetic.
- Vasoconstrictors provide hemostasis, increase duration of action, decrease systemic toxicity, and decrease required dose of the local anesthetic drug.
- Vasoconstrictors are adrenergic drugs and stimulate the "fight or flight" response of the sympathetic nervous system and increase heart rate and blood pressure.
- Endogenous release of epinephrine associated with stress in an anxious patient may compound the adverse effects of exogenous administration of epinephrine. This is of even greater concern for patients who are cardiovascularly compromised.
- Patients with a recent myocardial infarction, coronary bypass surgery, or cerebrovascular accident within the past 6 months, and those with uncontrolled hypertension, angina, arrhythmias, and hyperthyroidism should not be given an anesthetic with a vasoconstrictor until their medical condition is under control.
- Mepivacaine 3% and prilocaine 4% plain have the lowest vasodilating properties of all the local anesthetic agents and are good alternatives for patients who are unable to receive a vasoconstrictor.
- Prilocaine plain (block anesthesia) is the only intermediate acting local anesthetic in dentistry without a vasoconstrictor.
- Epinephrine once in the bloodstream is rapidly inactivated by adrenergic nerves.
- Patients with relative contraindications to vasoconstrictors can receive 0.04 mg of epinephrine per appointment.
- More diluted formulations of epinephrine (1:200,000) are safer for patients who are cardiovascularly compromised or elderly patients sensitive to epinephrine.
- More concentrated formulations of epinephrine (1:50,000) provide the greatest bleeding control.
- As epinephrine begins to decline in the tissue, it produces rebound vasodilation, and can potentially lead to postoperative bleeding.
- There is no difference in pain control between 1:50,000, 1:100,000 or 1:200,000 dilutions.
- Sodium bisulfite is added to local anesthetic solutions that contain a vasoconstrictor to prevent the oxidation of the vasoconstrictor. Many individuals are allergic to sodium bisulfite and should not receive an anesthetic containing a vasoconstrictor.
- Epinephrine in high doses (1:1000) is an invaluable drug for treating acute asthmatic attacks and anaphylactic reaction, and should be in every dental emergency kit.
- Levonordefrin is only 15% as potent as epinephrine and therefore manufactured in a higher concentration. Levonordefrin has the same systemic actions as epinephrine but to a lesser degree.
- Levonordefrin provides less hemostasis than epinephrine.

CASE STUDY 4-1

Stella requires emergency treatment for a broken tooth

Stella is in today for emergency treatment of a broken tooth on #3. She is in severe pain and because of the severity of the breakage, the tooth cannot be saved. The dentist believes it will be an easy extraction. The dentist asks Vicki the dental hygienist to administer the anesthesia. Upon review of the patient's medical history and consultation with the patient's physician, it is determined that Stella has uncontrolled hyperthyroidism.

Critical Thinking Questions

Considering Stella's medical history, what type of anesthetic should be selected for the procedure and why?

CHAPTER REVIEW QUESTIONS

1. The activity of the sympathetic autonomic nervous system neurotransmitters are terminated mainly by:
   A. Hydrolysis by acetylcholinesterase
   B. Metabolism by monoamine oxidase (MAO)
   C. Metabolism by catecholamine-O-methyl transferase (COMT)
   D. Re-uptake by adrenergic nerves

2. Which of the following is a sign of an epinephrine toxicity?
   A. Fatigue
   B. Tachycardia
   C. Miosis
   D. Hypotension
   E. Sleepiness

3. The maximum recommended dose of epinephrine per appointment for a patient with ischemic heart disease is?
   A. 0.02 mg
   B. 0.04 mg
   C. 0.2 mg
   D. 0.4 mg
   E. 2.0 mg

4. Epinephrine should be avoided in patients with:
   A. Untreated hyperthyroidism
   B. Hypotension
   C. Controlled diabetes
   D. Myocardial infarction or stroke within the prior 6 months
   E. Both A and D
   F. Both C and D

5. Epinephrine is used for:
   A. Seizures
   B. Angina pectoris
   C. Anaphylactic reactions
   D. Syncope
   E. Gout

6. An effect of epinephrine used in dentistry is to:
   A. Increase vasoconstriction and slow bleeding
   B. Decrease duration of anesthetic
   C. Calm down a nervous patient
   D. None of the above

7. Which of the following is a systemic effect of vasoconstrictors used with local anesthetics?
   A. Increased diastolic blood pressure
   B. Decreased systolic blood pressure
   C. Increased systolic blood pressure
   D. Decreased heart rate
   E. A and C above

8. Vasoconstrictors are added to local anesthetics to:
   A. Reduce bleeding
   B. Counteract the vasodilatory effects of local anesthetics
   C. Decrease possibility of an anesthetic overdose
   D. A and B
   E. B and C
   F. All of the above

9. Which of the following is the preservative added to local anesthetic solutions containing epinephrine to prevent its oxidation?
   A. Sodium bisulfite
   B. Sodium chloride
   C. Sodium bicarbonate
   D. None of the above

10. There is no difference in pain control when using a 1:50,000 or 1:100,000 concentration of epinephrine.
    A. True
    B. False

11. Epinephrine causes direct stimulation of which of the following adrenergic receptors resulting in cardiac stimulation?
    A. α
    B. β_1
    C. β_2
    D. None of the above; epinephrine does not stimulate the cardiovascular system

12. Which of the following vasoconstrictor can safely be administered to a patient with uncontrolled hyperthyroidism?
    A. Norepinephrine
    B. Phenylephrine
    C. Felypressin
    D. Levonordefrin

13. The half-life of epinephrine is approximately:
    A. 1–3 minutes
    B. 5–7 minutes

CHAPTER REVIEW QUESTIONS

C. 10–13 minutes

D. 15–20 minutes

14. What is a 1:1000 concentration of epinephrine used for?
    A. Increase hemostasis
    B. Increase duration of anesthetic
    C. Anaphylaxis
    D. Prevent systemic overdose

15. Levonordefin is added to which of the following local anesthetics?
    A. 2% Lidocaine
    B. 2% Mepivacaine
    C. 3% Mepivacaine
    D. 4% Prilocaine

16. Vasoconstrictor drugs are also known as:
    A. Sympathomimetic amines
    B. Catecholamines
    C. Adrenergic drugs
    D. All of the above
    E. None of the above

17. Epinephrine and norepinephrine are endogenous hormones excreted by:
    A. Adrenal gland
    B. Pituitary gland
    C. Parotid gland
    D. Pancreas

18. Which advenergic receptor causes epinephrine to have inhibitory actions that cause vasodilation and bronchodilation?
    A. α_1
    B. β_1
    C. β_2
    D. α_2

19. Which of the following concentrations is the most diluted?
    A. 1:50,000
    B. 1:100,000
    C. 1:200,000
    D. 1:1000

20. Signs and symptoms of a vasoconstrictor overdose manifests itself as:
    A. CNS depression
    B. CNS stimulation
    C. Cardiovascular depression
    D. Respiratory depression

REFERENCES

1. Malamed S: *Handbook of local anesthesia*, ed 5, St Louis, 2004, Mosby.
2. Ahlquist RP: A study of adrenotropic receptors, *Am J Physiol* 153:586-600, 1948.
3. Yagiela JA: Epinephrine and the compromised heart, *Orofacial Pain Management* 1:5-8, 1991.
4. Sisk A: Vasoconstrictors in local anesthesia for dentistry, *Anesth Prog* 39:187-193, 1992.
5. Darby M, Walsh M: *Dental hygiene theory and practice*, ed 3, St Louis, 2010, Saunders.
6. Jastak T, Yagiela J, Donaldson D: *Local anesthesia of the oral cavity*, St Louis, 1995, Saunders.
7. Management of dental problems in patients with cardiovascular disease: report of a working conference jointly sponsored by the American Dental Association and American Heart Association, *J Am Dent Assoc* 68:333-342, 1964.
8. Use of epinephrine in connection with procaine in dental procedures: report of the Speical Committee of the New York Heart Association, Inc., on the use of epinephrine in connection with procaine in dental procedures, *J Am Dent Assoc* 50:108, 1955.

ADDITIONAL RESOURCES

Becker D, Reed K: Essential of local anesthetic pharmacology, *Anesth Program* 53:98-109, 2006.

Finder RL, More PA: Adverse drug reactions to local anesthesia, *Dent Clin N Am* 46:447-457, 2002.

Paarmann C, Royer R: *Pain control for dental practitioners*. Baltimore, 2008, Lippincott Williams and Wilkins.

Malamed SF, Sykes P, Kubota Y, et al. Local anesthesia: a review, *Anesth Pain Control Dent* 1:11-24, 1992.

Haveles B: *Applied pharmacology for the dental hygienist*, ed 6. St Louis, 2011, Mosby.

Bahl R: Local anesthesia in dentistry, *Anesth Prog* 51:138-142, 2004.

Berecek KH, Brody MJ: Evidence for a neurotransmitter role for epinephrine derived from the adrenal medulla, *Am J Physiol* 242:H593-H601, 1982.

Tetzlaff JE: Clinical pharmacology of local anesthetics. Woburn, Butterworth-Heinemann.

Stiell IG, Hebert PC, Weitzman BN, et al. High-dose epinephrine in adult cardiac arrest, *N Engl J Med* 327(15):1045-1050, 1992.

Yagiela JA: Adverse drug interactions in dental practice: interactions associated with vasoconstrictors. Part V, *J Am Dent Assoc* 130:701-709, 1999.

Hargreaves K, Cohen S: *Cohen's pathways of the pulp*, ed 10, St Louis, 2011, Mosby.

Daniel S, Harfst S, Wilder R, et al. *Mosby's dental hygiene: concepts, cases and competencies*, ed 2, St Louis, 2008, Mosby.

CHAPTER 5

Local Anesthetic Agents

Demetra Daskalos Logothetis RDH, MS

CHAPTER OUTLINE

LEARNING OBJECTIVES

1. Define ester and amide local anesthetics.
2. List and describe the composition of local anesthetic solutions.
3. Discuss the properties and ionization factors of local anesthetics.
4. Discuss the biotransformation of each local anesthetic currently used in dentistry and how esters differ from amides.
5. List and discuss all ester and amide local anesthetics using their generic and proprietary names.
6. List the ester and amide local anesthetics and their formulations.
7. Discuss the selection considerations when choosing a local anesthetic.
8. Describe the factors that determine the duration of a local anesthetic.
9. Correctly complete the review questions and activities for this Chapter.

KEY TERMS

Absolute contrindication The offending drug should not be administered to the individual under any circumstances.

Amide A class of local anesthetics that are generally metabolized in the liver, and rarely produce an allergic reaction.

Ester A class of local anesthetics that are metabolized by plasma cholinesterase and commonly produce allergic reactions.

Generic A nonproprietary name.

Maximum recommended dose The maximum quantity of drug a patient can safely tolerate during an appointment based on their physical status.

Methemoglobinemia A rare hereditary condition characterized by the inability of the blood to bind to oxygen.

continued next page

KEY TERMS—cont'd

Methylparaben Bacteriostatic agent and preservative that was added to local anesthetics agents without vasoconstrictors before 1984 to prevent bacterial growth.

Nerve block Injection of local anesthetic in the vicinity of a nerve trunk to anesthetize the nerve's area of innervations providing a wider area of anesthesia, usually at a distance from the area of treatment.

Paresthesia Persistent anesthesia beyond the expected duration or altered sensation, such as tingling or itching beyond normal level.

Proprietary A brand name or trademark under which a proprietary product is marketed.

Relative contraindication The administration of the offending drug may be used judiciously.

Sodium bisulfite Preservative added to local anesthetics containing a vasoconstrictor to prevent deterioration.

Supraperiosteal injection Type of injection that anesthetizes a small area—one or two teeth and associated structures—when the local anesthetic agent is deposited near terminal nerve endings.

Vasoconstrictor Added to local anesthetic solutions to delay the absorption of local anesthetics causing a lower risk of systemic toxicity.

COMPOSITION OF LOCAL ANESTHETIC SOLUTIONS

Local anesthetics used in dentistry are manufactured in single-use cartridges, also referred to as carpules. Local anesthetic cartridges are designed to contain 2.0 mL of solution. However, when the silicone rubber stopper is added to the cartridge, it is capable of containing 1.8 mL of solution. Although most local anesthetic cartridges contain 1.8 mL of solution, not all are labeled as such. Some manufacturers label and market their anesthetics as containing 1.7 mL of solution. (See Box 5-1.) Local anesthetics are formulated in 2% solutions (36 mg per cartridge), 3% solutions (54 mg per cartridge), 4% solutions (72 mg per cartridge), and 0.5% solutions (9 mg per cartridge). (See Chapter 8 for dosaging facts and calculations.) In addition to the local anesthetic drug, the dental cartridge may contain several other ingredients such as:

- *Vasoconstrictor:* As discussed in Chapter 4, there are two vasoconstrictors currently added to local anesthetic solutions in the United States: epinephrine and levonordefrin. Epinephrine is available in 1:50,000, 1:100,000, and 1:200,000 dilutions, and levonordefrin is available in a 1:20,000 dilution and only with mepivacaine 2%. All local anesthetics are vasodilators, and vasoconstrictors are added to local anesthetic solutions to delay the absorption of local anesthetics, which reduces the potential for systemic toxicity and prolongs the duration of action. Because vasoconstrictors counteract the vasodilatory properties of local anesthetics, they are also beneficial for providing hemostasis.

- *Vasoconstrictor preservative:* Sodium bisulfite, metabisulfite, or acetone sodium bisulfite is only added to local anesthetic solutions that contain vasoconstrictors.[1] Since vasoconstrictors are unstable and have a short shelf life, sodium bisulfite is added to delay the deterioration of the vasoconstrictor. Sodium bisulfite is manufactured as an acid salt rendering it soluble in water and decreasing

BOX 5-1	Cartridge Variations of Anesthetic Volumes

Most local anesthetic cartridges contain 1.8 mL of solution. In some cases, manufacturer product inserts, and anesthetic labels identify the cartridge as containing 1.7 mL of solution. This variation is due to regulations set by the Food and Drug Administration to manufacturers dictating that cartridges should be labeled as containing 1.7 mL of solution if the manufacturer cannot guarantee that all cartridges contain 1.8 mL of solution. Since local anesthetic cartridges are filled by a machine and slight variations will occur, some manufacturers cannot guarantee that all cartridges contain 1.8 mL of solution and therefore are labeled as containing a minimum of 1.7 mL of solution. More manufacturers are likely to market and label their anesthetic in this manner. So, how does this affect drug calculations? Since there will be only a slight variation of +/− 0.1 between cartridges this should not alter the calculation formula of anesthetics labeled as 1.7 mL and will provide a margin of safety if 1.8 mL of solution is actually in the cartridge. (See Chapter 8 for dosing calculations.) However, some regional local anesthetic board examinations require licensure candidates to calculate doses based on 1.7 mL and 1.8 mL. Licensure candidates must be prepared to alter the calculation formulas with the specified amount of solution identified on the examination. Appendix 8-2 will provided drug calculation information based on 1.7 mL of solution.

the pH of the solution, making it significantly more acidic than the same solution without a vasoconstrictor. As discussed in Chapter 3, local anesthetic solutions that are more acidic have a greater quantity of charged cation molecules (RNH^+) than the uncharged base (anion) molecules (RH). This slows the efficiency of the local anesthetic solution to diffuse into the axoplasm, delaying the onset of action.

- Sodium hydroxide: Sodium hydroxide is a buffer that alkalinizes, or adjusts, the pH of the solution between 6 and 7.[2]

- Sodium chloride: Sodium chloride is a buffer which when added to a local anesthetic creates an injectable isotonic solution.

Methylparaben: Methylparaben is a bacteriostatic agent and preservative that was added to local anesthetics agents without vasoconstrictors before 1984 to prevent bacterial growth. Allergic reactions developed from repeated exposures to parabens led to the removal of this agent from dental anesthetic solutions. Dental patients who developed allergic reactions from local anesthetics containing methylparaben in the past may indicate on their medical history that they are allergic to local anesthetics. If this occurs, further dialogue is necessary to determine when the allergic reaction occurred. If the reaction occurred before 1984, it could indicate an allergy to methylparaben. Currently, no dental local anesthetic cartridges contain methylparaben.

SELECTION OF LOCAL ANESTHETIC AGENTS

There are two main classifications of local anesthetic agents: esters and amides. Esters are metabolized in the plasma by plasma cholinesterase, and most amides are metabolized in the liver, the exception being articaine which is metabolized in the blood similar to esters. Because there is a greater propensity of patients who are hypersensitive to injectable esters, all injectable local anesthetics manufactured for dentistry today are in the amide group. As discussed in Chapter 3, the intermediate hydrocarbon chain of the anesthetic molecule determines whether the anesthetic is classified as an ester or an amide. There are five generic classifications of amide local anesthetics available in North America for use in dentistry. Table 5-1 lists some generic and proprietary names. These amide local anesthetic preparations come in various concentrations, with or without vasoconstrictors. The preparations are as follows:

- Lidocaine: 2% Plain; 2% 1:50,000 epinephrine; 2% 1:100,000 epinephrine
- Mepivacaine: 3% Plain; 2% 1:20,000 levonordefrin
- Prilocaine: 4% Plain; 4% 1:200,000 epinephrine
- Articaine: 4% 1:100,000 epinephrine; 4% 1:200,000 epinephrine
- Bupivacaine: 0.5% 1:200,000 epinephrine

TABLE 5-1	Amide Local Anesthetics
GENERIC NAME	**PROPRIETARY NAME**
Lidocaine	Xylocaine, Alphacaine, Octocaine
Mepivacaine	Carbocaine, Arestocaine, Isocaine, Polocaine, Scandonest
Prilocaine	Citanest
Articaine	Septocaine, Zorcaine, Articadent
Bupivacaine	Marcaine

Modified from Darby M, Walsh M: *Dental hygiene theory and practice*, ed 3, St Louis, 2010, Saunders.

The selection of a local anesthetic agent should be determined by the dental hygienist on a patient-by-patient basis, taking into consideration the efficacy, safety, individual patient assessment, consultations, and the dental or dental hygiene care plan. Most dental hygiene care requiring the use of local anesthetics is typically nonsurgical periodontal treatment. However, dental practices in some states hire dental hygienists whose main responsibility in the practice is to administer local anesthetics for many of the procedures performed by the dentist. A dental hygienist may also be asked to administer the anesthesia for the dentist on a case-by-case basis. It is therefore essential for the dental hygienist to fully understand the need for pain control in all dental situations. The following are important considerations in determining the appropriate local anesthetic selection:

- The duration of pain control based upon the length of the procedure
- The need for post-treatment pain control
- The patient's health assessment, and current patient medications
- A local anesthetic, sodium bisulfite, or metabisulfite allergy
- The need for hemostasis

DURATION OF ACTION AND OPERATIVE PAIN CONTROL

As discussed in Chapter 3, there are several physical properties that determine the local anesthetic's onset and duration of action. Table 5-2 lists the properties for the local anesthetic agents that are currently available. The drug's pK_a determines the anesthetic's distribution of cations and anions. The lower the pK_a, the more anions are present in base form for better penetration through the lipid rich nerve, which provides a more rapid onset of action. The protein-binding capacity and the lipid solubility of the anesthetic are related to its duration of action. The lipid solubility also determines the anesthetic's potency. Bupivacaine has the highest percentage of protein binding and is the most lipid-soluble of all the local anesthetics; it therefore has the longest duration and is the most potent. However, bupivacaine has the highest pK_a and therefore the slowest onset of action. The vasodilating properties of anesthetics also play a significant role in both the potency and duration of action. Mepivacaine and prilocaine have the least vasodilating effects, allowing the anesthetic to remain in the area of disposition longer, especially following a nerve block[3,4] (Table 5-3). For this reason, both anesthetics are quite effective without a vasoconstrictor, and both are good alternatives when a vasoconstrictor is contraindicated.

The duration of local anesthetic agents is divided into three main categories, which are influenced by the presence or absence of a vasoconstrictor:

1. **Short-acting** anesthetics provide pulpal anesthesia of approximately 30 minutes and do not contain a vasoconstrictor. These include:

TABLE 5-2	Physical Properties of Local Anesthetics				
LOCAL ANESTHETIC	**PK$_A$***	**VASODILATING†**	**T ½‡**	**LIPID SOLUBILITY§**	**PROTEIN BINDING‖ (5%)**
Lidocaine	7.7	1	1.6	2.9	65
Mepivacaine	7.7	0.8	1.9¶	0.8	75
Prilocaine	7.7	0.5	1.6	0.9	55
Bupivacaine	8.1	2.5	3.5	27.5	95
Articaine	7.8	1¶	.75	1.5	54

*pK$_a$, Dissociation constant; rate of onset.
†Vasodilating lidocaine given value of 1.
‡Half-life (hours).
§Lipid solubility oil/water solubility; intrinsic potency, increased penetrability.
‖Protein binding duration of action
¶Estimated.
Modified from Haveles B: *Applied pharmacology for the dental hygienist*, ed 6, St Louis, 2011, Mosby.

TABLE 5-3	Duration of Pulpal Anesthesia of Local Anesthetics Without Vasoconstrictors by Injection Type	
LOCAL ANESTHETIC	**INFILTRATION (DURATION IN MINUTES)**	**NERVE BLOCK (DURATION IN MINUTES)**
Lidocaine 2%	5–10	10–20
Mepivacaine 3%	20	40
Prilocaine 4%	10–15	40–60

From Malamed SF: *Handbook of local anesthesia*, ed 5, St Louis, 2004, Mosby.

- Lidocaine 2%
- Mepivacine 3%
- Prilocaine 4%

2. **Intermediate-acting** anesthetics provide pulpal anesthesia of approximately 60 minutes and contain a vasoconstrictor, except for prilocaine 4% when administered as a nerve block. These include:
   - Lidocaine 2%; 1:50,000 epinephrine
   - Lidocaine 2%; 1:100,000 epinephrine
   - Mepivacaine 2%; 1:20,000 levonordefrin
   - Prilocaine 4% (intermediate only when administering a nerve block, may provide 60 minutes of pulpal anesthesia in some patients)
   - Prilocaine 4%; 1:200,000 epinephrine
   - Articaine 4%; 1:100,000 epinephrine
   - Articaine 4%; 1:200,000 epinephrine
3. **Long-acting** anesthetics provide pulpal anesthesia of approximately 90 minutes or more and contain a vasoconstrictor. Bupivacaine is the only long-acting anesthetic available in the United States.
   - Bupivacaine 0.5%; 1:200,000 epinephrine

Table 5-4 lists the local anesthetics by their duration of action categorized by short, intermediate, and long acting, and both pulpal and soft tissue anesthesia. Figure 5-1 illustrates the duration of action for soft tissue anesthesia

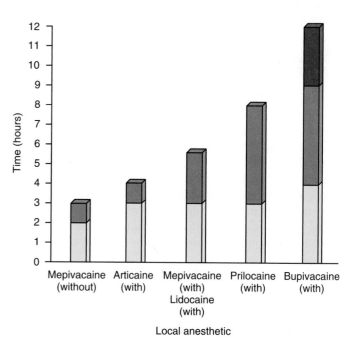

Figure 5-1 ■ Duration of anesthesia in soft tissue after a nerve block. (From Haveles B: *Applied pharmacology for the dental hygienist*, ed 6, St Louis, 2011, Mosby.)

following the administration of a nerve block, and Figure 5-2 illustrates the duration of action for pulpal anesthesia following the administration of a nerve block.

Duration of anesthesia varies among patients depending on individual response to anesthetic, accuracy of anesthetic administration, vascularity of tissue, variation of anatomic structure, and injection technique:

- *Individual response to anesthetic.* In general, individuals respond as expected to the onset and duration of action as listed in Table 5-4. However, some individuals are less or more sensitive to the administered anesthetic and expected duration is either decreased or increased, accordingly. Malamed[4] states that there are three types of individual responses to the administration of local anesthetics, *normal responders*, *hyper-responders*, and *hypo-responders*. These categories are utilized to determine the duration of action of a local anesthetic. Using lidocaine

TABLE 5-4	Categories of Duration of Action of Local Anesthetic Agents (Plain and with a Vasoconstrictor) Available in the United States

GENERAL CATEGORIES

SHORT DURATION (PULPAL = APPROXIMATELY 30 MIN)	INTERMEDIATE DURATION (PULPAL APPROXIMATELY 60 MIN)	LONG DURATION (PULPAL >90 MIN)
Lidocaine 2% plain	Lidocaine 2% 1:50,000 or 1:100,000 epinephrine	Bupivacaine 0.5% 1:200,000 epinephrine
Mepivacaine 3% plain (infiltration/nerve block)*	Mepivacaine 2% 1:20,000 levonordefrin	
Prilocaine 4% plain (infiltration)*†	Prilocaine plain (nerve block)*†	
	Prilocaine 4% 1:200,000 epinephrine‡	
	Articaine 4% 1:100,000 epinephrine‡	
	Articaine 4% 1:200,000 epinephrine	

PULPAL AND SOFT TISSUE ANESTHESIA

LOCAL ANESTHETICS	PULPAL (MIN)	SOFT TISSUE (MIN)
Lidocaine 2% plain	5–10	60–120
Lidocaine 2% 1:50,000 or 1:100,000 epinephrine	60	180–300
Mepivacaine 3% plain (infiltration/block)*	20 (infiltration) 40 (nerve block)	120–180
Mepivacaine 2% 1:20,000 levonordefrin	60	180–300
Prilocaine 4% plain (infiltration/block)*†	10–15 (infiltration) 40–60 (nerve block)	90–120 120–240
Prilocaine 4% 1:200,000 epinephrine†	60–90	180–480
Articaine 4% 1:100,000 epinephrine†	60–75	180–360
Articaine 4% 1:200,000 epinephrine	45–60	120–300
Bupivacaine 0.5% 1:200,000 epinephrine	90–180	240–540

*Mepivacaine plain is a short-acting anesthetic when administered by infiltration or nerve blocks, but the duration is increased with a nerve block.

*†Prilocaine plain administered as an infiltration is a short acting anesthetic. When administered as a nerve block it increases its duration to an intermediate action.

‡4% Prilocaine 1:200,000 and 4% articaine 1:100,000 are categorized as intermediate durations, but provides a slightly longer duration than the other intermediate drugs, extending the duration to 60–90 minutes.

Modified from Haveles B: *Applied pharmacology for the dental hygienist*, ed 6, St Louis, 2011, Mosby.

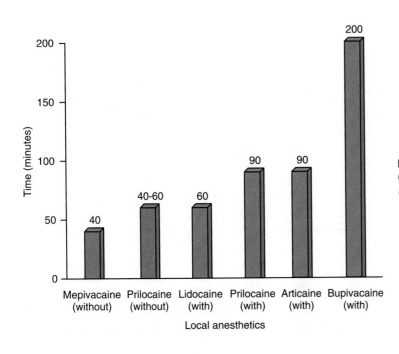

Figure 5-2 ■ Duration of pulpal anesthesia after a nerve block. (Modified from Haveles B: *Applied pharmacology for the dental hygienist*, ed 6, St Louis, 2011, Mosby.)

2% with epinephrine 1 : 100,000 as an example, approximately 70% of patients would fall in the *normal responder* category, representing a typical duration of 60 minutes of pulpal anesthesia. *Hyper-responders* represent approximately 15% of individuals who overly-respond to local anesthetics, and may have pulpal anesthesia of approximately 70 to 80 minutes or longer. *Hypo-responders* represent the final 15% of individuals who under-respond to local anesthetics and may have pulpal anesthesia of approximately 45 minutes or less. Individual patient responses should be anticipated from time to time. Once it is determined that a patient does not respond to the anesthetic drug as expected, a notation should be made in the patient's chart to signal the practitioner of the variation in the patient's response to the anesthetic and to document any modifications that were made to achieve appropriate duration of anesthesia (Box 5-2).

- *Accuracy of anesthetic administration.* Accuracy of anesthetic administration is most difficult when administering a nerve block, an injection of local anesthetic in the vicinity of a nerve trunk to anesthetize the nerve's area of innervations, such as with the inferior alveola (IA) block; it is least difficult when administering supraperiosteal injections, an injection that anesthetizes a small area by depositing anesthetic near the terminal nerve endings. To successfully achieve profound anesthesia of the IA block, the anesthetic solution should be deposited as close to the nerve trunk as possible. Because of the depth of penetration required for IA block, it is necessary to advance the needle through significant soft tissue, allowing a greater possibility for needle deflection, which can influence the accuracy of the injection.
- *Vascularity of tissue.* In healthy tissues, the onset of action and the duration of the anesthetic are more predictable. However, inflamed tissue has increased vascularity due to infection, slowing the onset of action and decreasing the duration because of rapid absorption.

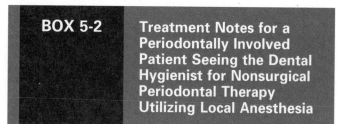

BOX 5-2   Treatment Notes for a Periodontally Involved Patient Seeing the Dental Hygienist for Nonsurgical Periodontal Therapy Utilizing Local Anesthesia

1/12/11
Nonsurgical periodontal therapy of the mandibular right quadrant: 36 mg of lidocaine 2% 1:100,000 epinephrine (0.018 mg) was administered for the IA, B blocks. No reaction to the anesthesia. Patient was still profoundly numb following the 60-minute appointment. At next visit ask patient how long the duration of anesthesia lasted and adjust anesthetic accordingly for hyper-responder.

D Logothetis

IA, inferior alveolar; *B,* buccal.

- *Variation of anatomic structure.* Anatomic variations are difficult to predict and often decrease the duration of local anesthetic action. Decreased anesthetic duration and effectiveness in the maxillae may be caused by[5]:
  - Density of bone. The density of the alveolar bone of the maxillae is typically less than the alveolar bone of the mandible, providing easy anesthetic diffusion and increased duration of pain control. Extra dense bone in this area decreases the success and duration of pain control.
  - Flaring of palatal roots of maxillary molars may affect the anesthetic's action.
  - A lower than normal zygomatic arch, commonly seen in children, may prevent or decrease the duration of the anesthetic's action in the maxillary molars.

Decreased anesthetic duration and effectiveness in the mandible may include the following[5]:
- The height of the mandibular foramen
- Width of the mandible
- Width and length of the ramus
- Volume of musculature and adipose tissue
- Injection technique. Soft tissue and pulpal anesthesia is increased when a nerve block rather than a supraperiosteal infiltration is administered.

POSTTREATMENT PAIN CONTROL

For effective pain management, the selection of an appropriate anesthetic agent for a dental procedure should take into consideration posttreatment pain control. For half mouth (two quadrants) nonsurgical periodontal therapy, profound anesthesia and a longer appointment time may be necessary. Although nonsurgical periodontal therapy usually does not require posttreatment pain control, long duration agents may be needed on occasion for some individuals if posttreatment discomfort is anticipated.[5] Most dental procedures performed by the dentist and dental hygienist fall within the intermediate range of pain control. Examples of procedures that may require postoperative pain control may include, but are not limited to, extractions (impacted third molars) and periodontal surgeries. If the dental hygienist is administering anesthesia for a non–dental hygiene procedure, consultation with the dentist before selecting the local anesthetic is appropriate. Anesthetics that provide longer posttreatment durations of pulpal and soft tissue anesthesia are 0.5% bupivacaine 1 : 200,000 epinephrine (long acting), and 4% prilocaine 1 : 200,000 epinephrine (which can provide intermediate to long) (see Table 5-4). Longer acting local anesthetic agents should be avoided for children and individuals with special needs to prevent the possibility of self-mutilation by accidentally biting or chewing on the lip or tongue.

PATIENT HEALTH ASSESSMENT AND CURRENT PATIENT MEDICATIONS

Local anesthetics used in dentistry today are reliable, and when administered correctly produce effective pain control with little toxicity.[6] However, certain medical conditions, such as cardiovascular disease, liver disease, hyperthyroidism, brittle diabetes, allergies, etc. and drug interactions, such as tricyclic antidepressants, cimetidine, beta blockers, etc. may influence the type and volume of anesthetic or vasoconstrictor that the patient may safely receive. The patient's medical history must be thoroughly evaluated and discussed at each dental hygiene appointment to determine if a relative or absolute contraindication exists for the local anesthetic agent or vasoconstrictor. A relative contraindication means that the administration of the offending drug may be used judiciously, and an absolute contraindication means the offending drug should not be administered to the individual under any circumstances. Once the dental hygienist determines if any contraindications exist utilizing consultations as needed, the maximum recommended dose (MRD) for the individual patient can be determined. The maximum recommended dose is the maximum quantity of drug a patient can safely tolerate during an appointment based on their physical status. Chapter 7 discusses in detail the relative and absolute contraindications to local anesthetic agents and vasoconstrictors based on the patient's physical status and current medications. Chapter 8 discusses the maximum recommended doses related to health conditions and medications.

LOCAL ANESTHETIC, SODIUM BISULFITE, AND METABISULFITE ALLERGY

The addition of the sodium bisulfite, metabisulfite preservative may cause allergic reactions in individuals who are sensitive to sulfites, including respiratory reactions in asthmatics (predominantly steroid-dependent asthmatics). It has been reported that up to 10% of the asthmatic population are allergic to bisulfites. Asthmatic patients who receive a local anesthetic with vasoconstrictor should be observed for signs and symptoms of an asthmatic attack.[1] Sulfites are one of the top food allergens. Sulfites are used in wine to prevent fermentation and oxidation, and are often used as a preservative in dried fruits and dried potato products. Individuals who are allergic to such foods or other sulfite-containing products should not be given an anesthetic with

a vasoconstrictor. Bisulfite allergies typically manifest as a severe respiratory allergy, commonly bronchospasm. Local anesthetic allergies are rare, and only 1% of reactions associated with the administration of anesthetic agents are true allergic reactions.[4] A documented drug allergy would indicate the need for an alternative drug selection and may represent an *absolute contraindication* to the offending drug. Sulfite sensitivities have been well documented[1,7-8] and may rule out anesthetic formulations that contain vasoconstrictors. Table 5-5 summarizes allergies that affect local anesthetic selection.

NEED FOR HEMOSTASIS

When vasoconstrictors are added to local anesthetic agents, there is no difference in pain control associated with the various vasoconstrictor dilutions. However, when hemostasis control is needed, adrenergic vasoconstrictors offer considerable value to the selection of an anesthetic, and the concentration of the vasoconstrictor is a significant factor in the amount of bleeding control they provide.[4,6] All local anesthetics containing a vasoconstrictor offer some degree of hemostasis. As discussed in Chapter 4, because epinephrine possesses both α and β actions with α receptors being less sensitive to epinephrine than β receptors, higher doses of epinephrine are needed to produce the vasoconstriction action of α receptors. Therefore, a 1:50,000 concentration provides the greatest hemostasis properties when compared to the 1:100,000 and 1:200,000 concentrations. For non-surgical periodontal therapy, a 1:100,000 epinephrine concentration will provide adequate hemostasis. In patients with heavy bleeding, the dental hygienist may consider using a 1:100,000 epinephrine concentration for pain control, and use small amounts of a 1:50,000 epinephrine concentration to infiltrate into papilla for bleeding control in the direct area of instrumentation. Levonordefrin is a selective α_2 agonist (75%) and produces vasoconstriction in low systemic concentrations. Although levonordefrin has significant effects on α receptors, it does not provide the same powerful vasoconstiction of the peripheral vasculature as epinephrine. Therefore epinephrine provides better bleeding control than levonordefrin.

TABLE 5-5	Allergies that Affect the Selection of Local Anesthetic Agents or Vasoconstrictors.			
REPORTED ALLERGY	**TYPE OF CONTRAINDICATION**	**DRUGS TO AVOID**	**POTENTIAL PROBLEM(S)**	**ALTERNATIVE DRUG**
Local anesthetic allergy, documented	Absolute	All local anesthetics in same chemical class (esters vs. amides)	Allergic response, mild (e.g., dermatitis, bronchospasm) to life-threatening reactions	Local anesthetics in different chemical class (esters vs. amides)
Sodium bisulfate or metabisulfite	Absolute	Local anesthetics containing a vasoconstrictor	Severe bronchospasm, usually in asthmatics	Local anesthetic without vasoconstrictor

Modified from Darby M, Walsh M: *Dental hygiene theory and practice,* ed 3, St Louis, 2010, Saunders, Elsevier.

AMIDE LOCAL ANESTHETICS

LIDOCAINE

Lidocaine was the first amide local anesthetic suitable for nerve blocks in dentistry and because of its reliabilty is currently the most commonly used local anesthetic solution in dentistry in the United States. It has become the standard to which other local anesthetics are compared. Pharmacologically, lidocaine is a xylidine derivative. It is approximately two times more potent than the ester procaine, and when injected intraorally, produces greater depth of anesthesia.[6]

Because lidocaine is a potent vasodilator it only offers pulpal anesthesia of 5-10 minutes, and therefore is rarely used in dentistry without a vasoconstrictor. However, when the commonly used formulation of 1 : 100,000 epinephrine is used, it provides profound pulpal anesthesia of approximately 60 minutes and soft tissue anesthesia of up to 5 hours with low risk of systemic toxicity and no documented allergic reactions.[6] The 1 : 50,000 formulation provides no further pain control than the 1 : 100,000 formulation and increases the risk for of adverse cardiovascular reactions. Elderly patients are more likely to be hyper-responders to vasoconstrictors, and in these individuals the 1 : 100,000 formulation should be used.[4] However, the 1 : 50:000 formulation does provide greater vasoconstriction offering better hemostasis than the 1 : 100,000 formulation, and therefore should be reserved for procedures that require bleeding control.[6]

Lidocaine has anticonvulsant properties and may be used to terminate or decrease the duration of grand mal and petit mal seizures. These anticonvulsant properties occur at blood levels below that of which lidocaine produces seizure activity in an overdose. Lidocaine decreases the excitability of neurons due to its depressant actions on the central nervous system (CNS) thus raising seizure thresholds.[4] In addition, patients may experience initial sedative effects from lidocaine compared to other local anesthetic agents. During toxic overdose reactions from local anesthetics, initial CNS stimulation is followed by CNS depression (see Figure 5-3). With lidocaine, the stimulation phase may be nonexistent or brief, displaying signs and symptoms of initial CNS depression rather than CNS stimulation.[2] (See Figure 5-3.)

Lidocaine is also an effective topical anesthetic and is currently the only topical amide anesthetic on the market. (See Chapter 6.) Lidocaine is metabolized in the liver through a complex pattern that uses several hepatic enzymes, and less than 10% of lidocaine is excreted unchanged by the kidneys.[4]

Lidocaine is available in three different formulations: 2% plain, 2% 1 : 50,000 epinephrine, and 2% 1 : 100,000 epinephrine. Table 5-6 lists the main properties of lidocaine, and Tables 5-7 through 5-9 give helpful tips for anesthetic selection and precautions for lidocaine formulations. (Also see Chapter 7 for specific guidelines related to the precautions for local anesthetics and vasoconstrictors.)

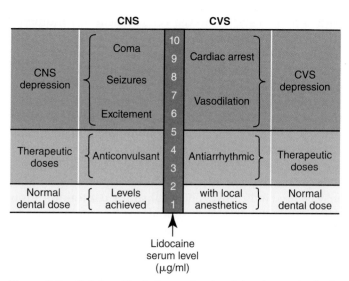

Figure 5-3 ■ Relationship between levels of local anesthesia in serum and the pharmacologic and adverse effects. *CNS*, Central nervous system, *CVS* cardiovascular system. (From Haveles B: *Applied pharmacology for the dental hygienist*, ed 6, St Louis, 2011, Mosby.)

The maximum recommended dose (MRD) for lidocaine is 2.0 mg/lb or 4.4 mg/kg, and the absolute MRD is 300 mg. (See Table 5-10 for lidocaine MRDs and Chapter 8 for calculation guidelines.)

MEPIVACAINE

Pharmacologically like lidocaine, mepivacaine is a xylidine derivative. Mepivacaine is similar to lidocaine in its onset of action, duration, potency, toxicity, and no reported allergic reactions. Mepivacaine is available in two different formulations: 3% mepivacaine plain, and 2% mepivacaine 1 : 20,000 levonordefrin. Because mepivacaine produces less vasodilation than lidocaine, it is an effective anesthetic without a vasoconstrictor and is supplied in this manner only in the 3% formulation. It can be used for short appointments providing pulpal anesthesia of approximately 20 minutes via infiltration injections, and 40 minutes via nerve blocks, and 2 to 3 hours of soft tissue anesthesia when profound pulpal anesthesia is not necessary. It is therefore a good alternative if the use of a vasoconstrictor is contraindicated. However, caution should be taken to avoid systemic toxicity related to using plain anesthetics. Two percent mepivacaine is the only anesthetic that is formulated with levonordefrin as its vasoconstrictor in the United States, and it provides equivalent depth and duration of pulpal (60 minutes) and soft tissue (3 to 5 hours) anesthesia as lidocaine with epinephrine. Levonordefrin, however, does not provide the same intensity of hemostasis as epinephrine. Similar to lidocaine, mepivacaine also has anticonvulsant properties.

Mepivacaine is not effective as a topical anesthetic. Like lidocaine, mepivacaine is metabolized in the liver using several hepatic enzymes, and variable excretion of

TABLE 5-6	Lidocaine

Chemical formula
2-(diethylamino)-2′,6′–acetoxylidide hydrochloride

Proprietary names	Xylocaine, Alphacaine, Octocaine
Formulations in dentistry	2% plain 2% lidocaine 1:50,000 epinephrine 2% lidocaine 1:100,000 epinephrine
Vasoactivity	Lidocaine plain is a potent vasodilator Significantly less vasodilatory properties compared to procaine Causes more vasodilation than mepivacaine and prilocaine
Duration of action (See Tables 5-3 and 5-4)	Short pulpal duration plain 5–10 min Intermediate pulpal duration with epinephrine 60 min
Potency	Equal potency to mepivacaine and prilocaine 2/3 as potent as articaine 1/4 as potent as bupivacaine
Toxicity	Similar toxicity to mepivacaine and articaine 60% more toxic than prilocaine Less toxic than bupivacaine about 1/4
Metabolism	Liver
Excretion	Kidneys, less than 10% excreted unchanged
pK_a	7.7
pH	Plain 6.5 Vasoconstrictor added 3.3–5.5
Onset of action	2–3 min
Half-life	Approximately 96 min (1.6 hours)
Dosage	4.4 mg/kg 2 mg/lb
Maximum recommended dose	300 mg
Pregnancy category	B, safe during lactation

Sources: Jastak T, Yagiela J, Donaldson D: *Local anesthesia of the oral cavity.* St Louis, 1995, Saunders; and Malamed S: *Handbook of local anesthesia,* ed 5, St Louis, 2004, Mosby.

unchanged mepivacaine from zero to 16% by the kidneys. Table 5-11 describes the main properties of mepivacaine, and Tables 5-12 and 5-13 give helpful tips for anesthetic selection and precautions for mepivacaine formulations. (Also see Chapter 7 for specific guidelines related to the precautions for local anesthetics and vasoconstrictors.)

The maximum recommended dose for mepivacaine is 2.0 mg/lb or 4.4 mg/kg, and the absolute MRD is 300 mg. (See Table 5-14 for mepivacaine MRDs and Chapter 8 for calculation guidelines.)

PRILOCAINE

Pharmacologically, prilocaine is similar to both lidocaine and mepivacaine. Chemically, prilocaine is a toluidine derivative, and lidocaine and mepivacaine are xylidine derivatives. Prilocaine is equal in potency to lidocaine and mepivacaine, and two-thirds as potent as articaine. Prilocaine is much less toxic (approximately half) than lidocaine, and slightly less toxic than mepivacaine and articaine. It is the least toxic anesthetic currently available, and minimally affects the CNS and CVS. When compared to lidocaine with a similar IV dose, CNS toxicity following the administration of prilocaine is shorter and less severe.[4]

Like mepivacaine, prilocaine produces very little vasodilation and is an effective plain anesthetic. In fact, when 4% prilocaine is administered as a nerve block it increases its duration from short to intermediate action providing pulpal anesthesia for approximately 40-60 minutes and soft tissue anesthesia for approximately 2 to 4 hours.[4] (See Table 5-4.)

Prilocaine is especially effective when slightly longer duration of action is needed than that of mepivacaine and lidocaine. Prilocaine plain has a slightly longer duration than mepivacaine plain, and prilocaine with 1:200,000 epinephrine has a slightly longer duration than lidocaine 1:100,000 epinephrine. Prilocaine 1:200,000 is also useful when a lower concentration of epinephrine is needed for patients with cardiovascular disease (such as ASA III) who are epinephrine-sensitive. The epinephrine concentration of 1:200,000 is half the potency of the 1:100,000 concentration; therefore patients with cardiovascular disease can receive twice as many cartridges (4.4) of prilocaine with epinephrine as they can cartridges (2.2) of lidocaine 1:100,000 epinephrine.

Prilocaine is metabolized more easily by the liver than lidocaine and mepivacaine, because much of the drug is already metabolized by alternate sites in the lungs and kidneys before it reaches the liver.[6] It is metabolized by hepatic amidases into orthotoluidine and *N*-propylalnine. The primary limiting factor for clinical use of prilocaine is methemoglobinemia, which can occur when prilocaine is metabolized to *ortho*-toluidine. Methemoglobinemia is characterized by the presence of a higher than normal level of methemoglobin in the blood that does not bind to oxygen. In large doses of prilocaine (more than the MRD), clinical cyanosis of the lips and mucous membranes can be observed. This is a relative contraindication to the use of prilocaine, and minimal doses should be administered to patients at risk for methemoglobinemia, or patients with oxygenation difficulties. (See Chapter 7 for more information.)

Topical uses of prilocaine can be found in combination with lidocaine in products such as Oraquix (Dentsply Pharmaceutical) and EMLA (AstraZeneca). (See Chapter 6.) Table 5-15 lists the main properties of prilocaine, and Tables 5-16 and 5-17 give helpful tips for anesthetic selection and precautions for prilocaine formulations. (Also see

Text continued on p. 78

TABLE 5-7	Lidocaine 2%

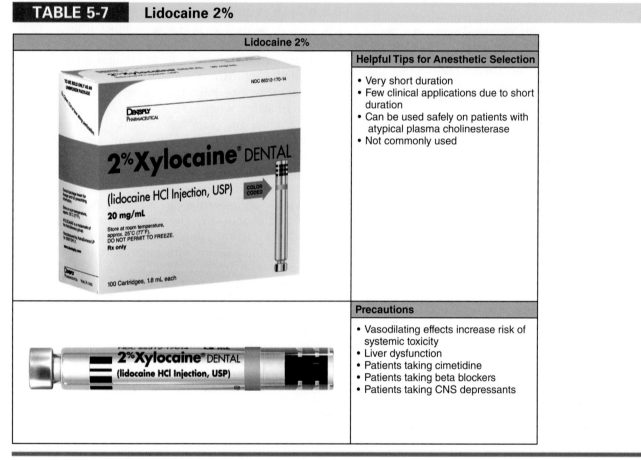

Lidocaine 2%	
	Helpful Tips for Anesthetic Selection
	• Very short duration • Few clinical applications due to short duration • Can be used safely on patients with atypical plasma cholinesterase • Not commonly used
	Precautions
	• Vasodilating effects increase risk of systemic toxicity • Liver dysfunction • Patients taking cimetidine • Patients taking beta blockers • Patients taking CNS depressants

Images courtesy of Dentsply Pharmaceutical, York, PA.

TABLE 5-8	Lidocaine 2% 1 : 50,000 epinephrine

Lidocaine 2% 1:50,000 epinephrine	
	Helpful Tips for Anesthetic Selection • Intermediate duration • Low risk of systemic toxicity • Best choice for bleeding control (recommended to infiltrate small amount directly into areas requiring hemostasis) • No difference in pain control compared to the 1:100,000 or 1:200,000 formulations • Can be used safely on patients with atypical plasma cholinesterase • Can be used (but not recommended) for significant cardiovascular disease at decreased dose of 0.04 mg per appointment (1.1 cartridge) • Worst choice for patients with significant cardiovascular disease or elderly patients sensitive to epinephrine
	Precautions • Patients with significant cardiovascular disease or elderly patients sensitive to epinephrine • Liver dysfunction • Patients taking cimetidine • Patients taking beta blockers • Patients taking CNS depressants • Patients allergic to sodium bisulfite • Steroid-dependent asthmatics • Patients taking tricyclic antidepressants • Patients taking phenothiazines • Cocaine and methamphetamine abusers • Patients with brittle diabetes • Patients with hyperthyroidism • Patients with hypertension • Patients with glaucoma • Patients with recent myocardial infarction • Patients with recent cerebrovascular accident • Patients with recent coronary bypass surgery • Patients with angina

Images courtesy of Dentsply Pharmaceutical, York, PA.

TABLE 5-9   Lidocaine 2% 1 : 100,000 epinephrine

Lidocaine 2% 1:100,000 epinephrine	
	Helpful Tips for Anesthetic Selection • Most commonly used local anesthetic • Intermediate duration • Low risk of systemic toxicity • Effective bleeding control but less than 1:50,000 formulation • Can be used safely on patients with atypical plasma cholinesterase • Best choice for pregnancy (category B) • Can be used for significant cardiovascular disease at decreased dose of 0.04 mg per appointment (2.2 cartridges) • Contains half as much epinephrine compared to the 1:50,000 dilution
	Precautions • Patients with significant cardiovascular disease • Liver dysfunction • Patients taking cimetidine • Patients taking beta blockers • Patients taking CNS depressants • Patients allergic to sodium bisulfite • Steroid-dependent asthmatics • Patients taking tricyclic antidepressants • Cocaine and methamphetamine abusers • Patients with brittle diabetes • Patients with hyperthyroidism • Patients with hypertension • Patients with glaucoma • Patients with recent myocardial infarction • Patients with recent cerebrovascular accident • Patients with recent coronary bypass surgery • Patients with angina

Images courtesy of Dentsply Pharmaceutical, York, PA.

TABLE 5-10 Lidocaine Maximum Recommended Doses Healthy Patient

Lidocaine Maximum Recommended Doses Healthy Patient (Based on 1.8 mL of solution)					
2% plain			**2% 1:50,000**		**2% 1:100,000**
Maximum milligrams and cartridges based upon body weight 2% solution = 36 mg/cartridge 4.4 mg/kg 2 mg/lb Absolute Maximum Recommended Dose = 300 mg Limiting drug "anesthetic" except for 1:50,000 formulation					
Weight kg	**Maximum mg (4.4 mg/kg)**	**Maximum cartridges**	**Weight lbs**	**Maximum mg (2 mg/lb)**	**Maximum cartridges**
10	44	1.2	30	60	1.6
20	88	2.4	50	100	2.7
30	132	3.6	70	140	3.8
40	176	4.8	90	180	5.0
50	220	6.1	110	220	6.1
60	264	7.3	130	260	7.2
65	286	7.9	140	280	7.7
70	308 (300 max)	8.5 (8.3 max)	150	300	8.3
80	352 (300 max)	9.7 (8.3 max)	170	340 (300 max)	9.4 (8.3 max)
90	396 (300 max)	11.0 (8.3 max)	190	380 (300 max)	10.5 (8.3 max)
100	440 (300 max)	12.0 (8.3 max)	210	420 (300 max)	11.6 (8.3 max)
Above absolute maximum dose of 300 mg and 8.3 cartridges			Above absolute maximum dose of 300 mg and 8.3 cartridges		
Absolute maximum dose for 2% lidocaine 1:50,000 is 5 cartridges The vasoconstrictor is the limiting drug in 1:50,000 epinephrine formulation for patients weighing more than 90 pounds					

TABLE 5-11   Mepivacaine

Chemical formula
1-methyl-2',6'–pipecoloxylidide hydrochloride

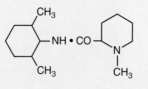

Proprietary names	Carbocaine, Arestocaine, Isocaine, Polocaine, Scandonest	
Formulations in dentistry	3% Mepivacaine plain	
	2% Mepivacaine 1:20,000 levonordefrin	
Vasoactivity	Weak vasodilator	
Duration of action (See Tables 5-3 and 5-4)	Short pulpal duration plain	20 min infiltration
		40 min block
	Intermediate pulpal duration with vasoconstrictor	60 min
Potency	Equal potency to lidocaine and prilocaine	
	2/3 as potent as articaine	
	1/4 as potent as bupivacaine	
Toxicity	Similar toxicity to lidocaine and articaine	
	Twice as toxic as prilocaine	
	Less toxic than bupivacaine about 1/4	
Metabolism	Liver	
Excretion	Kidneys, up to 16% excreted unchanged	
pK_a	7.6–7.7	
pH	Plain	4.5–6.8
	Vasoconstrictor added	3–3.5
Onset of action	1.5–2 min	
Half-life	Approximately 114 min (1.9 hours)	
Dosage	4.4 mg/kg	
	2 mg/lb	
Maximum recommended dose	300 mg	
Pregnancy category	C, safe during lactation	

Sources: Jastak T, Yagiela J, Donaldson D: *Local anesthesia of the oral cavity.* St Louis, 1995, Saunders; and Malamed S: *Handbook of local anesthesia,* ed 5, St Louis, 2004, Mosby.

TABLE 5-12   Mepivacaine 3%

Mepivacaine 3%	
	Helpful Tips for Anesthetic Selection
3% Polocaine® DENTAL (Mepivacaine HCl Injection, USP) 30 mg/mL	• Short duration • Provides slightly longer duration with nerve block • Can be used safely on patients with atypical plasma cholinesterase • Good choice when a vasoconstrictor is contraindicated utilizing nerve block
	Precautions
3% Polocaine® DENTAL (mepivacaine HCl Injection, USP)	• Increased risk of systemic toxicity without vasoconstrictor • Liver dysfunction • Patients taking beta blockers • Patients taking CNS depressants

Images courtesy of Dentsply Pharmaceutical, York, PA.

TABLE 5-13	Mepivacaine 2% 1 : 20,000 Levonordefrin

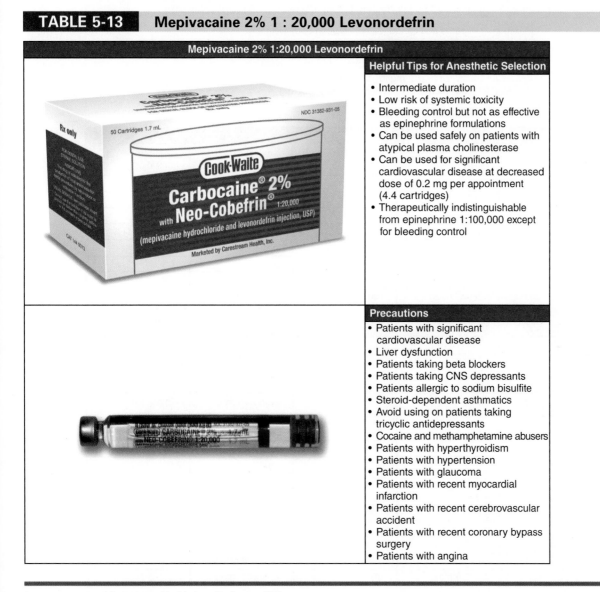

Mepivacaine 2% 1:20,000 Levonordefrin

Helpful Tips for Anesthetic Selection

- Intermediate duration
- Low risk of systemic toxicity
- Bleeding control but not as effective as epinephrine formulations
- Can be used safely on patients with atypical plasma cholinesterase
- Can be used for significant cardiovascular disease at decreased dose of 0.2 mg per appointment (4.4 cartridges)
- Therapeutically indistinguishable from epinephrine 1:100,000 except for bleeding control

Precautions

- Patients with significant cardiovascular disease
- Liver dysfunction
- Patients taking beta blockers
- Patients taking CNS depressants
- Patients allergic to sodium bisulfite
- Steroid-dependent asthmatics
- Avoid using on patients taking tricyclic antidepressants
- Cocaine and methamphetamine abusers
- Patients with hyperthyroidism
- Patients with hypertension
- Patients with glaucoma
- Patients with recent myocardial infarction
- Patients with recent cerebrovascular accident
- Patients with recent coronary bypass surgery
- Patients with angina

Images courtesy of Carestream Health, Inc., Rochester, N.Y.

TABLE 5-14	Mepivacaine Maximum Recommended Doses Healthy Patient

Mepivacaine Maximum Recommended Doses Healthy Patient (Based on 1.8 mL of solution)					
Maximum milligrams and cartridges based upon body weight 2% solution = 36 mg/cartridge 3% solution = 54 mg/cartridge 4.4 mg/kg 2 mg/lb Absolute Maximum Recommended Dose = 300 mg Limiting drug "anesthetic"					
2% 1:20,000 levonordefrin					
Weight kg	Maximum mg (4.4 mg/kg)	Maximum cartridges	Weight lbs (2 mg/lb)	Maximum mg	Maximum cartridges
10	44	1.2	30	60	1.6
20	88	2.4	50	100	2.7
30	132	3.6	70	140	3.8
40	176	4.8	90	180	5
50	220	6.1	110	220	6.1
60	264	7.3	130	260	7.2
65	286	7.9	140	280	7.7
70	308 (300 max)	8.5 (8.3 max)	150	300	8.3
80	352 (300 max)	9.7 (8.3 max)	170	340 (300 max)	9.4 (8.3 max)
90	396 (300 max)	11.0 (8.3 max)	190	380 (300 max)	10.5 (8.3 max)
100	440 (300 max)	12.0 (8.3 max)	210	420 (300 max)	11.6 (8.3 max)
Above absolute maximum dose of 300 mg and 8.3 cartridges			Above absolute maximum dose of 300 mg and 8.3 cartridges		
3% plain					
Weight kg	Maximum mg (4.4 mg/kg)	Maximum cartridges	Weight lbs (2 mg/lb)	Maximum mg	Maximum cartridges
10	44	0.81	30	60	1.1
20	88	1.6	50	100	1.8
30	132	2.4	70	140	2.5
40	176	3.2	90	180	3.3
50	220	4.0	110	220	4.0
60	264	4.8	130	260	4.8
65	286	5.2	140	280	5.1
70	308 (300 max)	5.7 (5.5 max)	150	300	5.5
80	352 (300 max)	6.5 (5.5 max)	170	340 (300 max)	6.2 (5.5 max)
90	396 (300 max)	7.3 (5.5 max)	190	380 (300 max)	7.0 (5.5 max)
100	440 (300 max)	8.1 (5.5 max)	210	420 (300 max)	7.7 (5.5 max)
Above absolute maximum dose of 300 mg and 5.5 cartridges			Above absolute maximum dose of 300 mg and 5.5 cartridges		

TABLE 5-15	Prilocaine

Chemical formula
2-(propylamino)-o-propionotoluidine hydrochloride

Proprietary names	Citanest	
Formulations in Dentistry	4% plain	
	4% Prilocaine 1:200,000 epinephrine	
Vasoactivity	Produces slight vasodilation	
Duration of action	Short pulpal duration plain (infiltration)	10–15 min
(See Tables 5-3 and 5-4)	Intermediate pulpal duration plain (block)	40–60 min
	Intermediate pulpal duration with vasoconstrictor	60-90 min
Potency	Equal potency to mepivacaine and lidocaine	
	2/3 as potent as articaine	
	1/4 as potent as bupivacaine	
Toxicity	40% less toxic than lidocaine	
	1/5 as toxic as bupivacaine	
Metabolism	Simpler hepatic metabolism than lidocaine and mepivacaine	
	Most of the drug is metabolized by the lungs before it reaches the liver	
Excretion	Kidneys, small fraction unchanged in urine	
pK$_a$	7.7–7.9	
pH	Plain	4.5–6.8
	Vasoconstrictor added	3–4
Onset of action	2 min	
Half-life	Approximately 96 minutes (1.6 hours)	
Dosage	6 mg/kg	
	2.7 mg/lb	
Maximum recommended dose	400 mg	
Pregnancy category	B, unknown safety during lactation	

Sources: Jastak T, Yagiela J, Donaldson D: *Local anesthesia of the oral cavity*. St Louis, 1995, Saunders; Malamed S: *Handbook of local anesthesia*, ed 5, St Louis, 2004, Mosby, and product monographs.

TABLE 5-16	Prilocaine 4%

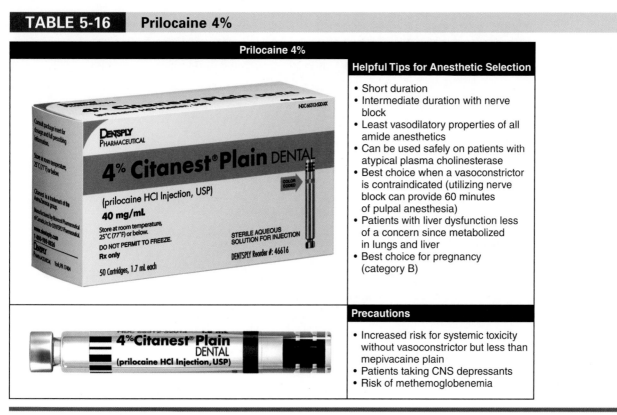

Prilocaine 4%

Helpful Tips for Anesthetic Selection

- Short duration
- Intermediate duration with nerve block
- Least vasodilatory properties of all amide anesthetics
- Can be used safely on patients with atypical plasma cholinesterase
- Best choice when a vasoconstrictor is contraindicated (utilizing nerve block can provide 60 minutes of pulpal anesthesia)
- Patients with liver dysfunction less of a concern since metabolized in lungs and liver
- Best choice for pregnancy (category B)

Precautions

- Increased risk for systemic toxicity without vasoconstrictor but less than mepivacaine plain
- Patients taking CNS depressants
- Risk of methemoglobenemia

Images courtesy of Dentsply Pharmaceutical, York, PA.

Chapter 7 for specific guidelines related to the precautions for local anesthetics and vasoconstrictors.)

The MRD for prilocaine is 2.7 mg/lb or 6 mg/kg, and the absolute MRD is 400 mg. (See Table 5-18 for prilocaine MRDs and Chapter 8 for calculation guidelines.)

ARTICAINE

Articaine (Septocaine) 1 : 100,000 epinephrine was approved for use in the United States in 2000. It is one-third as potent as lidocaine, and relatively equal in toxicity to lidocaine and mepivacaine. It provides intermediate duration of action of approximately 60-75 minutes of pulpal anesthesia and 3 to 6 hours of soft tissue anesthesia. (See Table 5-4.)

Pharmacologically, articaine is derived from thiophene, which makes it different from other amide anesthetics and allows better lipid solubility. Another basic property of articaine that differs among the other amides is that it contains an extra ester linkage. This causes articaine to be hydrolyzed by plasma esterase as well as enzymes in the liver. Ninety percent to 95% of articaine is metabolized in the blood, and only 5% to 10% is metabolized in the liver. This feature is clearly demonstrated when the half-life of articaine is compared with that of lidocaine. The elimination half-life for lidocaine is approximately 90 minutes; that for articaine is 45 minutes. Amides that are primarily metabolized in the liver have a longer half-life, increasing the risk for systemic toxicity. Articaine's major metabolite is articainic acid. It is inactive as a local anesthetic, and

systemic toxicity has not been observed.[7] This finding is important because an active metabolite may affect toxicity and may exert undesirable side effects. In comparison, lidocaine has active metabolites. Because of articaine's rapid metabolism and its inactive metabolites, it may be a safer drug to readminister later during a dental visit if more anesthetic is necessary. Only about 2% of articaine is excreted unchanged by the kidneys. Like prilocaine, articaine has been reported during regional anesthesia purposes to cause methemoglobinemia if administered IV in very high doses. However, there have been no reported cases of this at the recommended dose used in dentistry.[4]

Articaine contains a thiophene ring instead of benzene as lidocaine does. This gives the molecule better diffusion properties than lidocaine.[9] Some dentists who use articaine claim that they seldom miss an IA block and that buccal infiltration in the maxillary arch often was enough before an extraction of a molar. In addition, some studies have demonstrated that pulpal anesthesia can occur after a buccal infiltration in the mandible because of articaine's bone penetration properties.[10,11]

Since the FDA approval of articaine in 2000, some clinicians have been concerned about the frequent reports of paresthesia.[4,9] Paresthesia can be defined as persistent anesthesia beyond the expected duration or altered sensation, such as tingling or itching, beyond a normal level. Articaine is delivered as a 4% solution, whereas lidocaine is delivered as a 2% solution. One possible disadvantage

TABLE 5-17	Prilocaine 4% 1 : 200,000 Epinephrine

Prilocaine 4% 1:200,000 Epinephrine	
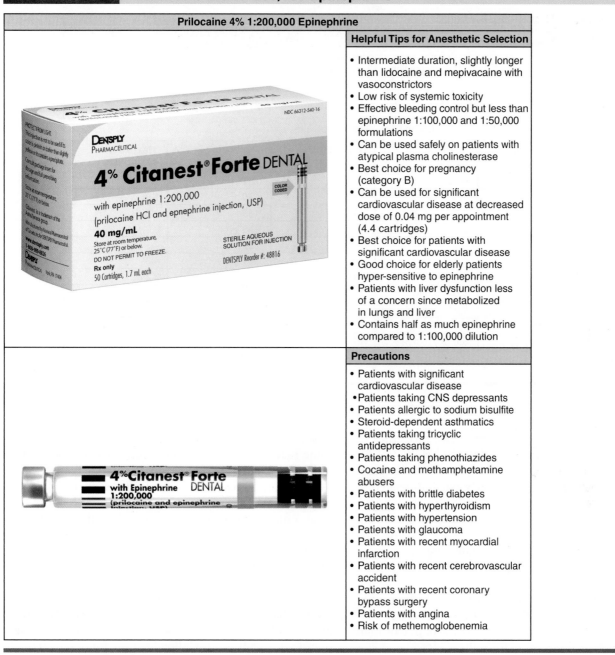	**Helpful Tips for Anesthetic Selection** • Intermediate duration, slightly longer than lidocaine and mepivacaine with vasoconstrictors • Low risk of systemic toxicity • Effective bleeding control but less than epinephrine 1:100,000 and 1:50,000 formulations • Can be used safely on patients with atypical plasma cholinesterase • Best choice for pregnancy (category B) • Can be used for significant cardiovascular disease at decreased dose of 0.04 mg per appointment (4.4 cartridges) • Best choice for patients with significant cardiovascular disease • Good choice for elderly patients hyper-sensitive to epinephrine • Patients with liver dysfunction less of a concern since metabolized in lungs and liver • Contains half as much epinephrine compared to 1:100,000 dilution
	Precautions • Patients with significant cardiovascular disease • Patients taking CNS depressants • Patients allergic to sodium bisulfite • Steroid-dependent asthmatics • Patients taking tricyclic antidepressants • Patients taking phenothiazides • Cocaine and methamphetamine abusers • Patients with brittle diabetes • Patients with hyperthyroidism • Patients with hypertension • Patients with glaucoma • Patients with recent myocardial infarction • Patients with recent cerebrovascular accident • Patients with recent coronary bypass surgery • Patients with angina • Risk of methemoglobenemia

Images courtesy of Dentsply Pharmaceutical, York, PA.

of the higher concentration of the local anesthetic solution is that it has been determined that local anesthetic-induced nerve injury is concentration dependent, with injuries increasing as concentration increases.[4,12-15] Some authors[9,12] have made recommendations to avoid using articaine for IA block because of the potential for paresthesia. Paresthesia has also been reported with 4% prilocaine. However, since most reported occurrences of paresthesia occur following the IA block and most commonly in association with the lingual nerve and are known to occur from injection technique and not the anesthetic agent, avoiding these nerve blocks with articaine is premature since questions

still remain without documented explanations. It is essential that the dental hygienist remain abreast of the current research of all anesthetics, and only administer a drug if the benefits outweigh the risks. For more information regarding paresthesia, see Chapter 14.

In August 2006, articaine 4% 1:200,000 was approved for use in the United States. Studies have shown that the duration and pulpal effectiveness is comparable to the 1:100,000 formulation. However, this formulation of articaine provides another alternative for patients with significant cardiovascular disease and for patients who are taking medications that enhance the systemic effect of

TABLE 5-18	Prilocaine Maximum Recommended Doses Healthy Patient

Prilocaine Maximum Recommended Doses Healthy Patient (Based on 1.8 mL of solution)					
4% plain			**4% 1:200,000 epinephrine**		
Maximum milligrams and cartridges based upon body weight 4% solution = 72 mg/cartridge 6 mg/kg 2.7 mg/lb Absolute Maximum Recommended Dose = 400 mg Limiting drug "anesthetic"					
Weight kg	**Maximum mg (6 mg/kg)**	**Maximum cartridges**	**Weight lbs**	**Maximum mg (2.7 mg/lb)**	**Maximum cartridges**
10	60	0.83	30	81	1.1
20	120	1.6	50	135	1.8
30	180	2.5	70	189	2.6
40	240	3.3	90	243	3.3
50	300	4.1	110	297	4.1
60	360	5.0	130	351	4.8
65	390	5.4	140	378	5.2
70	420 (400 max)	5.8 (5.5 max)	150	405 (400 max)	5.6 (5.5 max)
80	480 (400 max)	6.6 (5.5 max)	170	459 (400 max)	6.3 (5.5 max)
90	540 (400 max)	7.5 (5.5 max)	190	513 (400 max)	7.1 (5.5 max)
100	600 (400 max)	8.3 (5.5 max)	210	567 (400 max)	7.8 (5.5 max)
Above absolute maximum dose of 400 mg and 5.5 cartridges			Above absolute maximum dose of 400 mg and 5.5 cartridges		

epinephrine. Table 5-19 describes the main properties of articaine, and Tables 5-20 and 5-21 describe helpful tips for anesthetic selection, and precautions for articaine formulations. (Also see Chapter 7 for specific guidelines related to the precautions for local anesthetics and vasoconstrictors.)

The MRD for articaine is 3.2 mg/lb or 7 mg/kg, and the absolute MRD is 500 mg. (See Table 5-22 for articaine MRDs and Chapter 8 for calculation guidelines.)

BUPIVACAINE

Bupivacaine is the most potent and toxic of all amide anesthetics. It is four times more potent than lidocaine, mepivacaine, and prilocaine, and three times more potent than articaine. It is four times more toxic than lidocaine, mepivacaine, and articaine, and six times more toxic than prilocaine.[4] Pharmacologically, bupivacaine is structurally similar to mepivacaine, except the butyl group in bupivacaine is exchanged for the methyl group in mepivacaine. This substitution allows for a fourfold increase in potency, allows for toxicity, and provides bupivacaine with a major advantage of increased duration of action compared with other amides.[4,6] Bupivacaine is the only anesthetic that provides a long duration of action, and does so despite its intense vasodilating properties, second only to procaine and significantly more than lidocaine, and is therefore only formulated with 1:200,000 epinephrine. Bupivacaine is highly lipid soluable, and binds powerfully to protein receptor sites in the sodium channels. It provides approximately 1.5 to 3 hours of pulpal anesthesia, and 4 to 9 hours

of soft tissue anesthesia. Due to its long duration, bupivacaine may not be clinically practical for many dental procedures, including nonsurgical periodontal therapy. In an overdose, bupivacaine has equal effects on the CNS and cardiovascular system. Bupivacaine's long half-life (3.5 hours) further increases the risk for systemic toxicity.

The use of bupivacaine is indicated when long pulpal anesthesia is needed (greater than 1.5 hours) and/or postoperative pain control is expected to be needed (e.g., periodontal surgery, endodontics, oral surgery). In many situations, it may be prudent to administer after long procedures have been completed and immediately prior to the patient's discharge from the office. This provides the benefit of extended pain control, allowing time for oral pain medications to take effect. In addition, it is a good alternative when profound anesthesia has been difficult to attain with other anesthetic formulations. With the highest pK$_a$ of the amide anesthetics, bupivacaine has a slightly slower onset of action, but the duration of anesthesia is almost twice that of lidocaine. Bupivacaine is not recommended for use on patients who are prone to self-mutilation (patients with special needs and young children). It is metabolized by liver enzymes in the same manner as lidocaine and mepivacaine, and up to 16% is excreted unchanged by the kidneys. Table 5-23 lists the main properties of bupivacaine, and Table 5-24 gives helpful tips for anesthetic selection and precautions for bupivacaine. (Also see Chapter 7 for specific guidelines related to the precautions for local anesthetics and vasoconstrictors.)

TABLE 5-19	Articaine

Chemical formula
3-N-Propylamino-proprionylamino-2-carbomethoxy-4-methylthiophene hydrochloride

Proprietary names	Septocaine, Articadent	
Formulations in dentistry	4% Articaine 1:100,000 epinephrine 4% Articaine 1:200,000 epinephrine	
Vasoactivity	Equal to lidocaine	
Duration of action (See Tables 5-3 and 5-4)	Intermediate pulpal duration with epinephrine	60–75 min (1:100,000) 45–60 min (1:200,000)
Potency	1/3 more potent than lidocaine, mepivacaine and prilocaine 1/3 as potent as bupivacaine	
Toxicity	Similar to lidocaine and mepivacaine	
Metabolism	95% in plasma and 5% in liver—amide anesthetic that also contains ester component	
Excretion	Kidneys, less than 10% excreted unchanged	
pK_a	7.8	
pH	Vasoconstrictor added	4.4–5.2
Onset of Action	Infiltration (1:200,000) Block Infiltration (1:100,000) Block	1–2 min 2–3 min 1–2 min 2–2½ min
Half-life	45 min	
Dosage	7 mg/kg 3.2 mg/lb	
Maximum recommended dose	500 mg	
Pregnancy category	C, Unknown safety during lactation	

Sources:Jastak T, Yagiela J, Donaldson D: *Local anesthesia of the oral cavity*. St Louis, 1995, Saunders; Malamed S: *Handbook of local anesthesia*, ed 5, St Louis, 2004, Mosby, and product monographs.

The MRD for bupivacaine is 0.6 mg/lb or 1.3 mg/kg, and the absolute MRD is 90 mg. (See Table 5-25 for bupivacaine MRDs and Chapter 8 for calculation guidelines.)

ESTER LOCAL ANESTHETIC

Due to the high degree of hypersensitivity to injectable esters, all injectable local anesthetics manufactured for dentistry (in single use dental cartridges) today are in the amide group. Since injectable ester anesthetics are no longer used in dentistry, only procaine is discussed here because it is still available for use in medicine. Table 5-26 lists the ester local anesthetics of para-aminobenzoic acid (PABA) and benzoic acid.

PROCAINE

Although injectable esters are not available for use in dentistry, procaine is still available in multidose vials and is used as an antiarrhythmic. Formulations include: 2% procaine plain, 4% procaine plain, 2% procaine with 1:100,000 epinephrine, and 4% procaine with 1:100,000

epinephrine. Procaine is significantly less potent and toxic compared with all other amide local anesthetics. Procaine (Novocain) was the first injectable local anesthetic and was used routinely in dentistry until amide local anesthetics became available. Procaine produces the greatest vasodilating properties of all local anesthetics and provides no pulpal anesthesia.[4] Procaine's high degree of allergic reactions and its vasodilating properties made it less desirable, and its use was discontinued. Procaine is metabolized via plasma cholinesterase to PABA, which is the major metabolic by-product responsible for allergic reactions.

BUFFERING OF LOCAL ANESTHETICS

As discussed in chapter 3, chemically, amide local anesthetics are weak bases. They are combined with an acid to form a salt (hydrochloride salt) to render them water-soluble, creating a stable, injectable anesthetic solution. The pH (the acid-base balance) of the solution is manipulated by the manufacturer to complement the specific molecular

TABLE 5-20	Articaine 4% 1:100,000 Epinephrine

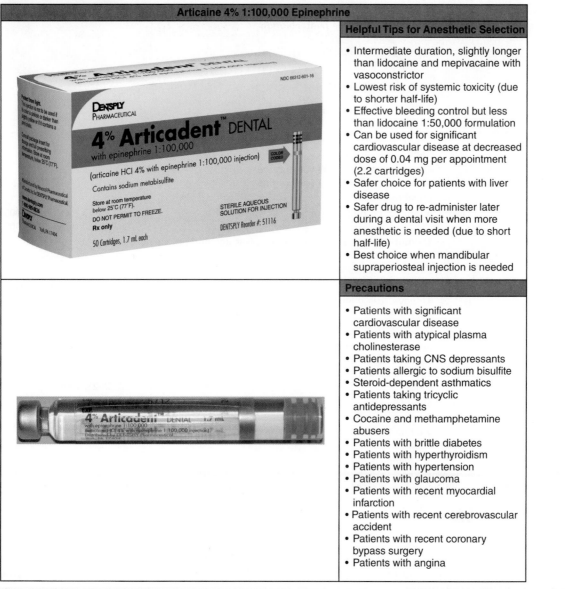

Articaine 4% 1:100,000 Epinephrine

Helpful Tips for Anesthetic Selection

- Intermediate duration, slightly longer than lidocaine and mepivacaine with vasoconstrictor
- Lowest risk of systemic toxicity (due to shorter half-life)
- Effective bleeding control but less than lidocaine 1:50,000 formulation
- Can be used for significant cardiovascular disease at decreased dose of 0.04 mg per appointment (2.2 cartridges)
- Safer choice for patients with liver disease
- Safer drug to re-administer later during a dental visit when more anesthetic is needed (due to short half-life)
- Best choice when mandibular supraperiosteal injection is needed

Precautions

- Patients with significant cardiovascular disease
- Patients with atypical plasma cholinesterase
- Patients taking CNS depressants
- Patients allergic to sodium bisulfite
- Steroid-dependent asthmatics
- Patients taking tricyclic antidepressants
- Cocaine and methamphetamine abusers
- Patients with brittle diabetes
- Patients with hyperthyroidism
- Patients with hypertension
- Patients with glaucoma
- Patients with recent myocardial infarction
- Patients with recent cerebrovascular accident
- Patients with recent coronary bypass surgery
- Patients with angina

Images courtesy of Dentsply Pharmaceutical, York, PA.

structure of each anesthetic. However, all local anesthetic solutions are acidic before injection. Local anesthetic solutions without vasoconstrictors range in pH from approximately 5 to more than 6; generally, preparations with vasoconstrictors are more acidic than plain formations because of the presence of sodium bisulfite and the pH ranges from approximately 3.8 to 5. Due to the acidic nature of the local anesthetic, there are several disadvantages such as: stinging or burning sensation on injection, post-injection tissue injury, and the reliability of local anesthetic action in the presence of infection and inflammation. The pH of the solution is important because it affects the way anesthetic works. The unionized (base) form that is lipophilic readily penetrates the nerve membrane to enter

the nerve axon, where the anesthetic attaches to receptors on the sodium channels, resulting in a blockade of nerve conduction. After injection, tissue buffering raises the pH and a percentage of the drug dissociates to become free bases, the amount depending upon the *dissociation constant* of the individual anesthetic, allowing the free base to penetrate the lipid cell membrane to reach the interior of the axon where a portion of the anesthetic re-ionizes. The re-ionized portion enters and plugs the sodium channels so that sodium ions cannot depolarize. As a result, action potentials are neither generated nor propagated and conduction block occurs.

Anesthetic buffering provides the practitioner a way to neutralize the anesthetic immediately before the injection

TABLE 5-21	Articaine 4% 1:200,000 Epinephrine

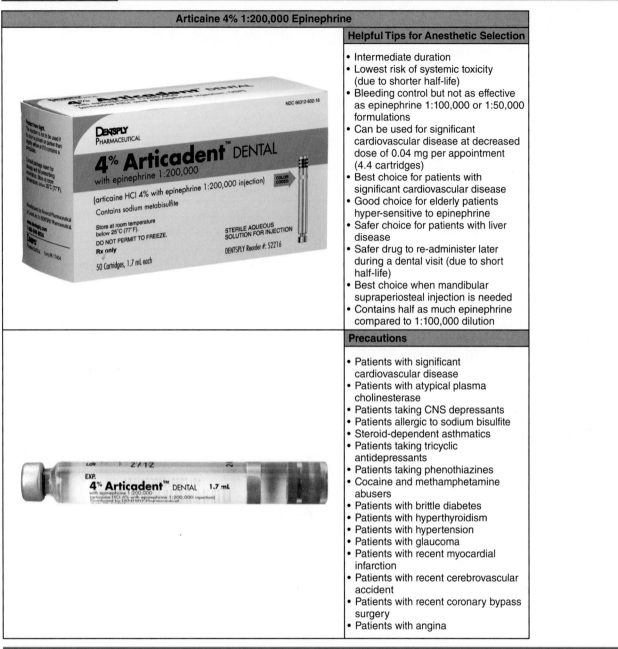

Articaine 4% 1:200,000 Epinephrine

Helpful Tips for Anesthetic Selection

- Intermediate duration
- Lowest risk of systemic toxicity (due to shorter half-life)
- Bleeding control but not as effective as epinephrine 1:100,000 or 1:50,000 formulations
- Can be used for significant cardiovascular disease at decreased dose of 0.04 mg per appointment (4.4 cartridges)
- Best choice for patients with significant cardiovascular disease
- Good choice for elderly patients hyper-sensitive to epinephrine
- Safer choice for patients with liver disease
- Safer drug to re-administer later during a dental visit (due to short half-life)
- Best choice when mandibular supraperiosteal injection is needed
- Contains half as much epinephrine compared to 1:100,000 dilution

Precautions

- Patients with significant cardiovascular disease
- Patients with atypical plasma cholinesterase
- Patients taking CNS depressants
- Patients allergic to sodium bisulfite
- Steroid-dependent asthmatics
- Patients taking tricyclic antidepressants
- Patients taking phenothiazines
- Cocaine and methamphetamine abusers
- Patients with brittle diabetes
- Patients with hyperthyroidism
- Patients with hypertension
- Patients with glaucoma
- Patients with recent myocardial infarction
- Patients with recent cerebrovascular accident
- Patients with recent coronary bypass surgery
- Patients with angina

Images courtesy of Dentsply Pharmaceutical, York, PA.

in vitro (outside the body) rather than the in vivo buffering process, which relies on the patient's physiology to buffer the anesthetic. Some authors suggest that bringing the pH of the anesthetic toward physiologic before injection may improve patient comfort by eliminating the sting, may reduce tissue injury, may reduce anesthetic latency, and may provide more effective anesthesia in the area of infection.[15-17] For example, buffering lidocaine with epinephrine raises the pH from 3.5 to 7.4 and produces a 6000 fold increase in active ionized anesthetic.[17] Other authors were unable to demonstrate any improvement.[19-20] Anesthetic

buffering is well documented in medicine,[15-18] and has recently been provided as an option for use in dentistry with lidocaine epinephrine combinations by Onpharma® using a mixing pen and cartridge connectors to provide an automated way to adjust the pH of lidocaine with epinephrine cartridges at chair side immediately prior to injection (Figure 5-4).

The buffering process uses a sodium bicarbonate solution that is mixed with the cartridge of local anesthetic like lidocaine with epinephrine. The interaction between the sodium bicarbonate ($NaHCO_3$) and the hydrochloric acid

TABLE 5-22	Articaine Maximum Recommended Doses Healthy Patient

Articaine Maximum Recommended Doses Healthy Patient (Based on 1.8 mL of solution)					
4% 1:100,000 epinephrine			4% 1:200,000 epinephrine		
Maximum milligrams and cartridges based upon body weight 4% solution = 72 mg/cartridge 7 mg/kg 3.2 mg/lb Absolute Maximum Recommended Dose = 500 mg Limiting drug "anesthetic"					
Weight kg	Maximum mg (7 mg/kg)	Maximum cartridges	Weight lbs	Maximum mg (3.2 mg/lb)	Maximum cartridges
10	70	0.97	30	96	1.3
20	140	1.9	50	160	2.2
30	210	2.9	70	224	3.1
40	280	3.8	90	288	4.0
50	350	4.8	110	352	4.8
60	420	5.8	130	416	5.7
65	455	6.3	140	448	6.2
70	490	6.8	150	480	6.6
80	560 (500 max)	7.7 (6.9 max)	170	544 (500 max)	7.6 (6.9 max)
90	630 (500 max)	8.7 (6.9 max)	190	608 (500 max)	8.4 (6.9 max)
100	700 (500 max)	9.7 (6.9 max)	210	672 (500 max)	9.3 (6.9 max)
Above absolute maximum dose of 500 mg and 6.9 cartridges			Above absolute maximum dose of 500 mg and 6.9 cartridges		

TABLE 5-23	Bupivacaine

Chemical formula
l-Butyl-1',6'–pipecoloxylidide hydrochloride

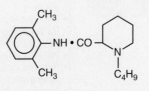

Proprietary names	Marcaine	
Formulations in dentistry	0.5% 1:200,000 epinephrine	
Vasoactivity	Greater than lidocaine, mepivacaine, prilocaine, but less than procaine	
Duration of action (See Tables 5-3 and 5-4)	Long pulpal duration with epinephrine	90–180 min
Potency	Four times more potent than lidocaine, mepivacaine, and prilocaine Three times more potent than articaine	
Toxicity	Four times more toxic than lidocaine and mepivacaine Six times more toxic than prilocaine	
Metabolism	Liver	
Excretion	Kidneys, 16% excreted unchanged	
pK$_a$	8.1	
pH	Vasoconstrictor added	3–4.5
Onset of action	5–8 min	
Half-life	210 minutes (3.5 hours)	
Dosage	1.3 mg/kg 0.6 mg/lb	
Maximum recommended dose	90 mg	
Pregnancy category	C, unknown safety during lactation	

TABLE 5-24	Bupivacaine 0.5% 1:200,000 Epinephrine

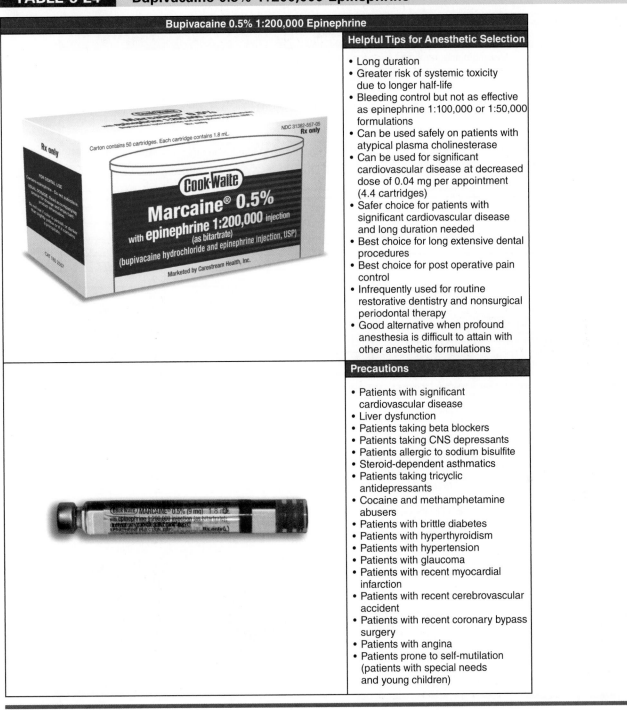

Bupivacaine 0.5% 1:200,000 Epinephrine

NDC 31382-557-05
Rx only

Carton contains 50 cartridges. Each cartridge contains 1.8 mL.

Rx only

FOR DENTAL USE

Cook-Waite

Marcaine® 0.5%
with **epinephrine 1:200,000** injection
(as bitartrate)
(bupivacaine hydrochloride and epinephrine injection, USP)

Marketed by Carestream Health, Inc.

Helpful Tips for Anesthetic Selection

- Long duration
- Greater risk of systemic toxicity due to longer half-life
- Bleeding control but not as effective as epinephrine 1:100,000 or 1:50,000 formulations
- Can be used safely on patients with atypical plasma cholinesterase
- Can be used for significant cardiovascular disease at decreased dose of 0.04 mg per appointment (4.4 cartridges)
- Safer choice for patients with significant cardiovascular disease and long duration needed
- Best choice for long extensive dental procedures
- Best choice for post operative pain control
- Infrequently used for routine restorative dentistry and nonsurgical periodontal therapy
- Good alternative when profound anesthesia is difficult to attain with other anesthetic formulations

Precautions

- Patients with significant cardiovascular disease
- Liver dysfunction
- Patients taking beta blockers
- Patients taking CNS depressants
- Patients allergic to sodium bisulfite
- Steroid-dependent asthmatics
- Patients taking tricyclic antidepressants
- Cocaine and methamphetamine abusers
- Patients with brittle diabetes
- Patients with hyperthyroidism
- Patients with hypertension
- Patients with glaucoma
- Patients with recent myocardial infarction
- Patients with recent cerebrovascular accident
- Patients with recent coronary bypass surgery
- Patients with angina
- Patients prone to self-mutilation (patients with special needs and young children)

Images Courtesy of Carestream Health, Inc., Rochester, N.Y.

(HCL) in the local anesthetic creates water (H_2O) and carbon dioxide (CO_2).[21] The CO_2 diffuses out of solution immediately and continues after the solution has been injected.[22] Catchlove concluded that the CO_2 in combination with lidocaine potentiates the action of lidocaine by a direct depressant effect of CO_2 on the axon concentrating the local anesthetic inside the nerve trunk through ion trapping thus changing the charge of the local anesthetic inside the nerve axon.[18] As with any new product, more research is needed to determine the advantages, disadvantages and consistency of results. Dental hygienists are encouraged to periodically review the companion Evolve Website for updated information on this product and others in the *content update section*.

TABLE 5-25	Bupivacaine Maximum Recommended Doses Healthy Patient

Bupivacaine Maximum Recommended Doses Healthy Patient (Based on 1.8 mL of solution)					
0.5% 1:200,000 epinephrine					
Maximum milligrams and cartridges based upon body weight 0.5% solution = 9 mg/cartridge 1.3 mg/kg 0.6 mg/lb Absolute Maximum Recommended Dose = 90 mg Limiting drug "anesthetic"					
Weight kg	**Maximum mg (1.3 mg/kg)**	**Maximum cartridges**	**Weight lbs (0.6 mg/lb)**	**Maximum mg**	**Maximum cartridges**
10	13	1.4	30	18	2.0
20	26	2.8	50	30	3.3
30	39	4.3	70	42	4.6
40	52	5.7	90	54	6.0
50	65	7.2	110	66	7.3
60	78	8.6	130	78	8.6
65	84	9.3	140	84	9.3
70	91	10.0	150	90	10.0
80	104 (90 max)	11.5 (10 max)	170	102 (90 max)	11.3 (10 max)
90	117 (90 max)	13.0 (10 max)	190	114 (90 max)	12.6 (10 max)
100	130 (90 max)	14.4 (10 max)	210	126 (90 max)	14.0 (10 max)
Above absolute maximum dose of 90 mg and 10 cartridges			Above absolute maximum dose of 90 mg and 10 cartridges		

TABLE 5-26	Ester Local Anesthetics

ESTERS OF PARA-AMINOBENZOIC ACID	ESTERS OF BENZOIC ACID
Procaine (Novocaine 2%)	Butacaine Piperocaine
Propoxycaine (0.4%): used in combination with procaine until its removal from the U.S. market in January 1996.	Benzocaine (Ethyl amino benzoate)
Ravocaine = procaine 2% propoxycaine 0.4% and levophed 1:30,000 or neo-cobefrin 1:20,000	Cocaine
Chloroprocaine	Hexylcaine Piperocaine Tetracaine

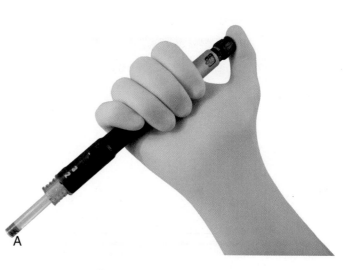

A

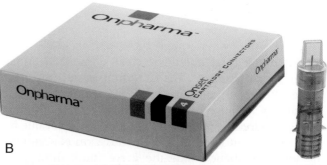

B

Figure 5-4 ■ **A,** Assembled mixing pen is a compounding and dispensing device used to mix two solutions together. Once assembled, the pen enables the precise transfer of fluid of sodium bicarbonate from a standard 3 mL size cartridge into the 1.8 mL anesthetic cartridge, allowing the two solutions to be mixed. **B,** The cartridge connector is used for the transfer of sterile solutions from one sealed container into a second sealed container and provides a reservoir for collecting excess solution displaced from the second sealed container during the transfer process. Images courtesy Onpharma Inc., Los Gatos, CA

DENTAL HYGIENE CONSIDERATIONS

- Local anesthetic cartridges containing a vasoconstrictor contain the preservative sodium bisulfite, which may cause allergic reactions including respiratory reactions in asthmatics (predominantly steroid dependent asthmatics).
- Methylparaben is a bacteriostatic agent/preservative added to local anesthetic cartridges before 1984 and is known to cause allergic reactions. Currently no anesthetic cartridges contain methylparaben.
- Ester anesthetics are no longer manufactured for use in dentistry.
- The selection of the local anesthetic drug should be determined by the dental hygienist on an individual patient basis taking into consideration the efficacy, safety, individual patient assessment, and the dental or dental hygiene care plan.
- Intermediate action anesthetics are most commonly used for regular restorative dentistry and nonsurgical periodontal therapy.
- Lidocaine is the standard by which all other local anesthetics are compared.
- Lidocaine is the most commonly used anesthetic in dentistry in the United States; it provides profound anesthetic without extensive duration.

- There is no difference in pain control between a 1:50,000, 1:100,000, or 1:200,000 formulations of epinephrine.
- Mepivacaine and prilocaine have the least vasodilating properties and are effective when a vasoconstrictor is contraindicated. Prilocaine may have intermediate duration when administered as a nerve block.
- Lidocaine, mepivacaine, and bupivacaine are metabolized in the liver by amidases.
- Prilocaine is metabolized in the liver and additionally by the lungs and kidneys as alternative sites.
- Because of prilocaine's metabolite orthotoluidine, when administered in high doses some individuals may develop methemoglobinemia by reducing the blood's oxygen-carrying capacity. This is a relative contraindication for at-risk patients.
- Articaine is the only amide anesthetic that has an ester component attached to the aromatic ring structure. It is metabolized primarily in the plasma by plasma cholinesterase, and therefore has the shortest half-life and the lowest risk for systemic toxicity.
- Bupivacaine is the only long-acting local anesthetic available in the United States.

CASE STUDY 5-1

Debbie is nervous about her extraction

Debbie is in your office for an impacted third molar extraction of tooth number 1. The dentist asks the dental hygienist Peggy to administer the local anesthesia. Debbie's blood pressure is 110/85 mm Hg and her weight is 102 lb. She has a history of atypical plasma cholinesterase, and she is very nervous about her dental appointment.

Critical Thinking Questions:

- What are the medical considerations when choosing a local anesthetic?
- Choose and justify an appropriate local anesthetic for this patient.

CHAPTER REVIEW QUESTIONS

1. The most important advantage of amide over ester local anesthetics is:
   A. Quicker onset
   B. Longer duration
   C. Less allergenicity
   D. Cheaper cost
2. Which local anesthetic is the longest acting?
   A. Lidocaine
   B. Procaine
   C. Bupivacaine with epinephrine
   D. Prilocaine with epinephrine
   E. Articaine with epinephrine
3. Which local anesthetic has the least vasodilatory effect when used without epinephrine?

   A. Mepivacaine
   B. Lidocaine
   C. Cocaine
   D. Procaine
4. Which local anesthetic has the greatest vasodilatory effect when used without epinephrine?
   A. Mepivacaine
   B. Lidocaine
   C. Articaine
   D. Procaine
5. One cartridge of anesthetic contains how much solution?
   A. 1.8 mL
   B. 1.8 g

   C. 1.8 mg
   D. 1.8 L

6. Factors in selection of local anesthetic for a patient include all of the following except:
   A. Length of time pain control is necessary
   B. Presence of any contraindication (absolute or relative) to the local anesthetic solution selection for administration
   C. Requirement for hemostasis
   D. Vitamin intake

7. Which of the following is false:
   A. Esters of para-aminobenzoic acid are not commercially available
   B. Procaine is an ester
   C. Topical benzocaine is an amide
   D. Prilocaine is an amide

8. Which of the following local anesthetics is metabolized in the plasma and liver?
   A. Lidocaine
   B. Bupivacaine
   C. Prilocaine
   D. Articaine

9. Which of the following is an advantage of having a local anesthetic metabolized in the plasma and liver?
   A. Increased duration of action of drug
   B. Shorter half-life of drug
   C. Decreased vasoactivity of drug
   D. Easy excretion of metabolites

10. Which of the following local anesthetics is metabolized in the lungs and liver?
   A. Mepivacaine
   B. Bupivacaine
   C. Prilocaine
   D. Articaine

11. Methylparaben is a:
   A. Local anesthetic preservative that prevents oxidation of epinephrine
   B. Bacteriostatic agent that is no longer added to dental cartridges due to high incidence of allergic reactions
   C. Buffer that alkalinizes the anesthetic solution
   D. Buffer that creates an isotonic solution

12. How is 3% mepivacaine formulated?
   A. 3% plain
   B. 3% 1:20,000 levonordefrin
   C. 3% 1:100,000 epinephrine
   D. 3% 1:200,000 epinephrine

13. Which of the following is a concern when selecting bupivacaine?

   A. Patient self-mutilation
   B. Decreased risk of toxicity
   C. Concentration of anesthetic
   D. Ease of biotransformation

14. Which of the following local anesthetics is the best option for readministration of anesthetic to provide a lessened likelihood of blood concentration buildup?
   A. Lidocaine
   B. Mepivacaine
   C. Prilocaine
   D. Articaine
   E. Bupivacaine

15. The lower the pK_a of a drug, the more cations are present, which decreases the onset of action.
   A. True
   B. False

16. Which of the following is not a factor in the duration of a local anesthetic?
   A. Individual response to anesthetic
   B. Anatomic structure
   C. Patient health assessment
   D. Injection technique

17. Which of the following local anesthetics used without a vasoconstrictor provides intermediate duration of action when administering a block injection?
   A. Lidocaine
   B. Mepivacaine
   C. Prilocaine
   D. Bupivacaine

18. Which of the following is the best reason for choosing a local anesthetic that provides a long duration?
   A. Need for postoperative pain control
   B. Medical status of patient
   C. Dense bone in the area of administration
   D. Infection in the area

19. When is lidocaine 1:50,000 epinephrine most effective?
   A. When postoperative pain control is needed
   B. When hemostasis is needed
   C. When treating a cardiovascularly-involved patient
   D. When more profound pain control is needed

20. Where is procaine metabolized?
   A. Liver
   B. Lungs
   C. Plasma
   D. Plasma and liver

REFERENCES

1. Stevenson DD, Simon RA: Sensitivity to ingested metabisulfites in asthmatic subjects, *J Allergy Clin Immunol* 68: 26-32, 1981.
2. Haveles B: *Applied pharmacology for the dental hygienist,* ed 6, St Louis, 2011, Mosby.
3. Bahl R: Local anesthesia in dentistry, *Anesth Prog* 51: 138-142, 2004.
4. Malamed S: *Handbook of local anesthesia,* ed 5, St Louis, 2004, Mosby.
5. Darby M, Walsh M: *Dental hygiene theory and practice,* ed 3, St Louis, 2010, Saunders, Elsevier.
6. Jastak T, Yagiela J, Donaldson D: *Local anesthesia of the oral cavity,* St Louis, 1995, Saunders.
7. Sher TH, Schwartz HJ: Bisulfite sensitivity manifesting an allergic reaction to aerosol therapy, *Ann Allergy* 54: 224-226, 1985.
8. Borghesan F, Basso D, Chieco Bianchi F. et al: Allergy to wine, *Allergy* 59: 1135-1136, 2004.
9. Isen DA: Articaine: pharmacology and clinical use of a recently approved local anesthetic, *Dent Today* 19: 72-77, 2000.
10. Mohammad DK, et al: Articaine and lidocaine mandibular buccal infiltration anesthesia: a prospective randomized double-blind cross-over study, *JOE* 32(4): 296-298, 2006.
11. Robertson D, et al: The anesthetic efficacy of articaine in buccal infiltration of mandibular posterior teeth, *J Am Dent Assoc* 138(8): 1104-12, 2007.
12. Oertel R, Rahn R, Kirch W: Clinical pharmacokinetics of articaine, *Clin Pharmacokinet* 33: 417-425, 1997.
13. Oertel R, Richter K: Plasma protein binding of the local anaesthetic drug articaine and its metabolite articainic acid, *Pharmazie* 53: 646-647, 1998.
14. Haas DA, Lennon D: A 21 year retrospective study of reports of paresthesia following local anesthetic administration, *J Can Dent Assoc* 61: 319-330, 1995.
15. Dower JS: A review of paresthesia, *Dent Today* 22: 64-69, 2003.
15. Bowles WH, Frysh H, Emmons R: Clinical Evaluation of Buffered Local Anesthetic, *General Dentistry* 43(2): 182, 1995.
16. Stewart JH, Cole GW, Klein JA: Neutralized lidocaine with epinephrine for local anesthesia, *J Dermatol Surg Oncol* 15(10): 1081, 1989.
17. Malamed S: Buffering local anesthetics in dentistry, *The Pulse* 44(1): 7-9, 2011.
18. Stewart JH, Cole GW, Klein JA: Neutralized Lidocaine with Epinephrine for Local Anesthesia, *J Dermatol Surg Oncol* 15(10): 1081, 1989.
19. Primosch RE, Robinson L: Pain elicited during intraoral infiltration with buffered lidocaine, *American Journal of Dentistry* 9(1): 5, 1996.
20. Whitcomb M, Drum M, Reader A, Nusstein M, Beck M: A prospective, randomized, double-blind study of the anesthetic efficacy of sodium bicarbonate buffered 2% lidocaine with 1:100,000 epinephrine in inferior alveolar nerve blocks, *Anesthesia progress* 57: 59, 2010.
21. Ackerman WE, Ware TR, Juneja M: The air-liquid interface and the pH and PCO2 of alkalinized local anaesthetic solutions, *Canadian Journal of Anaesthesiology* 39(4): 387, 1992.
22. Catchlove RFH: The influence of C02 and pH on local anesthetic action, *The Journal of Pharmacology and ExpTherap* 181(2): 298-309, 1972.

ADDITIONAL RESOURCES

Becker D, Reed K: Essentials of local anesthetic pharmacology. American Dental Society of Anesthesiology, *Anesth Program* 53: 98-109, 2006.

Hargreaves K, Cohen S: *Cohen's pathways of the pulp,* ed 10, St Louis, 2011, Mosby. 16. de Jong RH. Local anesthetics. St Louis: Mosby.

Finder RL, More PA: Adverse drug reactions to local anesthesia, *Dent Clin N Am* 46: 447-457, 2002.

Sisk A: Vasoconstrictors in Local Anesthesia for Dentistry, *Anesth Prog* 39: 187-193, 1992.

US Food and Drug Administration: Center for Food Safety and Applied Nutrition van der Meer, Auke Dirk MD; Burm, Anton G. L. MSc, PhD; Stienstra, Rudolf MD, PhD; van Kleef, Jack W. MD, PhD; Vletter, Arie A. BSc; Olieman, Wim; Pharmacokinetics of Prilocaine after Intravenous Administration in Volunteers: Enantioselectivity, Anesthesiology: April 1999, Volume 90, Issue 4, pp 988-992

Bartlett SZ: Clinical observation on the effect of injections of local anaesthetics preceded by aspiration, *Oral Surg* 33: 520-525, 1972.

Buckley JA, Ciancio SG, McMullen JA: Efficacy of epinephrine concentration in local aneshesia during periodontal surgery, *J Periodontol* 55: 653-657, 1984.

Isen DA: Articaine: Pharmacology and clinical use of a recently approved local anesthetic, *Dent Today* 19: 72-77, 2000.

Jacob W: Local anaesthesia and vasoconstrictive additional components, *Newslett Int Fed Dent Anesthesiol Soc* 2: 1-3, 1989.

Malamed SF, Gagnon S, Leblanc D: Efficacy of articaine: A new amide local anesthetic, *JAm Dent Assoc* 131: 635-642, 2000.

Malamed SF, Gagnon S, Leblanc D: A comparison between articaine HCL and lidocaineHCL in pediatric dental patients, *Am Acad Ped Dent* 22: 307-311, 2000.

Malamed SF, Gagnon S, Leblanc D: Articaine hydrochloride: a study of the safety of a new amide local anesthetic, *J Am Dent Assoc* 132: 177-184, 2001.

Haas DA, Harper DG, Saso MA, Young ER: Comparison of articaine and prilocaine anesthesia by infiltration in maxillary and mandibular arches, *Anesth Prog* 37: 230-237, 1990.

Jacob W: Local anaesthesia and vasoconstrictive additional components, *Newslett Int Fed Dent Anesthesiol Soc* 2: 1-3, 1989.

Jacobs W, Ladwig B, Cichon P, Oertel R, Kirch W: Serum levels of articaine 2 % and 4 % in children, *Anesth Prog* 42: 113-115, 1995.

Oertel R, Ebert U, Rahn R, Kirch W: The effect of age on the pharmacokinetics of the local anesthetic drug articaine, *Regional Anesth Pain Med* 24: 524-528, 1999.

Summary of Amide Local Anesthetic Agents and Vasoconstrictors

Generic name	Lidocaine			Mepivacaine		Prilocaine		Articaine	Bupivacaine
Available formulations	2% Plain Light Blue	2% 1:50,000 Epinephrine Green	2% 1:100,000 Epinephrine Red	3% Plain Plain Tan	2% 1:20,000 Levonordefrin Brown	4% Plain Black	4% 1:200,000 Epinephrine Yellow	4% 1:100,000 Epinephrine Gold 1:200,000 Silver	0.5% 1:200,000 Epinephrine Blue
ADA color coding band									
Other trade names/manufacturer	Lidocaine HCl Many Generics Xylocaine HCl Astra/Denstply Pharm.	Lidocaine HCl Many Generics Xylocaine HCl Astra/Denstply Pharm.	Lidocaine HCl Many Generics Xylocaine HCl Astra/Denstply Pharm.	Mepivacaine Many Generics Carbocaine Cook-Waite/Kodak Polocaine Astra/Denstply Pharm.	Mepivacaine Many Generics Carbocaine Cook-Waite/Kodak Polocaine Astra/Denstply Pharm. Scandonest Septodont	Citanest Plain Astra/Denstply Pharm.	Citanest Forte Astra/Denstply Pharm.	Septocaine Septodont Zorcaine Cook-Waite/Kodak Articadent Denstply	Marcaine Cook-Waite/Kodak Vivacaine Septodont
pKa	7.7	7.7	7.7	7.6-7.7	7.6-7.7	7.7-7.9	7.7-7.9	7.8	8.1
pH	6.5	3.3-5.5	3.3-5.5	4.5-6.8	3-3.5	4.5-6.8	3-4	4.4-5.2	3-4.5
Duration	Short	Intermediate	Intermediate	Short	Intermediate	Short infiltration Intermediate block	Intermediate	Intermediate	Long
Duration pulpal tissues	5-10 min.	60 min.	60 min.	20-40 min. (towards 40 min with block)	60-90 min.	Infiltration: 5-10 min. block: 40-60 min.	60-90 min.	1:100,000 60-75 min 1:200,000 45-60 min	90-180 min
Duration soft tissues	1-2 hours	3-5 hours	3-5 hours	2-3 hours	3-5 hours	Infiltration: 1.5-2 hours block: 2-4 hours	3-8 hours	3-6 hours	4-9 hours
MRD (mg/lb)	2.0	2.0	2.0	2.0	2.0	2.7	2.7	3.2	0.6
MRD (mg/kg)	4.4	4.4	4.4	4.4	4.4	6.0	6.0	7.0	1.3
MRD Absolute mg	300	300	300	300	300	400	400	500	90

CHAPTER 6

Topical Anesthetic Agents

Diana M. Burnham RDH, MS

CHAPTER OUTLINE

LEARNING OBJECTIVES

1. Define the key terms.
2. Discuss the purpose of topical anesthetics.
3. Identify ideal properties of topical anesthetics.
4. List common forms of topical anesthetics.
5. List and describe the methods for delivery of topical anesthetic drugs.
6. Identify and describe the common topical anesthetic agents used in dentistry.
7. Recognize and describe local and systemic signs and symptoms of adverse reactions to topical anesthetics.
8. Identify and describe topical anesthetic drug combinations used in dentistry.
9. Differentiate between products found over-the-counter and used by consumers and those that are applied by professionals and purchased through suppliers.
10. Correctly complete the review questions and activities for this chapter.

KEY TERMS

Benzocaine A common ester topical anesthetic.

Butamben An ester topical anesthetic; often combined with other topicals for use.

Dyclonine hydrochloride A ketone topical anesthetic.

Eutectic mixtures Mixture of two elements that have a lower melting point than any of their individual components.

Lidocaine An amide local anesthetic.

Methemoglobinemia A condition that prevents oxygen from being carried to body tissues effectively.

Tetracaine hydrochloride An ester anesthetic. Considered most potent and only used topically.

Topical Applied to body surface areas, such as skin or mucous membrane.

Transdermal Route of administration, delivered across the skin.

Transoral Route of administration, delivered via oral mucosa.

INTRODUCTION

One important component of the local anesthesia armamentarium is the topical anesthetic. Topical implies that the anesthetic will be applied to the body surface such as the skin or mucous membrane. In dentistry, topical anesthetics are used routinely to provide pain control before conventional local anesthetic injections. They contribute by minimizing the pain associated with needle insertion. Topical anesthetics are also frequently used for the treatment of minor injuries of the gingiva and oral mucosa, to increase comfort during minor dental and dental hygiene procedures, and to reduce the patient's gag reflex while taking radiographs and impressions.

Some topical anesthetic agents are also made available over-the-counter to the public and can be purchased at local food and drug stores (Figure 6-1). People of all ages use them to ease pain from teething, braces, apthous ulcers (canker sores), dentures, or toothaches.

Whether being applied professionally or in the comfort of your home (Tables 6-1 and 6-2), intraoral topical anesthetics should ideally be nonallergenic and produce no

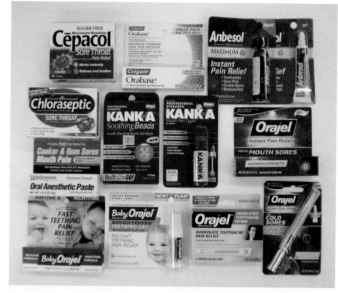

Figure 6-1 ■ Variety of topical anesthetic products that can be purchased over-the-counter in local food and drug stores.

TABLE 6-1			Common Topical Agents Administered Professionally						
PRODUCT NAME	**GEL**	**SPRAY**	**LIQUID**	**OINTMENT**	**PATCH**	**LOZENGE**	**CREAM**	**SINGLE UNIT DOSE**	**ACTIVE INGREDIENT**
Americaine	X	X							Benzocaine 20%
Anacaine				X					Benzocaine 10%
Benzo-Jel	X								Benzocaine 20%
CaineTips								X	Benzocaine 20%
Cetacaine	X	X	X						Benzocaine 14%, butamben 2%, tetracaine hydrochloride 2%
ComfortCaine	X								Benzocaine 20%
Cora-Caine				X					Benzocaine 16%
Denti-care	X								Benzocaine 20%
Gingicaine	X		X						Benzocaine 20%
HurriCaine	X	X	X					X	Benzocaine 20%
HurriPak			X						Benzocaine 20%
Kolorz	X								Benzocaine 20%
Lidocaine				X					Lidocaine 5%
Lollicaine								X	Benzocaine 20%
ProJel-20	X								Benzocaine 20%
One Touch Advanced	X								Benzocaine 14%, butamben 2%, tetracaine hydrochloride 2%
Oraqix	X								Lidocaine 2.5% and prilocaine 2.5%
Topex	X	X	X						Benzocaine 20%
Topex HandiCaine Stix								X	Benzocaine 20%
Topicale	X			X	X				Benzocaine gel and ointment 20%, patch 18%
Ultracare	X								Benzocaine 20%

TABLE 6-2 Common Topical Anesthetic Agents Self-Administered by Patients

PRODUCT NAME	GEL	SPRAY	LIQUID	OINTMENT	PATCH	LOZENGE	CREAM	SINGLE UNIT DOSE	ACTIVE INGREDIENT
Anbesol	X		X						Benzocaine: Baby 7.5%, Jr 10%, max strength 20%
BiZets						X			Benzocaine 15 mg
Cepacol		X				X			Benzocaine-spray 5% Lozenges 7.5 mg to 15 mg
Chloraseptic						X			Benzocaine 6 mg
Dentane	X								Benzocaine 7.5%
Dentapaine	X								Benzocaine 20%
HDA Toothache	X								Benzocaine 6.5%
Kank-A	X		X			X			Benzocaine-gel and liquid 20%, bead 3 mg
Orabase*									Benzocaine 20% *comes in a paste
Orajel Adult	X						X	X	Benzocaine-regular 10%, ultra and denture 15%, medicated swab 20%, PM max strength 20%
Orajel Baby	X		X					X	Benzocaine 7.5%, nighttime 10%, cooling cucumber 10%
Ora-Film*									Benzocaine 10% *comes in a thin film strip
Red Cross Canker				X					Benzocaine 20%
Sucrets						X			Dyclonine hydrochloride Children 1.2 mg, max strength 3 mg
Tanac			X						Benzocaine 10%
Thorets						X			Benzocaine 10 mg
Trocaine						X			Benzocaine 10 mg
Zilactin-B	X								Benzocaine 10%, max strength 20%

damage to the tissue to which it is applied. It should consist of a pain-free application, have an acceptable taste, and be able to remain at the site of application. Also, it must produce reliable effective anesthesia with a sufficient duration and not induce systemic toxicity (Box 6-1).

MECHANISM OF ACTION OF TOPICAL ANESTHETICS

The mechanism of action of topical anesthetics is similar to that of their injectable counterparts; however, topical anesthetics work by blocking nerve conductions at the surface of the skin or mucous membrane. The permeability of sodium ions to the nerve cell is decreased, resulting in

BOX 6-1 Ideal Properties of an Intraoral Topical Anesthetic

- Nonallergenic
- Produce no local damage to tissue
- Allow pain-free application
- Have an acceptable taste
- Remain at the site of application
- Produce reliable anesthesia
- Produce sufficient duration of anesthesia
- Produce no systemic toxicity

From Meechan JG. Intra-oral topical anaesthetics: a review. J Dent 2000;28;3-14.

decreased depolarization and an increased excitability threshold that, ultimately, blocks the conduction of the nerve impulse and produces a reversible loss of sensation.

TOPICAL ANESTHETIC FORMS AND METHODS OF DELIVERY

Topical anesthetic agents are available in a variety of commercial forms, including gels, ointments, sprays (both metered and unmetered), creams, liquids, and lozenges. The type of preparation can affect the efficacy. Depending on the form used, effective concentrations range from 0.2%–20%.[1,2] The methods of delivery include the use of cotton tip applicators, sprays, brushes, patches, blunted cannulas and/or syringes, and single-dose applicator swabs (Figure 6-2). When professionals apply topical anesthetics, each form and method of delivery is considered on an individual patient basis. Medical and dental histories should always be reviewed before the anesthetic is applied, and manufacturer's directions should be followed.

Usually when providing pain control before giving conventional local anesthetic injections, topical gels or ointments are applied with a cotton tip applicator. The site of penetration should first be dried using a 2 × 2 gauze square to increase visibility and accurate placement of the topical anesthetic (Figure 6-3). Only a small amount of the gel or ointment on the applicator tip is necessary to achieve the desired result (Figure 6-4). Many students and even clinicians apply excessive amounts of topical anesthesia, leading to an unnecessary effect on surrounding tissues. This excess mixes with the saliva and may anesthetize the tongue, soft palate, or pharynx. The topical agent should remain at the site of penetration for 1–2 minutes (depending on the concentration of the topical anesthetic) to ensure effectiveness (Figure 6-5). If these steps are followed, anesthesia should be achieved to a depth of approximately 2–3 mm into the tissue (Procedure 6-1). This helps provide comfort during the initial penetration of the local anesthetic needle.

Topical anesthetics in liquid form are also used in dentistry. Liquids provide anesthesia to a wide area. They are especially useful when trying to decrease a patient's gag reflex, making placement of impression materials or radiograph film more comfortable and tolerable. The use of a liquid for a more site-specific procedure requires an applicator. Cetacaine (Cetylite, Pennsauken, N.J.) which is available only by prescription, is administered by either a cotton pellet or via blunted cannula in order to deliver the anesthetic subgingivally (Figure 6-6). Another liquid, HurriPak

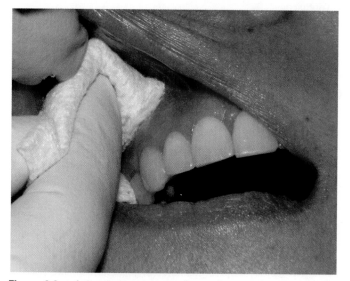

Figure 6-3 ■ A 2 × 2 gauze square is used to gently wipe and dry tissue at the site of needle penetration.

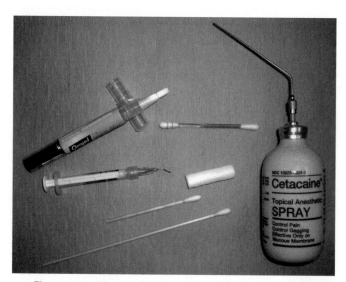

Figure 6-2 ■ Methods used to deliver topical anesthetics.

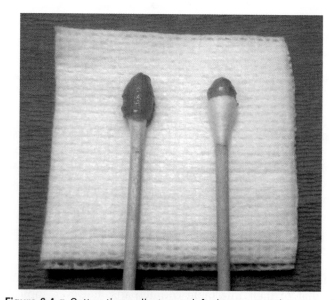

Figure 6-4 ■ Cotton tip applicator on left shows excessive amount of topical anesthesia. Cotton tip applicator on the right shows correct amount of topical anesthesia to be applied at each penetration site.

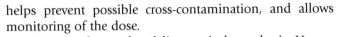

(Beutlich Pharmaceuticals) is designed primarily for the use of subgingival placement by using irrigation syringes with plastic tips (Figure 6-7). These are indicated when attempting to increase comfort during prophylaxis or non-surgical periodontal therapy procedures.

Gels, ointments, and liquids often come in multidose containers, but some products are packaged in single unit-dose applications. Lollicaine (Centrix), HandiCaine Stix (Topex Sultan Healthcare), and CaineTips (J Morita) are some of the products available through dental suppliers. These single unit-dose applications can also be found in over-the-counter products such as Orajel medicated tooth swabs (Figure 6-8). Individual packaging is less messy,

helps prevent possible cross-contamination, and allows monitoring of the dose.

Sprays are also used to deliver topical anesthesia. Unmetered sprays are not recommended because they do not allow control of the amount of anesthetic dispensed, nor are they easily contained at a specific site. However, the use of a metered spray with a disposable nozzle enables control over the amount of agent being dispensed, thus decreasing the risk for systemic toxicity (Figure 6-9). Both the Institute of Safe Medication Practices (ISMP) and the U.S. Food and Drug Administration (FDA) have released advisory statements informing the public of the association between benzocaine sprays and methemoglobinemia, wherein methemoglobin builds up in the blood, hindering the effective transport of oxygen to body tissues.

Patch delivery of topical anesthetic is advantageous because the patch can be placed directly on the delivery site and then adheres to the tissue. Transdermal patches are used regularly in medicine on intact skin to administer certain medications or to provide local dermal analgesia.

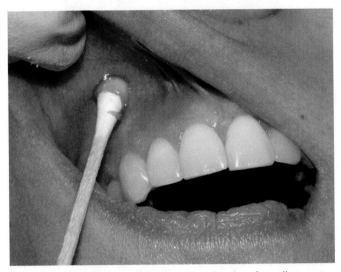

Figure 6-5 ■ Topical anesthetic placed at the site of needle penetration for 1–2 minutes.

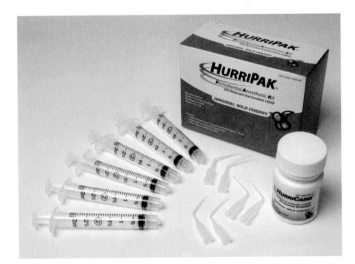

Figure 6-7 ■ HurriPak liquid topical anesthesia with plastic irrigation syringes and tips.

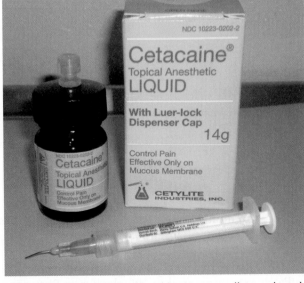

Figure 6-6 ■ Cetacaine liquid with cotton pellet and syringe applicator.

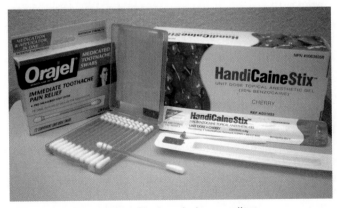

Figure 6-8 ■ Single unit-dose applicator.

PROCEDURE 6-1	Basic Topical Anesthesia Technique Before Giving Local Anesthesia Injection

STEP 1 Review medical and dental history.
STEP 2 Set-up armamentarium.

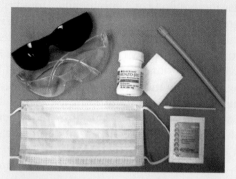

2 × 2 gauze
Cotton tip applicator
Saliva ejector
Topical anesthetic
Topical antiseptic (optional)
Personal protective equipment (PPE) and patient safety eyewear

STEP 3 Have on all PPE and make sure patient is wearing protective eyewear.
STEP 4 Place patient in supine position.
STEP 5 Prepare cotton tip applicator with proper amount of topical anesthetic.

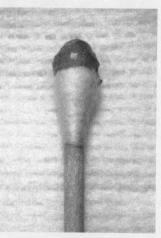

Remember: only a small amount is necessary to achieve the desired results.

STEP 6 Perform intraoral inspection of the areas where topical anesthesia is to be placed. Assess area for abrasions, lacerations, or any trauma that would affect absorption and increase risk for toxicity.

STEP 7 Identify landmarks. Using 2 × 2 gauze, gently wipe the area dry, removing any debris from the area.

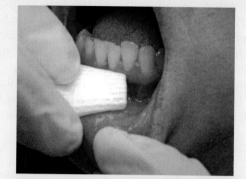

STEP 8 (Optional) Wipe area using a topical antiseptic such as Betadine (povidone-iodine). This step helps decrease the risk for infection, but is considered optional.

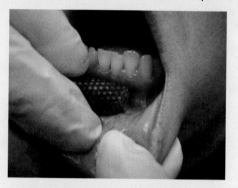

STEP 9 Place topical anesthesia at site of penetration. Leave in place for 1–2 minutes to ensure effectiveness.

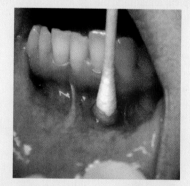

STEP 10 Remove cotton tip applicator, provide suction as necessary, and continue with the injection.

For example, Synera (ZARS Pharma, Salt Lake City, Utah) is an FDA-approved peel-and-stick topical anesthetic patch that numbs intact skin before minor needle procedures and superficial dermatologic procedures.[3] Lidoderm (Endo Pharmaceuticals, Chadds Ford, Pa.) is also an FDA-approved adhesive patch that provides pain relief from postherpetic neuralgia, commonly called after shingles pain.[4] These patches are not used intraorally, however.

Patches available for intraoral topical anesthesia are limited. The first FDA-approved transoral anesthetic patch, DentiPatch, was introduced in 1996 by Noven Pharmaceuticals, but the manufacturer discontinued the product.

Currently the only patch available for use intraorally is Topicale GelPatch (Premier Dental Co.) (Figure 6-10).

Regardless of the form and method of delivery, there is more than one option for delivering topical anesthetics to dental patients. Furthermore, dental hygienists must be aware that patients often self-medicate using these same drugs in over-the-counter formulations and should query their patients before administering any anesthetic agents.

COMMON TOPICAL AGENTS USED IN DENTISTRY

BENZOCAINE

Benzocaine is one of the more common and widely used topical anesthetics. It is available in gel, cream, ointment, lozenge, liquid solution, spray, and patch (Figure 6-11). It exists almost entirely in its base form, making absorption into circulation slow and therefore having a very low potential for systemic toxicity in healthy individuals.

- **Classification:** Benzocaine is an ester.
- **Available concentration:** The most commonly used concentration used in dentistry is 20%, although it is available in concentrations ranging from 6% to 20%.
- **Onset of action:** Rapid. Onset can occur as early as 30 seconds and have its peak effect at 2 minutes.
- **Duration:** 5–15 minutes.
- **Maximum recommended dose:** There is no published maximum dosage recommendations.[5]
- **Metabolism/excretion:** Benzocaine is metabolized via hydrolysis in the plasma and to a lesser extent in the liver by cholinesterase. Excretion occurs primarily through kidneys with only a small portion remaining unchanged in the urine.
- **Pregnancy/lactation:** FDA Category C/Excretion in breast milk unknown, use with caution.
- **Special considerations:** Methemoglobinemia has been reported following topical anesthesia use of benzocaine, particularly with higher concentrations of 14%–20% spray applications applied to the mouth and mucous membrane. Always apply as directed.[15,18,27]

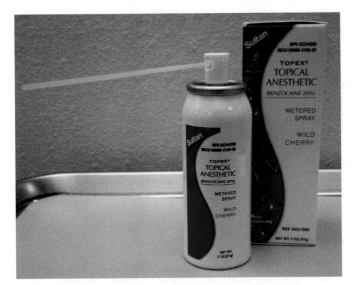

Figure 6-9 ■ Metered spray with disposable nozzle.

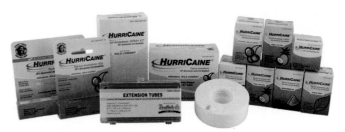

Figure 6-11 ■ Varieties of products used professionally that contain benzocaine.

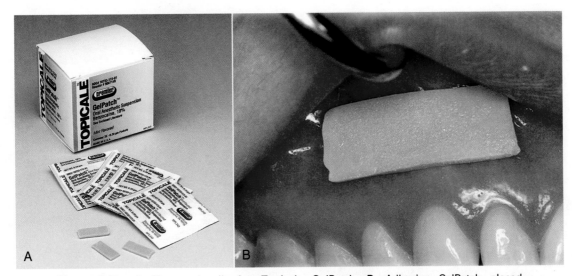

Figure 6-10 ■ **A,** Transoral adhesive Topicale GelPatch. **B,** Adhesive GelPatch placed intraorally.

LIDOCAINE

Lidocaine is a good alternative if a patient has sensitivity to esters. The most common topical preparation is an ointment (Figure 6-12), but it can be found as a patch, as a spray, and in a solution. It is available in two forms, as a base or a hydrochloride salt. The base form is poorly soluble in water and has poor penetration and absorption abilities. The hydrochloride salt form on the other hand is water soluble and can easily penetrate and be absorbed in the tissues, significantly increasing the risk of toxicity. The base form is preferred for application to mucous membranes and for covering large areas.

- **Classification:** Lidocaine is an amide.
- **Available concentration:** Most common in 2% or 5% preparations.
- **Onset of action:** Between 2 and 10 minutes.
- **Duration:** Depends on method of application; approximately 15–45 minutes.
- **Maximum recommended dose:** 200 mg (300 mg manufacturer recommendation).
- **Metabolism/excretion:** Metabolized in the liver and excreted via the kidney with less than 10% remaining unchanged.
- **Pregnancy/lactation:** FDA Category B/Enters breast milk in small amounts, use with caution.
- **Special considerations:** Always follow manufacturer's application directions and ask questions of physician staff if necessary.

DYCLONINE HYDROCHLORIDE

Dyclonine hydrochloride has a unique classification in that it is neither an ester nor an amide agent, but rather a ketone. This unique property is beneficial for patients with sensitivities to traditional topical anesthetics. As a topical anesthetic, dyclonine hydrochloride is available by prescription, and to patients it is available over-the-counter in Sucrets lozenges (Figure 6-13).

- **Classification:** Ketone.
- **Available concentration:** Formulated for use in dentistry as a 0.5% or 1% solution.
- **Onset of action:** Slow; may take up to 10 minutes to become effective.
- **Duration:** Average duration of 30 minutes; however, effects may last up to 1 hour.
- **Maximum recommended dose:** 200 mg (40 mL of 0.5% solution or 20 mL of a 1% solution).
- **Metabolism/excretion:** No information is available on the metabolism and excretion of dyclonine hydrochloride.
- **Pregnancy/lactation:** FDA Category C/Caution is recommended during lactation.

TETRACAINE HYDROCHLORIDE

Tetracaine hydrochloride is considered the most potent of the topical anesthetics. It is not made available for injection and with topical preparations is typically combined with other drugs.

- **Classification:** Tetracaine hydrochloride is an ester.
- **Available concentration:** 2% in topical preparations
- **Onset of action:** Slow; peak effects may take up to 20 minutes.
- **Duration:** Approximately 45 minutes.
- **Maximum recommended dose:** 20 mg for topical administration; 1 mL of a 2% solution.
- **Metabolism/excretion:** Metabolized by plasma pseudocholinesterase/excreted in the kidneys
- **Pregnancy/lactation:** FDA Category C/Caution is recommended during lactation.
- **Special considerations:** Highly soluble in lipids, making absorption into local tissues very rapid.

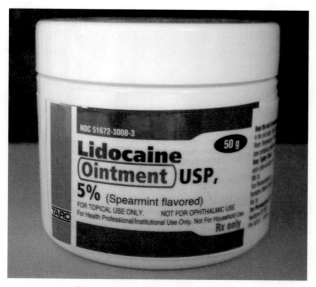

Figure 6-12 ■ Lidocaine products.

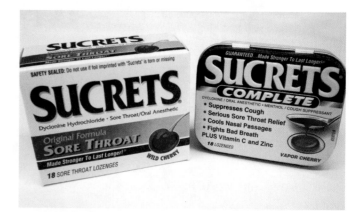

Figure 6-13 ■ Over-the-counter products containing dyclonine hydrochloride.

COMBINATIONS OF TOPICAL DRUGS

Topical anesthetic agents are also mixed and used in combinations in order to increase the anesthetic effect.

BENZOCAINE, BUTAMBEN, AND TETRACAINE

Cetacaine (Cetylite Industries) is the brand most often used in the dental office that contains the triple-action formula of benzocaine, butamben, and tetracaine. The benzocaine provides a quick onset while the properties of tetracaine allow deeper penetration of the agent, thus contributing to an increase in the duration of action. It is available by prescription only in spray, liquid, and gel forms (Figure 6-14).

- **Classification:** Benzocaine, butamben, and tetracaine are all esters.
- **Available concentration:** Triple-active formula of benzocaine 14%, butamben 2%, and tetracaine hydrochloride 2%.
- **Onset of action:** Rapid; approximately 30 seconds.
- **Duration:** Typically 30–60 minutes.
- **Maximum recommended dose:** Spray administered for 1 second. Gel and liquid 200 mg.
- **Metabolism/excretion:** hydrolysis via cholinesterase
- **Pregnancy/lactation:** FDA Category C/Use caution while nursing.
- **Special considerations:** Tetracaine is highly lipid-soluble, making absorption into local tissues very rapid. Not suitable for injection.

EUTECTIC MIXTURES

A eutectic mixture is a mixture of two elements that have a lower melting temperature than any of their individual components. This increases the concentration and enhances the drug's properties, resulting in a faster, more penetrating, longer-acting agent.

EMLA: 2.5% Lidocaine/2.5% Prilocaine Cream

The composition of 2.5% lidocaine and 2.5% prilocaine in a cream preparation is referred to as an EMLA: eutectic mixtures of local anesthetics. EMLA is distributed by AstraZeneca, but is also available in generic preparation. EMLA represents the first major breakthrough for surface anesthesia on intact skin. It should only be applied to intact skin and requires an occlusive dressing to allow the release of the drug into the epidermal and dermal layers. The onset, depth, and duration of dermal anesthesia depend primarily on the contact time during application. Satisfactory results should be achieved 1 hour after application, reach a maximum at 2–3 hours, and last for 1–2 hours after removal.[6] The combined use of lidocaine/prilocaine has been well recognized in the medical community, and has been used to provide efficacious topical anesthesia for a variety of medical procedures, such as venipuncture,

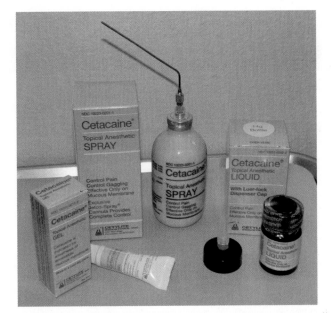

Figure 6-14 ■ Benzocaine, butamben, and tetracaine products available. Cetacaine (Cetylite Industries).

circumcision, and minor gynecologic procedures.[7,8] When used as directed, the risk of systemic toxicity remains low; however, if not used as prescribed, the systemic absorption of lidocaine and prilocaine can also become a side effect of the desired effect because the amount of drug absorbed depends on the surface area and the duration of the application. Although EMLA is FDA approved, the FDA released a Public Health Advisory in 2007 expressing concerns and warning the public of potential danger associated with the use of the topical anesthetic drug (Box 6-2).

The first documented use of lidocaine/prilocaine used in the oral cavity was done in 1985, by Holst and Evers.[9] Since then, many more studies have been conducted that show great promise for use of EMLA intraorally.[10-14] However, EMLA is currently approved by the FDA for use on intact, nonmucosal skin only.

- **Classification:** Lidocaine and prilocaine are both amides.
- **Available concentration:** 2.5% lidocaine and 2.5% prilocaine.
- None available for intraoral use.
- **Onset of action:** Satisfactory results achieved in 1 hour, with exception of genital mucosa which is 10–15 minutes. None reported for intraoral use.
- **Duration:** No information reported for intraoral use.
- **Maximum recommended dose:** No information for intraoral use.
- **Metabolism/excretion:** Primarily in the liver.
- **Pregnancy/lactation:** as a eutectic mixture, FDA Category B. Caution should be taken during lactation.

Oraqix: 2.5% Lidocaine/2.5% Prilocaine Gel

Even though studies do exist on the effectiveness of EMLA cream used intraorally, EMLA cream is not approved by the

Source: Cetacaine prescribing information.

Even though topical anesthetics are generally regarded as safe, if used improperly they can produce adverse reactions ranging in severity from mild to life-threatening or fatal. In 2007, the FDA released a Public Health Advisory alerting consumers of this potential risk by informing the public of two instances in which women, aged 22 and 25 years old, subsequently died of the toxic effects of the topical anesthetic drug. In order to lessen the pain of laser hair removal, both women were instructed to apply topical anesthetics to their legs and then wrap their legs in plastic wrap in order to increase the cream's numbing effect. Both women suffered seizures, fell into comas, and eventually died of the toxic effect of the anesthetic drugs. In 2009, the FDA released the Public Health Advisory again to remind the public of their concerns.

Full version of Public Health Advisory may be obtained at the FDA website: www.fda.gov/Drugs/DrugSafety/PostmarketDrugSafetyInformationfor PatientsandProviders/DrugSafetyInformationforHeathcareProfessionals/ PublicHealthAdvisories.
US Food and Drug Administration: Public Health Advisory: Life-Threatening Side Effects with the Use of Skin Products Containing Numbing Ingredients for Cosmetic Procedures (online press release): http://www.fda.gov/Drugs/ DrugSafety/PostmarketDrugSafetyInformationforPatientsandProviders/ DrugSafetyInformationforHeathcareProfessionals/PublicHealthAdvisories/ ucm054718.htm?sms_ss=email&at_xt=4d3d2191beaaa5a6%2C0.   Accessed January 31, 2011.

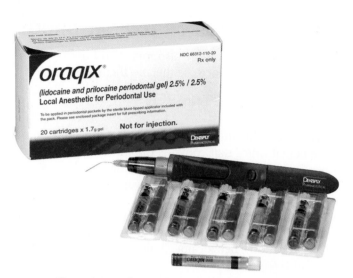

Figure 6-15 ▪ Oraqix delivery system applicator.

- **Pregnancy/lactation:** FDA Category B/Caution should be taken if administered to nursing mothers.
- **Special considerations:** Do not inject.

SPECIAL CONSIDERATIONS

The concentration of topical anesthetic agents is higher than that of their injectable counterparts. This is necessary in order to facilitate diffusion of the agent through the mucous membranes. In addition, topical anesthetics do not contain a vasoconstrictor. With these higher concentrations and the lack of vasoconstricting abilities, the risk of local and systemic absorption increases, thus increasing the risk of toxicity.

High plasma concentrations of topical anesthetics can produce adverse effects and results when patients are exposed to excessive amounts of the drugs. Children, older adults, and medically compromised individuals are more susceptible to the adverse reactions of topical anesthetics.

Possible localized adverse effects include irritation, stinging or burning at the site of application, sloughing, tissue discoloration, and temporary alteration in taste perception. The most prominent of the systemic effects of topical anesthetics are on the central nervous system and cardiovascular system. Excitatory effects of the central nervous system are often displayed at the initial signs and symptoms of overdose. Some of these signs and symptoms include dizziness, visual disturbances, tinnitus, disorientation, unusual nervousness or apprehension, and localized involuntary muscular activity. The excitatory manifestations may be very brief or not occur at all, in which case the first manifestation would be a depressant response, such as slurred speech, drowsiness, and respiratory impairment. Toxic overdoses

FDA for intraoral use. However, there is a prescription eutectic mixture available for use in the oral cavity that consists of a 2.5% lidocaine and 2.5% prilocaine gel called Oraqix (Dentsply Pharmaceuticals, York, Pa.). Oraqix is a microemulsion in which the oil phase is a eutectic mixture in a ratio of 1:1 weight. Oraqix can only be administered by means of a special applicator and does not work with standard dental syringes (Figure 6-15). While at room temperature in the cartridge, Oraqix remains in the liquid form; it begins to thicken into a gel upon application into the periodontal pocket and reaching body temperature. Even though pulpal anesthesia is not achieved, Oraqix is indicated to provide comfort to the gingival tissues during prophylaxis, periodontal assessment, and nonsurgical periodontal therapy. Assembly of the dispenser is quick and easy, making it available for use within seconds (Procedure 6-2).

- **Classification:** Lidocaine and prilocaine are amides.
- **Available concentration:** 5% periodontal gel (2.5% lidocaine and 2.5% prilocaine).
- **Onset of action:** Occurs by 30 seconds. Longer wait time does not enhance the anesthetic effect.
- **Duration:** Approximately 20 minutes (average, 14–31 minutes)
- **Maximum recommended dose:** Five cartridges at one treatment session.
- **Metabolism/Excretion:** Mainly metabolized in the liver

Source: Oraqix prescribing information. Dentsply Pharmaceuticals, York, Pa. www.oraqix.com.

STEP 1   Parts of the applicator include the body (right) and the tip (left). The blunt tip applicator and cartridge of Oraqix come packaged together in a blister pak.

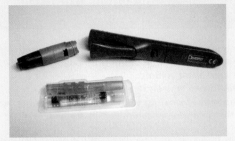

STEP 2   Remove blunt-tip applicator and cartridge of Oraqix from the blister pak.

STEP 3   Twist to break the seal of blunt tip applicator cap and attach it into the tip of the Oraqix dispenser. Twist to lock in place.

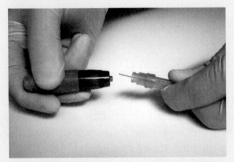

STEP 4   With thumb, press the mechanism-reset button down toward the back end of the body.

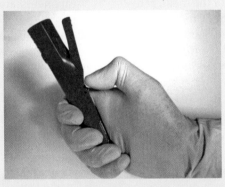

STEP 5   Load the Oraqix cartridge into the body of the dispenser. The side with the rubber stopper should be placed into the body of the dispenser.

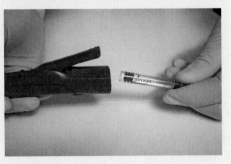

STEP 6   Join together the tip and the body of the dispenser. Twist and lock in place.

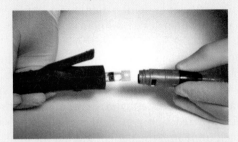

STEP 7   Remove applicator cap. Use the cap to bend the applicator tip. Use a double-bend technique if a bend greater than 45 degrees is desired.

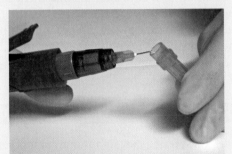

STEP 8   Using a modified pen grasp, begin dispensing Oraqix by pressing down on the paddle.

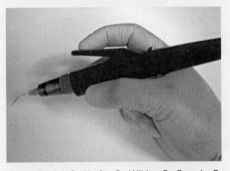

(From Daniel S, Harfst S, Wilder R, Francis B, Mitchell S: *Dental hygiene concepts, cases and competencies*, ed 2, St Louis, 2008, Mosby)

STEP 9   Apply Oraqix in two steps: first to the gingival margin around the selected teeth, then after 30 seconds, to the base of the periodontal pockets. Wait 30 seconds to begin procedure.

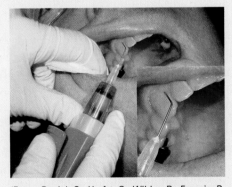

(From Daniel S, Harfst S, Wilder R, Francis B, Mitchell S: *Dental hygiene concepts, cases and competencies*, ed 2, St Louis, 2008, Mosby)

Adapted and summarized from http://www.dentsply.com. Full detailed dispenser directions available at http://www.dentsply.com/assets/DFU/oraqix_dfu.pdf.

result in seizures, unconsciousness, and respiratory arrest. In the cardiovascular system, patients may experience bradycardia and hypotension, leading to rare cases of cardiac arrest.

Allergic reactions associated with topical anesthetics are rare. Benzocaine and tetracaine are both esters, which increases their potential for an allergic reaction; however the risks are still low. Anaphylaxis is very rare with topical anesthetics. Any reaction would likely be delayed and not present itself until after the patient has left the dental office. Those mild allergic reactions can include swelling and raised welts on the skin, itching, or burning. Some allergic reactions occur up to 2 days after the anesthetic is given.

Although these adverse reactions are rare, the potential does exist. It is important to take all precautions necessary to minimize or avoid or prevent them (Box 6-3).

BOX 6-3	How to Avoid Toxic Reactions from Topical Anesthesia

1. Know the relative *toxicity* of the drug being used.
2. Know the *concentration* of the drug being used.
3. Use the *smallest* volume.
4. Use the *lowest* concentration.
5. Use the *least toxic* drug to satisfy clinical requirements.
6. Limit the *area of application* (avoid sprays).

From Haveles E: *Applied pharmacology for the dental hygienist*, ed 5, St Louis, 2011, Mosby.

DENTAL HYGIENE CONSIDERATIONS

- Topical anesthesia is an important component of the local anesthesia armamentarium and is used routinely in dentistry to provide pain control prior to conventional local anesthetic injections.
- Topical anesthesia comes in a variety of preparations including gels, ointments, creams, liquids, sprays and lozenges.
- Topical anesthesia is available as a prescription or over-the-counter with concentrations ranging from 0.2% to 20%.
- Be aware that products available over-the-counter can have concentrations just as high as those used professionally in the dental office.

- Only a minimal amount of topical anesthesia is needed to obtain the desired effect. Placing the topical anesthesia at a site for 1–2 minutes will provide anesthesia 2–3 mm into the tissue or mucosa.
- Even though adverse and allergic reactions are rarely noted with use of topical anesthetics, a thorough review of the medical history is always necessary before their application.
- With the many varieties of topical anesthesia available, it is important to select a product that is safe and will provide the most benefit for the patient.

CASE STUDY 6-1

Mrs. Ester Caine
  Age: 69 years
  Blood pressure: 140/90
  Mrs. Ester Caine presents to your office today to begin treatment. Upon reviewing her medical history you discover that she has a complex medical history. You determine that her ASA status is a class III, but there are no contraindications for treatment today.

She is to have four quadrants of nonsurgical periodontal therapy to remove moderate subgingival and supragingival calculus and to treat her severe inflammation. She expresses to you a great fear of needles. She asks if you can use "the gel on a cotton swab" like her sister had done at her office in Colorado. You agree and begin applying benzocaine gel on the upper right quadrant. Partially through the procedure she winces and asks you

to add more because she is still having some discomfort. You add more benzocaine and continue to work quadrant by quadrant. As you begin the final quadrant you notice that Mrs. Caine is becoming restless and appears strangely apprehensive. She tells you she hears ringing in her ears and you notice that her left cheek begins to twitch. You ask how she is feeling and she responds, "I feel very sleepy." Her speech is noticeably slurred. You immediately stop and assess Mrs. Caine more thoroughly.

Critical Thinking Questions
- What should you suspect is happening with Mrs. Caine as you are beginning the final quadrant?
- If no anesthesia was injected, how could this happen?
- What are some other treatment options that should have been offered to Mrs. Caine?

CHAPTER REVIEW QUESTIONS

1. Which of the following topical anesthetics is classified as an amide?
   A. Benzocaine
   B. Lidocaine
   C. Tetracaine
   D. Dyclonine

2. Benzocaine is available in which of the following preparations?
   A. Cream
   B. Gel
   C. Spray
   D. Patch
   E. All of the above

3. Which of the following statements is incorrect?
   A. Allergic reactions associated with topical anesthetics are rare
   B. Topical anesthetics are made available over-the-counter
   C. The more topical placed at the site of needle penetration the better
   D. Tetracaine hydrochloride is considered the most potent of the topical anesthetics

4. Which of the following topical anesthetics has an FDA pregnancy category B?
   A. Tetracaine hydrochloride
   B. Benzocaine
   C. Lidocaine/prilocaine
   D. Dyclonine hydrochloride
   E. All of the above

5. Which of the following would be an indication for use of a topical anesthetic?
   A. To minimize patient's gag reflex
   B. To numb patient's tongue so they will stop talking so much
   C. To achieve pulpal anesthesia
   D. All of the above

6. Which of the following is true regarding maximum recommended doses for topical anesthesia?
   A. It is difficult to monitor exact doses being given
   B. Patches are a good way to monitor exact doses
   C. Maximum recommended dose does not exist for all topical anesthetics
   D. All of the above

7. Concentrations available in over-the-counter products can be as high as those administered professionally in the dental office.
   A. True
   B. False

8. Which of following topical anesthetics do not require a prescription?
   A. EMLA
   B. Cetacaine
   C. Oraqix
   D. Benzocaine

9. All of the following are considered ideal properties of a topical anesthetic EXCEPT:
   A. It should produce no damage to the tissue
   B. It should have an acceptable taste
   C. It should not induce systemic toxicity
   D. It should be allergenic

10. Which method of delivery is recommended to decrease the risk of methemoglobinemia?
    A. Unmetered spray
    B. Metered spray
    C. Unmetered spray with disposable nozzle
    D. Metered spray with disposable nozzle

11. Topical anesthetics generally penetrate _____ into to the tissue.
    A. 1–2 mm
    B. 2–3 mm
    C. 3–4 mm
    D. 5–6 mm

12. Oraqix is composed of which of the following anesthetic agents?
    A. Lidocaine
    B. Prilocaine
    C. Procaine
    D. A and B
    E. A and C

13. The concentrations of topical anesthetics are greater than those of their injectable counterparts and they do not contain vasoconstrictors.
    A. The first part of statement is true; the second part of the statement is false
    B. The first part of the statement is false; the second part of the statement is true
    C. Both statements are true
    D. Both statements are false

14. Which of the following describes an advantage of single unit-dose applications?
    A. Prevents cross-contamination
    B. Doses administered can monitored
    C. Less messy
    D. All of the above

15. EMLA is approved for use on which of the following areas?
    A. Intact skin
    B. Mucous membranes
    C. Hard palate
    D. All of the above

16. Pulpal anesthesia can be achieved using 2.5% lidocaine and 2.5% prilocaine gel mixture.
    A. True
    B. False

17. Which of the following topical anesthetic agents is considered a ketone?
    A. Benzocaine
    B. Dyclonine hydrochloride

CHAPTER REVIEW QUESTIONS

C. Lidocaine
D. A and B
E. All of the above

18. If plasma concentrations in the body become too high, the most prominent systemic effect will occur in which of the following systems?
A. Respiratory system
B. Cardiovascular system
C. Central nervous system
D. B and C
E. All of the above

19. Allergic reactions associated with topical anesthetics are rare. It is not necessary to review a patient's medical history before applying a topical anesthetic agent.
A. The first statement is true; the second statement is false

B. The first statement is false; the second statement is true
C. Both statements are true
D. Both statements are false

20. Which of the following is a possible localized adverse reaction associated with topical anesthesia?
A. Burning or stinging
B. Sloughing
C. Tissue discoloration
D. A and B
E. All of the above

REFERENCES

1. Malamed SF: Clinical action of specific agents. In Malamed SF, ed. *Handbook of local anesthesia*, ed 5, St Louis, 2004, Mosby, 55-81.
2. Yagiela JA: Injectable and topical local anesthetics. In *American Dental Association guide to dental therapeutics*, ed 2. Chicago, 2000, Donnelley & Sons, 1-16.
3. SYNERA Complete Prescribing Information: *Salt Lake City*. Utah, May 2010, ZARS Pharma, www.synera.com.
4. LIDODERM Complete Prescribing Information: *Chadds Ford*. Pa, March 2010, Endo Pharmaceuticals, www.lidoderm.com
5. Yagiela JA: Injectable and topical local anesthetics. In Ciancio SG, ed. *American Dental Association guide to dental therapeutics*, ed 3, Chicago, 2003, ADA Publishing.
6. AstraZeneca. EMLA product information sheet. May 2005. www1.astrazeneca-us.com/pi/EMLA.pdf.
7. Zilbert A: Topical anesthesia for minor gynecological procedures: a review, *Obstet Gynecol Surv* 57: 171-177, 2002.
8. Mansell-Gregory M, Romanowski B: Randomised double trial of EMLA for the control of pain related to cryotherapy in the treatment of genital HPV lesions, *Sex Transm Infect* 74(4): 274-275, 1998.
9. Holst A, Evers H: Experimental studies of new topical anaesthetics on the oral mucosa, *Swed Dent J* 9: 185-191, 1985.
10. Nayak R, Sudah P: Evaluation of three topical anaesthetic agents against pain: a clinical study, *Ind J Dent Res* 17(4):155-160, 2006.
11. Abu M, Anderson L: Comparison of topical anesthetics (EMLA/Oraqix vs. benzocaine) on pain experienced during palatal needle injection, *Oral Surg Oral Med Oral Path Oral Radiol Endod* 103: 16-20, 2007.
12. Meechan JG: The use of EMLA for an intraoral soft tissue biopsy in a needle phobic: a case report, *Anesth Prog* 48: 32-42, 2001.
13. Vickers ER, Punnia-Moorthy A: A clinical evaluation of three topical anaesthetic agents, *Aust Dent J* 37: 266-270, 1992.
14. Svensson P, Petersen JK: Anesthetic effect of EMLA occluded with orahesive oral bandages on oral mucosa. A placebo-controlled study, *Anesth Progr* 39: 79-82, 1992.

ADDITIONAL RESOURCES

Bassett K, DiMarco A: Safety first, *Dimensions of dental hygiene* 5(10):20-25, 2007.
Cetacaine product information available from Cetylite Industries, Pennsauken, NJ. www.cetylite.com.
Kundu S, Achar S: Principles of office anesthesia: part II. Topical anesthesia, *Am Fam Physician* 66(1): 99-102, 2002.
Malamed SF: *Handbook of local anesthesia*, ed 5, St Louis, 2004, Mosby.
Meechan JG: Effective topical anesthetic agents and techniques, *Dent Clin North Am* 46: 759-766, 2002.

Oraqix: Product information available from Dentsply Pharmaceuticals, York, Pa. www.dentsplydental.com.
Overman P: Controlling the pain, *Dimensions of Dental Hygiene* 2(11): 10-14, 2004.
Meechan JG: Intra-oral topical anaesthetics: a review, *J Dent* 28: 3-14, 2000.
Haveles E: *Applied pharmacology for the dental hygienist*, ed 5, St Louis, 2007, Mosby.
Tetzlaff JE: *Clinical pharmacology of local anesthetics*, Woburn, Mass, 2000, Butterworth Heinemann.

Yagiela JA: *Pharmacology and therapeutics for dentistry*, ed 5, St Louis, 2004, Mosby.
Yagiela JA: Safely easing the pain for your patients, *Dimensions of Dental Hygiene* 3(5): 20-22, 2005.
Mosby's Dental Drug Reference, ed 9, St Louis, 2010, Mosby.

PART III

Patient Assessment

CHAPTER 7

Preanesthetic Assessment

Demetra Daskalos Logothetis RDH, MS

CHAPTER OUTLINE

LEARNING OBJECTIVES

1. Determine the relative risk presented by a patient prior to administering local anesthesia by interpretation of the medical history.
2. Differentiate between relative and absolute contraindications.
3. Discuss the role emotional status, blood pressure, and pulse have on selection/utilization of local anesthetics.
4. Evaluate blood pressure as it relates to administering local anesthesia.
5. List the concerns for patients with malignant hyperthermia, hyperthyroidism, methemoglobinemia, allergies, cocaine and methamphetamine addiction, heart conditions, stroke, liver or kidney disease, atypical plasmacholinesterase, and bleeding disorders when selecting local anesthetics and scheduling treatment.
6. Describe dental fear and how dental professionals deal with patient fears through

continued next page

KEY TERMS

Absolute contraindication The offending drug should not be administered to the individual under any circumstances.

Bradycardia Decreased heart rate

Cardiac dose A vasoconstrictor dose that can be administered safely to patients with ischemic heart disease.

Concomitant Two or more drugs in the systemic circulation at the same time

Dental phobia Unfounded fear or morbid dread of dental treatment.

Malignant hyperthermia An inherited syndrome triggered by exposure to the neuromuscular

blocking agent succinylcholine and to certain drugs used for general anesthesia.

Maximum recommended dose Highest amount of drug that can be safely administered per appointment.

Methemoglobinemia Rare hereditary condition characterized by the inability of the blood to bind to oxygen.

Pressor Exaggerated increase in blood pressure.

Relative contraindication The administration of the offending drug may be used judiciously (i.e., administration of a minimal effective dose).

Tachycardia Increased heart rate.

▌ INTRODUCTION

To meet the human need for safety, a thorough medical history evaluation utilizing appropriate dental and medical consultations of the patient's current health status is an essential requirement before providing dental hygiene care. The administration of local anesthetic and vasoconstricting agents provides an additional rationale for a thorough health history and health status review. This chapter will focus on further evaluating the patient's medical and psychological status to determine the appropriateness of administering local anesthetic and vasoconstrictor agents. This important preanesthetic information will assist the dental hygienist in choosing the appropriate technique, agent, and dosage to prevent or minimize local anesthetic complications or emergencies.[1] Most healthy patients can tolerate the standard recommended doses of local anesthetics without any adverse reactions. Other patients, including medically compromised patients, may also safely receive local anesthetics if all precautions are recognized and appropriate drug modifications are rendered. These modifications to treatment are categorized into relative contraindications, and absolute contraindications. (Discussed later.)

All drugs exert their actions on multiple body systems; local anesthetics and vasoconstrictors are no exception. Local anesthetics exert their actions by depressing excitable membranes of the central nervous system (CNS) and cardiovascular system (CVS). These actions are dependent upon the amount of local anesthetic agent in the systemic

circulation and are influenced by the administration technique (aspirating to prevent IV injection), and successful ability of the body to metabolize the drug in the liver (for most amides) and the plasma (for esters and articaine), and the ability of the kidneys to excrete any unmetabolized drug.[2] Other commonly observed responses due to the act of the administration of local anesthetics are due to psychological reactions and produce commonly observed reactions of syncopy, or hyperventillation, and other less common reactions such as tonic-clonic convulsions, bronchospasm, and angina pectoris.[2]

The dental hygienist must evaluate, through the health history, the patient's physical and psychological ability to tolerate the administration of a local anesthetic or vasoconstrictor, a history of anesthetic hypersensitivity, and current medications that may have an interaction with the anesthetic drug being administered. This preanesthetic evaluation should be determined utilizing a team approach of consultation with the dentist, patient's physician, and any specialists involved in the patient's medical care. For dental hygienists working in alternative settings such as nursing homes, hospitals, public health programs, collaborative dental hygiene practices, or other settings without the physical presence of a dentist it is of the utmost importance to utilize a multi-disciplinary approach to patient evaluation. The collection of preanesthetic data guides the dental hygienist in determining the:

- Appropriateness of administering a local anesthetic or vasoconstrictor

- Need for a medical consultation
- Need for modification of the dental hygiene care plan
- Type of anesthetic most appropriate for the patient's treatment
- Contraindications to any of the medications to be employed

The preanesthetic evaluation should include a complete medical/dental history, a dialogue history, and a physical and psychological examination.

MEDICAL, DENTAL, AND DIALOGUE HISTORY

The most common and efficient method of obtaining a medical/dental history in the dental office is by a printed questionnaire filled out by the patient followed by a dialogue history, allowing the dental hygienist to follow up on questions to gain further information. The health history questionnaire constitutes a legal document. In the case of a minor, this form must be completed by the parent or legal guardian. These medical history forms should be updated at each patient visit. Information gleaned from the patient's medical history should include information regarding current and past medical and dental conditions, current and past medications including over the counter drugs, herbs, and supplements, any adverse reactions to medications including local anesthetic agents, and any problems with past dental experiences.

Medications currently being taken by the patient are in their system when a local anesthetic is administered. This is referred to as concomitant: two or more drugs given at the same time, or in the same day.[3] This can alter the efficiency and safety of the administered local anesthetic by decreasing the efficiency of its metabolism and excretion. This may affect the type of anesthetic selected and its safe dosage level. The dental hygienist should utilize a current *Physicians' Desk Reference (PDR)* or other drug references to look up all drugs the patient is currently taking to determine the safest anesthetic drug selection, and the safest dosage a patient can tolerate.

The dialog history is invaluable in gaining more information regarding the patient's medical status as well as determining the patient's personal fears associated with local anesthetic administration. In addition, the dialog history provides and opportunity for the dental hygienist to assess the patient's individual response to local anesthetic agents categorized as *"normal," "hyper-responder,"* or *"hypo-responder."* (See Chapter 5.)

Many medical history forms are available, including one from the American Dental Association, www.ada.org. The content details of most medical history forms are essentially similar, and should be modified to meet the specific needs of individual dental practices. Appendix 7-1 is an example of a medical history form in English and in Spanish. Other multi-lingual medical history forms are available at www.metdental.com. Table 7-1 explains each medical history question and its implications on local anesthesia.

PHYSICAL EXAMINATION

VISUAL EXAMINATION

A simple visual examination can provide valuable information regarding the patient's general health and well being. For instance, observing the patient's posture, body movements, speech patterns, and skin can help to identify the anxious patient, which is an important consideration when administering local anesthetics.

VITAL SIGNS

Preanesthetic vital signs are important to provide the dental hygienist with baseline values to provide a standard of comparison in the event that an emergency situation should occur. Another benefit to obtaining vital signs is to identify diagnosed or undiagnosed conditions that may require modifications to treatment, drug selection, and dosage. Vital signs should be recorded on the patient's permanent record at each visit requiring anesthetic administration.

Blood Pressure

The administration of a local anesthetic agent will further elevate the existing blood pressure of patients, and to a greater extent in the anxious patient.[2] Obtaining a preanesthetic blood pressure provides valuable baseline information. Many local anesthetic emergencies alter a patient's blood pressure, and preanesthetic numbers are critical in assessing the severity of the emergency. Furthermore, the use of a vasoconstrictor may need to be limited or avoided in the presence of hypertension. See Table 7-2 for adult blood pressure guidelines for dental management of the hypertensive patient. An accurate blood pressure recording is essential. See Figure 7-1 for guidelines for proper blood pressure cuff size, and Box 7-1 for common errors in blood pressure assessment.

Pulse

The most common procedure for assessing the pulse rate is to palpate the radial artery on the thumb side of the wrist for 1 minute. (Figure 7-2). Tachycardia (>100 beats per minute) is an abnormally elevated heart rate and may be a sign of a cardiovascular disease or influenced by stress and anxiety. Bradycardia (<60 beats per minute) is a slow heart rate.[4] Table 7-3 lists the acceptable ranges of heart (pulse) rate, and Table 7-4 discusses the factors that influence heart (pulse) rate. Local anesthetics containing epinephrine are contraindicated in patients with uncontrolled cardiac dysrhythmias.

Respiration

Respiration can be evaluated before or after the pulse rate is assessed while the dental hygienist's fingers are in the pulse monitoring position. The rate and depth of the respiration is observed by the rise and fall of the resting patient's chest. Hyperventilation (breathing that is deeper and more rapid than normal) is a common occurrence in apprehensive patients, especially before the administration

TABLE 7-1	Medical History Questions Explained

MEDICAL HISTORY QUESTION	LOCAL ANESTHETIC IMPLICATIONS
Are you in good health?	Treatment modifications may be considered for patients who reveal a significant disability, medical or psychological condition. Significant medical conditions may contraindicate or limit the use of a local anesthetic or vasoconstrictor. Patients with special needs should not receive bupivacaine due to the possibility of self-mutilation.
Are you currently under the care of a physician?	Dental hygiene care modifications should be considered for a patient with a medically compromising condition. Significant medical conditions may contraindicate or limit the use of a local anesthetic or vasoconstrictor. Medical consultation with patient's general physician or specialist may be indicated before anesthetic selection and treatment.
Has there been any change in your general health within the past year?	A recent change may indicate needed treatment modifications that may influence anesthetic selection.
Have you had any serious illness, operation, or been hospitalized in the past 5 years?	Identify local anesthesia precautions that may be needed if there is a prior history of serious illness. Existing or chronic medical conditions may indicate the need for modifications in care. Stress reduction protocols implemented for patients with medical conditions that could be exacerbated by stress/anxiety from the administration of local anesthetics and dental hygiene care.
Have you had any problems with or during dental treatment?	Complications often are a source of patient dissatisfaction and fear; if possible avoid repeating the complication. Stress reduction for the anxious patient. Selection of local anesthetic of adequate duration for effective postoperative pain control.
Are you allergic or had any reaction to any medications (including local anesthetics)?	Allergic reactions to local anesthetics are rare and essentially non-existent. Evaluate further to determine if a true allergy exists. Patient should be referred to an allergist if there is still concern regarding a local anesthetic allergy if after questioning the patient, the dental hygienist is unsure if the patient has a true allergy to local anesthetics. If the patient has a true allergy to sulfites, vasoconstrictors should be avoided.
Any other allergies, such as metals, latex, food, or pollen?	Increase risk for a latex allergy from the rubber stopper and diaphragm of the glass cartridge. However, no documented allergies to latex from the anesthetic cartridge have been reported. Patients who have many allergies to foods, metals, or pollen may be more susceptible to allergic reactions to sulfites or ester topical anesthetics.
Artificial heart valves or shunts	The administration of local anesthetics does not require antibiotic prophylaxis, except for the periodontal ligament injection (PDL). However, nonsurgical periodontal treatment performed by the dental hygienist requires antibiotic prophylaxis. Nature of dental treatment will dictate the need for antibiotic prophylaxis. (See Appendix 7-2 for prophylaxis guidelines.) See Table 7-13 for premedication guidelines.
Cardiovascular disease, such as heart trouble, heart attack, angina, high blood pressure, hardening of the arteries, or stroke?	Heart attack: delay treatment for 6 months, after 6 months: decrease the amount of epinephrine to 0.04 mg per appointment, and levonordefrin to 0.2 mg per appointment. Unstable angina: ASA IV—increased risk of severe angina attack. Dental hygiene treatment should be postponed until condition is under control. Absolute contraindication to vasoconstrictors until condition is under control. Stable angina: ASA III—adequate pain control will decrease the risk of angina attack due to apprehension and nervousness. Vasoconstrictors can be administered, but at a decreased dose of 0.04 mg per appointment for epinephrine, and 0.2 mg for levonordefrin. Uncontrolled high blood pressure: dental hygiene treatment should be postponed until blood pressure is under control, absolute contraindication to vasoconstrictors until blood pressure is under control. Controlled blood pressure with beta blockers: relative contraindication to vasoconstrictors and amide local anesthetics. Monitor blood pressure after initial local anesthetic injection and post treatment for signs of increased blood pressure. Stroke: delay treatment for 6 months, after 6 months: decrease the amount of vasoconstrictors to 0.04 mg per appointment for epinephrine and 0.2 mg for levonordephrin. Avoid intravascular injections of vasoconstrictors.
Have you taken cortisone in the last 2 years?	Identify patients at risk for adrenal insufficiency. Stress reduction protocol, and consider nitrous oxide or IV sedation to further reduce stress.
Were you born with any heart problems?	Usually can safely receive dental care with the use of local anesthetics and vasoconstrictors. Medical consultation as needed.

TABLE 7-1	Medical History Questions Explained—cont'd

MEDICAL HISTORY QUESTION	LOCAL ANESTHETIC IMPLICATIONS
Sinus trouble, asthma, hayfever, or skin rashes?	Asthma: adequate pain control to not precipitate attack. Stress reduction protocol. Sodium bisulfite preservative for vasoconstrictors may cause respiratory reactions in asthmatics (predominantly steriod dependent asthmatics).
Fainting spells, seizures, epilepsy or convulsions?	Anxiety during injection. Adequate pain control to not precipitate seizure. Stress reduction protocol.
Diabetes?	Epinephrine is associated with the inhibition of peripheral glucose uptake by the tissues and opposes the action of insulin. Concentrations of epinephrine used in dentistry do not raise the glucose blood levels significantly. Uncontrolled "brittle" diabetes: dental hygiene treatment should be postponed until condition is under control. Use epinephrine with caution. Controlled diabetes: blood glucose levels should be evaluated prior to dental hygiene treatment. Morning appointments after a meal. Vasoconstrictors can be administered.
Hepatitis, yellow jaundice, cirrhosis, or liver disease?	Decreased liver function increases the half-life of the amides metabolized in the liver, increasing risk of overdose. Limit the dose of amides metabolized in the liver. Articaine may be a safer choice because it is predominantly metabolized in the blood.
AIDS or HIV infection?	Careful disposal of contaminated needles. Follow postexposure protocols (Chapter 15).
Thyroid problems (goiter)?	Hyperthyroid patients have an increased sensitivity to epinephrine. Uncontrolled hyperthyroidism: postpone dental hygiene treatment until condition is under control, absolute contraindication to vasoconstrictors. Controlled hyperthyroidism: vasoconstrictors can be administered, but use minimal effective dose. Pheochromocytoma (catecholamine producing tumor): postpone dental hygiene treatment until condition is under control. Absolute contraindication to vasoconstrictors. Liver function may be reduced: limit the dose of amides.
Respiratory problems, emphysema, bronchitis?	Stress reduction protocol.
Have you ever had a joint replacement?	The administration of local anesthetics does not require antibiotic prophylaxis, except for the PDL injection. However, nonsurgical periodontal treatment performed by the dental hygienist requires antibiotic prophylaxis. Nature of dental treatment will dictate the need for antibiotic prophylaxis. (See Appendix 7-2 for prophylaxis guidelines for joint replacements.)
Kidney trouble or dialysis treatment	Usual doses do not pose an increased risk. Significant renal disease: medical consultation needed. Limiting the amount of anesthetic is recommended depending upon severity.
Anemia or blood disorders?	Methemoglobinemia: substitute other amides for prilocaine, and topical lidocaine for topical benzocaine. Atypical plasma cholinesterase: substitute ester topical anesthetics with lidocaine and substitute articaine with other amides. Avoid block injections for clotting disorders.
Have you been diagnosed with alcoholism?	Decreased liver function increases the half-life of the amides metabolized in the liver, increasing risk of overdose. Limit the dose of amides. Articaine may be a safer choice because it is predominantly metabolized in the blood.
Do you use recreational drugs?	Vasoconstrictors administered the same day that a patient has used cocaine or methamphetamine can be life-threatening.
Are you pregnant or nursing a baby?	Elective dental hygiene care with anesthesia can be safely administered in any trimester, in consultation with the patient's physician. Conservative approach: avoid elective treatment with anesthesia until the second trimester. Choose local anesthetic that falls in category B. Choose safe anesthetic for lactation.
Are you taking any medications, including any nonprescription medications or natural supplements, such as birth control, calcium, ginseng, or garlic?	Decrease amount of amide local anesthetic for patients taking cimetidine, beta blockers, CNS depressants. Decrease amount of esters and articaine for patients taking sulfonamides and cholinesterase inhibitors. Decrease the amount of epinephrine per appointment for patient taking tricyclic antidepressants, beta blockers, phenothiazides, and digitalis glycosides. Avoid levonordefrin for patients taking tricyclic antidepressants.

TABLE 7-2	Adult Blood Pressure Guidelines Used in the Dental Hygiene Process of Care	
BLOOD PRESSURE (MM HG)	**ASA PHYSICAL STATUS CLASSIFICATION**	**DENTAL AND DENTAL HYGIENE THERAPY CONSIDERATION AND INTERVENTIONS RECOMMENDED**
<140 systolic and <90 diastolic	I	No unusual precautions related to patient management based on blood pressure readings. Recheck in 6 months.
140–159 systolic and/or 90–94 diastolic	II	No unusual precautions related to patient management based on blood pressure readings needed unless blood pressure remains above normal after three consecutive appointments. Recheck blood pressure prior to dental or dental hygiene therapy for three consecutive appointments; if all exceed these guidelines, seek medical consultation. Stress-reduction protocol if indicated, such as administration of nitrous oxide-oxygen analgesia, should be considered.
160–199 systolic and/or 95–114	III	Recheck blood pressure in 5 minutes; if still elevated, seek medical consultation prior to dental or dental hygiene therapy. No unusual precautions related to patient management based on blood pressure readings after medical approval is obtained. Stress-reduction protocol if indicated, such as administration of nitrous oxide-oxygen analgesia.
>200 systolic and/or >115 diastolic	IV	Recheck blood pressure in 5 minutes; immediate medical consultation if still elevated. Dental or dental hygiene therapy, routine, or emergency treatment may be performed if nitrous oxide-oxygen analgesia lowers the blood pressure below >200 systolic or >115 diastolic. If blood pressure is not reduced using nitrous oxide-oxygen analgesia, only (noninvasive) emergency therapy with drugs (analgesics, antibiotics) is allowable to treat pain and infection. Refer to hospital if immediate dental therapy is indicated.

From Darby M, Walsh M: *Dental hygiene theory and practice*, ed 3, St Louis, 2010, Saunders, Elsevier.

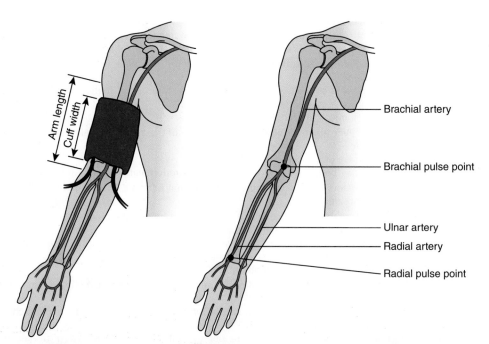

Figure 7-1 ◼ Proper placement of blood pressure cuff. Guidelines for cuff size: Cuff width = 20% more than upper arm diameter or 40% of circumference and two thirds of arm length. (From Darby M, Walsh M: *Dental hygiene theory and practice*, ed 3, St Louis, 2010, Elsevier.)

BOX 7-1	Common Errors in Blood Pressure Detection
False high readings	Bladder or cuff too narrow
	Cuff wrapped too loosely or unevenly
	Deflating cuff too slowly (false high diastolic reading)
	Arm below heart level
	Arm not supported
	Multiple examiners using different Korotkoff sounds
	Inflating too slowly or deflating too quickly (false high diastolic)
	Stethoscope that fits poorly or impairment of examiner's hearing causing sounds to be muffled (false high systolic)
	Repeating assessments too quickly (false high systolic)
False low reading	Failure to identify the auscultatory gap
	Bladder or cuff too wide
	Deflating cuff too quickly (false low systolic)
	Arm above heart level
	Stethoscope that fits poorly or impairment of examiner's hearing causing sounds to be muffled (false low systolic)
	Stethoscope pressed too firmly (false low diastolic)
	Inaccurate inflation level (false low systolic)

From Darby M, Walsh M: *Dental hygiene theory and practice*, ed 3, St Louis, 2010, Saunders, Elsevier.

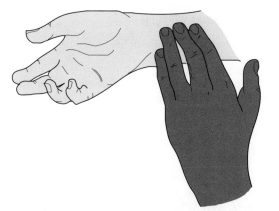

Figure 7-2 ■ Position of the fingers in measuring the radial pulse. (From Potter PA, Perry AG: *Fundamentals of nursing*, ed 7, St Louis, 2009, Mosby.)

TABLE 7-3	Acceptable Ranges of Heart (Pulse) Rate

AGE	HEART RATE (BEATS PER MINUTE)
Toddler	120–160
Preschooler	80–110
School-age child	75–100
Adolescent	60–100
Adult	60–100

Modified from Potter PA, Perry AG: *Fundamentals of nursing*, ed 7, St Louis, 2009, Mosby.

TABLE 7-4	Factors That Influence Heart (Pulse) Rate	
FACTOR	**INCREASED PULSE RATE**	**DECREASED PULSE RATE**
Exercise	Short-term exercise	A conditioned athlete who participates in long-term exercise will have a lower heart rate at rest
Temperature	Fever and heat	Hypothermia
Emotions and stress	Acute pain and anxiety increase sympathetic stimulation, affecting heart rate	Unrelieved severe pain increases parasympathetic stimulation, affecting heart rate; relaxation
Medications	Positive chronotropic drugs, e.g., epinephrine	Negative chronotropic drugs, e.g., digitalis, beta and calcium blockers
Hemorrhage	Loss of blood increases sympathetic stimulation	
Postural changes	Standing or sitting	Lying down
Pulmonary conditions	Diseases causing poor oxygenation such as asthma, chronic obstructive pulmonary disease (COPD)	

From Potter PA, Perry AG: *Fundamentals of nursing*, ed 7, St Louis, 2009, Mosby.

TABLE 7-5	Acceptable Ranges of Respiratory Rate According to Age

AGE	RATE (BREATHS PER MINUTE)
Toddler (2 years)	25–32
Child	18–30
Adolescent	12–19
Adult	12–20

Modified from Potter PA, Perry AG: *Fundamentals of nursing*, ed 7, St Louis, 2009, Mosby.

of a local anesthetic injection. (See Table 7-5 for acceptable ranges of respiratory rate, and Chapter 14 for signs, symptoms, and treatment of hyperventilation.)

WEIGHT

The weight of the patient is used before the administration of a local anesthetic to determine the patient's maximum recommended dose (MRD). Consideration should be given to lowering the MRD for children with excess weight.

BOX 7-2	Common Origins of Dental Fear

- Previously painful or negative dental experiences including careless comments made by dental professionals
- Severe discomfort with feeling helpless or out of control in the oral healthcare setting
- Embarrassment caused by dental neglect and fear of ridicule or belittlement
- Scary stories of negative dental experiences learned vicariously from family and friends
- Negative portrayals of dentists in movies, on television, or in printed materials
- A sense of depersonalization in the oral health care setting, intensified by the use of masks, gloves, and shields
- Fear of pain
- Fear of injections
- Fear the injection won't work
- Feelings of helplessness and loss of control
- Loss of personal space (i.e., physical closeness of practitioner to the client's face)
- A general fear of the unknown
- A previous bad experience that unknowingly has become associated with dentistry

From Darby M, Walsh M: *Dental hygiene theory and practice*, ed 3, St Louis, 2010, Saunders, Elsevier.

BOX 7-3	Clinical Signs of Moderate Anxiety

- Unnaturally stiff posture
- Nervous play
- White-knuckle syndrome
- Perspiration on forehead and hands
- Overwillingness to cooperate with clinician
- Nervous conversation
- Quick answers

Modified from Darby M, Walsh M: *Dental hygiene theory and practice*, ed 3, St Louis, 2010, Saunders, Elsevier.

BOX 7-4	Effects of Stress on the Body

- Dilated pupils
- Decreased salivation (tight dry throat)
- Chest pain
- High blood pressure
- Shortness of breath
- Increased heart rate
- Increased blood cholesterol and blood glucose
- Gastrointestinal disturbances
- Headache
- Back and neck aches
- Clenched jaws
- Grinding of teeth (bruxism)
- Indigestion
- Increased perspiration (e.g. sweaty hands, visible perspiration beads above upper lip)
- Insomnia
- Increased or decrease in weight
- Hives
- Dry mouth (xerostomia)
- Irritation of gastrointestinal tract lining (e.g., stomach ulcers)
- Decreased immune response

From Darby M, Walsh M: *Dental hygiene theory and practice*, ed 3, St Louis, 2010, Saunders, Elsevier.

In this situation, the MRD may allow a greater volume of anesthetic to be administered based upon the child's weight, but their immature liver may not be able to readily biotransform the anesthetic, putting the child at risk for an overdose. (See Chapter 8.)

PSYCHOLOGICAL EVALUATION

Dental phobia is any objectively unfounded fear or morbid dread of dental treatment. Dental phobia is a real affliction that affects many individuals, usually due to a traumatic, difficult, and/or painful dental experience (Box 7-2).

The evaluation of the patient's attitude and psychological fears is an important component to the preanesthetic assessment. The typical medical history form should include a few questions regarding the patient's past dental history and any previous trouble associated with the treatment. Further dialogue should be conducted by the dental hygienist to recognize possible stresses and anxiety that can exacerbate the patient's medical problems such as angina, asthma, hyperventilation, seizures, or vasodepressor syncopy.[1,2,4] Anxiety and fear can be recognized by increases in vital signs and visual observation of the patient's body movements, skin color (paleness), cold sweats, posture, trembling, and verbal communication (Box 7-3).

The body's response to fear provokes the stress response referred to as "fight-or-flight." These symptoms include a state of alarm and adrenaline production causing an increase in heart rate and blood pressure, as well as irritability, muscular tension, and the inability to concentrate (Box 7-4). These symptoms can be further intensified by the administration of exogenous epinephrine. (See Chapter 4.)

Fear and apprehension also lowers the patient's pain reaction threshold, and even minor, nonpainful procedures may be perceived as painful (Chapter 1). A stress reduction protocol is essential for the apprehensive patient and should start before the dental appointment and continue through the postoperative period if necessary[2] (Box 7-5).

ADEQUATE PAIN CONTROL AND THE FEAR OF THE NEEDLE

Adequate pain control is essential to provide thorough nonsurgical periodontal therapy, and is best accomplished by the administration of local anesthetics. The apprehensive patient who fears the dental needle may resist the administration of local anesthetics for nonsurgical periodontal theapy. The dental hygienist should explain the advantages of profound anesthesia during these procedures, and that care will be taken to reduce the discomfort of the injection (Box 7-6). (See Chapter 11 for basic injection techniques.)

BOX 7-5   Stress Reduction Protocol

- Recognize the patient's level of anxiety (be a good observer)
- Complete medical consultation before care, as needed
- Premedicate the evening before the dental appointment, as needed
- Premedicate immediately before the dental appointment, as needed
- Schedule the appointment in the morning
- Minimize the patient's waiting time
- Monitor and record preoperative vital signs and postoperative vital signs
- Consider psychosedation during therapy
- Consider appointment length for highly anxious and medically compromised patient; do not exceed the patient's limits of tolerance
- Select an anesthetic agent with appropriate posttreatment pain control
- Administer adequate pain control during therapy
- Follow up with postoperative pain and anxiety control
- Telephone the highly anxious or fearful patient later the same day that treatment was delivered

Modified from Darby M, Walsh M: *Dental hygiene theory and practice*, ed 3, St Louis, 2010, Saunders, Elsevier.

BOX 7-6   Benefits of Adequate Pain Control and Nonsurgical Periodontal Therapy

- Dental hygienist can provide more thorough treatment on a relaxed patient
- The periodontal therapy will be less traumatic for the patient
- The less traumatic the experience, the more likely the patient will return to complete treatment
- Without adequate pain control, sedation and stress reduction are impossible to achieve

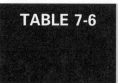

TABLE 7-6   American Society of Anesthesiologists (ASA) Physical Classification System

CLASSIFICATION	DESCRIPTION OF CLASSIFICATION
ASA I	A normal, healthy patient
ASA II	A patient with a mild systemic disease but this does not interfere with daily activity (e.g., a healthy patient with considerable anxiety; a healthy pregnant patient; a patient who has well-controlled type 2 diabetes, controlled epileptic, and/or well-controlled asthma)
ASA III	A patient with moderate to severe systemic disease that limits activity but is not incapacitating but may affect daily activity (e.g., stable angina, exercise-induced asthma, postmyocardial infarct or cerebrovascular accident more that 6 months before treatment, poorly controlled hypertension)
ASA IV	A patient with an incapacitating systemic disease that is a constant treat to life (e.g., myocardial infarction within past 6 months, or cerebrovascular accident within 6 months, uncontrolled epilepsy or uncontrolled diabetes, blood pressure greater than 200/115)
ASA V	A moribund patient not expected to survive 24 hours with or without an operation
ASA E	Emergency operation. The "E" precedes the number to indicate the patient's physical status, (e.g., ASAE-III)

From Little JW, Falace DA, Miller CS, Rhodus NL: *Dental management of the medically compromised patient*. St Louis, 2008, Mosby; Malamed SF: *Handbook of local anesthesia*, ed 5, St Louis, 2004, Mosby.

SELECTION OF LOCAL ANESTHETIC FOR THE ANXIOUS PATIENT

In order to reduce stress and anxiety during nonsurgical periodontal therapy, it is critical that adequate pain control be obtained. The potentially adverse actions of the released catecholamines on cardiovascular function in the patient with clinically significant heart or blood vessel disease warrant the inclusion of vasoconstrictors in the local anesthetic solution. Without adequate control of pain, sedation and stress reduction are impossible to achieve. Therefore, the anesthetic must outlast the dental treatment, and the inclusion of a vasoconstrictor is the best way to ensure this occurrence. In most situations, cardiovascularly involved patients may receive vasoconstrictors in limited doses. This is referred to as the cardiac dose, a safe dose of vasoconstricting drugs that can be administered to a patient with ischemic heart disease by limiting the amount of epinephrine to 0.04 mg per appointment, and 0.2 mg per appointment for levonordefrin. If the dental hygienist selects a vasoconstrictor concentration of 1 : 200,000, the patient can safely receive 4.4 cartridges of anesthetic with epinephrine, which should be adequate for most nonsurgical periodontal procedures. A 1 : 100,000 concentration can be safely administered but this patient should only receive 2.2 cartridges of anesthetic with epinephrine. (See Chapter 8 for dosage calculations.)

▌RISK ASSESSMENT

Once a thorough medical history and vital signs have been obtained, the data must be evaluated to determine whether a patient can, physiologically and psychologically, safely undergo dental treatment and receive local anesthetics. Based on this information, modifications to dental treatment or selection of an anesthetic may be required. The American Society of Anesthesiologists have developed a system to express the anxiety and medical risk of a patient receiving dental care regardless of the type of procedure or anesthesia used (Table 7-6). As the classification level increases, the risk for dental care increases as well.[3] Another helpful tool for determining the at-risk patient is evaluating the ABCs of risk assessment (Table 7-7).[3]

TABLE 7-7	ABCs of Risk Assessment
A:	Possible Issues
Antibiotics	Antibiotic requirement (prophylactic or therapeutic)?
Anesthesia	Any potential problems associated with local anesthetics or vasoconstrictors
Anxiety	Patient requirement for sedation
Allergy	Possible allergy to prescribed drug, or anesthetic?
B:	
Bleeding	Possibility of abnormal hemostasis
C:	
Chair position	Patient's tolerance to supine positioning
D:	
Drugs	Interactions, adverse effects, side effects, allergies
Devices	Prosthetic valves, prosthetic joints, stents, pace makers, A-V fistulas that may require consideration
E:	
Equipment	Potential problems or concerns associated with x-rays, ultrasonic scaler, electrosurgery, oxygen
Emergencies	Potential for occurrence

Modified from Little J, Falace D, Miller C, Rhodus N: *Dental management of the medically compromised patient*, ed 7, St Louis, 2008, Mosby.

CONTRAINDICATIONS TO LOCAL ANESTHESIA

Local anesthetic agents and vasoconstrictors are relatively safe drugs when administered utilizing the appropriate standard of delivery (see Chapter 11). However, certain medical conditions and drug interactions may necessitate limiting or avoiding their use. Modifications to the selection of a local anesthetic agent and the dental hygiene care plan are determined when the patient's assessment has been thoroughly reviewed and standard procedures are contraindicated. Contraindications to local anesthetics and vasoconstrictors are divided into two categories:

Absolute contraindication. The administration of the offending drug increases the possibility of a life-threatening situation and should not be administered to the individual under any circumstances.

Relative contraindication. The administration of the offending drug is preferably avoided because of the increased possibility of an adverse reaction to the drug. However, if an acceptable alternative drug is not available, the drug may be used judiciously (i.e., administration of a minimal effective dose).

VASOCONSTRICTOR DRUG-DRUG INTERACTIONS

Epinephrine and other vasoconstrictors may produce drug-to-drug interactions with prescribed medications the patient may be taking (Table 7-8). The dental hygienist should administer vasoconstrictors with great caution or eliminate them entirely when patients are taking the drugs described

BOX 7-7	Commonly Prescribed Tricyclic Antidepressants

- Amitriptyline (Elavil)
- Amoxapine (Asendin)
- Clomipramine (Anafranil)
- Desipramine (Norpramin, Pertofrane)
- Doxepin (Sinequan, Adapin)
- Nortriptyline (Pamelor)
- Imipramine (Tofranil)
- Protriptyline (Vivactil)
- Trimipramine (Surmontil)

in the following paragraphs. The dental hygienist should consult the patient's physician if uncertain that a vasoconstrictor can be safely administered.

TRICYCLIC ANTIDEPRESSANTS

Tricyclic antidepressants are prescribed for the management of severe depression, and when used in combination with exogenously administered vasoconstrictors, the patient's cardiovascular actions are enhanced.[4] An exaggerated increase in the pressor (increase in blood pressure) effects is likely to occur following the administration of local anesthetics with vasoconstrictors in patients taking tricyclic antidepressants.[4] The pressor effects of epinephrine are potentiated twofold, and the enhancement with levonordefrin and norepinephrine is fivefold. If the patient also has arrhythmias, the situation is of even greater concern.[4] For dental treatment, levonordefrin and norepinephrine should be avoided, and epinephrine should be administered at the lowest effective dose similar to that recommended for a cardiovascularly involved patient (0.04 mg per appointment for epinephrine). See Box 7-7 for commonly prescribed tricyclic antidepressants.

NONSELECTIVE β BLOCKERS

Nonselective β blockers are antihypertensive drugs used to lower systolic and diastolic blood pressure. However, when used with exogenously administered vasoconstrictors, especially epinephrine, the combined effect leads to blockade of β-adrenergic receptors in the skeletal muscles and may cause hypertension and reflex bradycardia. The antihypertensives listed in Box 7-8 may potentiate the action of epinephrine and other adrenergic amines by significantly increasing the pressor potency due to their unopposed α-adrenergic receptors. If vasoconstriction is needed, use with caution limiting their use to the lowest effective dose, otherwise avoid their use. If vasoconstrictors are administered, preanesthetic and postanesthetic vital signs should be monitored and documented. In addition, the patient should be monitored throughout treatment for symptoms of altered (increased) blood pressure.

CARDIAC DRUGS

Digitalis glycosides are used for the treatment of congestive heart failure. The combination of digitalis glycosides and epinephrine increases the potential for cardiac

TABLE 7-8	Modifications to The Use of Vasoconstrictors	
CONDITION	**SIGNIFICANCE**	**DOSE MODIFICATION**
Cardiovascular disease	ASA III patients are treatable with appropriate modifications	Limit vasoconstrictor to cardiac dose; 0.04 mg per appointment for epinephrine; 0.2 mg per appointment for levonordefrin; do not use 1:50,000 epinephrine
Patients taking tricyclic antidepressants	Increases effects of vasoconstrictor; both epinephrine and levonordefrin may cause acute hypertension and cardiac dysrhythmia but levonordefrin to a greater degree	Avoid levonordefrin; limit epinephrine to cardiac dose of 0.04 mg per appointment; do not use 1:50,000 epinephrine
Patients taking nonselective beta blockers	Increased hypertension resulting in rebound bradycardia; potential cardiac arrest	If vasonstriction is necessary, limit vasoconstrictor to cardiac dose; 0.04 mg per appointment for epinephrine; 0.2 mg per appointment for levonordefrin; do not use 1:50,000 epinephrine
Diabetes	Vasoconstrictors directly oppose effect of insulin, possible changes in blood levels of glucose; amounts used in dentistry are generally safe and do not significantly raise blood sugar levels	Limit the dose of vasoconstrictor for patients with uncontrolled "brittle" diabetes
Controlled hyperthyroidism	Sensitivity to vasoconstrictors increasing their effect	Surgically corrected or medication controlled respond normally to vasoconstrictors.
Phenothiazines	Haloperidol (Haldol): chlorpromazine (Thorazine) may reverse the pressor effect of vasoconstrictors resulting in an increased risk of hypotension, and have been noted to antagonize the peripheral vasoconstrictive effects of epinephrine	Limit vasoconstrictor to cardiac dose; 0.04 mg per appointment for epinephrine; 0.2 mg per appointment for levonordefrin; do not use 1:50,000 epinephrine
Digitalis glycosides	Epinephrine increases the potential for cardiac arrhythmias	Use epinephrine in consultation with patient's physician

BOX 7-8	Commonly Prescribed Nonselective Beta Blockers

- Propranolol (Inderal)
- Metoprolol (Lopressor)
- Atenolol (Tenormin)
- Timolol (Blocadren)
- Nadolol (Corgard)
- Pindolol (Visken)
- Betaxolol (Kerlone)
- Acebutolol (Sectral)
- Esmolol (Brevibloc)
- Bisoprolol (Zebeta)
- Penbutolol (Levatol)
- Sotalol (Betapace)
- Carteolol (Cartrol)

arrhythmias. Use epinephrine in consultation with the patient's physician.

PHENOTHIAZIDES

The drug interaction between epinephrine and phenothiazine occurs because phenothiazine is an α blocker that antagonizes the β effects of epinephrine. When this occurs, the β (vasodilatory) effects of epinephrine predominate. Phenothiazine such as haloperidol (Haldol), thioridazine (Mellaril) and chlorpromazine (Thorazine) may reverse the pressor effect of vasoconstrictors, resulting in an increased risk of hypotension. Phenothiazine has been noted to antagonize the peripheral vasoconstrictive effects of epinephrine. The minimal effective dose of epinephrine should

be administered similar to that recommended for a cardiovascularly involved patient (0.04 mg per appointment).

ILLEGAL (RECREATIONAL) DRUGS (COCAINE, METHAMPHETAMINE)

Cocaine is a local anesthetic drug that significantly stimulates the central nervous system (CNS) and cardiovascular system (CVS). Cocaine stimulates the release of norepinephrine and inhibits the adrenergic nerve reuptake, causing tachycardia, severe hypertension, and arrhythmias, for example.[4] Methamphetamine affects the neurotransmitter epinephrine by either increasing its release or stopping its metabolic breakdown and reuptake resulting in a hypertensive crisis. Vasoconstrictor should **not** be administered to a patient who is suspected of using cocaine or methamphetamine on the day of dental treatment; it may lead to a hypertensive crisis, stroke, or myocardial infarction.

VASOCONSTRICTORS AND SYSTEMIC DISEASE INTERACTIONS

Few health conditions absolutely contraindicate the administration of vasoconstrictors, and in these situations patients are not usually seen for elective dental procedures such as nonsurgical periodontal therapy until the systemic disease is under control. The dental hygienist must carefully weigh the benefits of the administration of vasoconstrictors with the risks involved to determine if a vasonconstrictor should be adminstered. Table 7-9 summarizes the vasoconstrictor contraindications.

TABLE 7-9	Absolute Contraindications—Do Not Use Vasoconstrictors
CONDITION	**SIGNIFICANCE**
Recent myocardial infarction within 6 months	Increase cardiovascular effects to dangerous levels; ASA IV until recuperation Avoid all dental care until condition is under control
Recent coronary bypass surgery within 6 months	Increase cardiovascular effects to dangerous levels; ASA IV until recuperation Avoid all dental care until condition is under control
Uncontrolled high blood pressure	Increase blood pressure to dangerous levels Avoid all dental care until condition is under control
Uncontrolled angina	Increase risk of severe angina attack Avoid all dental care until condition is under control
Uncontrolled arrhythmias	Increase cardiovascular effects to dangerous levels Avoid all dental care until condition is under control
Sulfite allergies	Avoid vasoconstrictor in true allergic reaction
Pheochromocytoma: catecholamine-producing tumors	Tumor of the adrenal gland, causes adrenal insufficiency Avoid all dental care until condition is under control
Uncontrolled hyperthyroidism	Risk of thyroid crisis, thyroid storm Avoid all dental care until condition is under control
Cocaine or methamphetamine abusers	Avoid use of vasopressors; may lead to myocardial infarction
Glaucoma	Vasoconstrictors increase the amount of ocular pressure Avoid use of vasopressors

CARDIOVASCULAR DISEASE

Stress provoked by dental procedures is likely to increase blood pressure, pulse, and possibly respiration (hyperventilation) in many patients. Patients with cardiovascular disease are more susceptible than healthy patients to these responses producing further adverse effects on their already compromised system. Therefore, authorities[2-6] recommend small amounts (cardiac dose) of epinephrine; 0.04 mg per appointment (2.2 cartridges containing 1:100,000) as compared to a maximum of 0.2 mg in a healthy adult (approximately 8.3 cartridges of lidocaine with epinephrine) to be administered to these patients for most dental procedures including nonsurgical periodontal therapy. Profound local anesthesia is indicated to minimize release of endogenous epinephrine in response to pain. Adequate aspiration is critical to prevent intravascular injection. The use of concentrated vasoconstrictors 1:50,000 epinephrine for bleeding control, is contraindicated.

Patients with significant cardiovascular disease should not receive elective dental procedures or vasoconstrictors until their disease is controlled. The following are absolute contraindications to the use of vasoconstrictors:

- Blood pressure greater than 200/115 mm Hg
- Within 6 months after a heart attack or stroke
- Severe cardiovascular disease
- Daily episodes of angina pectoris or unstable (preinfarction) angina
- Cardiac dysrhythmias despite appropriate therapy
- Within 6 months of coronary artery bypass surgery

HYPERTHYROIDISM

Patients with hyperthyroidism are sensitive to catecholamines and may precipitate an exaggerated response to vasoconstrictors, resulting in cardiac stimulation and risk of developing thyrotoxicosis more commonly known as *thyroid storm*. Uncontrolled hyperthyroidism is an absolute contraindication to vasoconstrictors because of the possibility of causing a thyroid crisis. Patients should not receive elective dental care or vasoconstrictors until the situation is controlled, and then only the minimal effective dose should be administered, not to exceed 0.04 mg per appointment for epinephrine, and 0.2 mg per appointment for levonordefrin.

ASTHMA

The addition of the sodium bisulfite, metabisulfite to prevent the oxidation of vasoconstrictors may cause respiratory reactions in asthmatics (predominantly steriod dependent asthmatics). It has been reported that up to 10% of the asthmatic population are allergic to bisulfites. Asthmatic patients who receive a local anesthetic with vasoconstrictor should be observed for signs and symptoms of an asthmatic attack. Bisulfite allergies typically manifest as a severe respiratory allergy, commonly bronchospasm.[6-8]

ALLERGIES

Amino esters are derivatives of para-aminobenzoic acid (PABA), which have been associated with acute allergic reactions. Amino amides are not associated with PABA and do not produce allergic reactions with the same frequency.

Since the removal of methylparaben, a local anesthetic preservative (structurally similar to PABA) from local anesthetic solutions, the possibility of an amide local anesthetic allergic reaction is extremely rare, and essentially nonexsistent.[4,5] Moreover, there are no confirmed cases of a true allergy to a pure amide anesthetic. However, patients often claim that they are allergic to local anesthetics. These patients must be further questioned to rule out the possibility of misinformation or misdiagnosis. Also, patients who may have experienced rapid adrenergic symptoms from the vasoconstrictor or experienced a local anesthetic overdose may confuse these symptoms with an allergic reaction. A well-documented allergic reaction to a local

TABLE 7-10	Allergies That Affect the Selection of Local Anesthetic Agents or Vasoconstrictors			
REPORTED ALLERGY	**TYPE OF CONTRAINDICATION**	**DRUGS TO AVOID**	**POTENTIAL PROBLEM(S)**	**ALTERNATIVE DRUG**
Local anesthetic allergy, documented	Absolute	All local anesthetics in same chemical class (esters vs. amides)	Allergic response, mild (e.g., dermatitis, bronchospasm) to life-threatening reactions	Local anesthetics in different chemical class (esters vs. amides)
Sodium bisulfate or metabisulfite	Absolute	Local anesthetic containing a vasoconstrictor	Allergic reaction Severe bronchospasm, usually in asthmatics	Local anesthetic without vasoconstrictor

Modified from Darby M, Walsh M: *Dental hygiene theory and practice*, ed 3, St Louis, 2010, Saunders, Elsevier.

anesthetic represents an absolute contraindication to that class of drugs, and an unrelated drug should be selected. A patient who has an allergic reaction to one agent is likely to experience hypersensitivity to another agent in the same group. Cross-hypersensitivity between esters and amides is unlikely.

As discussed in Chapter 4, local anesthetics with adrenergic vasoconstrictors contain the antioxidant sodium bisulfite, or metabisulfite. Documented allergic reactions have been reported to these agents.[6,7,8] Patients who have demonstrated a true allergy to sulfites should not receive a local anesthetic agent containing vasoconstrictors (an absolute contraindication). Table 7-10 summarizes allergies that affect the selection of local anesthetic agents.

ESTER DERIVATIVE LOCAL ANESTHETIC INTERACTIONS

Injectable esters are no longer available for use in dentistry because of their well documented risk of allergeic reactions. However, since the amide articaine is metabolized in the same manner as esters these interactions should be noted and discussed. Table 7-12 summarizes the ester derivative local anesthetic interactions.

CHOLINESTERASE INHIBITORS

Cholinesterase inhibitors are frequently prescribed for the treatment of myasthenia gravis and glaucoma. Patients taking cholinesterase inhibitors should not be given ester derivative local anesthetics, or the amide articaine. Ester derivatives and articaine are metabolized primarily in the bloodstream by plasma cholinesterase. If cholinesterase is inhibited, then the ester derivatives and articaine are more slowly broken down and systemic toxicity may result.[9] Avoid esters and the amide articaine.

SULFONAMIDES

Procaine and tetracaine undergo hydrolysis to PABA, a major metabolic by-product. Sulfonamides competitively inhibit PABA in microorganisms. PABA derivatives, therefore, may antagonize the antibacterial activity of sulfonamides, rendering them ineffective. Since the use of ester injectable local anesthetics is no longer available in dentistry this is unlikely to occur. However, ester topical anesthetics should not be given to a patient taking sulfonamides. Instead use lidocaine.

ATYPICAL PLASMA CHOLINESTERASE

Ester anesthetics and the amide articaine are metabolized in the plasma by cholinesterase enzymes. Some individuals, approximately 1 in every 2820, demonstrate an atypical form of plasma pseudocholinesterase.[4] This is an uncommon autosomal recessive genetic trait.[5] Amide local anesthetics, except for articaine, can be safely administered to these patients.

AMIDE LOCAL ANESTHETIC DRUG/DRUG INTERACTIONS

Only a few amide local anesthetic interactions occur with prescribed drugs. These typically manifest by delaying the metabolism of the local anesthetic agent. The importance of each interaction is summarized in Table 7-11.

HISTAMINE H_2 RECEPTOR BLOCKERS

Amide local anesthetics that are primarily metabolized in the liver have a potential for drug interactions with other drugs that influence hepatic metabolism. Tagamet (cimetidine) decreases hepatic blood flow and inhibits hepatic metabolism of amides, particularly lidocaine, by competing for binding to hepatic oxidative enzymes, and therefore increases the half-life of the amide anesthetic, increasing the risk for toxic overdose. Caution should be used when administering large doses of lidocaine. The interaction between lidocaine and cimetidine is of greater concern in patients with a history of congestive heart failure (ASA III or greater) due to the decrease in blood delivered to the liver, and an increase in blood delivered to the brain increases the risk of an anesthetic overdose.[2]

BETA BLOCKERS

Beta adrenergic blocking drugs, such as propranolol and metoprolol, share the same effect as cimetidine on amide biotransformation, particularly lidocaine. Beta blockers inhibit metabolism of amides by decreasing hepatic blood flow and interfere with the delivery of amide to the liver

TABLE 7-11	Modifications to the Use of Anesthetics	
CONDITION	**SIGNIFICANCE**	**ACTION OR ALTERNATIVE DRUG**
Patients taking H$_2$-receptor blocker cimetidine (Tagamet) on a regular basis	Drug reduces capacity of liver to metabolize lidocaine	Reduce dosage lidocaine; greater clinical significance in patients with CHF (ASA III or greater)
Patients taking beta blockers predominately Inderal (propranolol)	Inhibits metabolism of amides by decreasing hepatic blood flow increasing risk of toxic overdose	Reduce dosage of amides
Significant liver disease	Amides primarily metabolized in the liver increase possibility of toxic overdose	Reduce dosage of amides, articaine is preferred
Renal dysfunction	Slight risk of toxicity with severe renal dysfunction	Use local anesthetics but use judiciously
Malignant hyperthermia	Life-threatening syndrome caused by general anesthetics	Medical consultation is recommended; use amides but reduce dosage
Methemoglobinemia	Potential for clinical cynosis	Use amides but avoid prilocaine or topical benzocaine
Cholinesterase Inhibitors	Frequently prescribed for the treatment of myasthenia gravis and glaucoma	Should not be given ester derivative anesthetics or articaine
Atypical pseudo-cholinesterase	Inability of esters or amide articaine to be metabolized in the plasma by cholinesterase enzymes	Should not be given ester derivative anesthetics or articaine
Pregnancy	Anesthetics are not teratogenic and pose little danger to the fetus	For most conservative approach use category B anesthetics only after first trimester
CNS depressants (examples—opioids or opioid derivatives, antianxiety drugs, phenothiazines, and barbiturates)	Could potentiate drowsiness. Barbiturates induce hepatic microsomal enzymes that could alter the rate of amide type local anesthetic metabolism	Use amides in lower doses

for biotransformation.[5] An increasing risk for toxic overdose is possible. Caution should be used when administering large doses of lidocaine. Not all antihypertensives behave in this manner. Dental hygienists should utilize a current *Physician's Desk Reference (PDR)* for specific drug interactions.

OTHER AMIDE LOCAL ANESTHETIC INTERACTIONS

MALIGNANT HYPERTHERMIA

Malignant hyperthermia is an inherited syndrome triggered by exposure to certain drugs used for general anesthesia and the neuromuscular blocking agent succinylcholine. It is a rare occurrence in approximately 1:15,000 in children and approximately 1:50,000 in adults.[5] It can produce drastic uncontrolled skeletal muscle oxidative metabolism, which overwhelms the body's capacity to supply oxygen, remove carbon dioxide, and regulate body temperature, eventually leading to circulatory collapse and death if not treated quickly.

The trait may never be identified in many individuals, and may occur only after several episodes of anesthetic administration. Symptoms are characterized by a high fever, tachycardia, cardiac dysrhythmias, and cyanosis. Complications may be life-threatening and are associated with the administration of general anesthesia.[4,5]

Although general anesthetics are known to trigger the episode, the ability for amide local anesthetics to act in the same manner is controversial. It is therefore recommended that a medical constulation be conducted prior to treating

these patients, and when treating these patients the guidelines from the Malignant Hyperthermia Association of the United States (MHAUS) should be followed.[5,6,10-14]

METHEMOGLOBINEMIA

Prilocaine (and possibly topical benzocaine) administered in high doses may produce methemoglobinemia, a rare hereditary condition characterized by the inability of the blood to bind to oxygen. Prilocaine is metabolized to *ortho-toluidine* and is characterized by the presence of higher than normal levels of methemoglobinemia in the blood, that does not bind to oxygen. Clinical cyanosis of the lips and mucous membranes may be observed. Substitute other amide anesthetics as an alternative anesthetic, and topical lidocaine for benzocaine.

LIVER DISEASE

Significant liver disease (ASA III) such as cirrhosis and hepatitis B could interrupt the biotransformation of the amides that are primarily metabolized in the liver. Interruption of their biotransformation could lead to systemic toxicity. Liver disease represents a relative contraindication to amides, and the minimal effective dose should be administered. Because articaine is primarily metabolized in the plasma, this anesthetic may provide a better choice over lidocaine, mepivacaine, and bupivacaine in some situations.

KIDNEY DISEASE

Only a small percentage of unmetabolized local anesthetics are excreted in the urine, and usual doses of anesthetics do not pose any additional risk. Toxic serum levels of anesthetic could develop in patients with significant renal dysfunction, but this occurrence is rare.

PREGNANCY

Local anesthetics administered during pregnancy are not teratogenic and pose little danger to the fetus. Pregnancy is represented as a temporary contraindication relative to elective dental hygiene care, with the administration of local anesthetics.[4,5] Pregnant women can receive elective dental hygiene care with anesthesia in any trimester, in consultation with the patient's physician.[4] The conservative approach when administering local anesthetics to a pregnant patient is to wait until the second trimester and to choose a drug in the category B pregnancy risk classification of drugs (Table 7-12).

BLEEDING DISORDERS

A patient with a blood clotting disorder should be assessed for the potential to develop excessive bleeding as a result of puncturing a blood vessel. Local anesthetic injection techniques that pose a greater risk of positive aspirations are the posterior superior alveolar (PSA) block, inferior alveolar (IA) block, and the infraorbital (IO) block and should be avoided in favor of supraperiosteal, and periodontal ligament injections, or other techniques that do not pose a threat of excessive bleeding.

TABLE 7-12	**Pregnancy Risk Classification of Local Anesthetics**	
ANESTHETIC	**PREGNANCY RISK CATEGORY**	**LACTATION CATEGORY**
Lidocaine	B (Caution advised)	Safe
Mepivacaine	C (Weigh risk vs. benefit)	Unknown (caution recommended)
Prilocaine	B (Caution advised)	Unknown (caution recommended)
Articaine	C (Weigh risk vs. benefit)	Unknown (caution recommended)
Bupivacaine	C (Weigh risk vs. benefit)	Unknown (caution recommended)

Food and Drug Administration (FDA) www.fda.gov

TABLE 7-13	**American Heart Association Recommendations for Prophylactic Antibiotic Coverage Regimen for Select Dental Procedures in Adults and Children with High and Moderate Risk for Infective Endocarditis**		
SITUATION	**AGENT**	**CHILD OR ADULT**	**REGIMEN**
Standard prophylaxis for persons not allergic to penicillin	Amoxicillin (oral)	Adult	2 g orally 1 hour before the procedure
		Child	50 mg/kg orally 1 hour before the procedure
Allergic to penicillin	Clindamycin (oral) or	Adult Child	600 mg orally 1 hour before the procedure 20 mg/kg orally 1 hour before the procedure
	Azithromycin (oral) or clarithromycin (oral)	Adult Child	500 mg orally 1 hour before the procedure 15 mg/kg orally 1 hour before the procedure
Unable to take oral medications	Ampicillin (IM or IV)	Adult Child	2 g within 30 minutes before the procedure 50 mg/kg within 30 minutes before the procedure
Allergic to penicillin and unable to take oral medications	Clindamycin (IV)	Adult Child	600 mg within 30 minutes before the procedure 20 mg/kg within 30 minutes before the procedure

Adapted from Dajani AS, et al: Prevention of bacterial endocarditis, *JAMA* 277(22):1798, 1997.

DENTAL HYGIENE CONSIDERATIONS

- The dental hygienist must evaluate through a comprehensive medical history the patient's physical ability to tolerate the administration of a local anesthetic or vasoconstrictor.
- The evaluation of the patient's attitude and psychological fears are important components to the preanesthetic assessment. Fear and anxiety provoke the "fight-or-flight" response.
- Medical consultation with the patient's physician or specialist should be completed as necessary before the administration of the local anesthetic agent.
- Maximum recommended doses for the selected local anesthetic drug must be calculated before administration of the agent. These doses are dependent upon the patient's medical condition(s).

- Stress reduction protocols must be implemented for patients with medical conditions that could be exacerbated by stress and anxiety.
- True allergic reactions to a pure amide local anesthetic agent are extremely rare. If an allergic reaction exists, it will most likely be due to the vasoconstrictor preservative, sodium bisulfite.
- Many patients confuse signs and symptoms of an anesthetic or vasoconstrictor overdose with an allergic reaction. Dialog with the patient is invaluable in gaining more information regarding the patient's medical status.
- Treatment should be delayed if the patient has had a heart attack or stroke within 6 months of treatment.

DENTAL HYGIENE CONSIDERATIONS—cont'd

- Decreased liver function increases the half-life of the amides metabolized in the liver, increasing the risk for overdose.
- Vasoconstrictors administered the same day a patient has used cocaine or methamphetamines can be life threatening.
- Preanesthetic baseline vital signs are essential to provide a standard of comparison in an emergency.
- The proper duration of anesthetic for treatment and postoperative pain control is important to reduce patient stress and anxiety. Patients who feel pain during the procedure or on the way home could have potentially adverse reactions to endogenous release of catecholamines.

- An absolute contraindication means that the drug should not be administered under any circumstances.
- A relative contraindication means that the drug can be administered but precautions should be taken, and the drug should be used judiciously.
- The dental hygienist should be familiar with all absolute and relative contraindications to local anesthetic and vasoconstrictor drugs. These contraindications should be reviewed periodically during practice.
- Nerve blocks (PSA, IO, IA) should be avoided in patients with bleeding disorders. Supraperiosteal and PDL injections are less likely to produce a hematoma and excessive bleeding.

CASE STUDY 7-1

Travis comes to your office for nonsurgical periodontal therapy of the mandibular right quadrant. He is very sensitive and local anesthesia will be needed. His blood pressure is 150/100 mm Hg and his weight is 180 lb. He has a history of chronic asthma and is taking Tagamet for an ulcer. Everything else is within normal limits (WNL).

Critical Thinking Questions
- What are the medical considerations when choosing a local anesthetic?

- Choose an appropriate local anesthetic for this patient.
- What treatment modifications should be made for this patient if any?
- Are any dosage modifications indicated for the drug selected?

CASE STUDY 7-2

Soula is in your office for nonsurgical periodontal therapy. Her blood pressure is 135/90 mm Hg and her weight is 128 lb. She has a history of malignant hyperthermia, and she is taking Elavil. Everything else is WNL.

Critical Thinking Questions
- What are the medical considerations when choosing a local anesthetic?

- Choose an appropriate local anesthetic for this patient.
- What treatment modifications should be made for this patient, if any?
- Are any dosage modifications indicated for the drug selected?

CASE STUDY 7-3

Matia is in your office for nonsurgical periodontal therapy. She is very sensitive and local anesthesia will be needed. Her blood pressure is 130/85 mm Hg and her weight is 150 lb. Matia has diabetes, which is controlled. She has a history of hypertension and is taking Tenormin.

Critical Thinking Questions
- What are the medical considerations when choosing a local anesthetic?

- Choose an appropriate local anesthetic for this patient.
- What treatment modifications should be made for this patient, if any?
- Are any dosage modifications indicated for the drug selected?

CHAPTER REVIEW QUESTIONS

1. Which drug is most likely to exhibit a drug interaction with epinephrine?
   A. Sulfonamides
   B. Monoamine oxidase inhibitors
   C. Tricyclic antidepressants
   D. Serotonin specific reuptake inhibitors
   E. Acetaminophen

2. Before injecting a patient with a local anesthetic with or without a vasoconstrictor, the dental hygienist should:
   A. Review the patient's health history
   B. Take the patient's blood pressure
   C. Determine if a patient has a history of allergies
   D. Determine if any contraindications exsist to the selected anesthetic
   E. All of the above

3. Patients with bleeding disorders will most likely be susceptible to:
   A. Technique of anesthetic administration
   B. Vasoconstrictors
   C. Ester anesthetics
   D. Amide anesthetics

4. Following the administration of a local anesthetic with a vasoconstrictor, the patient experiences mild itching and a slight rash. This is most likely due to:
   A. The amide anesthetic
   B. Methylparaben
   C. Sodium bisulfite
   D. The epinephrine

5. Patients with an artificial heart valve need premedication before a local anesthetic injection:
   A. True
   B. False

6. Which of the following is an absolute contraindication to the use of vasoconstrictors?
   A. Blood pressure 175/95 mm Hg
   B. Heart attack 5 months ago
   C. Use of Tricyclic antidepressants
   D. Controlled diabetes

7. Which of the following drugs is the best choice to administer when a patient has a history of hepatitis B?
   A. Mepivacaine
   B. Lidocaine
   C. Bupivacaine
   D. Articaine

8. Which of the following anesthetics should be avoided if a patient has methemoglobinemia?
   A. Bupivacaine
   B. Prilocaine
   C. Lidocaine
   D. Procaine

9. Which anesthetic falls under the pregnancy risk category B?
   A. Lidocaine
   B. Bupivacaine
   C. Articaine
   D. Mepivacaine

10. It is recommended to monitor a patient's blood pressure throughout treatment for symptoms of altered (increased) blood pressure when a patient is taking which of the following medications:
    A. Phenothiazines
    B. Monoamine oxidase inhibitors
    C. Nonspecific beta blockers
    D. Insulin
    E. Barbiturates

11. When a patient is taking a tricyclic antidepressant and is also given levonordefrin, blood pressure enhancement is fivefold greater than with levonordefrin alone?
    A. True
    B. False

12. Select the local anesthetic that is most likely to inhibit the antibacterial activity of sulfonamides:
    A. Lidocaine
    B. Prilocaine
    C. Articaine
    D. Procaine
    E. Bupivacaine

13. Patients with atypical plasma cholinesterase should not receive which classification of drugs?
    A. All amides
    B. All esters
    C. Vasoconstrictors
    D. Sulfonamides

14. Methemoglobinemia is caused by the metabolite:
    A. Ortho-toludine
    B. Benzene
    C. Para-amino benzoic acid
    D. Xylidine

15. Which of the following treatment modifications are important for patients with alcoholism?
    A. Avoid amide local anesthetics
    B. Administer the minimal effective dose of articaine
    C. Administer the minimal effective dose of lidocaine, mepivacaine, or bupivicaine
    D. No treatment modifications are necessary for all amides
    E. Administer the minimal effective dose of epinephrine

16. Patients taking Elavil should:
    A. Not receive amide local anesthetics
    B. Receive amide local anesthetic when administed in the minimal effective dose
    C. Not receive ester local anesthetics
    D. Receive lowest effective dose of epinephrine similar to that recommended for a cardiovascularly involved patient

17. ASA II describes a patient:
    A. With a mild systemic disease that does not interfere with daily activity
    B. With a mild systemic disease that interferes with daily activity
    C. With moderate to severe systemic disease that limits activity but is not incapacitating
    D. Who is healthy

18. Which of the following can cause a false high blood pressure reading?
    A. Blood pressure cuff is too narrow
    B. Bladder or cuff is too wide
    C. Cuff is deflated too quickly
    D. Arm is above heart level

19. Which of the following is a relative contraindication to the use of an amide local anesthetic?
    A. Patient is taking tricyclic antidepressants
    B. Patient is taking Tagamet
    C. Patient is taking monoamine oxidase inhibitors
    D. Patient has diabetes and is taking antidiabetic medication
    E. All of the above

20. A patient is considered to have tachycardia if beats per minute is greater than 80.
    A. True
    B. False

REFERENCES

1. Darby M, Walsh M. *Dental hygiene theory and practice*, ed 3, St Louis, 2010, Saunders.
2. Malamed SF: *Medical Emergencies in the Dental Office*, ed 6, St. Louis, 2007, Mosby.
3. Haveles, B: *Applied Pharmacology for the Dental Hygienist*, ed 6, St. Louis, 2011, Mosby.
4. Little JW, Falace DA, Miller CS, Rhodus NL: *Dental Management of the Medically Compromised Patient*, St. Louis, 2008, Mosby.
5. Malamed SF: *Handbook of Local Anesthesia*, ed 5, St Louis, 2004, Mosby.
6. Jastak T, Yagiela J, Donaldson D: *Local Anesthesia of the Oral Cavity*, St. Louis, 1995, Saunders.
7. Schwartz HJ, Sensitivity to injected metabisulfites; variation in the clinical presentation, *J Allergy Clin Immunol* 71:487, 1983.
8. Simon RA, Green L., Stevenson DD: The incidence of ingensted metabisulfite sensitivity in an asthmatic population, *J Allergy Clin Immunol* 69-118, 1982.
9. Oertel R, Rahn R, Kirch W. Clinical pharmacokinetics of articaine. *Clin Pharmacokinet* 33:417-425, 1997.
10. Becker, D, Reed, K: *Essentials of Local Anesthetic Pharmacology*. American Dental Society of Anesthesiology. Anesthesia Program, 53, 2006.
11. de Jong RH: *Local anesthetics*, St Louis, 1994, Mosby.
12. Bahl, R: Local Anesthesia in Dentistry, *Anesth Prog* 51:138-142 2004 by the American Dental Society of Anesthesiology.
13. Finder RL., More PA: Adverse drug reactions to local anesthesia, *Dent Clin N Am* 46:447-457, 2002.
14. Litman R, Rosenberg H: Malignant hyperthermia: update on susceptibility testing, *JAMA* 293(23):2918–2924, 2005.

ADDITIONAL RESOURCES

Sisk A: Vasoconstrictors in Local Anesthesia for Dentistry, *Anesth Prog* 39:187-193, 1992.

US Food and Drug Administration: Center for Food Safety and Applied Nutrition van der Meer, Auke Dirk MD; Burm, Anton G. L. MSc, PhD; Stienstra, Rudolf MD, PhD; van Kleef, Jack W. MD, PhD; Vletter, Arie A. BSc; Olieman, Wim; Pharmacokinetics of Prilocaine after Intravenous Administration in Volunteers: Enantioselectivity, *Anesthesiology* 90(4):988-992, April 1999.

Bartlett SZ. Clinical observation on the effect of injections of local anesthetics preceded by aspiration, *Oral Surg* 33: 520-525, 1972.

Buckley JA, Ciancio SG, McMullen JA. Efficacy of epinephrine concentration in local aneshesia during periodontal surgery, *J Periodontol* 55:653-657, 1984.

Isen DA. Articaine: Pharmacology and clinical use of a recently approved local anesthetic, *Dent Today* 19:72-77, 2000.

Jacob W. Local anaesthesia and vasoconstrictive additional components, *Newslett Int Fed Dent Anesthesiol Soc* 2:1-3, 1989.

Jacob W. Local anaesthesia and vasoconstrictive additional components, *Newslett Int Fed Dent Anesthesiol Soc* 2:1-3, 1989.

Jacobs W, Ladwig B, Cichon P, Oertel R, Kirch W: Serum levels of articaine 2 % and 4 % in children. *Anesth Prog* 42:113-115, 1995.

Oertel R, Ebert U, Rahn R, Kirch W. The effect of age on the pharmacokinetics of the local anesthetic drug articaine, *Regional Anesth Pain Med* 24:524-528, 1999.

Adams V, Marley J, McCarroll C: Prilocaine induced methaemoglobinaemia in a medically compromised patient. Was this an inevitable consequence of the dose administered? *Br Dent J* 203(10): 585–587, 2007.

Sample Medical History Form in English/Spanish

MEDICAL ALERT Sample Medical History Form in English/Spanish

Date/Fecha

Name/Nombre

Last Apellido	**First** Nombre	**Initial** Inicial	**Soc. Sec. #** Num. de Seguro Social	**Home Phone** Teléfono	**Business Phone** Teléfono del Trabajo

Address Dirección	**City** Ciudad	**State** Estado	**Zip code** Código Postal	**Occupation** Ocupación	**Employer** Empleador

Dr.

Birthdate Fecha de Nacimiento	**Sex** Sexo	**Height** Estatura	**Weight** Peso	**Marital Status** Estado Civil	**Previous Dentist's Name** Nombre de su Dentista	**Previous Dentist's Phone** Núm. Telefónico de su Dentista

Dr.

Physician's Name Nombre de su Doctor	**Phone #** Número de Teléfono	**Person to contact in case of emergency** Persona a llamar en caso de emergencia	**Phone #** Num. Telefónico

For the following questions, check yes or no, whichever applies. Your answers will be considered confidential. Please note that during each of your visits you will be asked questions about your responses to this questionnaire and there may be additional questions concerning your health.

Para las siguentes preguntas, marque si o no para la respuesta que mejor aplique. Sus respuestas serán consideradas confidenciales. Por favor note que durante su visita inicial será cuestionado sobre sus respuestas a ésta forma y posiblemente habrá preguntas adicionales relacionadas con su salud.

Yes SI	No No	**Check each item.** Marque cada pregunta	**Provider's comments** Comentarios del Proveedor
		Are you in good health? ¿Está en buena salud?	
		Are you currently under the care of a physician? If not, when was your last visit? ¿Está bajo cuidado médico?	
		Has there been any change in your general health within the past year? ¿Hubo algún cambio en su salud durante el año pasado?	
		Have you had any serious illness operation, or been hospitalized? ¿Ha tenido una enfermedad seria, operación o ha sido hospitalizado?	
		Have you had any problems with or during dental treatment? ¿Ha tenido algún problema durante un tratamiento dental?	
		Are you allergic to or had reactions to any medications including local anesthetics? If yes, please list. ¿Sufre de alergias o ha tenido alguna reacción alérgica a alguna medicina, incluyendo la anestesia local?	
		Do you have any other allergies (metals, latex, food, pollen, etc.)?	
		Please check below if you have or had any of the following diseases or problems. *Por favor marque en las lineas debajo si padece o ha padecido de alguna enfermedad o problema mencionado.*	
		Artificial heart valves or shunts? Válvulas cardiacas dañadas, válvulas cardiacas artificiales, marca pasos, soplo de corazón o fiebre reumática	
		Cardiovascular disease (heart trouble, heart attack, angina, high blood pressure, hardening of the arteries, stroke, etc.) Enfermedad cardiovascular como problemas del corazón, ataque cardiaco, angina de pecho, alta presión, endurecimiento de las arterias, infarto, etc.	
		Have you taken Cortisone in the last two years?	

Yes SI	No No	Check each item. Marque cada pregunta	Provider's comments Comentarios del Proveedor
		Were you born with any heart problems? ¿Nació con algún problema cardiaco (del corazón)?	
		Sinus trouble Problemas de sinusitis	
		Asthma, hayfever or skin rashes? Asma o catarro asmático	
		Fainting spells, seizures, epilepsy or convulsions Desmayos, convulsiones o ataques epilépticos	
		Persistent diarrhea, weight loss or vomiting Diarrea persistente, pérdida de peso o vómitos	
		Diabetes (sugar problems) Diabetis (azúcar alta en la sangre)	
		Hepatitis, yellow jaundice, cirrhosis, or liver disease Hepatitis, itericia, cirrosis u alguna otra enfermedad hepática(del higado)	
		AIDS or HIV infection SIDA (Sindrome de Immunodeficiencia Adquirida) or VIH (Virus de Immunodeficiencia Humana)	
		Thyroid problems (goiter) Problemas con las glándulas tiroides	
		Respiratory problems, emphysema, bronchitis, black lung, etc. Problemas respiratorios, enfisema, bronquitis, etc.	
		Arthritis or painful swollen joints Artritis o inflamación en las coyonturas	
		Have you ever had a joint replacement? Utiliza prótesis (ex: coyonturas, válvulas, aparatos auditivos, implantes, etc.) además de la dentadura	
		Kidney trouble or dialysis treatment Algún problema con los riñones o le han hecho diálisis	
		Tuberculosis or positive TB skin test Tuberculosis o ha salido positivo en un examen de tuberculosis	
		Anemia or blood disorders Anemia o alguna otra enfermedad sanguinea (de la sangre)	
		Gonorrhea, syphilis, herpes or other similar diseases Gonorrea, sífilis, herpes u otra enfermedad parecida	
		Problems with mental health or nerves Trastornos mentales o nerviosos	
		Cancer Cáncer	
		Stomach ulcer, hyperacidity or other GI problems Úlceras estomacales, acidez u otros problemas gastrointestinales	
		Do you use Tobacco or snuff products? ¿Fuma o mastica tabaco?	
		Have you been diagnosed with alcoholism? ¿Ha sido diagnosticado(a) con alcoholismo o esta recuperandose del mismo?	
		Do you have vision or hearing problems? Problemas visuales o auditivos	
		Do you use recreational drugs? ¿Usa drogas recreativas?	
		Are you pregnant or nursing a baby? ¿Está embarazada o amamantando?	

Are you taking any medicine(s), including any non-prescription medicine or natural remedies? If yes, please list below in left column.
¿Está tomando algún medicamento, incluyendo medicinas sin receta médica o suplementos naturales? (ejemplo; pastillas anticonceptivas, calcio, ginseng ajo etc.)

Medication Name:	Condition Used For:	Dental Implications: (Provider Comments)	Resource: (Provider Comments)

I certify that I have read and understand the above questionnaire, and have answered the questions willingly, truthfully, and to the best of my ability.
Yo certifico que he leído y comprendido este cuestionario y que mi condición médica puede afectar mi salud y tratamiento dental. He respondido a las preguntas voluntariamente, con sinceridad y a lo mejor de mi abilidad.

_____

Signature of Patient or Legal Guardian
Firma del Paciente o Tutor Legal

Date
Fecha

_____

Signature of Dental Provider
Firma del Dentista o Profesorado

Date
Fecha

Vital signs: Blood Pressure _____ **Pulse** _____ **Respiration** _____

From the University of New Mexico, Division of Dental Hygiene

Antibiotic Premedication Guidelines for Professional Oral Healthcare

CONDITIONS	PROPHYLAXIS RECOMMENDED	PROPHYLAXIS NOT RECOMMENDED
Dental procedures	Dental extractions Periodontal procedures including surgery, scaling and root planning, probing, and maintenance care (supportive periodontal therapy) Dental implant placement and reimplantation or avulsed teeth Endodontic (root canal) instrumentation or surgery only beyond the apex Subgingival placement of antibiotic fibers or strips Initial placement of orthodontic bands but not brackets Intraligamentary local anesthetic injections Every attempt should be made to complete procedures/services in as few appointments as possible Follow-up appointments should be scheduled at least 9 days apart if patient is premedicated	Restorative dentistry (operative and prosthodontic with or without retraction cord) Local anesthetic injections (nonintraligamentary) Intracanal endodontic treatment; post placement and buildup Placement of rubber dams Postoperative suture removal Placement of removal prosthodontic or orthodontic appliances Taking of oral impressions Fluoride treatments Taking of oral radiographs Orthodontic appliance adjustment Shedding of primary teeth
Cardiac Conditions	**High-Risk Category** Prosthetic cardiac valves, including bioprosthetic and hemograft valves A history of infective endocarditis Certain specific, serious congenital (present from birth) heart conditions, including: Unrepaired or incompletely repaired cyanotic congenital heart disease, including those with palliative shunts and conduits A completely repaired congenital heart defect with prosthetic material or device, whether placed by surgery or by catheter intervention, during the first six months after the procedure Any repaired congenital heart defect with residual defect at the site or adjacent to the site of a prosthetic patch or a prosthetic device A cardiac transplant that develops a problem in a heart valve.	
Orthopedic conditions	**Joint Replacement Patients** Within the first 2 years of joint replacement History of previous prosthetic joint infection Joint replacement patients who are immunocompromised/immunosuppressed by: Any disease, drug, or radiation-induced immunosuppression Inflammatory arthropathics (rheumatoid arthritis, systemic lupus erythematosus)	Not routinely indicated for most patients with joint replacements after two years of replacement or with plates, pins, or screws
Other conditions	Renal transplants/dialysis Immunosuppressive therapy (i.e., cyclosporine)	

Adapted from American Dental Association, American Academy of Orthopaedic Surgeons: Advisory statement: antibiotic prophylaxis for dental patients with total hip joint replacements, *J Am Dent Assoc* 134:895, 2003; Wilson W, Taubert KA, Gewitz M, et al: 2007 American Heart Association Guidelines, *J Am Dent Assoc* 138:739, 2007.

CHAPTER 8

Determining Drug Doses

Demetra Daskalos Logothetis RDH, MS

CHAPTER OUTLINE

LEARNING OBJECTIVES

1. Calculate maximum recommended doses (MRDs) for local anesthetic.
2. Calculate MRDs for vasoconstrictors for a healthy patient and a medically compromised patient.
3. Successfully complete review questions and activities for this chapter.

KEY TERMS

Absolute maximum dose The absolute maximum dose that any patient can receive per appointment, regardless of their weight.

Cardiac dose A vasoconstrictor dose that can be administered safely to patients with ischemic heart disease.

Limiting drug The drug that limits the total amount of volume delivered based upon the patient's medical status.

Maximum recommended dose Highest amount of drug that can be safely administered per appointment to a patient depending on their physical health.

▌INTRODUCTION

To increase the safety of the patient during the administration of local anesthetics and vasoconstrictors, the dental hygienist must always administer the smallest clinically effective dose. This is especially critical when administering anesthetics and vasoconstrictors to the medically compromised patient. Each cartridge of solution may contain either one drug (the anesthetic) or two drugs (the anesthetic and vasoconstrictor, including a preservative). The maximum recommended dose (MRD) of the solution that contains both the anesthetic and vasoconstrictor is dependent upon which of the two drugs reaches its MRD first. The drug that limits the total amount of volume delivered is referred to as the limiting drug. (See Box 8-1.)

All drugs have maximum dose levels, including local anesthetics and vasoconstrictors, which are determined by the manufacturer based on results from animal and human studies. These doses can be found in the product inserts. The maximum doses determined by the manufacturer have been reviewed by the Council on Dental Therapeutics of the American Dental Association and the United States Pharmacopeial (USP) Convention.[1,2] Dosage guidelines for local anesthetics and vasoconstrictors are also offered by recognized experts in the field, such as Malamed[3], and are usually more conservative doses than those recommended by the ADA council, the USP, or the manufacturer.[3] The dental hygienist must decide which maximum dose is the appropriate level based on the treatment to be delivered, and the health status of the patient. The information presented in this chapter assists the dental hygienist in determining the appropriate dosage to be administered.

MAXIMUM RECOMMENDED DOSES OF LOCAL ANESTHETICS

The MRD for a local anesthetic is defined as the highest amount of an anesthetic drug that can be safely administered without complication to a patient while maintaining its efficacy. MRDs should also be adjusted to consider the patient's overall health and any mitigating medical factors that could hamper the patient's recovery. These amounts are determined based on maximum dosage for each appointment. The dosage calculation is based on the patient's weight, and can be calculated based on milligrams per pound (mg/lb) or milligrams per kilogram (mg/kg). As discussed previously, each practitioner should determine which recommendation to follow. This author recommends, and will follow, the more conservative guidelines[3]. Table 8-1 provides the MRD per appointment for each local anesthetic recommended in this text.

CALCULATION OF MAXIMUM RECOMMENDED DOSE FOR LOCAL ANESTHETICS

All MRDs per appointment are calculated first based on milligrams (See Box 8-2 for dosing facts). Information needed to complete the MRD calculation is:
1. Patient's weight
2. The drug concentration expressed as a percentage, 0.5%, 2%, 3%, or 4%
3. Amount of local anesthetic in a standard cartridge
4. The maximum recommended dose for the selected anesthetic based upon milligrams per pound or mg per kilogram. (See Table 8-1.)

For clinical practicality, this amount can then be converted to maximum number of cartridges per appointment and maximum number of milliliters per appointment. The following are steps for calculating MRDs (Box 8-3).

Step 1: Obtain necessary patient information

The dental hygienist must first obtain the necessary patient information before beginning the drug calculation. The

TABLE 8-1	Maximum Recommended Doses of Local Anesthetic Agents per Appointment for Healthy Patients*

ANESTHETIC	mg/lb	mg/kg	MAXIMUM mg PER APPOINTMENT
Lidocaine	2.0	4.4	300 mg
Mepivacaine	2.0	4.4	300 mg
Prilocaine	2.7	6.0	400 mg
Articaine	3.2	7.0	500 mg
Bupivacaine	0.6	1.3	90 mg

*MRD listed for the local anesthetic drug is determined for anesthetic drug only, not the vasoconstrictor; dosages must be reduced for children, older adults, and medically compromised patients.

BOX 8-2	Dosing Facts for Anesthetic Drugs

1 cartridge = 1.8 mL of solution
Some cartridges are marketed as a minimum of 1.7 mL of solution. In these cases 1.8 mL will be used in all formulas.
1 cc = 1 mL
1.8 cc = 1.8 mL
1 kilogram (kg) = 2.2 pounds (lb)
1 g = 1000 mg
2% solution = 2 g/100 mL so 2% = 2000 mg/100 mL or 20 mg/1 mL
3% solution = 3 g/100 mL so 3% = 3000 mg/100 mL or 30 mg/1 mL
4% solution = 4 g/100 mL so 4% = 4000 mg/100 mL or 40 mg/1 mL
0.5% solution = 0.5 g/100 mL so 0.5% = 500 mg/100 mL or 5 mg/1 mL

BOX 8-1	Limiting Drug

The limiting drug of the anesthetic solution is determined when an anesthetic drug and a vasoconstrictor drug are combined into one cartridge. The limiting drug is the drug (local anesthetic or vasoconstrictor) that reaches its MRD first based upon the patient's medical status. As a rule of thumb, for **healthy** patients, the anesthetic drug in most situations reaches its MRD dose before the vasoconstrictor in all drug concentrations except for one. The exception is when lidocaine 2% 1:50,000 epinephrine is used. In this situation, the vasoconstrictor **may** be the limiting drug.

selection of the anesthetic drug that will be administered will be determined by the treatment to be rendered and the patient's medical history (see Chapter 7). Once the drug is determined, the dental hygienist must obtain the patient's weight to determine the local anesthetic calculation.

Step 2: Calculate milligrams (mg) of selected anesthetic in one cartridge

The number of milligrams of anesthetic solution in one cartridge is determined by the percentage of local anesthetic per milliliter of solution. Most standard local anesthetic cartridges are designed to contain 1.8 mL of solution, some manufacturers label their cartridges as containing a minimum of 1.7 mL of solution (See Box 8-4.)

This small variance will not alter the calculation formula. Therefore, 1.8 mL will be used in all dosing formulas even for cartridges labeled as containing 1.7 mL. Some regional local anesthesia board examinations are currently requiring the candidate to calculate drug doses based on both 1.7 mL and 1.8 mL. A special appendix has been included at the end of this chapter to assist licensure candidates who will be taking these examinations. (See Appendix 8-2 and Box 8-4.)

All anesthetics are labeled with a percentage concentration. A 100% local anesthetic solution contains 1 g (1000 mg) of anesthetic per milliliter of solution, a 10% local anesthetic solution contains 0.1 g (100 mg) of anesthetic per milliliter of solution, and 1% local anesthetic solution contains 0.01 g (10 mg) of local anesthetic per milliliter of solution. You can therefore calculate the number of milligrams of local anesthetic per milliliter by multiplying the percent concentration of local anesthetic agent by 10 mg. A 2% lidocaine solution contains 2×10 mg/mL = 20 mg/mL of lidocaine and a 3% mepivacaine solution contains 3×10 mg/mL = 30 mg/mL of mepivacaine. Because there is 1.8 mL of solution in one cartridge, the dental hygienist should multiply the number of milligrams in 1 mL by 1.8. to get the maximum mg of the selected anesthetic per cartridge.

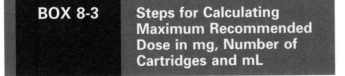

$$2\% \ lidocaine \ 2 \times 10 \ mg/mL$$
$$= 20 \ mg/mL \times 1.8 \ mL \ per \ cartridge = 36 \ mg$$

Table 8-2 lists the local anesthetic concentrations in percentage of solution, mg/mL, and total number of milligrams per cartridge.

BOX 8-3	Steps for Calculating Maximum Recommended Dose in mg, Number of Cartridges and mL

Step 1: Obtain necessary patient information

Step 2: Take the percentage of solution and multiply by 10. Take the answer and multiply by 1.8 = mg of anesthetic per cartridge.

Step 3: Convert pounds to kilograms if using this unit of measurement lb ÷ 2.2 = kg.

Multiply pounds by mg/lb or kilograms by mg/kg (memorize Table 8-1). This number may be different for each anesthetic and gives the MRD in mg.

Step 4: Divide the MRD (step 3) by the number of mg of anesthetic per cartridge (step 2) = maximum number of cartridges.

Step 5 (Optional): Multiply maximum number of cartridges (step 4) by 1.8 (mL in one cartridge) = maximum number of milliliters.

(This unit of measurement is not always needed.)

BOX 8-4	Volume of Anesthetic Per Cartridge

Most standard local anesthetic cartridges distributed in North America are designed to contain 1.8 mL of solution, and drug calculations are based upon this amount. Some manufacturers market their anesthetics as 1.7 mL of solution. This variation is in compliance with the FDA regulations stating that manufacturers must label their anesthetics with a guaranteed amount of solution. Since local anesthetic solutions are filled on by a machine on a conveyor belt there will be slight solution variations of +/- 0.1. Therefore, some manufacturers will guarantee and label their anesthetics with a *minimum* of 1.7 mL of solution. This will not alter the calculation formula of an anesthetic labeled as 1.7 mL and will provide a margin of safety if 1.8 mL of solution is actually in the cartridge. All drug calculations in this chapter will be based upon 1.8 mL of solution in one cartridge of anesthetic.

Some regional local anesthesia board examinations are currently requiring candidates to calculate drug doses based upon the labeled amount of solution: 1.7 mL or 1.8 mL depending on the manufacturer. Licensure candidates must be prepared to alter the calculation formulas with the specified amount of solution identified on the examination. Therefore a special appendix has been included with this chapter that will provide calculation information and dosage tables to assist licensure candidates who will be taking these examinations. (See Appendix 8-2.)

| TABLE 8-2 | Calculation of mg per Cartridge for Varying Anesthetic Concentrations |

LOCAL ANESTHETIC CONCENTRATION (%)	NUMBER OF mg/mL	MULTIPLY BY mg IN ONE CARTRIDGE OF ANESTHETIC	NUMBER OF mg/CARTRIDGE
2%	20	1.8	36
3%	30	1.8	54
4%	40	1.8	72
0.5%	5	1.8	9

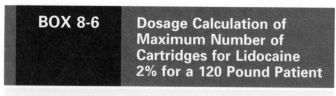

BOX 8-5	Dosage Calculation of MRD for Lidocaine 2% for a 120 Pound Patient

MRD can be calculated based on mg/lb or mg/kg as listed on table 8-1

To calculate milligrams of drug per unit of body weight, *milligrams per pound (mg/lb)*

$$120 \text{ lb} \times 2 \text{ (mg/lb)} = 240 \text{ mg (MRD)}$$

To calculate milligrams of drug per unit of body weight, *milligrams per kilogram (mg/kg)*
To convert pounds to kilograms divide the pounds by 2.2.

$$120 \div 2.2 = 54.5 \text{ kg} \times 4.4 \text{ (mg/kg)} = 240 \text{ mg (MRD)}$$

BOX 8-6	Dosage Calculation of Maximum Number of Cartridges for Lidocaine 2% for a 120 Pound Patient

2% = 36 mg per cartridge (see Table 8-2 and Box 8-2)
MRD = 240 mg (see Box 8-5)
Divide MRD (240 mg) by number of mg per cartridge (36 mg):
240/36 = 6.6 cartridges

BOX 8-7	Dosage Calculation of Maximum Number of Milliliters for Lidocaine 2% for a 120 Pound Patient

Calculating this dose is optional and only needed if maximum mL is required.
2% = 36 mg per cartridge (see Table 8-2 and Box 8-2)
MRD = 240 mg (see Box 8-5)
Maximum cartridges = 6.6 cartridges (see Box 8-6)
Multiply number of cartridges (6.6) by 1.8 mL of solution in one cartridge: 6.6 × 1.8 = 11.8 mL

Step 3: Calculate patient's MRD of anesthetic in mg

The patient's MRD is the dose in mg that can be delivered to a patient in one appointment. For most dental hygiene procedures requiring anesthesia, this dose will most likely never be reached. The dosage calculation for the MRD is based on the patient's weight, and can be calculated based on maximum milligrams per pound (mg/lb) or maximum milligrams per kilogram (mg/kg) (see Table 8-1). To calculate the number of milligrams the patient can receive of the chosen anesthetic, multiply the patient's weight (lbs or kgs) by the MRD (mg/lb or mg/kg) listed in Table 8-1. (See Box 8-5 for dosage calculation example.) The absolute MRD is the absolute maximum dose that any patient can receive per appointment, regardless of their weight. For example, a 200-lb patient can receive only 300 mg of lidocaine 2% even though the calculated number based upon his weight is higher. These MRDs are typically based on healthy adult patients weighing 150 pounds, with only a few exceptions. For lidocaine and mepivacaine the MRD per appointment is 300 mg, and any patient weighing more than 150 pounds should receive no more than 300 mg. of either of these drugs. (Table 8-1 lists MRDs for each local anesthetic drug.)

Step 4: Convert MRD of anesthetic to cartridges

Because local anesthetic solutions are administered in single-use cartridges, the dental hygienist must convert the MRD in milligrams (described in step 3) to the maximum number of cartridges to make this clinically practical. This is accomplished by dividing the MRD in milligrams (step 3) by the number of milligrams per cartridge of anesthetic (step 2). (See Box 8-6 for dosage calculation example).

Step 5 (Optional): Convert maximum cartridges of anesthetic to milliliters

In one cartridge of solution there is 1.8 mL. To convert the maximum number of cartridges to maximum number of milliliters, multiply the number of cartridges by 1.8. (See Box 8-7 for dosage calculation example.) This step is optional and only necessary if the clinician would like to know the maximum number of mL.

CALCULATING MILLIGRAMS OF ANESTHETIC ADMINISTERED

To calculate the milligrams of anesthetic administered, multiply the number of cartridges administered by the number of milligrams of anesthetic in each cartridge. If the dental hygienist administered two cartridges of a 3% drug (mepivacaine):

$$2 \text{ (cartridges)} \times 54 \text{ mg/cartridge (see Table 8-2)}$$
$$= 108 \text{ mg of 3\% mepivacaine was administered.}$$

Then, the number of milligrams administered is the measurement that should be used for chart documentation. Therefore, the dental hygienist should document that the patient received 108 mg of 3% mepivacaine. If the dental hygienist administered less than an entire cartridge, the dental hygienist should determine how much of the cartridge was administered. Helpful tips follow:

- Some manufacturers place volume indicators on the anesthetic cartridges, allowing the clinician to deposit precise volumes of anesthetic or to determine precisely how much anesthetic was delivered (Figure 8-1).
- If the cartridge does not have a volume indicator label, the clinician can determine the local anesthetic volume by the width of the rubber stopper. Each

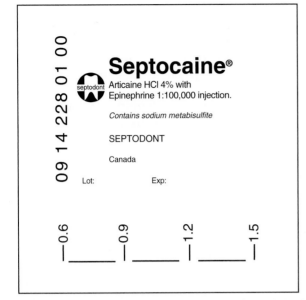

Figure 8-1 ■ Volume indicator label. (Courtesy Septodont, New Castle, Del.)

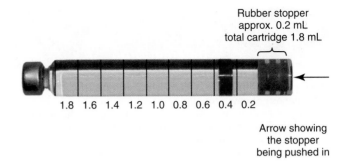

Figure 8-2 ■ Volume of anesthetic deposited by the width of the rubber stopper.

rubber stopper deposits approximately 0.2 mL of solution from a 1.8 mL cartridge (Figure 8-2).

- If the dental hygienist deposited one cartridge and three stoppers of the second cartridge of mepivacaine 3%, the calculation of administered drug would be as follows:

$$1.6 \ (cartridges) \times 54 \ mg/cartridge = 86.4 \ mg \ of \ mepivacaine$$
3% was administered.

CALCULATING ADDITIONAL DOSES OF THE SAME DRUG

If the patient weighs 120 lbs, and the dental hygienist will be administering 3% mepivacine, the patient's MRD is 240 mg.

$$120 \times 2 \ mg/lb = 240 \ mg \ MRD$$

or

$$120 \times 4.4 \ mg/kg = 240 \ MRD$$

As discussed earlier, if the dental hygienist administered two cartridges of 3% mepivacaine, the patient received 108 mg of the MRD of 240 mg. To determine how many more milligrams of drug (mepivacaine) this patient can receive, subtract the MRD (240 mg) by the dose administered (108 mg).

$$240 \ mg - 108 \ mg = 132 \ mg$$

The patient can receive 132 more mg of mepivacaine 3%.

To determine how many more cartridges this patient can receive, divide 132 mg by 54 mg (3% mepivacaine in one cartridge):

$$132 \div 54 \ mg/cartridge = 2.4 \ cartridges$$

The patient can receive 2.4 additional cartridges of 3% mepivacaine.

CALCULATING ADDITIONAL DOSES OF DIFFERENT DRUGS

In some instances, the dental hygienist may need to administer a different anesthetic drug to a patient after a drug has already been administered. Although this is uncommon, the situation may arise, and the dental hygienist must know how to calculate the amount of the new drug he or she can safely administer. There is no guaranteed formula to calculate this number.[3] However, a commonly used method to ensure that the total dose of the two drugs does not exceed the MRD of the most toxic drug, the lower of the two individual MRDs should be used to calculate the amount of the second drug.[3] The following steps describe this method for a 130-lb healthy patient using 2% lidocaine as drug number one (two cartridges already administered) and switching to 4% prilocaine as drug number two as an example: (See Box 8-8 for summary of steps.)

Step 1: Determine a second anesthetic drug that the patient may safely receive. At this point it is important to again consider the patient's medical history to ensure that the patient does not have any contraindications to the new drug. (For this example, prilocaine is drug number two.)

Step 2: Determine how much anesthetic of drug number one (2% lidocaine) has been administered. In this example 2 cartridges of 2% lidocaine was administered.

$$2\% \ solution = 20 \ mg/mL \times 1.8 \ mL \ per \ cartridge$$
$$= 36 \ mg \ in \ one \ cartridge$$

$$2 \ cartridges \ already \ administered: 2 \times 36 \ mg/cartridge$$
$$= 72 \ mg \ of \ 2\% \ lidocaine \ was \ administered$$

Step 3: Calculate the MRD of drug number two (4% prilocaine), and use the lower of the two MRDs as the new MRD. The MRD for lidocaine (260 mg for the 130 pound patient) should have already been determined. This example will be utilizing maximum mg/kg to determine MRD.

$$130\ lbs \div 2.2 = 59\ kg \times 6\ mg/kg\ (for\ prilocaine)$$
$$= 354\ mg\ MRD$$

$$130\ lbs \div 2.2 = 59\ kg \times 4.4\ mg/kg\ (for\ lidocaine)$$
$$= 260\ mg\ MRD$$

Lidocaine is the lower of the two MRDs, and will be used for the remainder of the calculation.

Step 4: Subtract the MRD (260 mg, step 3) by the number of milligrams already administered (step 2):

$$260\ mg - 72\ mg = 188\ mg\ of\ prilocaine\ may\ be\ administered.$$

Step 5: To make this clinically practical, the number of cartridges of prilocaine that can be administered should be calculated. Therefore divide the new MRD (188 mg) by the number of milligrams in one cartridge of 4% prilocaine:

$$4\%\ solution = 40\ mg/mL \times 1.8\ mL\ per\ cartridge$$
$$= 72\ mg\ in\ one\ cartridge$$

$$188\ mg \div 72\ mg = 2.6\ cartridges\ of\ 4\%\ prilocaine\ may\ be\ administered.$$

When might it be needed to switch to a different anesthetic drug during treatment? Although it is usually uncommon to switch anesthetic drugs during treatment, the following are a few examples of when it might be needed to switch to a different drug:

- A cardiac patient may be receiving treatment with lidocaine 2% 1:100,000 epinephrine using the cardiac dose described in chapter 7 for epinephrine. More

anesthetic is needed for treatment, but the MRD for epinephrine for this medically compromised patient (0.04 mg) has been exceeded. The dental hygienist may safely switch to a local anesthetic drug without a vasoconstrictor (such as 3% mepivacaine or 4% prilocaine).

- The dental hygienist administers a local anesthetic drug, but has no more on hand for another dose. The dental hygienist should select a different anesthetic to complete treatment.
- Inadequate anesthesia due to a "bad batch" of anesthetic. This is highly unlikely to occur. Inadequate anesthesia is usually due to improper technique, anatomic variations, or a too-low volume of administered anesthetic. The dental hygienist should attempt to readminister the anesthetic, adjusting his or her technique. If anesthesia is still inadequate after utilizing troubleshooting techniques described in Chapters 12 and 13, the dental hygienist may wish to ask another dental hygienist or dentist in the office to attempt the anesthesia. This should not discourage the dental hygienist. Anatomic variations may make it difficult to achieve successful anesthesia, and a different practitioner using a slightly different technique may be able to successfully achieve anesthesia in the patient.

MAXIMUM RECOMMENDED DOSE OF ANESTHETIC FOR MEDICALLY COMPROMISED PATIENTS, ELDERLY PATIENTS, OR CHILDREN

MRDs of the local anesthetic agent should be decreased for patients with medically compromised situations (see Chapter 7), elderly patients, and children (Table 8-3).

Certain medical conditions described in Table 8-3 may significantly increase the half-life of the administered drug, causing an increase in blood plasma levels of the drug, increasing the risk of an overdose. Moreover, older patients' organ functions may be reduced, decreasing the effectiveness of the organs to biotransform the administered anesthetic and increasing the risk of overdose. There is no guaranteed formula to calculate this number. Therefore the lowest effective dose should be administered, significantly lowering the MRD based on body weight. The dental hygienist should review the dental hygiene care plan, taking into consideration the necessity of lowering the patient's MRD.[3]

The care plan should minimize the extent of treatment completed in one appointment. For example, an appointment for nonsurgical periodontal therapy for two quadrants that could normally be completed in one appointment could be completed in two shorter appointments rather than one longer appointment. This would decrease the amount of local anesthetic needed per appointment, providing safer treatment to the medically compromised or elderly patient.

In contrast, children's organ function may be immature, decreasing the effectiveness of the organs to biotransform

TABLE 8-3	MRD Should Be Decreased in the Following Medically Compromised Situations	
CONDITION	**SIGNIFICANCE**	**MODIFICATION OR ALTERNATIVE DRUG**
Patients taking cimitadine (Tagamet) on a regular basis	Drug reduces capacity of liver to metabolize lidocaine, increasing the half-life of the drug.	Reduce dosage of lidocaine or administer other amides.
Patients taking beta blockers	Inhibits metabolism of amides by decreasing hepatic blood flow, increasing risk of toxic overdose.	Reduce dosage of lidocaine, mepivacaine, or bupivacaine. Articaine may be a safer choice.
Significant liver disease	Inhibits metabolism of amides by decreasing hepatic blood flow, increasing risk of toxic overdose.	Reduce dosage of lidocaine, mepivacaine, or bupivacaine. Articaine may be a safer choice.
Renal dysfunction	Slight risk of toxicity with severe renal dysfunction.	Use esters or amides but use judiciously.
Malignant hyperthermia	Life-threatening syndrome caused by general anesthetics.	Use amides but reduce dosage.
Methemoglobinemia	Potential for clinical cyanosis.	Use amides but do not use prilocaine or topical benzocaine.
Cholinesterase Inhibitors	Inability of esters to be metabolized in the plasma by cholinesterase enzymes. Inability of articaine (amide) to be metabolized in the plasma by cholinesterase enzymes.	Avoid or reduce the dosage of articaine, or use other amides at full dose. Do not use topical esters such as benzocaine or tetracaine; use topical amide lidocaine as a substitution.
Atypical pseudocholinesterase	Inability of esters to be metabolized in the plasma by cholinesterase enzymes. Inability of articaine (amide) to be metabolized in the plasma by cholinesterase enzymes.	Avoid or reduce the dosage of articaine, or use other amides at full dose. Do not use topical esters such as benzocaine or tetracaine; use topical amide lidocaine as a substitution.
Central nervous system depressants (e.g., opioids, opioid derivatives, antianxiety drugs, phenothiazines, barbiturates)	Could potentiate drowsiness. Barbiturates induce hepatic microsomal enzymes and could alter the rate of amide-type local anesthetic metabolism.	Decrease the dosage of amides.

the administered anesthetic, increasing the risk of overdose. In addition, calculating the child's MRD based on their weight may indicate that an overweight child could receive 300 mg (approximately a 150-lb child) of lidocaine. This amount of anesthetic may not be biotransformed effectively due to immature organs. Again, there is no guaranteed formula to calculate this number. Therefore the lowest effective dose should be administered in this situation, significantly lowering the MRD based on body weight.

The dental hygienist should review the dental hygiene care plan, taking into consideration the necessity of lowering the patient's MRD.[3] The care plan should minimize the extent of treatment completed in one appointment.

The need for local anesthesia to be administered by the dental hygienist to a pediatric patient is rare, since these patients typically do not require nonsurgical periodontal therapy. However, in some instances, the dentist performing restorative work on children may ask the dental hygienist to administer the local anesthetic. Moreover, if a pediatric patient has a back-to-back appointment, first with the dental hygienist and second with the dentist for restorative work, it may be more time efficient for the dental hygienist to administer the local anesthesia for the restorative work prior to moving the patient into the dentist's chair.

■ VASOCONSTRICTOR DOSES

When administering local anesthetics with vasoconstrictors, the local anesthetic solution will have two potentially limiting drugs: (1) the dose of local anesthetic agent, and (2) the dose of the accompanying vasoconstrictor. Either of these agents may be the limiting drug in determining maximum dose of any particular local anesthetic depending upon the patient's medical status (see Box 8-1).

You will recall that local anesthetics are frequently labeled with two concentrations of drugs. Lidocaine 2% with 1:100,000 epinephrine means that the concentration of lidocaine in the cartridge is 2% and the concentration of epinephrine is 1 gram in 100,000 mL of solution. These two different concentrations are in no way related and each must be considered independently.

VASOCONSTRICTOR CONCENTRATIONS

Vasoconstrictor concentrations are always expressed as a ratio. It is necessary to be able to convert this ratio to the number of milligrams of vasoconstrictor per milliliter of solution because the maximum doses are expressed in milligram amounts. For example, the maximum dose of epinephrine for a healthy adult is 0.2 mg (discussed next).

TABLE 8-4	Volume of Vasoconstrictor Drug	
CONCENTRATION 1 g/mL OF SOLUTION	MILLIGRAMS PER MILLILITER	MILLIGRAMS PER CARTRIDGE mg/mL × 1.8
1:20,000	0.05	0.09
1:50,000	0.02	0.036
1:100,000	0.01	0.018
1:200,000	0.005	0.009

TABLE 8-5	Recommended Maximum Dosages of Vasoconstrictors			
CONCENTRATION	MAXIMUM RECOMMENDED DOSE PER APPOINTMENT HEALTHY PATIENT	NUMBER OF CARTRIDGES HEALTHY PATIENT (ASA I)	MAXIMUM RECOMMENDED DOSE PER APPOINTMENT PATIENT WITH CARDIOVASCULAR DISEASE (ASA III OR IV)	NUMBER OF CARTRIDGES PATIENT WITH CARDIOVASCULAR DISEASE
1:50,000 Epinephrine	0.2 mg	5.5	0.04 mg	1.1
1:100,000 Epinephrine	0.2 mg	11.1	0.04 mg	2.2
1:200,000 Epinephrine	0.2 mg	22.2	0.04 mg	4.4
1:20,000 Levonordefrin	1.0 mg	11.1	0.2 mg	2.2

It is necessary to understand that 1:1000 means that there is 1 g (1000 mg) of vasoconstrictor in 1000 mL of solution or 1 mg of vasoconstrictor in 1 mL of solution. A 1:10,000 solution contains 1 mg vasoconstrictor in 10 mL of solution or 0.1 mg of vasoconstrictor in 1 mL of solution, and a 1:100,000 solution contains 0.01 mg of vasoconstrictor in 1 mL of solution (Table 8-4).

MAXIMUM RECOMMENDED DOSE FOR VASOCONSTRICTOR DRUGS

The maximum doses for vasoconstrictor drugs are based on recommendations from the American Heart Association and the New York Heart Association.[3,4] Maximum doses of vasoconstrictors are calculated based on the recommended dose for a "healthy" individual and a "compromised" individual, and are not dependent upon the patient's weight as determined in the calculation of MRDs for the local anesthetic drug. For healthy individuals the MRD for epinephrine is 0.2 mg per appointment, and 1.0 mg for levonordefrin. When limits of vasoconstrictors are needed for patients with ischemic heart disease, this is referred to as the cardiac dose. The cardiac dose for epinephrine is 0.04 mg per appointment, and 0.2 mg for levonordefrin. See Table 8-5 for the maximum recommended doses of vasoconstrictors. See Chapter 7 for information on "healthy" verses "compromised" conditions affecting the selection and dosage of local anesthetics and vasoconstrictors.

BOX 8-9	Dosing Facts for Vasoconstrictors

1 Cartridge = 1.8 mL of solution
Some cartridges are marketed as a minimum of 1.7 mL of solution. In these cases 1.8 mL will be used in all formulas.
1 cc = 1 mL
1.8 cc = 1.8 mL
1 g = 1000 mg
Max dose of epinephrine for a healthy patient = 0.2 mg
Max dose of epinephrine for a patient with significant cardiovascular disease = 0.04 mg (cardiac dose)
Max dose of levonordefrin for a healthy patient = 1.0 mg
Max dose of levonordefrin for a patient with significant cardiovascular disease = 0.2 mg (cardiac dose)

CALCULATING VASOCONSTRICTOR DRUG DOSES

Several easy steps to follow in calculating drug doses for vasoconstrictors are described in the following sections (Boxes 8-9 and 8-10).

Step 1: Obtain necessary patient information

The dental hygienist must first obtain the necessary patient information before beginning the drug calculation. The selection of the drug to be administered will be determined by the treatment to be rendered and the patient's medical history (see Chapter 7). From the patient's medical history, the dental hygienist determines whether the patient requires the cardiac dose of vasoconstrictor or the dose for a healthy patient. Once this is determined, the dental hygienist can calculate the safe dose of the selected vasoconstrictor.

Step 2: Calculate milligrams of vasoconstrictor in one cartridge of anesthetic

Using a $1:100,000$ epinephrine concentration as an example, this ratio contains 1 g, or 1000 mg, of vasoconstrictor diluted in 100,000 mL of solution. The ratio must be converted to the amount of vasoconstrictor per milliliter of solution because the maximum doses are expressed in milligram amounts. Because there is 1.8 mL of solution in one cartridge, this number must be multiplied by 1.8 to calculate the number of milligrams in one cartridge. In this example there are 0.018 mg of vasoconstrictor drug per cartridge. Calculation and unit conversions for each of the vasoconstrictor concentrations used in dentistry are listed in Table 8-6.

Step 3: Obtain MRD of vasoconstrictor

Because the dose calculation for vasoconstrictors is not dependent upon the patient's weight, there is no need to calculate the MRD as shown earlier in step 3 of the anesthetic drug calculation. There are only two MRDs for vasoconstrictors: (1) healthy patient (MRD 0.2 mg per appointment for epinephrine and 1.0 mg for levonordefrin); (2) patients with significant cardiovascular disease (MRD 0.04 mg per appointment for epinephrine and 0.2 mg for levonordefrin). (See table 8-5 for maximum doses of vasoconstrictors.)

Step 4: Convert MRD of vasoconstrictor to cartridges

Because local anesthetic solutions with vasoconstrictors are administered in single-use cartridges, the dental hygienist must convert the MRD in milligrams (described in step 3) to the maximum number of cartridges to make this application clinically practical. This is accomplished by dividing the MRD in milligrams (step 3) by the number of milligrams of vasoconstrictor per cartridge of anesthetic (step 2).

For a healthy patient receiving 1:100,000 epinephrine :

0.2 mg (MRD) ÷ 0.018 mg/cartridge = 11.1 cartridges

For patients with significant cardiovascular disease receiving 1:100,000 epinephrine:

0.04 mg (MRD) ÷ 0.018 mg/cartridge = 4.4 cartridges

Table 8-7 lists dosage calculations of each vasoconstrictor concentration. Since these calculations are not dependent upon the patient's weight, these numbers should be memorized for the healthy and cardiac doses.

Step 5 (Optional): Convert maximum cartridges of vasoconstrictor to milliliters

In one cartridge of solution, there is 1.8 mL. To convert the maximum number of cartridges to the milliliters, multiply the number of cartridges by 1.8. (Example $1:100,000$ epinephrine healthy patient: 11.1 cartridges maximum × 1.8 mL = 19.98 mL maximum.)

CALCULATING MILLIGRAMS OF VASOCONSTRICTOR ADMINISTERED

Calculating the milligrams of vasoconstrictor administered utilizes the same principles as used for calculating the milligrams administered for the anesthetic. Multiply the number of cartridges administered by the number of

---

BOX 8-10 — Calculating Vasoconstrictor Maximum Drug Doses

Step 1: Obtain necessary patient information utilizing the patient's medical history form.
Step 2: Calculate the milligrams (mg) of vasoconstrictor in one cartridge of the anesthetic. (See Tables 8-4 and 8-6.)
Step 3: Obtain the MRD (healthy vs. cardiac dose).
Step 4: Convert MRD to cartridges. Divide the MRD (step 3) by the number of mg per cartridge (step 2) = maximum number of cartridges.
Step 5 (Optional): Convert maximum cartridges to milliliters Multiply maximum number of cartridges (step 4) by 1.8 (maximum mL per cartridge) = maximum number of mL.

TABLE 8-6 — Calculation and Unit Conversions of Vasoconstrictor Concentrations

RATIO	UNIT CONVERSION TO mg/mL	MILLIGRAMS PER CARTRIDGE
1:20,000	$\frac{1000 \text{ mg}}{20,000 \text{ mL}} = \frac{1 \text{ mg}}{20 \text{ mL}} = \frac{0.05 \text{ mg}}{1 \text{ mL}}$ of solution	0.05 mg/mL × 1.8 mL = 0.09 mg
1:50,000	$\frac{1000 \text{ mg}}{50,000 \text{ mL}} = \frac{1 \text{ mg}}{50 \text{ mL}} = \frac{0.02 \text{ mg}}{1 \text{ mL}}$ of solution	0.02 mg/mL × 1.8 mL = 0.036 mg
1:100,000	$\frac{1000 \text{ mg}}{100,000 \text{ mL}} = \frac{1 \text{ mg}}{100 \text{ mL}} = \frac{0.01 \text{ mg}}{1 \text{ mL}}$ of solution	0.01 mg/mL × 1.8 mL = 0.018 mg
1:200,000	$\frac{1000 \text{ mg}}{200,000 \text{ mL}} = \frac{1 \text{ mg}}{200 \text{ mL}} = \frac{0.005 \text{ mg}}{1 \text{ mL}}$ of solution	0.005 mg/mL × 1.8 mL = 0.009 mg

1 gram = 1000 mg

TABLE 8-7	Conversion of MRD Vasoconstrictors to Maximum Number of Cartridges

Conversion of MRD (Healthy Patient = 0.2 mg) of Epinephrine to Maximum Number of Cartridges

CONCENTRATION	mg/CARTRIDGE	CONVERSION TO MAXIMUM NUMBER OF CARTRIDGES MRD ÷ mg PER CARTRIDGE
1:50,000	0.036	0.2 mg ÷ 0.036 mg = 5.5 cartridges
1:100,000	0.018	0.2 mg ÷ 0.018 mg = 11.1 cartridges
1:200,000	0.009	0.2 mg ÷ 0.009 mg = 22.2 cartridges

Conversion of MRD (Cardiac Dose = 0.04 mg) of Epinephrine to Maximum Number of Cartridges

CONCENTRATION	mg/CARTRIDGE	CONVERSION TO MAXIMUM NUMBER OF CARTRIDGES MRD ÷ mg PER CARTRIDGE
1:50,000	0.036	0.04 mg ÷ 0.036 mg = 1.1 cartridges
1:100,000	0.018	0.04 mg ÷ 0.018 mg = 2.2 cartridges
1:200,000	0.009	0.04 mg ÷ 0.009 mg = 4.4 cartridges

Conversion of MRD (Healthy Patient = 1.0 mg) of Levonordefrin to Maximum Number of Cartridges

CONCENTRATION	mg/CARTRIDGE	CONVERSION TO MAXIMUM NUMBER OF CARTRIDGES MRD ÷ mg PER CARTRIDGE
1:20,000	0.09	1.0 mg ÷ 0.09 mg = 11.1 cartridges

Conversion of MRD (Compromised Patient = 0.2 mg) of Levonordefrin to Maximum Number of Cartridges

CONCENTRATION	mg/CARTRIDGE	CONVERSION TO MAXIMUM NUMBER OF CARTRIDGES MRD ÷ mg PER CARTRIDGE
1:20,000	0.09	0.2 mg ÷ 0.09 mg = 2.2 cartridges

milligrams of vasoconstrictor in each cartridge. If the dental hygienist administered two cartridges of 2% lidocaine 1:100,000, then:

$$2\ (cartridges) \times 36 = 72\ mg\ of\ lidocaine\ administered.$$

$$2\ (cartridges) \times 0.018 = 0.036\ mg\ of\ epinephrine\ administered.$$

CALCULATING ADDITIONAL DOSES OF THE SAME VASOCONSTRICTOR

If the patient's MRD of epinephrine is 0.2 mg and the dental hygienist administered two cartridges of 2% lidocaine 1:100,000 epinephrine, then the patient received 0.036 mg of the MRD of 0.2 mg. To determine how many more milligrams of drug this patient can receive, subtract the MRD by the total dose delivered:

$$0.2 - 0.036 = 0.164\ mg$$

The patient can receive 0.164 mg more of epinephrine 1:100,000.

To determine how many more cartridges this patient can receive, divide the remaining amount of epinephrine the patient can receive (0.164 mg) by the number of milligrams of vasoconstrictor in each cartridge (0.018 mg):

$$0.164 \div 0.018 = 9.1\ cartridges$$

The patient can receive 9.1 additional cartridges of 1:100,000 epinephrine.

DETERMINING THE LIMITING DRUG

As previously discussed, when a local anesthetic agent and a vasoconstrictor are combined in an anesthetic cartridge, the dental hygienist must determine which of the two drugs is the limiting drug. The limiting drug will be the drug that limits the amount of solution that can be safely administered based upon the patient's medical status. For example, the absolute maximum recommended dose of 2% lidocaine, 1:100,000 epinephrine for a healthy patient is 300 mg or 8.3 cartridges of lidocaine, and 0.2 mg or 11.1 cartridges of epinephrine. Since 8.3 cartridges is the lower number, in this example the local anesthetic is the limiting drug. In contrast, for a patient with ischemic heart disease, the MRD for epinephrine is 0.04 mg or 2.2 cartridges, and 300 mg or 8.3 cartridges of lidocaine. Since 2.2 cartridges is the lower number, in this example the vasoconstrictor is the limiting drug.

DENTAL HYGIENE CONSIDERATIONS

- The MRD of an anesthetic containing a vasoconstrictor is dependent upon which of the two drugs reaches its MRD first.
- The limiting drug is the drug that limits the total amount of volume delivered.
- The anesthetic agent is usually the limiting drug for healthy patients unless lidocaine 2% 1 : 50,000 is used, and then the vasoconstrictor may be the limiting drug.
- The dental hygienist must obtain necessary medical history information before determining the MRD.
- The MRD for epinephrine for a healthy patient is 0.2 mg per appointment and 0.04 mg per appointment for patients with significant cardiovascular disease.

- The MRD for levonordefrin for a healthy patient is 1.0 mg per appointment and 0.2 mg per appointment for patients with significant cardiovascular disease.
- MRDs of local anesthetic agents should be decreased for patients with medically compromised health, older adults, and children. There is no guaranteed formula; therefore the minimal effective dose should be administered.
- Local anesthetic drugs are expressed in percentages, and vasoconstrictor drugs are expressed in ratios.

CASE STUDY

Dr. Colvin asks the dental hygienist to switch anesthetics

A patient is in your office for restorative work. The dentist you work for cannot achieve numbness in the patient, because he says the anesthetic is "bad." He asks the dental hygienist for assistance. He administered two cartridges of prilocaine 4% 1 : 200,000 and tells you to switch to 2% lidocaine 1 : 100,000. The patient's blood pressure is 128/90 mm Hg and her weight is 140 lb. She has a history of hepatitis B 10 years ago.

Critical Thinking Questions:
- What medical history issues should be considered for lidocaine?
- How many more milligrams and cartridges of lidocaine can be safely administered to this patient?
- Should the dental hygienist switch the anesthetic? Why or why not?

CHAPTER REVIEW QUESTIONS

1. The cardiac dose of epinephrine is:
   A. 0.02 mg
   B. 0.04 mg
   C. 0.2 mg
   D. 0.4 mg
   E. 2 mg
2. What does 2% local anesthetic solution mean?
   A. 2 mg per 100 mL
   B. 2000 mg per 100 mL
   C. 20 mg per 1 mL
   D. All of the above
3. The dental hygienist administered 2.3 cartridges of 3% mepivacaine. How many cc were administered?
   A. 3.24 cc
   B. 4.80 cc
   C. 4.14 cc
   D. 3.98 cc
4. What is the MRD dose of 2% lidocaine for a 120-lb patient?
   A. 240 mg
   B. 280 mg

   C. 230 mg
   D. 300 mg
5. How many cartridges of lidocaine 2% 1 : 100,000 epinephrine can be safely administered to a 120 pound patient taking tricyclic antidepressants?
   A. 1.1 cartridges
   B. 2.2 cartridges
   C 3.3 cartridges
   D. 4.4 cartridges
6. How many cartridges of prilocaine 4% can a healthy 150 pound patient receive?
   A. Three cartridges
   B. Four cartridges
   C. Five cartridges
   D. Six cartridges

For questions 7–13 use the following information to answer the questions.

A 140 lb healthy patient received 2.5 cartridges of 2% lidocaine 1 : 100,000 epinephrine. The dental hygienist reaches for another cartridge and realizes there is no more 2% lidocaine. The dental hygienist

CHAPTER REVIEW QUESTIONS

decides to switch to 4% articaine 1:200,000 epinephrine.

7. What is the MRD for lidocaine?
   A. 289 mg
   B. 269 mg
   C. 280 mg
   D. 299 mg

8. How many milligrams of lidocaine did the dental hygienist administer?
   A. 80 mg
   B. 90 mg
   C. 75 mg
   D. 85 mg

9. What is the MRD for articaine?
   A. 400 mg
   B. 420 mg
   C. 445 mg
   D. 435 mg

10. How many more milligrams of articaine can be administered to this patient?
    A. 190 mg more
    B. 179 mg more
    C. 169 mg more
    D. 199 mg more

11. How many more cartridges of articaine can be administered to this patient?
    A. 2.6 cartridges
    B. 2.5 cartridges
    C. 2.7 cartridges
    D. 2.8 cartridges

12. How many more milliliters of articaine can be administered?
    A. 4.7 mL
    B. 4.4 mL
    C. 4.9 mL
    D. 5.0 mL

13. Assuming the maximum dose was administered, how many milligrams of epinephrine were administered to this patient?
    A. 0.055 mg of epinephrine
    B. 0.099 mg of epinephrine
    C. 0.068 mg of epinephrine
    D. 0.088 mg of epinephrine

14. What is the cardiac dose for levonordefrin?
    A. 0.2 mg
    B. 0.04 mg

C. 0.02 mg
D. 1 mg

15. How many milligrams are in one cartridge of 4% articaine?
    A. 72 mg
    B. 68 mg
    C. 54 mg
    D. 9 mg

16. What is the absolute maximum dose of bupivacaine?
    A. 80 mg
    B. 70 mg
    C. 100 mg
    D. 90 mg

17. How many cartridges of prilocaine 4% with epinephrine can a 130-lb patient with significant cardiovascular disease receive?
    A. 2.2 cartridges
    B. 4.9 cartridges
    C. 4.4 cartridges
    D. 5.9 cartridges

18. The dental hygienist administered three cartridges of mepivacaine 3% to a 170-lb patient. How many more cartridges of mepivacaine can the dental hygienist administer to complete the treatment?
    A. 2.5 more
    B. 3.2 more
    C. 3.8 more
    D. 1.8 more

19. What is the absolute number of milligrams of epinephrine 1:50,000 a patient with significant cardiovascular disease may receive?
    A. 0.072 mg
    B. 0.029 mg
    C. 0.039 mg
    D. 0.049 mg

20. What is the MRD for 0.5% bupivacaine for a 102-lb patient?
    A. 70 mg
    B. 60 mg
    C. 80 mg
    D. 50 mg

REFERENCES

1. ADA Council on Scientific Affairs: *ADA guide to dental therapeutics*, ed 2, Chicago, 2000, American Dental Association.

2. USP DI Updates On-line, United States Pharmacopeial Convention, Inc., www.usp.org.

3. Malamed S: *Handbook of local anesthesia*, ed 5, St Louis, 2004, Mosby.

4. Special Committee of the New York Heart Association: Use of epinephrine with procaine in dental procedures, *J Am Dent Assoc* 50:108, 1955.

Summary of Local Anesthetics Agents and Vasoconstrictors

Anesthetic	Concentration of anesthetic agent (expressed in percentage)	Amount of anesthetic agent (mg/ml)	Amount of anesthetic agent per cartridge (mg/cartridge) (mg per 1 mL x 1.8)	Maximum dose of anesthetic agent (mg/lb)	Maximum dose of anesthetic agent (mg/kg)	Maximum recommended dose (MRD) anesthetic per appointment	Number of cartridges needed to reach MRD of limiting agent (healthy patient)	Vasoconstrictor formulations (expressed in ratios)
Lidocaine (Xylocaine) Many generics	2%	20 mg/ml	36 mg	2.0 mg/lb	4.4 mg/kg	300 mg	8.3	Plain / 1:50,000 epinephrine / 1:100,000 epinephrine
Mepivacaine (Carbocaine or Polocaine)	3%	30 mg/ml	54 mg	2.0 mg/lb	4.4 mg/kg	300 mg	5.5	No vasoconstrictor in this concentration
Mepivacaine (Carbocaine, Polocaine)	2%	20 mg/ml	36 mg	2.0 mg/lb	4.4 mg/kg	300 mg	8.3	Levonordefrin or Neo-Cobefrin in 1:20,000
Prilocaine (Citanest)	4%	40 mg/ml	72 mg	2.7 mg/lb	6 mg/kg	400 mg	5.5	No vasoconstrictor in Citanest Plain / 1:200,000 epinephrine in Citanest Forte
Articaine (Septocaine)	4%	40 mg/ml	72 mg	3.2 mg/lb	7 mg/kg	500 mg	6.9	1:100,000 epinephrine / 1:200,000 epinephrine
Bupivacaine (Marcaine)	0.5%	5 mg/ml	9 mg	0.6 mg/lb	1.3 mg/kg	90 mg	10	1:200,000 epinephrine

Dosing Information for Regional Board Examinations Requiring Calculations Based on 1.7 mL of Solution

Some regional local anesthesia board examinations are currently requiring candidates to calculate drug doses based upon the labeled amount of solution: 1.7 mL or 1.8 mL depending on the manufacturer. Licensure candidates must be prepared to alter the calculation formulas with the specified amount of solution identified on the examination. Drug dosing information for regional local anesthesia board examinations requiring calculations based on 1.7 mL of solution are provided in this appendix. Appendix Table 8-1 provides step by step drug calculation information, and

Appendix Table 8-2 provides a drug calculation example. Appendix Tables 8-4–8-8 provide dosage information for each local anesthetic agent.

Board examination testing requirements are reviewed annually by examination committees, and changes are made annually for local anesthetic board examinations. The companion Evolve Website will provided updated information in the *content update section* and the *board examinations section* of the website. Licensure candidates should review the website periodically for new updates.

APPENDIX TABLE 8-1	Steps for Calculating Maximum Recommended Dose in mg, Number of Cartridges and mL Based on 1.7 mL of Solution

Step 1: Determine the number of mg in one cartridge of solution
Take the percentage of solution and multiply by 10
Take the answer and multiply by 1.7 = mg per cartridge (See also Appendix Table 8-3)
Step 2: Convert pounds to kilograms if using this unit of measurement lb ÷ 2.2 = kg
Multiply pounds by mg/lb or kilograms by mg/kg (memorize Table 8-1). This number may be different for each anesthetic and gives the MRD in mg.
Step 3: Divide the MRD (step 2) by the number of mg per cartridge (step 1) = maximum number of cartridges
Step 4: (Optional) Multiply maximum number of cartridges (step 3) by 1.7 (mL in one cartridge) = maximum number of milliliters

APPENDIX TABLE 8-2	Example Dosage Calculation of MRD in mg, Number of Cartridges and mL Based on 1.7 mL of Solution for Lidocaine 2% for a 120 Pound Patient

Step 1: Determine the number of mg in one cartridge of solution
2% solution = 2 × 10 = 20 × 1.7 = 34 mg in one cartridge (see Appendix Table 8-3)
Step 2: Calculate the MRD
MRD can be calculated based on mg/lb or mg/kg as listed on Table 8-1
To calculate milligrams of drug per unit of body weight, *milligrams per pound (mg/lb)*
120 lb × 2 (mg/lb) = 240 mg (MRD)
To calculate milligrams of drug per unit of body weight, *milligrams per kilogram (mg/kg)*
To convert pounds to kilograms divide the pounds by 2.2.
120 ÷ 2.2 = 54.5 kg × 4.4 (mg/kg) = 240 mg (MRD)
2% = 34 mg per cartridge
Step 3: Determine the maximum number of cartridges
Divide MRD (240 mg) by number of mg per cartridge (34 mg)
240/34 = 7.0 cartridges
Step 4: (Optional) Determine the maximum number of mL
Multiply number of cartridges (7.0) by number of mL in one cartridge (1.7)
7.0 × 1.7 = 11.9 mL

APPENDIX TABLE 8-3	Calculation of mg per Cartridge for Varying Anesthetic Concentrations Based on 1.7 mL of Solution

LOCAL ANESTHETIC CONCENTRATION (%)	NUMBER OF mg/mL	MULTIPLY BY mg IN ONE CARTRIDGE OF ANESTHETIC	NUMBER OF mg/CARTRIDGE
2%	20	1.7	34
3%	30	1.7	51
4%	40	1.7	68
0.5%	5	1.7	8.5

APPENDIX TABLE 8-4	Lidocaine Maximum Recommended Doses Healthy Patient Based on 1.7 mL of Solution

Lidocaine Maximum Recommended Doses Healthy Patient Based on 1.7 mL of Solution						
2% plain			2% 1:50,000 epinephrine		2% 1:100,000 epinephrine	
Maximum milligrams and cartridges based upon body weight 2% solution = 34 mg/cartridge 4.4 mg/kg 2 mg/lb Absolute Maximum Recommended Dose = 300 mg Limiting drug "anesthetic" except for 1:50,000 formulation						
Weight kg	Maximum mg (4.4 mg/kg)	Maximum cartridges	Weight lbs	Maximum mg (2 mg/lb)	Maximum cartridges	
10	44	1.3	30	60	1.7	
20	88	2.5	50	100	2.9	
30	132	3.8	70	140	4.1	
40	176	5.1	90	180	5.2	
50	220	6.4	110	220	6.4	
60	264	7.7	130	260	7.6	
65	286	8.4	140	280	8.2	
70	308 (300 max)	9.0 (8.8 max)	150	300	8.8	
80	352 (300 max)	10.3 (8.8 max)	170	340 (300 max)	10.0 (8.8 max)	
90	396 (300 max)	11.6 (8.8 max)	190	380 (300 max)	11.1 (8.8 max)	
100	440 (300 max)	12.9 (8.8 max)	210	420 (300 max)	12.3 (8.8 max)	
Above absolute maximum dose of 300 mg and 8.8 cartridges			Above absolute maximum dose of 300 mg and 8.8 cartridges			
Absolute maximum dose for 2% lidocaine 1:50,000 is 5 cartridges The vasoconstrictor is the limiting drug in 1:50,000 epinephrine formulation						

APPENDIX TABLE 8-5	Mepivacaine Maximum Recommended Doses Healthy Patient Based on 1.7 mL of Solution

Mepivacaine Maximum Recommended Doses Healthy Patient Based on 1.7 mL of Solution

Maximum milligrams and cartridges based upon body weight
2% solution = 34 mg/cartridge
3% solution = 51 mg/cartridge
4.4 mg/kg
2 mg/lb
Absolute Maximum Recommended Dose = 300 mg

Limiting drug "anesthetic"

2% 1:20,000 levonordefrin					
Weight kg	Maximum mg (4.4 mg/kg)	Maximum cartridges	Weight lbs	Maximum mg (2 mg/lb)	Maximum cartridges
10	44	1.3	30	60	1.7
20	88	2.5	50	100	2.9
30	132	3.8	70	140	4.1
40	176	5.1	90	180	5.2
50	220	6.4	110	220	6.4
60	264	7.7	130	260	7.6
65	286	8.4	140	280	8.2
70	308 (300 max)	9.0 (8.8 max)	150	300	8.8
80	352 (300 max)	10.3 (8.8 max)	170	340 (300 max)	10.0 (8.8 max)
90	396 (300 max)	11.6 (8.8 max)	190	380 (300 max)	11.1 (8.8 max)
100	440 (300 max)	12.9 (8.8 max)	210	420 (300 max)	12.8 (8.8 max)
Above absolute maximum dose of 300 mg and 8.8 cartridges			Above absolute maximum dose of 300 mg and 8.8 cartridges		
3% plain					
Weight kg	Maximum mg (4.4 mg/kg)	Maximum cartridges	Weight lbs (2 mg/lb)	Maximum mg	Maximum cartridges
10	44	0.9	30	60	1.2
20	88	1.7	50	100	1.9
30	132	2.5	70	140	2.7
40	176	3.4	90	180	3.5
50	220	4.3	110	220	4.3
60	264	5.1	130	260	5.0
65	286	5.6	140	280	5.4
70	308 (300 max)	6.0 (5.8 max)	150	300	5.8
80	352 (300 max)	6.9 (5.8 max)	170	340 (300 max)	6.6 (5.8 max)
90	396 (300 max)	7.7 (5.8 max)	190	380 (300 max)	7.4 (5.8 max)
100	440 (300 max)	8.6 (5.8 max)	210	420 (300 max)	8.2 (5.8 max)
Above absolute maximum dose of 300 mg and 5.8 cartridges			Above absolute maximum dose of 300 mg and 5.8 cartridges		

APPENDIX TABLE 8-6	Prilocaine Maximum Recommended Doses Healthy Patient Based on 1.7 mL of Solution

Prilocaine Maximum Recommended Doses Healthy Patient Based on 1.7 mL of Solution

4% plain			4% 1:200,000 epinephrine		
Maximum milligrams and cartridges based upon body weight 4% solution = 68 mg/cartridge 6 mg/kg 2.7 mg/lb Absolute Maximum Recommended Dose = 400 mg Limiting drug "anesthetic"					
Weight kg	Maximum mg (6 mg/kg)	Maximum cartridges	Weight lbs	Maximum mg (2.7 mg/lb)	Maximum cartridges
10	60	0.88	30	81	1.2
20	120	1.7	50	135	1.9
30	180	2.6	70	189	2.7
40	240	3.5	90	243	3.5
50	300	4.4	110	297	4.3
60	360	5.2	130	351	5.1
65	390	5.7	140	378	5.5
70	420 (400 max)	6.1 (5.8 max)	150	405 (400 max)	5.9 (5.8 max)
80	480 (400 max)	7.0 (5.8 max)	170	459 (400 max)	6.7 (5.8 max)
90	540 (400 max)	7.9 (5.8 max)	190	513 (400 max)	7.5 (5.8 max)
100	600 (400 max)	8.8 (5.8 max)	210	567 (400 max)	8.3 (5.8 max)
Above absolute maximum dose of 400 mg and 5.8 cartridges			Above absolute maximum dose of 400 mg and 5.8 cartridges		

APPENDIX TABLE 8-7	Articaine Maximum Recommended Doses Healthy Patient Based on 1.7 mL of Solution

Articaine Maximum Recommended Doses Healthy Patient Based on 1.7 mL of Solution

4% 1:100,000 epinephrine			4% 1:200,000 epinephrine		
Maximum milligrams and cartridges based upon body weight 4% solution = 68 mg/cartridge 7 mg/kg 3.2 mg/lb Absolute Maximum Recommended Dose = 500 mg Limiting drug "anesthetic"					
Weight kg	Maximum mg (7 mg/kg)	Maximum cartridges	Weight lbs	Maximum mg (3.2 mg/lb)	Maximum cartridges
10	70	1.0	30	96	1.4
20	140	2.0	50	160	2.3
30	210	3.0	70	224	3.2
40	280	4.1	90	288	4.2
50	350	5.1	110	352	5.1
60	420	6.1	130	416	6.1
65	455	6.6	140	448	6.5
70	490	7.2	150	480	7.0
80	560 (500 max)	8.2 (7.3 max)	170	544 (500 max)	8.1 (7.3 max)
90	630 (500 max)	9.2 (7.3 max)	190	608 (500 max)	8.9 (7.3 max)
100	700 (500 max)	10.2 (7.3 max)	210	672 (500 max)	9.8 (7.3 max)
Above absolute maximum dose of 500 mg and 7.3 cartridges			Above absolute maximum dose of 500 mg and 7.3 cartridges		

APPENDIX TABLE 8-8	Bupivacaine Maximum Recommended Doses Healthy Patient Based on 1.7 mL of Solution

Bupivacaine Maximum Recommended Doses Healthy Patient Based on 1.7 mL of Solution					
0.5% 1:200,000 epinephrine					
Maximum milligrams and cartridges based upon body weight 0.5% solution = 8.5 mg/cartridge 1.3 mg/kg 0.6 mg/lb Absolute Maximum Recommended Dose = 90 mg Limiting drug "anesthetic"					
Weight kg	Maximum mg (1.3 mg/kg)	Maximum cartridges	Weight lbs	Maximum mg (0.6 mg/lb)	Maximum cartridges
10	13	1.5	30	18	2.1
20	26	3.0	50	30	3.5
30	39	4.5	70	42	4.9
40	52	6.1	90	54	6.3
50	65	7.6	110	66	7.7
60	78	9.1	130	78	9.1
65	85	10.0	140	84	9.8
70	91	10.7	150	90	10.5
80	104 (90 max)	12.2 (10.5 max)	170	102 (90 max)	12.0 (10.5 max)
90	117 (90 max)	13.7 (10.5 max)	190	114 (90 max)	13.4 (10.5 max)
100	130 (90 max)	15.2 (10.5 max)	210	126 (90 max)	14.8 (10.5 max)
Above absolute maximum dose of 90 mg and 10.5 cartridges			Above absolute maximum dose of 90 mg and 10.5 cartridges		

APPENDIX TABLE 8-9	Volume of Vasoconstrictor Drug

CONCENTRATION 1 g/mL OF SOLUTION	MILLIGRAMS PER MILLILITER	MILLIGRAMS PER CARTRIDGE mg/mL × 1.7
1:20,000	0.05	0.085
1:50,000	0.02	0.034
1:100,000	0.01	0.017
1:200,000	0.005	0.008

APPENDIX TABLE 8-10	Recommended Maximum Dosages of Vasoconstrictors

CONCENTRATION	MAXIMUM RECOMMENDED DOSE (MRD) PER APPOINTMENT HEALTHY PATIENT	NUMBER OF CARTRIDGES HEALTHY PATIENT (ASA I) BASED ON 1.7 mL OF SOLUTION	MAXIMUM RECOMMENDED DOSE (MRD) PER APPOINTMENT PATIENT WITH CARDIOVASCULAR DISEASE (ASA III OR IV)	NUMBER OF CARTRIDGES PATIENT WITH CARDIOVASCULAR DISEASE BASED ON 1.7 mL OF SOLUTION
1:50,000 Epinephrine	0.2 mg	5.8	0.04 mg	1.2
1:100,000 Epinephrine	0.2 mg	11.7	0.04 mg	2.3
1:200,000 Epinephrine	0.2 mg	25	0.04 mg	5
1:20,000 Levonordefrin	1.0 mg	11.7	0.2 mg	2.3

As described in the chapter content for local anesthetic agents that contain a vasoconstrictor, an additional calculation to determine the maximum number of cartridges based on the vasoconstrictor needs to be determined. When administering local anesthetics with vasoconstrictors the local anesthetics will have two potentially limiting drugs: (1) the dose of local anesthetic agent and (2) the dose of the accompanying vasoconstrictor. Either of these agents may be the limiting drug in determining maximum dose of any particular local anesthetic depending upon the patient's medical status. Appendix Table 8-9 provides the volume of vasoconstrictor drug in each concentration based on 1.7 mL of solution. Appendix Table 8-10 provides recommended doses of vasoconstrictors for healthy and cardiovascularly involved patients, and maximum number of cartridges for each based on 1.7 mL of solution.

PART IV

Local Anesthetic Techniques for the Dental Hygienist

CHAPTER 9

Armamentarium/Syringe Preparation

Demetra Daskalos Logothetis RDH, MS

CHAPTER OUTLINE

LEARNING OBJECTIVES

1. Describe and assemble all equipment necessary to deliver local anesthetics before dental or dental hygiene procedures.
2. Demonstrate appropriate aseptic procedures for discarding anesthetic needles and cartridges.
3. Recognize manufacturer color codes for needle gauge and discuss the parts of the needle.
4. Recognize American Dental Association standard color codes for anesthetic cartridges.
5. List and describe the seven types of syringes used in anesthetic procedures and the advantages and disadvantages of each.
6. Discuss care and handling of the syringe, needle, and cartridge.
7. Describe the cartridge inspection process and the ramifications of the following:
   • Cracked cartridge
   • Bubbles in cartridge
   • Corroded/rusted caps
   • Outdated anesthetic solution
   • Extruded plunger
8. Discuss problems relative to the needle, which may occur during anesthetic procedures.
9. List and describe the parts of the cartridge and role of each.
10. Define the following: harpoon, gauge, bevel, deflection.
11. Successfully complete review questions and activities for this chapter.

KEY TERMS

Armamentarium Local anesthetic supplies, materials, and devices needed to successfully administer a local anesthetic.

Aspiration test Negative pressure placed on the anesthetic syringe prior to the deposition of anesthetic to determine if the tip of the needle rests within a blood vessel, observed by absence or entry of blood into the cartridge.

Bevel The angled surface of the needle tip.

Breech-loading Allows the glass anesthetic cartridge to be inserted into the syringe through the side of the barrel.

Cartridge Contains the sterile local anesthetic drug and other contents.

Computer-controlled local anesthetic delivery device (CCLAD) Computerized local anesthetic delivery system that controls the amount and rate of administered anesthetic.

Deflection The deviation in direction of the anesthetic needle from its intended path.

Finger grip Winged or wingless component of the syringe that allows the clinician to hold and control the syringe.

Gauge The diameter of the tubular lumen (channel) of the needle.

Harpoon Sharp tip attached to the internal end of the piston of an aspirating syringe that embeds into the silicone rubber stopper allowing retraction for an aspiration test.

Negative pressure Produced when the thumb ring of a syringe is pulled back, causing retraction of the rubber stopper producing an aspiration test.

Hemostat Instrument used in dentistry to retrieve small items, such as broken needles.

Hub The location of the shaft of the needle that joins and secures the needle to the syringe adaptor.

Jet injector Needleless syringe that delivers anesthesia to mucous membranes at high pressure.

Lumen Inner tubular (channel) area of an anesthetic needle.

Needle adaptor Threaded tip of the syringe that allows the attachment of the needle to the barrel of the syringe.

Needle shields Covers that protect the needle that is inserted in the tissue, as well as the cartridge penetrating end of the needle.

Penetrating end The part of the needle shaft that passes through the hub and penetrates the rubber diaphragm of the cartridge.

Piston Solid metallic cylinder of the anesthetic syringe attached to the thumb ring that displaces anesthetic solution when positive pressure is exerted on the thumb ring.

Positive aspiration Blood entering the cartridge following an aspiration test indicating the needle tip is within a blood vessel.

Safety syringe Plastic disposable syringe that decreases the risk of accidental exposure to the clinician from contaminated needles.

Shaft The length of the needle comprised of long tubular metal.

Silicone rubber stopper Located at the bottom of the anesthetic cartridge, where the harpoon is embedded.

Syringe adaptor Plastic or metal adaptor that provides a means to attach the needle to the syringe.

Syringe barrel The part of the local anesthetic syringe that hold the glass cartridge.

Thumb ring Attached to the external end of the piston allowing the clinician to advance or retract the piston.

Topical antiseptic Antimicrobial substance applied to tissue to reduce the risk of infection.

INTRODUCTION

The administration of safe and effective local anesthesia depends on the anesthetic delivery devices. There are three main components to the armamentarium of anesthetic equipment and supplies: the aspirating syringe, the disposable hypodermic needle, and the single-dose anesthetic cartridge. When handled correctly, this equipment will ensure that the dental hygienist can precisely administer the local anesthetic agent to the patient without risk of intravascular injection and cross-contamination. In addition to the syringe, needle, and cartridge, supplemental equipment includes topical antiseptic, topical anesthetic, applicator sticks, gauze, hemostat or cotton pliers, and needle capping aids, all of which are also important to the effective delivery of local anesthetic agents (Figure 9-1).

SYRINGES

The first intraoral local anesthetic syringe was introduced by Cook Laboratories in 1921, and considerable improvements have been made since then, with the most important improvement being the addition of the aspirating harpoon. The harpoon allows the anesthetic syringe to engage the silicone rubber stopper of the anesthetic cartridge. This addition introduced the important concept of aspirating prior to injecting local anesthetic solution to assess whether the location of the needle tip is within a blood vessel. Intravascular injections rapidly produce high blood levels of

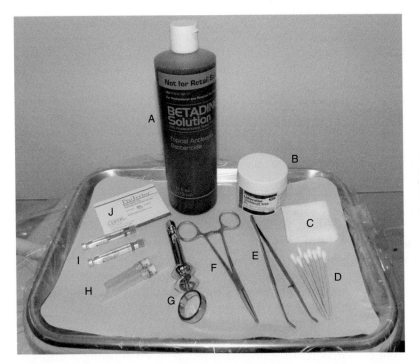

Figure 9-1 ■ Local anesthetic armamentarium. **A,** Betadine antiseptic. **B,** Topical anesthetic. **C,** Gauze. **D,** Cotton tip applicators. **E,** Cotton pliers. **F,** Hemostat. **G,** Aspirating syringe. **H,** Long and short needles. **I,** Anesthetic cartridges. **J,** Needle sheath prop.

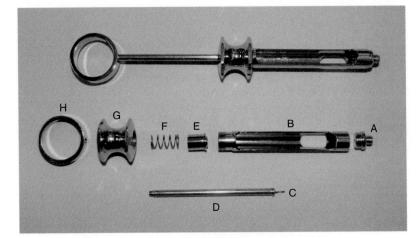

Figure 9-2 ■ Components of a standard local anesthetic syringe. **A,** Needle adaptor. **B,** Syringe barrel. **C,** Harpoon. **D,** Piston. **E,** Guide gearing. **F,** Spring. **G,** Finger grip. **H,** Thumb ring.

drug potentially resulting in an anesthetic overdose. Intravascular injections can be prevented by performing an aspiration test. Aspiration tests are accomplished by pulling back on the thumb ring of the syringe to create negative pressure within the cartridge. This action determines if the needle tip rests within a blood vessel, as observed by the absence or entry of blood into the cartridge.[1,2]

Certain criteria have been developed by the Council on Dental Material and Devices of the American Dental Association for the acceptance of local anesthetic syringes that include the following[3,4]:

- Syringes must be durable and able to withstand repeated sterilization without damage. (If the unit is disposable, it should be packaged in a sterile container.)
- Syringes should be capable of accepting a wide variety of cartridges and needles of different manufacturers and permit repeated use.

- Syringes should be inexpensive, self-contained, lightweight, and simple to use with one hand.
- Syringes should provide for effective aspiration and be constructed so that blood may be easily observed in the cartridge.

COMPONENTS OF THE ANESTHETIC SYRINGE

Needle Adaptor

The needle adaptor (Figure 9-2A), is located at the top of the syringe and is attached to the barrel of the syringe. The threaded tip allows the attachment of the needle to the barrel of the syringe. The needle is attached by passing it through the needle adaptor to the barrel and properly screwing it to the adaptor. The needle penetrates the diaphragm at the top of the local anesthetic cartridge. Care should be taken when removing the needle from the needle adaptor. The needle adaptor can be easily unscrewed when the needle is removed and can be inadvertently disposed of with the contaminated needle into the sharps container (Figure 9-3).

Syringe Barrel

The breech-loading syringe barrel (Figure 9-2B) allows the glass anesthetic cartridge to be inserted into the syringe through the side of the barrel. The barrel has a "large window" and a "small window" on opposite sides (Figure 9-4). The large window provides adequate room for breech-loading cartridges to be inserted into the syringe and provides the clinician with direct vision of the cartridge during anesthetic administration. This is an important feature because any positive aspiration that occurs during the injection can be seen. The large window should always be in view of the clinician during administration of local anesthetics (see Chapter 11).

Piston and Harpoon

The piston (Figure 9-2D) passes through the finger grip and attaches to the thumb ring of the syringe. The spring (Figure

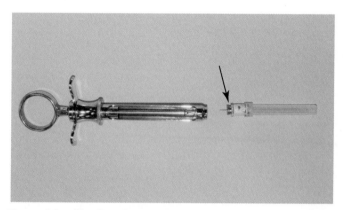

Figure 9-3 ■ Needle adaptor can be inadvertently disposed of in sharps container.

9-2F) allows the piston to be pulled back during the insertion of the cartridge, and during aspiration tests. The harpoon (Figure 9-2C) of the aspirating syringe is a sharp tip attached to the internal end of the piston. Advancing the piston allows the clinician to embed the harpoon into the silicone rubber stopper at the bottom of the cartridge. The advantage and purpose of the harpoon is to provide negative pressure inside the anesthetic cartridge when the thumb ring is pulled back, causing the rubber stopper to retract producing an aspiration test. If the tip of the needle is within a blood vessel, blood will enter the cartridge signaling the clinician of a positive aspiration. (See Chapter 11.)

Finger Grip

The finger grip (Figure 9-2G) attaches to the barrel of the syringe, and allows the piston to pass through and attach to the thumb ring. Clinicians hold the syringe using the finger grip with the index and middle fingers, providing the clinician stability and control of the syringe. There are two basic types of finger grips, winged and wingless; these may be silicone-coated to aid in establishing a firm grip (Figure 9-5).

Thumb Ring

The purpose of the thumb ring (Figure 9-2H) is to add control over the syringe, and to advance or retract the piston. The thumb ring is attached to the external end of the piston. Applying pressure to the thumb ring advances the piston to embed the harpoon into the silicone rubber stopper, and pushes the anesthetic solution out of the cartridge through the needle. Pulling back on the thumb ring provides negative pressure by retracting the silicone rubber stopper and producing an aspiration. Syringes are available with different sizes of thumb rings to accommodate varying hand sizes (Figure 9-6). The dental hygienist must be able to stretch his or her fingers to effectively pull back on the

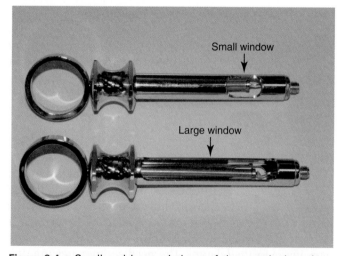

Figure 9-4 ■ Small and large windows of the anesthetic syringe. The large window should be facing up toward the clinician during the administration of the local anesthetic.

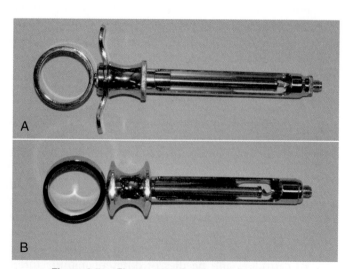

Figure 9-5 ■ Finger grips **A,** Winged. **B,** Wingless.

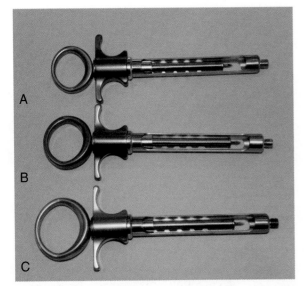

Figure 9-6 ■ Thumb ring sizes. **A**, Small (petite). **B**, Medium. **C**, Large.

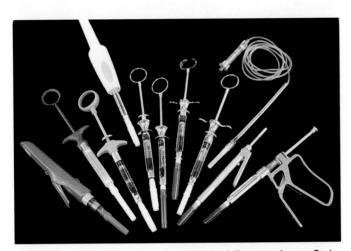

Figure 9-7 ■ Variations of local anesthetic delivery syringes. Styles are numerous: metal, plastic, computerized, pressurized, and topical anesthetic delivery. (From Daniel S, Harfst S, Wilder R, et al: *Dental hygiene concepts, cases and competencies*, ed 2, St Louis, 2008, Mosby.)

thumb ring and should select an appropriate syringe to fit his or her hand size.

TYPES OF LOCAL ANESTHETIC SYRINGES

There are several styles of syringes manufactured to be used for local anesthetic administration (Figure 9-7) with different sizes of thumb rings to accommodate various hand sizes, and personal preference dictates the size and type of thumb ring to use (Figure 9-6). They are as follows[2]:

- Reusable breech-loading metallic cartridge-type aspirating syringe
- Reusable breech-loading metallic cartridge-type self-aspirating syringe

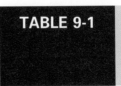

TABLE 9-1	Advantages and Disadvantages of Metallic, Breech-loading, Aspirating Syringe

ADVANTAGES	DISADVANTAGES
Readily visible cartridge through large window to detect positive aspirations and to observe the rate of solution deposition	Heavy weight of the syringe
	Size may be too large for smaller hands
Ease of aspiration with one hand	Harpoon disengagement may occur during aspiration, necessitating the clinician to remove the syringe, reengage the harpoon, and repeat the procedure
Autoclavable	
Rust resistant	
Long-lasting	

- Reusable breech-loading plastic cartridge-type aspirating syringe
- Pressure syringe for periodontal ligament injection
- Jet injector
- Computer-controlled local anesthetic delivery devices
- Disposable safety syringes

REUSABLE BREECH-LOADING METALLIC CARTRIDGE-TYPE ASPIRATING SYRINGE

The most commonly used syringe for the administration of intraoral local anesthetics is the reusable breech-loading metallic cartridge-type aspirating syringe (Figure 9-2). Single-use cartridges of anesthetic are inserted into the syringe through the large window. The harpoon is embedded in the silicone rubber stopper, and the needle is affixed to the needle adaptor. The device is then ready to be used (discussed later).

The advantages and disadvantages of using the metallic breech-loading aspirating syringe are listed in Table 9-1. To help accommodate the differences in hand sizes, newer syringes have been manufactured to include choices of smaller syringes with smaller thumb rings to facilitate the smaller-handed clinician in performing sufficient aspiration techniques (Figure 9-6). The disadvantage of the smaller syringe is that the entire cartridge of anesthetic cannot be deposited. A small portion of the anesthetic remains in the cartridge and is unusable (Figure 9-8).

Disengagement of harpoon during the injection can occur when the clinician retracts the thumb ring to achieve an aspiration. This can be due to a dull harpoon, excessive pull on the thumb ring, or improper engagement of the harpoon during syringe set up. This frequently produces a "popping" noise, alerting the clinician to the disengagement. However, the dental hygienist should check to make certain that the harpoon is fully engaged during aspiration to ensure that the proper technique has been accomplished. If the harpoon becomes disengaged during the aspiration, the negative aspiration cannot be guaranteed and the dental hygienist must remove the syringe from the patient's mouth,

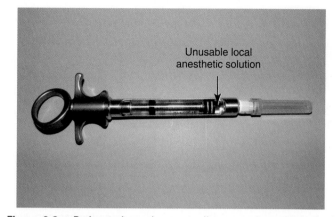

Figure 9-8 ■ Petite syringe does not allow complete removal of anesthetic solution from the cartridge compared to the standard syringe. Unusable remaining anesthetic is enough to administer buccal block to achieve complete anesthesia of a quadrant following the inferior alveolar block.

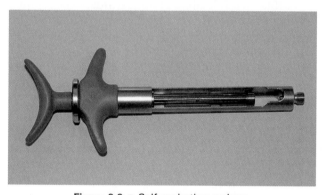

Figure 9-9 ■ Self-aspirating syringe.

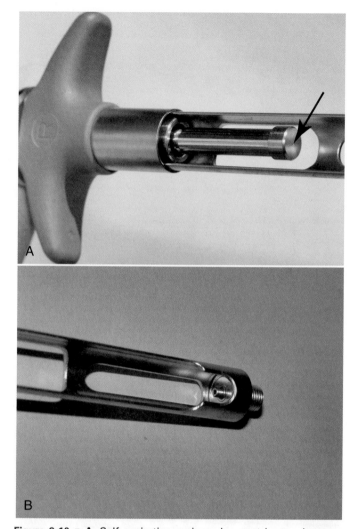

Figure 9-10 ■ **A,** Self aspirating syringe does not have a harpoon attached to the piston. **B,** Metallic sleeve of self-aspirating syringe is located at the base of the syringe and comes in contact with the diaphram of the cartridge, stretching it to produce the necessary negative pressure within the cartridge to produce an aspiration test.

remove the needle, and reengage the harpoon into the silicone rubber stopper. The needle must be placed back on the syringe, and the injection repeated.

REUSABLE BREECH-LOADING METALLIC CARTRIDGE-TYPE SELF-ASPIRATING SYRINGE

The importance of aspirating before anesthetic deposition and the potential hazards associated with intravascular injections are widely known and accepted. The breech-loading metallic cartridge-type self-aspirating syringe aids the clinician in performing this procedure without difficulty (Figure 9-9).

The self-aspirating syringe achieves the negative pressure necessary for an aspiration without a harpoon (Figure 9-10A). Instead, the negative pressure is achieved by a metallic sleeve at the base of the syringe that surrounds the needle-penetrating end and rests on the rubber diaphragm in the cartridge (Figure 9-10B). There are two types of thumb rings available—one with a half-moon and one with a thumb ring (Figure 9-11A). When the dental hygienist exerts pressure on the thumb ring, the entire cartridge moves forward, causing the elasticity of the rubber diaphragm to come in contact with the metallic sleeve and

stretches the diaphragm. When the thumb ring is released, the cartridge springs back slightly, producing negative pressure within the cartridge to achieve an aspiration (Figure 9-11B). An alternative method, using a self-aspirating syringe, uses a thumb disk that when pressed and released produces the negative pressure in a similar fashion as the thumb ring (Figure 9-11C). Table 9-2 lists the advantages and disadvantages of a self-aspirating syringe.

REUSABLE BREECH-LOADING PLASTIC CARTRIDGE-TYPE ASPIRATING SYRINGE

A plastic version of the cartridge-type aspirating syringe is available for intraoral administration of local anesthetics. The syringe is autoclavable and chemically sterilizable. The same concepts apply as for the metallic version. Advantages and disadvantages are listed in Table 9-3.

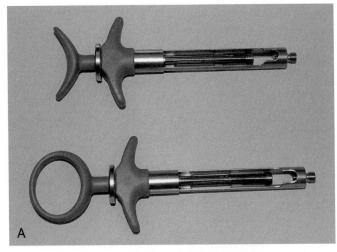

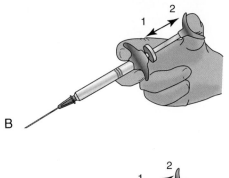

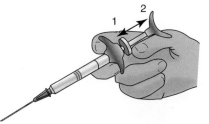

Figure 9-11 ■ **A,** Self-aspirating syringe with half-moon and thumb ring. **B,** Aspiration using thumb ring. (1, Apply pressure on thumb ring. 2, Release thumb ring.) **C,** Aspiration using thumb disk. (1, Apply pressure on the thumb disk. 2, Release thumb disk.)

TABLE 9-2	Advantages and Disadvantages of Metallic, Self-Aspirating Syringe

ADVANTAGES	DISADVANTAGES
Readily visible cartridge through large window to detect positive aspirations and to observe the rate of solution deposition	Heavy weight of the syringe
Ease of aspiration with small hands	Size may be too large for smaller hands
No disengagement of harpoon from rubber stopper can occur	Thumb must be moved from thumb ring to thumb disk
Autoclavable	Insecurity of clinician accustomed to harpoon type syringe
Rust resistant	
Long-lasting	

TABLE 9-3	Advantages and Disadvantages of Plastic, Breech-Loading, Aspirating Syringe

ADVANTAGES	DISADVANTAGES
Readily visible cartridge through large window to detect positive aspirations and to observe the rate of solution deposition	Size may be too large for smaller hands
Lighter weight	Harpoon disengagement may occur during aspiration, necessitating the clinician to remove the syringe, reengage the harpoon, and repeat the procedure
The look may be less threatening to the patient than the metallic version	Discoloration of plastic from autoclave
Ease of aspiration with one hand	
Autoclavable	
Rust resistant	
Long lasting with proper maintenance	
Lower cost	

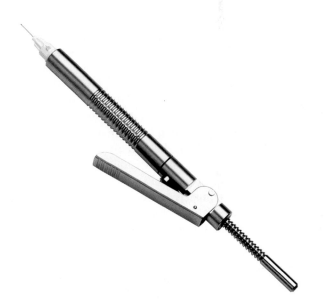

Figure 9-12 ■ Pressure type syringe. (Courtesy of Septodont, New Castle, Del.)

PRESSURE-TYPE SYRINGES

The pressure-type syringe is used for periodontal ligament (PDL) or intraligamentary injections, and provides reliable anesthesia for one tooth in the mandible (Figure 9-12). This allows the clinician to achieve anesthesia of a single tooth in the mandible where field blocks are unsuccessful because of bone density, and an inferior alveolar block, or Gow-Gates mandibular nerve block anesthetizes more teeth than needed for the procedure. (See Chapter 13.) Standard syringes can be used for this injection but the tissue resistance necessitates more muscle strength to administer. The advantage of a pressure syringe is that it administers a measured dose of 0.2 mL of anesthetic, making it easier to

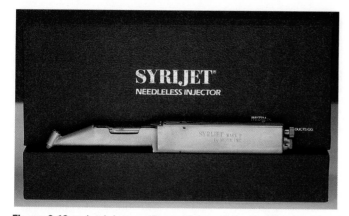

Figure 9-13 ■ Jet injector. (From Malamed S: *Handbook of local anesthesia*, ed 5, St Louis, 2004, Mosby.)

express the solution against the tissue resistance. The disadvantage is the higher cost, and may cause trauma to surrounding tissues when anesthetic is delivered under pressure.

JET INJECTOR SYRINGE

The dental hygienist may encounter the jet injector syringe (see Figure 9-13), which is used primarily for topical anesthesia of soft tissues before needle insertion or mucosal anesthesia of the palate. The jet injector syringe delivers the anesthesia in measured doses of 0.05–0.2 mL to the mucous membranes at high pressure (2000 psi) through small orifices called *jets*. It delivers the anesthetic without the use of a needle, and due to the high pressure associated with the anesthetic administration, the patient may be startled by the force by which the anesthetic is delivered. For complete pulpal anesthesia, nerve blocks or supraperiosteal injections must be administered after the jet injector is used. Topical anesthetics can accomplish the same result as the jet injector at a fraction of the cost.[2]

COMPUTER-CONTROLLED LOCAL ANESTHETIC DELIVERY DEVICES

In 1997, Milestone Scientific Inc. introduced the first computer-controlled local anesthetic delivery (CCLAD) system as the Wand System. This device was designed to replace the standard breech-loading aspirating syringe and deliver a "virtually painless" injection of local anesthetic.[5,6] The clinician holds a feather-light "wand" handpiece as if holding a pen, which gives superior ergonomic control. Clinicians with small hands may find the wand headpiece easier to use because of the design and ultralightweight features. A penlike grasp allows clinicians to rotate the handpiece back and forth, using a birotational insertion technique that eliminates needle deflection during needle penetration into tissues, resulting in accurate needle placement.[5,6] The handpiece can be less intimidating for the patient and can help alleviate the patient's fear associated with the standard large metal syringe.

Recently, Milestone Scientific Inc. introduced the next generation to CCLAD systems with the introduction of the

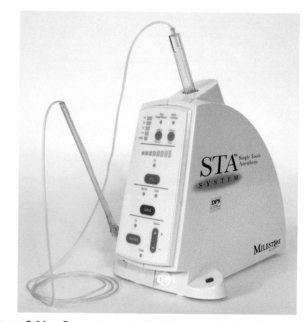

Figure 9-14 ■ Computer-controlled local anesthetic delivery device. STA Single Tooth Anesthesia System. (Courtesy of Milestone Scientific.)

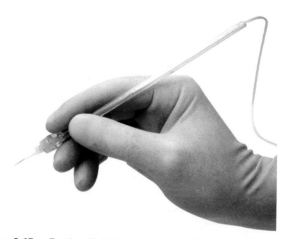

Figure 9-15 ■ Feather-light handpiece provides ergonomic control.

STA Single Tooth Anesthesia System (Figure 9-14). The STA system incorporates dynamic pressure-sensing (DPS) technology to provide real-time continuous pressure feedback during the injection. The STA system guides the clinician with audible and visual feedback, enabling him or her to identify the optimal location to perform a PDL injection. The STA system can be used to perform all the standard dental injections, as well as newer-described injections such as the AMSA, P-ASA, and STA-intraligamentary.

The STA and Wand systems precisely regulate the flow rate of the local anesthetic solution administered via a computer-controlled module. In addition, the DPS technology regulates and monitors the pressure of the anesthetic solution. These systems are activated by foot control, allowing the clinician to delicately hold the Wand handpiece (Figure 9-15). The rate of flow can be set as precisely as 1 drop every other second (slow rate), or the clinician can use

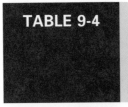 **TABLE 9-4**	**Advantages and Disadvantages of Computer-Controlled Local Anesthetic Delivery System**

ADVANTAGES	DISADVANTAGES
Precise control of anesthetic flow and pressure	Cost
Provides setting for slow (1 drop every other second) flow rate to create a numbing pathway for the needle	
Automatic aspiration	
Lightweight handpiece requires activation of fine muscles of the hand rather than larger muscles, resulting in less hand fatigue	
Rotational needle insertion minimizes needle deflection for more accurate deposition at target site	

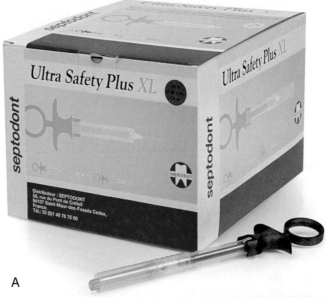

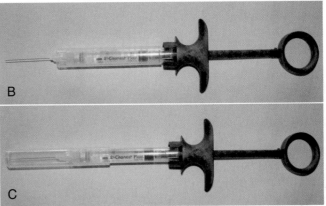

Figure 9-16 ■ **A,** UltraSafety Plus XL, aspirating syringe. (Ultra Safety Plus System courtesy of Septodont, New Castle, Del.) **B,** UltraSafety Plus XL, aspirating syringe ready for injection, **C,** UltraSafety Plus XL, aspirating syringe sheathed to prevent needlestick injury.

the foot pedal to set the control rate at various settings, including "cruise control." Patients typically experience painless injection. Although there is still a minimal sensation of the needle insertion, the actual medication administration is precisely controlled and painless. The advantages and disadvantages of this system are listed in Table 9-4.

DISPOSABLE SAFETY SYRINGES

Due to concerns regarding the risk of accidental exposure to the clinician from contaminated needles following the administration of local anesthetics, the safety syringe was developed, such as the UltraSafety Plus XL (Figure 9-16A), as an alternative to the standard breech-loading aspirating syringe. The safety syringe is a plastic, single use, or partially disposable syringe. A plastic sheath on the syringe is retracted when the clinician is ready to administer an injection (Figure 9-16B), and the sheath locks over the needle upon removal from the tissue; the mechanism is activated by the clinician easily with one hand (Figure 9-16C). This provides an added advantage over standard syringes by decreasing the risk of accidental exposure.

ROUTINE MAINTENANCE OF REUSABLE SYRINGES

Routine maintenance of reusable syringes is required to ensure the long-term efficiency of the device. Manufacturer recommendations include:

- Thorough cleaning and sterilization following appropriate infection control guidelines after each patient.
- Following repeated autoclaving, the dental hygienist should dismantle and lubricate, with a light oil, all the threaded joints.
- To ensure reliable aspiration, the piston and harpoon should be replaced if the harpoon readily disengages from the rubber stopper of the cartridge or if the harpoon is bent.

▌NEEDLE

The needle delivers the anesthetic solution from the cartridge to the surrounding tissues. The type of injection, how much tissue needs to be penetrated, and individual preference, will determine whether a short or long needle should be used. All needles manufactured for dentistry are stainless steel, presterilized, and disposable.

NEEDLE COMPONENTS
Bevel

The bevel of the needle (Figure 9-17A) is the angled surface of the needle tip that is directed into the tissue. Patient discomfort can be minimized by the sharpness of the bevel. The bevels may be configured by manufacturers as short, medium, or long (Figure 9-18). The angle of the bevel in relation to the long axis of the needle may have an effect on the amount of needle deflection when significant tissue is penetrated, such as with the inferior alveolar block. The

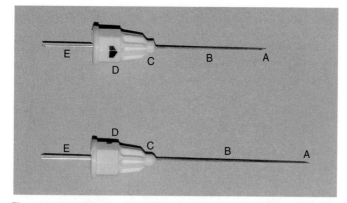

Figure 9-17 ■ Components of the needle. **A,** Bevel. **B,** Needle shaft. **C,** Hub. **D,** Needle adaptor. **E,** Cartridge penetrating end.

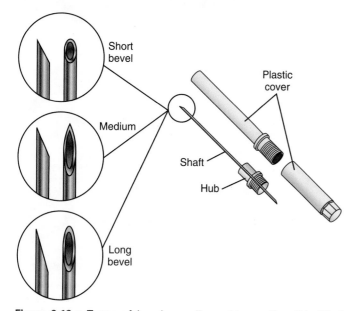

Figure 9-18 ■ Types of bevels on disposable needles. (Modified from Jastak T, Yagiela J, Donaldson D: *Local anesthesia of the oral cavity.* St Louis, 1995, Saunders.)

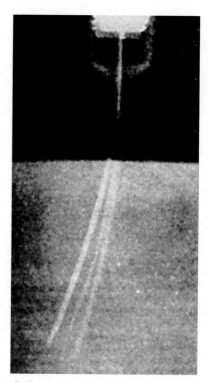

Figure 9-19 ■ Deflection of needle. (From Robison SE, et al: Comparative study of deflection characteristics and fragility of 25-, 27- and 30-gauge short dental needles, *J Am Dent Assoc* 109:920-924, 1984.)

greater the angle of the bevel, the greater the degree of needle deflection[2] (Figure 9-19). To increase patient comfort during injections that are administered in close proximity to the periosteum, the bevel of the needle should be turned toward the bone (Figure 9-20). To assist the clinician in determining the location of the bevel, several manufacturers are placing indicators of the bevel location on the hub of the needle (Figure 9-21).

Shaft

The shaft of the needle (Figure 9-17B) is the length of the needle that is comprised of long tubular metal extending from the tip of the needle through the hub (discussed next) to the piece (cartridge-penetrating end) that penetrates the diaphragm of the cartridge. Needle breakage is rare; however, needle breakage usually occurs when the entire shaft of the needle is inserted up to the hub. This primarily occurs from exerted lateral pressure against the shank or sudden movement of the syringe or patient.

The significant components of the shaft are the length and the gauge. The gauge is the diameter of the tubular lumen (channel) of the needle. (Discussed later.)

Hub

The hub and syringe adaptor (Figure 9-17C–D) are made of plastic or metal and provides a means to attach the needle to the syringe. The syringe adaptor and hub are frequently referred to as "the hub." The metal syringe adaptor has a prethreaded interior that allows for easy attachment to the syringe. A disadvantage to the metal syringe adaptor is that it can easily be unscrewed, and when fully screwed is seated in one position securing the bevel of the needle in one direction, making it difficult to properly align the bevel toward the bone. The plastic syringe adaptor is not prethreaded and the dental hygienist must simultaneously push and screw the needle onto the syringe. The advantages of the plastic syringe adaptor include easy adaptation and bevel alignment with most syringes. The hub of the needle is the point where the shaft of the needle joins and secures the needle to the syringe adaptor. The needle shank should never be inserted into tissue up to the hub of the needle.

Cartridge-Penetrating End

The cartridge penetrating end (Figure 9-17E) is the part of the shaft that passes through the hub and penetrates the rubber diaphragm of the cartridge, lying within the anesthetic solution of the cartridge.

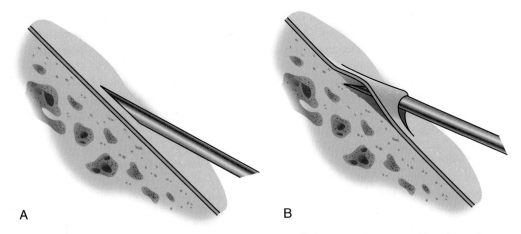

A   B

Figure 9-20 ■ **A,** Correct bevel placement against bone. **B,** Incorrect placement of bevel, causing the tip to scrape the bone.

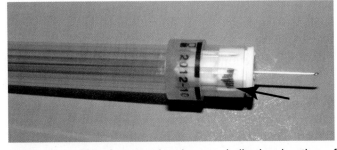

Figure 9-21 ■ Manufacturer placed arrow indicating location of bevel.

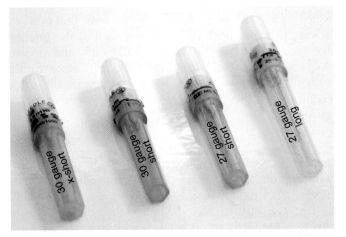

Figure 9-22 ■ Color-coding by needle gauge. (Courtesy of Septodont, New Castle, Del.)

Needle Shields

Needle shields protect the needle that is inserted in the tissue, as well as the cartridge-penetrating end of the needle. Various colors are used by manufacturers to determine the designated length and gauge of the needle that is inserted in the tissue. The shield that covers the cartridge-penetrating end is clear. There are no uniform guidelines for the color of needle shields. However, manufacturers are consistent with their own color-coding system (Figure 9-22).

Gauge

Needles used for intraoral injection are available in gauge sizes of 25, 27, and 30. The gauge is the diameter of the lumen of the needle. The smaller the gauge number, the larger the diameter of the needle. Therefore the 25-gauge needle has the largest diameter, followed by the 27-gauge, and so on. The needle with the smallest diameter lumen is the 30-gauge (Table 9-5). The gauge selection is determined by the depth of tissue penetration and the risk of intravascular injection. The 25-gauge needle is the recommended needle for areas of high risk for positive aspiration, such as the inferior alveolar block, and posterior superior alveolar block. A common belief among practitioners is that the 30-gauge needle causes less discomfort to the patient

TABLE 9-5	Common Needle Gauges Used For Intra-oral Injections	
GAUGE	**OUTSIDE DIAMETER (mm)**	**LUMEN DIAMETER (mm)**
25	0.51	0.25
27	0.41	0.20
30	0.31	0.15

than the 25-gauge needle. However, numerous comparisons over the years have demonstrated that patients cannot discern the difference between a 25-gauge needle and a 30-gauge needle. The 25-gauge needle is safer for the patient because the lumen is larger, providing easier access for blood to enter the cartridge during the aspiration procedure.[7,8]

Larger gauge needles (25 gauge) have several significant advantages over smaller gauge needles (30 gauge). Due to the rigidity of the larger gauge needles, less deflection occurs during significant tissue penetration (Figure 9-19). This provides greater accuracy to the target location and increases the likelihood of success of the injection. This is of particular importance for the inferior alveolar (IA) block. Moreover, because the shaft of the 25-gauge needle is significantly stronger than its thinner counterparts, needle breakage is considerably minimized. Although it is possible to aspirate with smaller gauge needles, the smaller lumen does significantly impede the bloodflow into the cartridge. It also requires more pressure by the clinician to adequately aspirate through the narrow lumen of smaller gauge needles. This makes it difficult to achieve a reliable aspiration, increases the possibility of needle movement away from the target location, and increases the likelihood that the harpoon will disengage from the rubber stopper during aspiration. Therefore it is recommended that the dental hygienist use a 25-gauge needle for injections that pose an increased risk for positive aspirations such as the inferior alveolar, posterior superior alveolar and mental and incisive blocks. However, the 27-gauge needle may be more readily available, and is also acceptable. The 30-gauge needle is not recommended. See Box 9-1 for the advantages of larger gauge needles.

Length

There are two commonly used needle lengths for the intraoral injection: long and short. The short needle is approximately 20 mm, and the long needle is approximately 32 mm, as measured from the hub to the tip of the needle (Figure 9-23A). Ultrashort needles, approximately 12 mm, are available in 30 gauge (Figure 9-23B). The needle length selection is based on the amount of tissue that needs to be penetrated to reach the target location and to deposit the anesthetic successfully. Long needles are required for injections, such as the inferior alveolar block, that require significant needle penetration of thick tissue to reach the nerve. Short needles are preferred for injections that require less soft tissue penetration to reach the target location, such as supraperiosteal injections.

For safety reasons, the needle should never be inserted to the hub. Although needle breakage is rare, a sufficient

length of the shaft for both lengths must be visible in the oral cavity during insertion to permit retrieval of the needle fragment in case of breakage. Long needles are required for the inferior alveolar block, the Gow Gates mandibular block, and preferred for the infraorbital (IO) block. This allows for adequate tissue penetration to reach the target and allows for sufficient length of the shaft to be visible.

CARE AND HANDLING OF NEEDLES

Proper care and handling of contaminated needles will reduce the risk of needle exposure to the patient and clinician. The following recommendations should be followed by the dental hygienist to minimize the risk of cross contamination:

- Needles are presterilized by the manufacturer and are disposable. They should never be used on more than one patient.
- For patient comfort, the needle should be changed after approximately three to four injections in the same patient. The stainless steel of the needle becomes dull after three to four needle penetrations, causing tissue trauma and pain on insertion with each subsequent injection. The patient may also experience soreness when sensation returns.
- Needles should be immediately covered by the protective shield, using the one-handed scoop method with

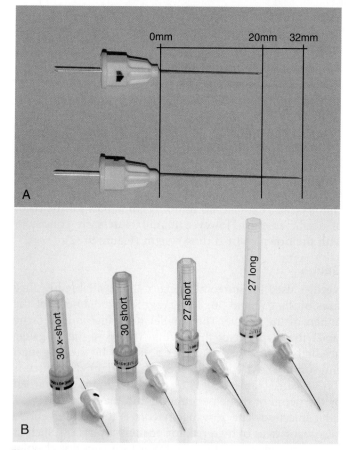

Figure 9-23 ■ **A,** Length of dental needles short verses long. **B,** various needle lengths according to gauge. (**B,** Courtesy of Septodont, New Castle, Del.)

| BOX 9-1 | Advantages of Larger Gauge Needle over Smaller Gauge Needles |

- Less deflection from intended path as needle is penetrated through significant tissue
- Greater accuracy in achieving target location
- Increased success of the injection
- Less chance of needle breakage
- Aspiration is easier to achieve and more reliable
- No difference in patient comfort

a needle sheath prop or other recapping aids (discussed later), following the administration of the injection to prevent accidental needlestick with the contaminated needle.

- Several recapping devices are available to assist the dental hygienist in recapping the contaminated needle (Figure 9-24).
- The dental hygienist should scoop the contaminated needle into the shield using one hand, as demonstrated in Figure 9-25.
- The dental hygienist should know the location of the uncovered needle tip at all times whether inside or outside of the patient's mouth. This will prevent needle injury to both the patient and clinician. This will also prevent accidental needle contamination by the clinician in case the needle tip touches any extra-oral surface. If needle contamination occurs, the dental hygienist should recap the needle using the method described above and discard it in the appropriate container. A new sterilized needle should be placed to complete the injection.

- Contaminated needles should be properly disposed of after use in an approved sharps containers (Figure 9-26). The sharps containers should be properly disposed of according to federal, state, and local regulations.

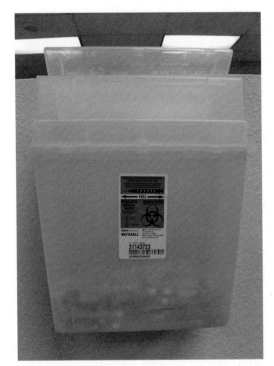

Figure 9-26 ■ Needle disposal in approved sharps containers.

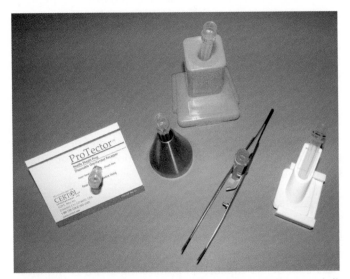

Figure 9-24 ■ Recapping devices. Needle capping devices are available in many forms to assist the dental hygienist to safely cap the contaminated needle utilizing a one-handed technique.

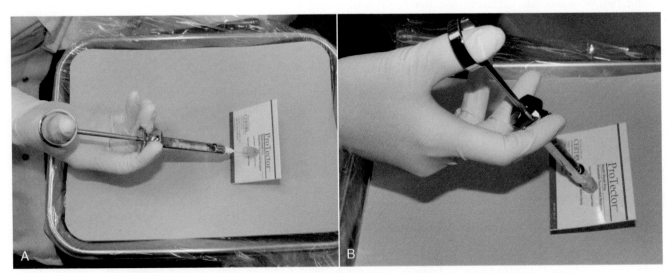

Figure 9-25 ■ Scoop method with a needle sheath prop to safely cap contaminated needle.
A, One-handed scoop technique. **B,** Secure the needle using one hand.

NEEDLE PROBLEMS

The dental hygienist should be aware that several needle problems can occur during or after the injection.

Pain on Insertion

Patients may complain of pain during needle insertion. This is usually due to dull needles following repeated needle penetrations. To prevent this problem, the dental hygienist should change the needle after three to four needle penetrations.

Pain on Withdrawal

The patient may complain of pain when the needle is withdrawn from the tissue. This is usually due to barbs on the needle tip. Barbs can occur during manufacturing, but are most likely to occur if the needle contacts bone forcefully during the injection. To prevent this, the needle should never be forced against any hard surface during the injection.

Needlestick Exposure to the Administrator

To prevent accidental needlestick exposure to the clinician, the one-handed scoop method with needle sheath prop should be used immediately following the injection to cap the needle in the protective shield. Needlestick injuries typically occur from inattention by the clinician or unexpected patient movement. (See Chapter 15 for needlestick protocol.)

Needle Breakage

Although needle breakage is rare when needles are properly used, the incidence of needle breakage is increased in the following situations:

- *Bending the needle prior to the injection.* If the injection is administered properly, there is no need to bend the needle to reach the target location. Bending the needle compromises the integrity of the needle and increases the risk of breakage. Therefore the needle should never be bent by the dental hygienist. The only exception is during intraligamentary injection techniques, because the needle is not in deep tissue.
- *Sudden direction changes.* Needle breakage can occur if sudden direction changes are made during the administration of the anesthetic, especially when the needle is deeply embedded in tissue. If the needle must be redirected during the injection (e.g., with the inferior alveolar block; see Chapter 13), the needle should be withdrawn almost completely from the tissue and the change in direction can be safely made. The needle can then be re-advanced to the target location.
- *Forcing the needle against resistance.* Needles are not designed to penetrate bone and should never be forced against resistance.
- *Inserting the needle to the hub.* Breakage of the needle is more likely to occur at the hub (the weakest portion of the needle) if sudden movement of the syringe or

patient occurs. The likelihood of needle breakage increases when the needle is inserted into tissue all the way to the hub. Moreover, if the needle breaks at the hub during the injection, the needle fragment will be embedded in tissue and impossible to retrieve.

- *Using 30-gauge needles.* According to Malamed, the majority of needle breakage incidences have occurred with 30-gauge short or ultrashort needles.[2] It is recommended that the dental hygienist use 25-gauge needles for all injections that penetrate significant soft tissue. (See Chapters 12 and 13.)

ANESTHETIC CARTRIDGES

The glass local anesthetic cartridge (also referred to as a *carpule,* a trademark term of Cook-Waite Laboratories) contains the sterile local anesthetic drug and other contents in a convenient single use dose. Each cartridge consists of a glass cylinder with a rubber diaphragm enclosed in a metal cap at the top of the cartridge (Figure 9-27B) and a silicone rubber stopper at the bottom of the cartridge (Figure 9-27D). The glass tube allows the dental hygienist adequate visibilty of delivered doses and aspiration tests.

CARTRIDGE COMPONENTS

The standard local anesthetic cartridge is prefilled with up to 1.8 mL of sterile anesthetic solution and consists of several components.

The Glass Cylinder

The glass cylinder (Figure 9-27A) is the body of the cartridge and contains the anesthetic solution. (See Chapter 5 for the composition of the local anesthetic solution.) The glass cylinder is capable of containing 2 mL of solution. However, once the rubber stopper is added, the net volume of anesthetic is reduced to a maximum 1.8 mL for all local anesthetic agents.

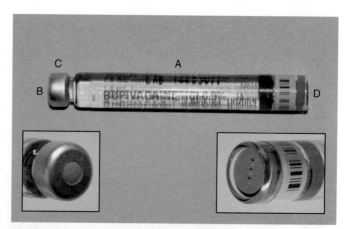

Figure 9-27 ■ Components of local anesthetic cartridge. **A,** Glass cylinder containing anesthetic solution. **B,** Diaphragm. **C,** Aluminum cap. **D,** Silicone rubber stopper slightly indented from glass rim.

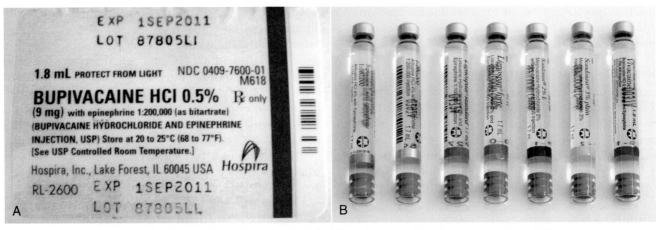

Figure 9-28 ■ **A,** ADA Mylar label standard. **B,** ADA color-coated bands on anesthetic cartridge identifies drug.

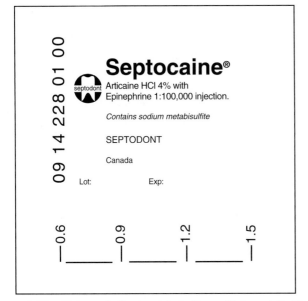

Figure 9-29 ■ Volume indication label. (From Malamed S: *Handbook of local anesthesia*, St Louis, 2004, Mosby. Courtesy of Septodont, New Castle, Del.)

TABLE 9-6	American Dental Association Color Coding of Local Anesthetic Cartridges

Local Anesthetic Drug	ADA Color Coded Band
Lidocaine 2%	Light blue
Lidocaine 2% 1:50,000 epinephrine	Green
Lidocaine 2% 1:100,000 epinephrine	Red
Mepivacaine 3%	Plain Tan
Mepivacaine 2% 1:20,000 levonordefrin	Brown
Prilocaine 4%	Yellow
Prilocaine 4% 1:200,000 epinephrine	Black
Articaine 4% 1:100,000 epinephrine	Silver
Articaine 4% 1:200,000 epinephrine	Gold
Bupivacaine 0.5% 1:200,000 epinephrine	Blue

Source: American Dental Association June 2003 color coding of local anesthetic cartridges

Cartridge Labeling

On the body of the glass cylinder, a Mylar plastic label is applied by the manufacturer that lists the contents of the cartridge, the trade and generic drug names, drug concentrations, vasoconstrictor dilutions, expiration date, and the manufacturer's name (Figure 9-28A). Some manufacturers may include volume indicators on the label to assist in determining the amount of solution deposited (Figure 9-29). A color-coded band on the Mylar plastic label on the glass cylinder also identifies the anesthetic drug contained in the cartridge. The standardized color-coded bands are required by the American Dental Association for all local anesthetic cartridges to receive the ADA Seal of Approval (Table 9-6 and Figure 9-28B). The Mylar plastic label also serves as protection to the patient and administrator in the event of glass breakage during the administration of anesthetic.

Silicone Rubber Stopper

The silicone rubber stopper (or plunger) is located at the bottom of the anesthetic cartridge and is slightly indented from the rim of the glass barrel (Figure 9-27D). This is an important feature for the dental hygienist to observe when examining the cartridges prior to syringe setup. Cartridges that have rubber stoppers that are not indented slightly should be discarded because sterility of the solution cannot be guaranteed. The harpoon of the aspirating syringe is embedded into the rubber stopper, providing the clinician a means to aspirate. Recently many manufacturers are using nonlatex materials for the rubber stoppers and rubber diaphrams (discussed next) due to latex allergies becoming more common. The local anesthetic solution is administered by pressure on the thumb ring, creating movement of the rubber stopper forward into the glass cylinder. The width of each rubber stopper expels approximately 0.2 mL of solution providing a means to determine the amount of anesthetic deposited when an entire cartridge is not administered (Figure 9-30).

Diaphragm

The rubber diaphragm is made of semipermeable material and is located at the top of the cartridge where the needle is inserted into the center of the rubber (Figure 9-27B). Because the rubber is semipermeable, if the cartridge is improperly stored (e.g., in disinfecting solution), the anesthetic solution can be contaminated by diffusion of the disinfecting solution into the cartridge.

Aluminum Cap

The silver colored aluminum cap fits securely around the rubber diaphragm, keeping it in place (Figure 9-27C).

CARE AND HANDLING OF THE CARTRIDGE

Local anesthetic cartridges are packaged in boxes containing *blister packs* of 5 or 10 units of 10 sealed cartridges (Figure 9-31). Local anesthetic cartridges should be stored in their original container at room temperature in a dark place. This keeps the cartridges clean and uncontaminated, and prevents premature deterioration of the solution, particularly the oxidation of the vasoconstrictor drug due to prolonged exposure to heat or direct sunlight.

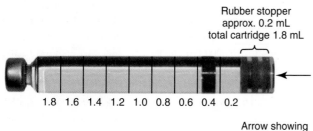

Rubber stopper
approx. 0.2 mL
total cartridge 1.8 mL

1.8 1.6 1.4 1.2 1.0 0.8 0.6 0.4 0.2

Arrow showing
the stopper
being pushed in

Figure 9-30 ■ Volume of anesthetic deposited by the width of the rubber stopper.

Commercially available cartridge warmers keep the local anesthetic solution at body temperature. It has been assumed by many dental professionals that this promotes patient comfort during the administration of the anesthetic solution. These warmers are not necessary or recommended. Overheating of the cartridge can cause a burning sensation during injection of anesthetic solution and destroy the heat-sensitive vasoconstrictor drug and decrease the duration of action.[9]

The local anesthetic cartridge does not need to be prepared before use if stored properly. The anesthetic solution is presterilized during manufacturing, and bacterial cultures taken from the exterior cartridge immediately after opening the container have not demonstrated any bacterial growth.[2] If the dental hygienist is concerned about the exterior surfaces of the cartridge, he or she can wipe all the surfaces with an approved ADA disinfectant. The local anesthetic cartridge should never be placed in alcohol or sterilizing solutions because the rubber diaphragm is permeable. This can cause contamination of the local anesthetic solution and corrode the aluminum cap.

The expiration date of the anesthetic is located on the box or canister, and is also located on each individual cartridge. Local anesthetic cartridges should be discarded and not used past the expiration date. The reliability of the solution cannot be guaranteed, and the administration of an expired solution may result in patient discomfort.

The manufacturer inserts product identification information in every local anesthetic container. This provides the clinician with important information concerning the anesthetic agent, including dosages, warnings, precautions, care and handling, and more. Practitioners should review the product inserts periodically (Figure 9-32).

CARTRIDGE PROBLEMS

Problems with the cartridge are rarely observed; however, the dental hygienist may encounter the following.

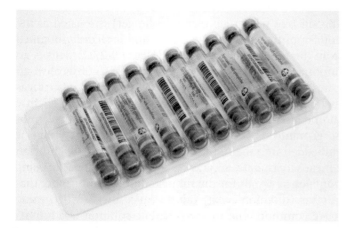

Figure 9-31 ■ Blister pack of cartridges. (Courtesy of Septodont, New Castle, Del.)

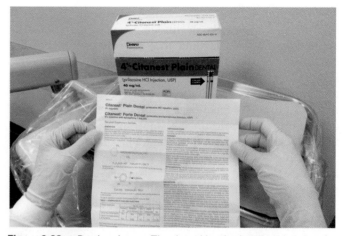

Figure 9-32 ■ Product insert: The dental hygienist should review for drug information.

Bubble in the Cartridge

During manufacturing, bubbles can be trapped in the cartridge and are either small or large.

- *Small bubble.* Nitrogen gas is used during manufacturing of the anesthetic solution to prevent oxygen from being trapped in the cartridge potentially destroying the vasoconstrictor. Small bubbles (1–2 mm in diameter) are harmless and produced by nitrogen gas bubbled into the solution during this process (Figure 9-33A).
- *Large bubble.* Bubbles in the cartridge that are larger than 2 mm are a warning that the anesthetic cartridge has been frozen. They can be present in the cartridge with or without the rubber stopper extended beyond the glass rim. These cartridges should not be used and should be discarded because the sterility of the anesthetic solution cannot be guaranteed (Figure 9-33B-C).

Extruded Stopper

If the rubber stopper is extruded beyond the glass rim and accompanied with a large bubble it is an indication the cartridge has been frozen and should not be used (Figure 9-33B). An extruded stopper without a large bubble is an indication that the cartridge has been placed in disinfecting solution (see Figure 9-33D). The disinfecting solution can be diffused through the diaphragm into the anesthetic solution, causing the stopper to extrude past the glass rim. The sterility of the anesthetic solution cannot be guaranteed. These cartridges should not be used and should be discarded.

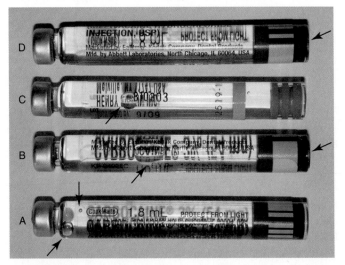

Figure 9-33 ■ **A,** Insignificant small nitrogen bubbles. **B,** Large bubble with extruding stopper indicating the cartridge has been frozen and should be discarded. **C,** Large bubble without extruded stopper indicating the cartridge has been frozen and should be discarded. **D,** Extruded stopper without a bubble indicates the cartridge has been placed in disinfecting solution and should be discarded.

Sticky Stopper

A sticky stopper is due to paraffin being employed during manufacturing. This has become less of a problem since most manufacturers are currently treating the rubber stopper with silicone. Storing cartridges at room temperature can minimize this problem.

Burning on Injection

Burning sensations can be experienced by the patient for the following reasons:

- *pH of the drug.* This is a normal reaction due to the anesthetic solution having a lower pH (5–6) than the tissues (7.4) in which it is administered. The sensation only lasts a couple of seconds until the anesthetic takes effect and is noted primarily on sensitive patients and when the anesthetic is deposited on anterior teeth.
- *Cartridge contains a vasoconstrictor drug.* The use of a vasoconstrictor and the sodium bisulfite preservative lowers the pH of the anesthetic even further than the anesthetic without a vasoconstrictor to between 3.8 and 5, which causes a burning sensation.
- *Overheated cartridges.* Overheating of cartridges causes burning sensations upon administration. Warmers are not recommended, and local anesthetic solution should be kept at room temperature.
- *Expired solutions.* The burning sensation from local anesthetic solutions, especially those that contain a vasoconstrictor, are enhanced when an expired solution is used. This can be avoided by carefully checking the expiration date before use.
- *Cartridge containing disinfecting solution.* Cartridges contaminated with disinfecting solution and subsequently injected into the mucous membranes can produce an intense burning sensation. This can also cause other problems such as paresthesia and tissue edema (see Chapter 14). Cartridges should never be placed in disinfecting solution.

Corroded Cap

The dental hygienist may observe a corroded aluminum cap (white debris) if it has been immersed in quaternary compounds such as benzalkonium chloride used for "cold sterilization." Disinfection of the cartridge can be accomplished by using an approved ADA disinfectant lightly applied to a gauze square. Never immerse the cartridge into disinfecting solutions.

Rust on Cap

Red rust on the cartridge is an indication that a cartridge contained in the metal container has broken, depositing the anesthetic solution on the other cartridges within the container. This cartridge should not be used and should be discarded, and all other cartridges within the same container should be evaluated for rust.

Leakage during Injection

This is due to the off center perforation of the needle penetrating end into the rubber diaphragm of the anesthetic cartridge, producing an oval puncture. When the anesthetic solution is administered, leakage through the diaphragm may occur. The dental hygienist should carefully insert the needle into the diaphragm to avoid this problem.

Broken Cartridge

A broken cartridge can be a result of the following situations:

- *Breakage during shipping and handling.* Cartridges arriving in damaged containers should be examined carefully for possible fractures or chips in the cartridges. Hairline fractures may not be easily identified. However, the Mylar plastic label also serves as a protective shield by reinforcing the glass in case the cartridge fractures during administration.
- *Excessive force during harpoon engagement.* The harpoon should be gently engaged into the rubber stopper during syringe set up. Exerting excessive force may fracture the cartridge.
- *Bent needle is not properly perforating the diaphragm.* Anesthetic equipment and supplies should be carefully examined by the dental hygienist before syringe setup, and care should be taken when attaching the needle to the cartridge diaphragm. Leakage of anesthetic solution into the patient's mouth can occur if the needle does not properly penetrate the diaphragm.

▌ SUPPLEMENTARY ARMAMENTARIUM

In addition to the syringe, needle, and cartridge, supplemental equipment includes topical antiseptic, topical anesthetic, applicator sticks, gauze, and hemostat or cotton pliers, and needle capping aids.

TOPICAL ANTISEPTIC

A topical antiseptic (Betadine or merthiolate) may be applied to the tissue to reduce the possibility of surface microorganisms from entering the soft tissues, which could result in a postinjection infection[2] (Figure 9-34). This step is optional, and prior to application the patient must be first screened for a possible allergy to iodine. However, the use of topical antiseptic prior to the administration should be considered for patients who are immunosuppressed.[2] Another method to reduce the surface bacteria prior to the injection is wiping the surface with gauze.

TOPICAL ANESTHETIC

Topical anesthetic agents are applied to the mucous membranes before needle insertion to provide soft tissue anesthesia of the terminal nerve endings for patient comfort. They are most effective if applied to the dry mucous

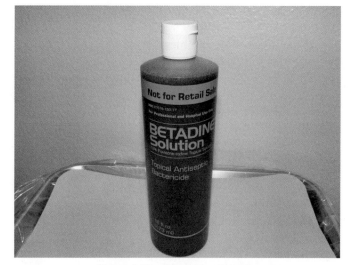

Figure 9-34 ■ Topical antiseptic.

membrane for 1–2 minutes. Topical anesthetics do not contain vasoconstrictors and are absorbed rapidly when applied to the mucous membranes. The concentration of topical anesthetics is high compared to injectable anesthetics to facilitate diffusion through the mucous membranes (approximately 2–3 mm).[9] Because of the rapid absorption and higher concentrations, only small amounts should be used and caution should be taken to avoid toxic reactions from surface applications (Figure 9-35 and see Chapter 6).

APPLICATOR STICKS

Cotton-tipped applicator sticks are used in the application of topical antiseptics and anesthetics. They are also recommended to provide pressure anesthesia during palatal injections (Figure 9-36).

GAUZE

Gauze 2 × 2 squares are used to dry the mucous membranes prior to the application of topical antiseptic and anesthetic. They are also used to dry the tissues prior to needle insertion, and although not as effective, can serve as an alternative to the application of topical antiseptic. The gauze squares can assist in retraction, visibility, and stabilization.

HEMOSTAT OR COTTON PLIERS

Hemostat or cotton pliers should be a part of the local anesthetic armamentarium in the rare incidence of a needle breakage. The hemostat, or cotton pliers, can aid in the retrieval of the needle fragment (Figure 9-37).

▌ PREPARATION OF THE BREECH LOADING-ASPIRATING SYRINGE

Proper evaluation and setup of the anesthetic equipment and supplies is important to minimize the occurrence of complications during the administration of the local

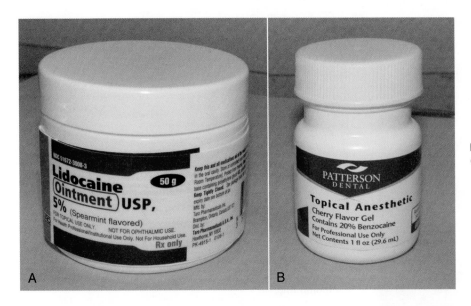

Figure 9-35 ■ Topical anesthetic. **A,** Lidocaine (amide). **B,** Benzocaine (ester).

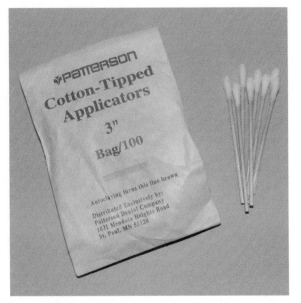

Figure 9-36 ■ Cotton-tipped applicator sticks.

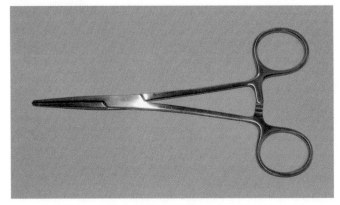

Figure 9-37 ■ Hemostat.

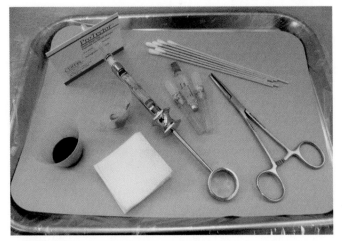

Figure 9-38 ■ Typical local anesthetic armamentarium setup.

anesthetic. The dental hygienist should follow the following recommended steps for the preparation of equipment.

STEP 1

Based on the treatment to be performed and the patient's medical history, the appropriate local and topical anesthetics should be selected, and the appropriate equipment should be assembled. Figure 9-38 shows a typical local anesthetic setup.

The equipment should include:
- Personal protective equipment
- Anesthetic syringe
- Anesthetic cartridge
- Needle (length and gauge selected according to injection to be administered)
- Topical antiseptic (optional)
- Topical anesthetic
- Gauze
- Cotton-tip applicators
- Hemostat or cotton pliers

STEP 2

The dental hygienist should carefully evaluate the local anesthetic cartridge (Figure 9-39):

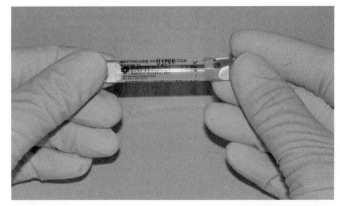

Figure 9-39 ■ The dental hygienist should evaluate the cartridge.

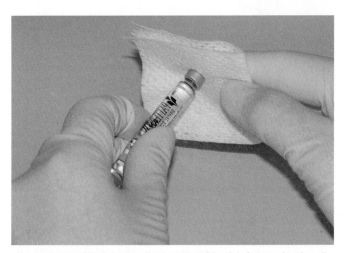

Figure 9-40 ■ Wiping the diaphragm with disinfectant (optional).

- Check the selected anesthetic to ensure that the proper drug has been selected.
- Check that anesthetic drug is not outdated.
- Check for large bubbles that might be present in the cartridge.
- Check for an extruded stopper that extends beyond the glass rim.
- Check for any corrosion of rust on the cartridge.
- Check the cartridge for any hairline fractures or chipped glass.

STEP 3 (OPTIONAL)

If the dental hygienist feels it is necessary, he or she can wipe the rubber diaphragm with a disinfectant applied to a gauze square (Figure 9-40).

STEP 4

Retract the piston of the syringe by pulling back on the thumb ring (Figure 9-41).

STEP 5

Insert the cartridge with the rubber stopper going into the syringe first toward the piston (Figure 9-42).

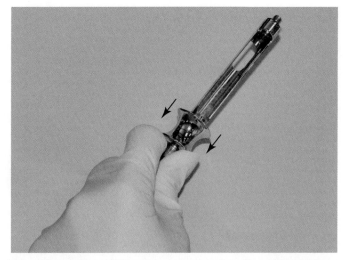

Figure 9-41 ■ Retract the piston of the syringe by pulling back on the thumb ring.

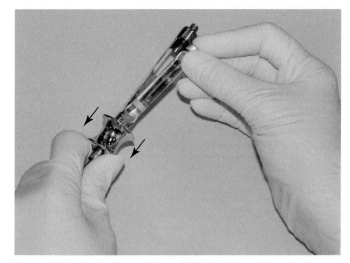

Figure 9-42 ■ Insert the cartridge with the rubber stopper going into the syringe first toward the piston.

STEP 6

Engage the harpoon into the plunger with gentle finger pressure exerted on the thumb ring (Figure 9-43). Do not exert extreme force on the rubber stopper; the glass cartridge may break (Figure 9-44).

STEP 7

Attach the needle. Remove the shield from the needle penetrating end (Figure 9-45A). If the seal is intact, it should require snapping the seal as the shield is twisted. Seals that are not intact should be discarded. Attach the needle adaptor to the needle of the syringe. If a plastic hub is being used, the dental hygienist must simultaneously push and screw the needle into position. The needle should always be attached to the syringe after the cartridge has been inserted. The harpoon is too difficult to engage into the rubber stopper when the needle is already in place, causing excessive force to be applied to the thumb rings to engage the harpoon (Figure 9-45B).

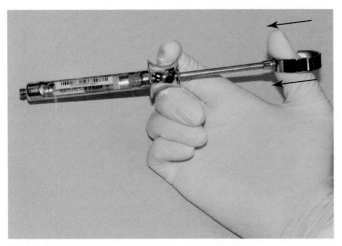

Figure 9-43 ■ Engage the harpoon into the rubber stopper with gentle finger pressure exerted on the thumb ring.

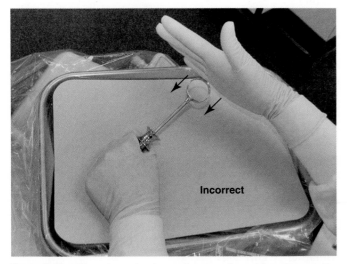

Incorrect

Figure 9-44 ■ Do not exert extreme force on the rubber stopper; the glass may break.

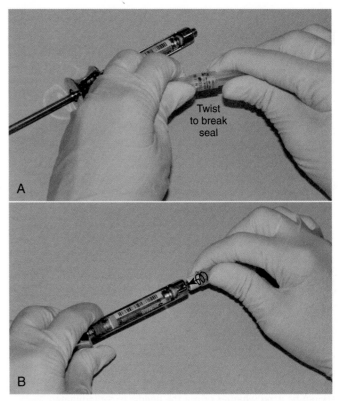

Twist to break seal

A

B

Figure 9-45 ■ Attach the needle. **A,** Remove the shield from the needle penetrating end by twisting to snap the seal and attach to the needle adaptor of the syringe. **B,** If a plastic hub is being used, the dental hygienist must simultaneously push and screw the needle into position. The needle should always be placed onto the syringe after the cartridge has been inserted and the harpoon is engaged. The harpoon is too difficult to engage if the needle is already in place, causing excessive force to be applied to the thumb ring to engage the harpoon.

STEP 8

Carefully uncap the colored plastic shield for the needle and expel a few drops of anesthetic to ensure the proper flow of solution (Figure 9-46).

STEP 9

Scoop the protective shield back onto the needle using the one-handed scoop technique with a needle sheath prop to protect the needle until it is ready for use. The scoop technique should be used whether or not the needle is contaminated (Figure 9-47).

Recapping the needle should be accomplished using the scoop technique immediately after the needle is removed from the tissues. The protective shield should remain on the needle at all times when the syringe is not in use (Figure 9-48). Needle capping devices are available in many forms (Figure 9-24). Individual preference will determine the aid that is appropriate.

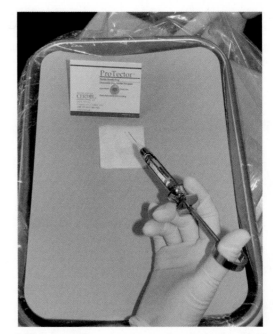

Figure 9-46 ■ Carefully uncap the colored plastic shield of the needle and expel a few drops of anesthetic to ensure the proper flow of solution.

UNLOADING THE BREECH-LOADING ASPIRATING SYRINGE

Following the completion of the anesthetic injection, and once the needle is safely capped, the dental hygienist should follow the following steps for dismantling the anesthetic syringe.

STEP 1

Take the syringe to the appropriate sharps container. Carefully remove the needle (Figure 9-49A) and immediately discard in the approved sharps container (Figure 9-49B). It is recommended that the cartridge penetrating end of the needle not be recapped and left on the anesthetic tray before discarding because there is the possibility that the used needle could be mistaken for an unused needle and be reused on another patient. This technique ensures that the needle cannot accidentally be used on another patient and protects the clinician from needlestick exposure from the needle penetrating end. For dental hygiene students or practicing dental hygienists taking the Western Regional Anesthesia Board Examination, this is the required method of needle disposal by not recapping the cartridge end of the needle.

When discarding the needle, care should be taken to avoid inadvertently discarding the needle adaptor (Figure 9-50).

If the needle adaptor remains on the needle, it can be safely removed with cotton pliers (Figure 9-51A). Never attempt to remove the needle adaptor with unprotected hands (Figure 9-51B).

STEP 2

Retract the piston by pulling back on the thumb ring (Figure 9-52).

STEP 3

Remove the cartridge (Figure 9-53A) and dispose in separate sealed container (Figure 9-53B), or in approved sharps container (Figure 9-26).

Occasionally the rubber stopper may be lodged on the harpoon. It can be safely removed with cotton pliers (Figure 9-54).

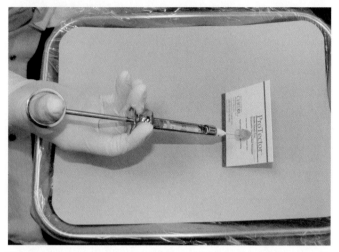

Figure 9-47 ■ Scoop the protective shield back onto the needle using the one-handed scoop technique with a needle sheath prop to protect the needle until it is ready for use. The scoop technique should be used whether or not the needle is contaminated.

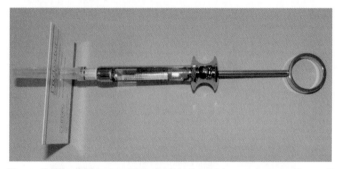

Figure 9-48 ■ The protective shield should be on the needle at all times when the syringe is not in use.

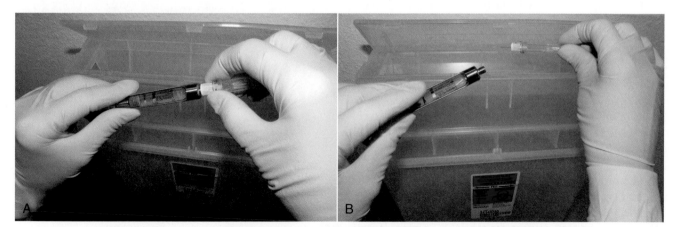

Figure 9-49 ■ Take the syringe to the appropriate sharps container. **A,** Carefully remove the needle. **B,** Immediately discard in the approved sharps container. (Remember that the cartridge penetrating end of the needle shaft is contaminated after use.)

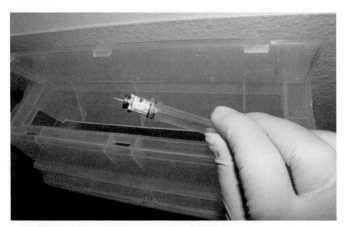

Figure 9-50 ■ When discarding the needle, care should be taken to avoid inadvertently discarding the needle adaptor.

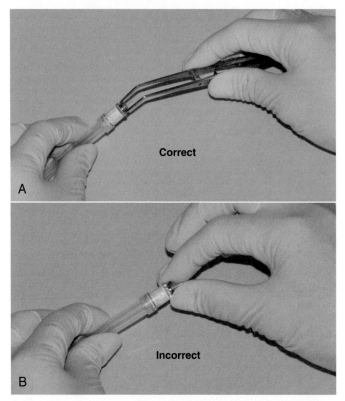

Correct

A

Incorrect

B

Figure 9-51 ■ **A,** If the needle adapter remains on the needle, it can be safely removed with cotton pliers. **B,** Never attempt to remove the needle adapter with unprotected hands.

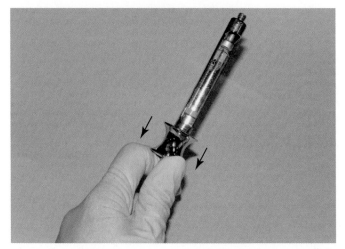

Figure 9-52 ■ Retract the piston by pulling back on the thumb ring.

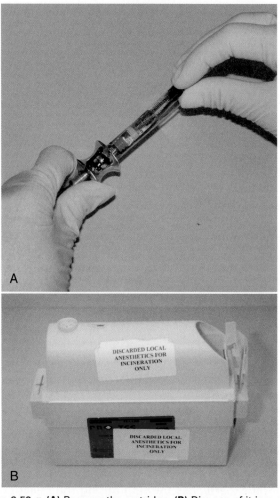

A

B

DISCARDED LOCAL
ANESTHETICS FOR
INCINERATION
ONLY

DISCARDED LOCAL
ANESTHETICS FOR
INCINERATION
ONLY

Figure 9-53 ■ **(A)** Remove the cartridge, **(B)** Dispose of it in a separate sealed container. (From Malamed S: *Handbook of local anesthesia*, St Louis, 2004, Mosby.)

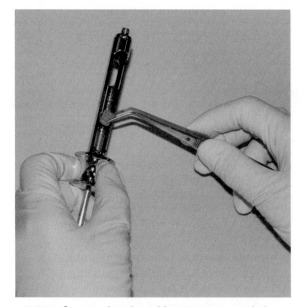

Figure 9-54 ■ On occasion the rubber stopper may lodge on the harpoon. It can be safely removed with cotton piers. Never attempt to remove with fingers.

DENTAL HYGIENE CONSIDERATIONS

- It is critical for the dental hygienist to administer local anesthetics with an aspirating syringe. If the tip of the needle is within a blood vessel, blood will enter the cartridge through the lumen of the needle following a successful aspiration.
- The dental hygienist should select a syringe that accommodates his or her hand size for ease of aspiration and stability of the syringe.
- Disengagement of the harpoon during aspiration frequently produces a "popping" noise. Should this occur, the dental hygienist must remove the needle from the tissue, reengage the harpoon, and re-do the procedure.
- The bevel of the needle should be toward the bone when administering injections in close proximity to the periosteum.
- The smaller the gauge number, the larger the diameter of the lumen.
- A 25-gauge needle is recommended for areas of high risk for positive aspiration (inferior alveolar block, posterior superior alveolar block, mental and incisive blocks).

- Long needles should be used when penetrating significant thick tissue (inferior alveolar, Gow-Gates mandibular block, and infraorbital blocks).
- The dental hygienist should know the location of an uncovered needle at all times whether the needle is inside or outside the mouth.
- Using the one-handed scoop method with a needle sheath prop, the dental hygienist should immediately cap the needle following the injection.
- The dental hygienist should never bend the needle before use except for intraligamentary injections.
- The dental hygienist should never insert the needle to the hub and should not make any sudden direction changes while the needle is embedded in tissue.
- The dental hygienist should not use cartridges that contain large bubbles, extruded stoppers, corroded caps, rust on the cap, or expired solutions.
- The dental hygienist should discard contaminated needles in an approved sharps container.

CASE STUDY 9-1

Gloria experiences burning during the injection
Gloria is in the office today for nonsurgical periodontal therapy. Stacey, the dental hygienist, is assembling the equipment when she drops the anesthetic cartridges on the floor. Concerned that she has contaminated the cartridges, she drops them into the disinfecting solution to clean them before she loads a cartridge in the syringe. Approximately 30 minutes later, Stacey removes the cartridges from the disinfecting solution and loads the syringe. Stacey administers an ASA block to the patient who immediately demonstrates signs of extreme discomfort. Stacey removes and safely caps the needle, and

questions Gloria regarding the discomfort. Gloria expresses that she has never experienced such an intense burning sensation before when she received a local anesthetic. A few minutes later Stacey notices some swelling in the area of the injection.

Critical Thinking Questions
- Why was the patient experiencing burning during the injection?
- How could Stacey have avoided this response?
- Why did the swelling occur?

CHAPTER REVIEW QUESTIONS

1. What is the most important improvement that has been made to the local anesthetic syringe?
   A. Recapping devices to prevent needle sticks
   B. The addition of the aspirating harpoon
   C. Adding weight for better grasp
   D. Various thumb ring sizes
2. Which of the following are important criteria for an acceptable local anesthetic syringe?
   A. Inexpensive, self-contained, and able to withstand repeated sterilization without damage
   B. Able to withstand repeated sterilization, light weight, and expensive
   C. Not self-contained, inexpensive, and able to withstand repeated sterilization without damage

   D. Not self-contained, heavy in weight, and able to withstand repeated sterilization without damage
3. What is the purpose of applying negative pressure to the harpoon?
   A. To ensure the rubber stopper does not move
   B. To advance the piston
   C. To evaluate whether needle is within a blood vessel
   D. To evaluate whether the needle is within a nerve
4. Computer-controlled anesthetic devices are beneficial because they deliver exact amounts of anesthetic at a controlled rate, but they are less ergonomic for the clinician.

CHAPTER REVIEW QUESTIONS

A. Both statements are true
B. Both statements are false
C. First statement is true, second statement is false
D. First statement is false, second statement is true

5. What is the definition of the needle bevel?
   A. The diameter of the needle lumen
   B. The lumen of the needle
   C. The angled point or tip of the needle
   D. The plastic or prethreaded metal adapter

6. Which of the following intraoral needle gauges used in dentistry are listed from smallest to the largest?
   A. 16, 20, 30
   B. 25, 27, 30
   C. 30, 27, 16
   D. 30, 27, 25

7. It is safe to insert the needle to the hub, because the hub of the needle is the strongest part of the needle.
   A. Both statements are true
   B. Both statements are false
   C. First statement is true, but the reasoning is false
   D. First statement is false, but the reasoning is true

8. Larger needle gauges have what advantages over smaller gauge needles?
   A. Less deflection
   B. Greater accuracy
   C. Increased injection success
   D. B and C
   E. All of the above

9. The bevel of the needle should:
   A. Never touch the bone
   B. Be turned away from the bone
   C. Be turned toward the bone
   D. All of the above

10. What are the two commonly used needle lengths for intraoral injections?
    A. 16 mm, 24 mm
    B. 25 mm, 30 mm
    C. 30 mm, 32 mm
    D. 20 mm, 32 mm

11. All are acceptable ways to recap a needle, EXCEPT:
    A. The use of recapping devices
    B. Single-handed scoop method
    C. Using cotton pliers to recap the needle
    D. Using fingers to recap the needle when the needle has NOT entered the patient's mouth

12. All are ways that increase the risk of needle breakage, EXCEPT:
    A. Using a 25-gauge needle
    B. Inserting to the hub
    C. Bending the needle
    D. Sudden directional changes

13. The color-coded band on the anesthetic cartridges identifies what?
    A. Drug inside the cartridge
    B. Amount of solution

C. Expiration date
D. Location of the bevel

14. Warming the anesthetic solution is recommended for patient comfort because it can activate the vasoconstrictor, causing an increase in the duration of action.
    A. Both statements are true
    B. Both statements are false
    C. First statement is true, but the reasoning is false
    D. First statement is false, but the reasoning is true

15. Which of the following indicate that the cartridge should be used?
    A. Small bubbles less than 2 mm
    B. Large bubbles more than 2 mm
    C. Extruded stopper
    D. Extruded stopper with a large bubble

16. What causes the burning sensation when the anesthetic is injected into the tissues?
    A. The anesthetic is more acidic than the tissues
    B. The low pH
    C. Vasoconstrictors
    D. All of the above
    E. None of the above

17. What are characteristics of topical anesthetics?
    A. Provide soft tissue anesthesia
    B. Diffuse 5 mm into the mucous membrane
    C. Less concentrated than injectable anesthetic solutions
    D. A and B
    E. All of the above

18. What is optional when preparing to give an intraoral injection?
    A. Personal protective equipment
    B. Anesthetic syringe, cartridge, and needle
    C. Topical antiseptic
    D. Hemostat

19. How should a clinician properly dispose of anesthetic needles?
    A. Recapping utilizing the scoop method and placing in the garbage
    B. Bending the needle, recapping, and disposal in an approved sharps container
    C. Recapping utilizing the scoop method and disposal in an approved sharps container
    D. Bending the needle, recapping, and disposal in a biohazard container

20. Which of the following are ways to decrease pain during injections?
    A. Change needle after 3–4 tissue penetrations
    B. Withdraw the needle quickly
    C. Use a vasoconstrictor
    D. Advance the needle quickly

REFERENCES

1. Jastak T, Yagiela J, Donaldson D: *Local anesthesia of the oral cavity*, St Louis, 1995, Saunders.
2. Malamed S: *Handbook of local anesthesia*, ed 5, St Louis, 2004, Mosby.
3. Council on Dental Materials and Devices: New American National Standard Institute/American Dental Association Specification No. 34 for Dental Aspirating Syringes, *J Am Dent Assoc* 97:236-238, 1978.
4. Council on Dental Materials, Instruments, and Equipment. Addendum to American National Standard Institute/ American Dental Association Specification No. 34 for Dental Aspirating Syringes, *J Am Dent Assoc* 104:69-70, 1982.
5. Friedman MJ, Hochman MN: 21st century computerized injection for local pain control, *Compendium of Continuing Education in Dentistry* 18:995-1003, 1997.
6. Hochman MN, Chiarello D, Hochman CB, et al: Computerized local anesthesia delivery vs. traditional syringe technique, *NYS Dent J* 63:24, 29, 1997.
7. Fuller NP, Menke RA, Meyers WJ: Perception of pain to three different intraoral penetrations of needles, *J Am Dent Assoc* 99:822-824, 1979.
8. Brownbill JW, Walker PO, Bourcy BD, Keenan KM, Comparison of inferior dental nerve block injections in child patients using 30 gauge and 25 gauge short needles, *Anesth Prog* 34:215-219, 1987.
9. Darby M, Walsh M: *Dental hygiene theory and practice*, ed 3, St Louis, 2010, Saunders.

ADDITIONAL RESOURCES

Daniel S, Harfst S, Wilder R, et al: *Dental hygiene concepts, cases and competencies*, ed 2, St Louis, 2008, Mosby.

CHAPTER 10

Anatomic Considerations for the Administration of Local Anesthesia

Margaret Fehrenbach RDH, MS

CHAPTER OUTLINE

LEARNING OBJECTIVES

1. Define and pronounce the key terms and anatomic terms in this chapter.
2. Locate and identify the skull bones of the head that are relevant to the administration of local anesthesia.
3. Describe in detail and indicate the various parts and landmarks of the maxillae, palatine bones, and mandible on a diagram, skull, and patient.
4. Identify and trace the routes of the blood vessels of the head and neck that are relevant to the administration of local anesthesia on a diagram, skull, and patient.

5. Locate the glandular tissue of the head and neck that are relevant to the administration of local anesthesia on a diagram, skull, and patient.
6. Integrate an understanding of head and neck anatomy into the technique of local anesthesia administration for clinical dental hygiene dental practice.
7. Successfully complete review questions for this chapter.

KEY TERMS

Anastomosis/Anastomoses Connecting channel(s) among the blood vessels.

Arteriole Smaller vessels of the artery.

Artery Component of the vascular system that arises from the heart, carrying blood away from it.

Canal Opening in bone that is long, narrow, and tubelike.

Capillary Smaller vessels of the arterioles that form a network.

Condyle Oval bony prominence usually involved in joints.

Dental plexus A network of vessels or nerves.

Foramen/foramina Short, windowlike opening in bone.

Fossa/fossae Depression on a bony surface.

Line Straight, small ridge of bone.

Notch Indentation at the edge of a bone.

Process General term for any prominence on a bony surface.

Tuberosity Large, often rough prominence on the surface of bone.

Vein Component of the vascular system that carries blood to the heart.

Venous sinuses Blood-filled spaces between the two layers of tissue.

INTRODUCTION

The management of pain with hemostatic control through local anesthesia during dental hygiene care requires a thorough understanding by the dental hygienist of the anatomy of the relevant regions of the skull and the trigeminal and facial nerves, as well as adjacent structures. This chapter discusses the anatomic considerations for local anesthesia.

SKULL BONES

The skull bones involved in local anesthetic administration are the maxillae, palatine bones, and mandible. Soft tissue of the face and oral cavity may serve the dental hygienist as initial landmarks to visualize and then palpate before local anesthesia administration, as discussed in Chapters 12 and 13. However, there are many variations in soft tissue topographic anatomy among patients. Thus to increase the reliability of the local anesthesia, the dental hygienist must learn to rely mainly on the visualization and palpation of the bony landmarks while injecting patients.

The prominences and depressions on the bony surface of the skull are landmarks for the attachments of associated muscles, tendons, and ligaments as well as for the administration of local anesthesia. A general term for any prominence on a bony surface is a process. One specific type of prominence located on the bony surface is a condyle, which is usually involved in joints. Another large, often rough prominence is a tuberosity. A line is a straight, small ridge. One type of depression on the bony surface is a notch, an indentation at the edge of the bone. A generally deeper depression on a bony surface is a fossa (plural, fossae).

The openings in the bone are also landmarks where various nerves and blood vessels enter or exit, which is important when administering local anesthesia. A foramen (plural, foramina) is a short windowlike opening in the bone. A canal is a longer, narrow tubelike opening in the bone.

MAXILLAE

The upper jaw, or maxillae, consists of paired maxilla or maxillary bones that are fused together at the intermaxillary suture (Figure 10-1). Each maxilla includes a body and four processes: frontal, zygomatic, palatine, and alveolar processes. The body of the maxilla has orbital, nasal, infratemporal, and facial surfaces. The bodies contain air-filled spaces or paranasal sinuses, the maxillary sinuses.

From an anterior view, each frontal process of the maxilla articulates with the frontal bone and forms the medial orbital rim with the lacrimal bone on its anterior surface (Figures 10-2 and 10-3). Each maxilla's orbital surface is separated from the sphenoid bone by the inferior orbital fissure (Table 10-1; Figure 10-1). The inferior orbital fissure carries the infraorbital and zygomatic nerves, infraorbital

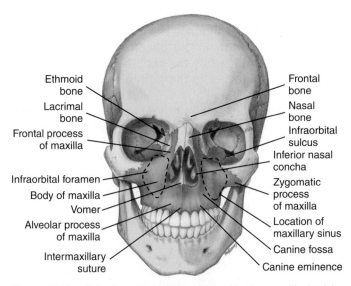

Figure 10-1 ■ Anterior view of the skull with the maxilla and its associated landmarks highlighted. (From Fehrenbach MJ, Herring SW: *Illustrated anatomy of the head and neck*, ed 3, St Louis, 2007, Saunders.)

Labels in figure: Ethmoid bone; Lacrimal bone; Frontal process of maxilla; Infraorbital foramen; Body of maxilla; Vomer; Alveolar process of maxilla; Intermaxillary suture; Frontal bone; Nasal bone; Infraorbital sulcus; Inferior nasal concha; Zygomatic process of maxilla; Location of maxillary sinus; Canine fossa; Canine eminence

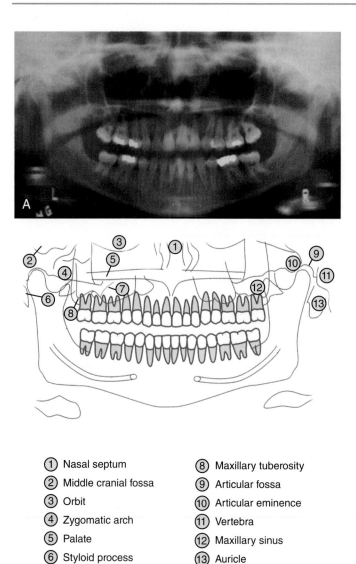

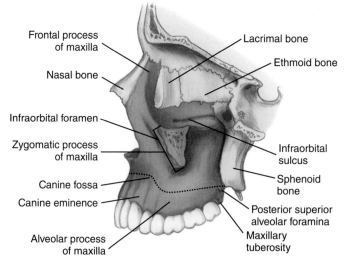

① Nasal septum
② Middle cranial fossa
③ Orbit
④ Zygomatic arch
⑤ Palate
⑥ Styloid process
⑦ Septa in maxillary sinus

⑧ Maxillary tuberosity
⑨ Articular fossa
⑩ Articular eminence
⑪ Vertebra
⑫ Maxillary sinus
⑬ Auricle

B

Figure 10-2 ■ **A,** Panoramic radiograph. **B,** Panoramic anatomy of the midface. (**A,** From Bath-Balogh M, Fehrenbach M: *Illustrated dental embryology, histology, and anatomy*, ed 3, St Louis, 2010, Saunders. **B,** Modified from Olson SS: *Dental radiography laboratory manual*, Philadelphia, 1995, Saunders; and in Fehrenbach MJ, Herring SW: *Illustrated anatomy of the head and neck*, ed 3, St Louis, 2007, Saunders.)

Figure 10-3 ■ Cutaway view of the lateral aspect of the skull with the maxilla highlighted. (From Fehrenbach MJ, Herring SW: *Illustrated anatomy of the head and neck*, ed 3, St Louis, 2007, Saunders.)

artery, and inferior ophthalmic vein (see later discussion). The groove in the floor of the orbital surface is the infraorbital sulcus.

The infraorbital sulcus becomes the infraorbital canal and then terminates on the facial surface of each maxilla as the infraorbital foramen (see Figures 10-3 and 10-19 and Table 10-1). It is located approximately 2 cm inferior to the midpoint of the inferior margin of the orbit, in a vertical line with the supraorbital and notch, which is superior to it. This foramen transmits the infraorbital nerve and blood vessels (discussed later). Palpation of the infraorbital foramen will cause soreness on the patient. The infraorbital foramen is a landmark for the administration of the infraorbital block (see Chapter 12).

Inferior to the infraorbital foramen is an elongated depression, the canine fossa. The canine fossa is just posterosuperior to the roots of the maxillary canine teeth. Each tooth of the maxillary arch is covered by a prominent facial ridge of bone, a part of the alveolar process of the maxilla (Table 10-2; Figures 10-3 and 10-19). The facial ridge over the maxillary canine, the canine eminence is especially prominent, making it a landmark for the administration of the anterior superior alveolar block (see Chapter 12).

The maxillary bone over the facial surface of the maxillary teeth is less dense and more porous than the mandibular bone over similar teeth as can be viewed on a panoramic radiograph (see Figure 10-2). This allows a greater incidence of clinically adequate local anesthesia for the maxillary teeth when the local anesthetic agent is administered as a supraperiosteal injection or local infiltration than would occur with similar teeth on the mandibular arch (see Chapters 12 and 13).

From the lateral view, each zygomatic process of the maxilla articulates with the zygomatic bone laterally, completing the infraorbital rim (Figures 10-2, 10-3, and 10-17 and Table 10-2).

On the posterior part of the body of the maxilla is a rounded, roughened elevation, the maxillary tuberosity, just posterior to the most distal molar of the maxillary dentition (Figures 10-2, 10-4, and 10-19). The superolateral part of the maxillary tuberosity is perforated by one or more posterior superior alveolar foramina, where the posterior superior alveolar nerve and blood vessel branches enter the bone from the back (see later discussion). The maxillary tuberosity and posterior superior alveolar foramina are landmarks for the administration of the posterior superior alveolar block (see Chapter 12).

On the inferior surface, each palatine process of the maxilla articulates with the other to form the major or

TABLE 10-1	Bony Openings in the Skull and Contents Related to the Trigeminal Nerve	
BONY OPENING	**LOCATION**	**CONTENTS**
Foramen ovale	Sphenoid bone	Mandibular division of the fifth cranial or trigeminal nerve and vessels
Foramen rotundum	Sphenoid bone	Maxillary nerve of the fifth cranial or trigeminal nerve and vessels
Greater palatine foramen	Palatine bone	Greater palatine nerve and vessels
Incisive foramen	Maxillae	Both right and left nasopalatine nerves and branches of the sphenopalatine artery
Inferior orbital fissure	Sphenoid bone and maxillae	Infraorbital and zygomatic nerves, infraorbital artery, and ophthalmic vein
Infraorbital foramen and canal	Maxilla	Infraorbital nerve and vessels
Lesser palatine foramen	Palatine bone	Lesser palatine nerve and vessels
Mandibular foramen	Mandible	Inferior alveolar nerve and vessels
Mental foramen	Mandible	Mental nerve and vessels
Superior orbital fissure	Sphenoid bone	Ophthalmic nerve of the fifth cranial or trigeminal nerve and vessels

TABLE 10-2	Maxillary and Mandibular Processes and Associated Structures	
PROCESSES OF SKULL	**SKULL BONES**	**ASSOCIATED STRUCTURES**
Alveolar process	Mandible	Contains roots of mandibular teeth
Alveolar process	Maxilla	Contains roots of maxillary teeth
Coronoid process	Mandible	Part of ramus
Frontal process	Maxilla	Forms medial infraorbital rim
Palatine processes	Maxilla	Forms anterior part of hard palate
Zygomatic process	Maxilla	Forms lateral part of infraorbital rim

TABLE 10-3	Sutures of Maxillae and Palatine Bones	
SUTURE	**BONY ARTICULATIONS**	
Intermaxillary suture	Maxillae	
Median palatine suture	Anterior part: maxillae Posterior part: palatine bones	
Transverse palatine suture	Maxillae and palatine bones	

anterior part of the hard palate (Figure 10-4; see Figure 10-2 and Table 10-2). There are a number of small pores in the maxillary bone of the anterior hard palate. The suture between these two palatine processes of the maxilla is the anterior part of the median palatine suture (see Table 10-3). In the patient, this suture is covered by the median palatine raphe, a midline fibrous band of tissue, which is a landmark along with the pores for the administration of the anterior middle superior alveolar block (see Chapter 12).

In the anterior midline between the two articulating palatine processes of the maxillae, just posterior to the maxillary central incisors, is the incisive foramen (see Table 10-1 and Figure 10-20). This foramen carries both branches of the right and left nasopalatine nerves and blood vessels from the nasal cavity to the palate (see later discussion). The incisive papilla is the soft tissue that bulges over the incisive foramen. The incisive foramen and incisive papilla are both landmarks for the administration of the nasopalatine block (see Chapter 12).

The alveolar process of the maxilla usually contains the roots of the maxillary teeth (see Figures 10-2 and 10-4 and Table 10-2). The apices of these roots on both the facial

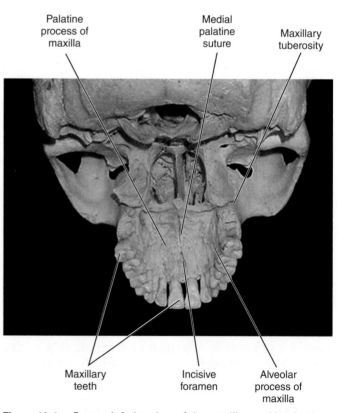

Palatine process of maxilla

Medial palatine suture

Maxillary tuberosity

Maxillary teeth

Incisive foramen

Alveolar process of maxilla

Figure 10-4 ■ Posteroinferior view of the maxillae and hard palate. (From Fehrenbach MJ, Herring SW: *Illustrated anatomy of the head and neck*, ed 3, St Louis, 2007, Saunders.)

and lingual surface of the maxillary alveolar process are landmarks for the administration of most of the maxillary injections (see Chapter 12). The maxillary alveolar process can become resorbed in a patient who is completely edentulous in the maxillary arch (resorption occurs to a lesser extent in partially edentulous cases). However, the more superior body of the maxilla is not resorbed with tooth loss, but its walls may become thinner in this case.

PALATINE BONES

The palatine bones are paired bones, each of which consists of two plates, the horizontal and vertical plates. Both the horizontal and vertical plates can be seen from a posterior

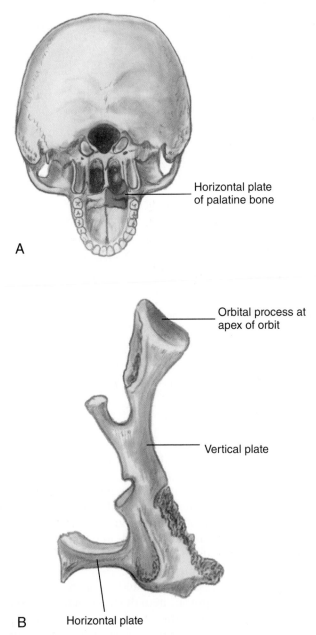

A

B   Horizontal plate

Horizontal plate
of palatine bone

Orbital process at
apex of orbit

Vertical plate

Figure 10-5 ■ Posterior view of the right palatine bone with its location demonstrated on a posterior-inferior view of the skull. (From Fehrenbach MJ, Herring SW: *Illustrated anatomy of the head and neck*, ed 3, St Louis, 2007, Saunders.)

view of the palatine bone (Figure 10-5). The horizontal plates of the palatine bones form the lesser or posterior part of the hard palate. The vertical plates of the palatine bones form a part of the lateral walls of the nasal cavity, and each plate contributes a small lip of bone to the orbital apex.

The palatine bones serve as a link between the maxillae and the sphenoid bone with which they articulate, as well as with each other. The two horizontal plates articulate with each other at the posterior part of the median palatine suture and with the maxillae at the transverse palatine suture (see Figure 10-4 and Table 10-3).

Two important foramina in the palatine bones, the greater and lesser palatine foramina (Figure 10-6; see Figure 10-20 and Table 10-1), transmit nerves and blood vessels to this region (discussed later). The larger greater palatine foramen is located in the posterolateral region of each of the palatine bones, usually at the apex of the maxillary third molar. The greater palatine foramen transmits the greater palatine nerve and blood vessels and is a landmark for the administration of the greater palatine block (see Chapter 12).

The smaller opening nearby, the lesser palatine foramen, transmits the lesser palatine nerve and blood vessels to the soft palate and tonsils. The lesser palatine nerve within this foramen can sometimes inadvertently become anesthetized with the greater palatine block due to close proximity to the greater palatine foramen and its nerve, making the patient feel uncomfortable as their soft palate become anesthetized. Both foramina are openings of the pterygopalatine canal that carries the descending palatine nerves and blood vessels from the pterygopalatine fossa to the palate.

MANDIBLE

The lower jaw, or mandible, is the only freely movable bone of the skull (Figures 10-7 and 10-8). The mandible has a movable articulation with the temporal bones at each temporomandibular joint. The single mandible also articulates with both of the maxilla by way of their contained respective lower and upper dental arches.

From an anterior view of the mandible, there are many important landmarks (Figures 10-9 and 10-11). The mental

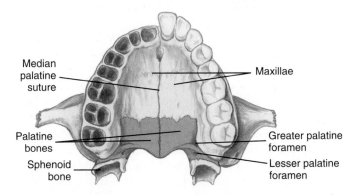

Median
palatine
suture

Maxillae

Palatine
bones

Greater palatine
foramen

Sphenoid
bone

Lesser palatine
foramen

Figure 10-6 ■ Inferior view of the hard palate with the palatine bones highlighted. (From Fehrenbach MJ, Herring SW: *Illustrated anatomy of the head and neck*, ed 3, St Louis, 2007, Saunders.)

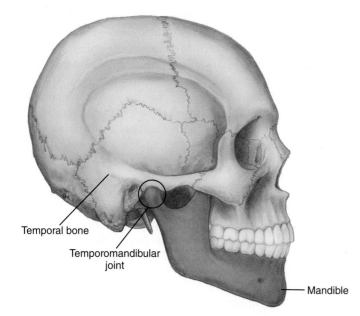

Figure 10-7 ■ Lateral view of the skull showing the mandible and the temporomandibular joint. (From Fehrenbach MJ, Herring SW: *Illustrated anatomy of the head and neck*, ed 3, St Louis, 2007, Saunders.)

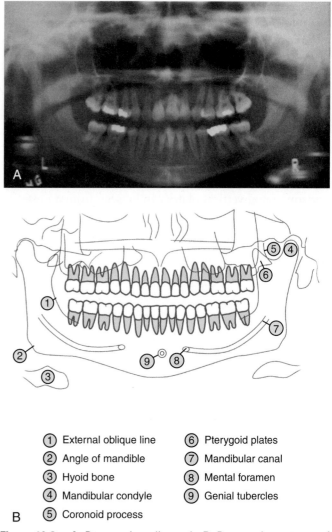

①	External oblique line	⑥	Pterygoid plates
②	Angle of mandible	⑦	Mandibular canal
③	Hyoid bone	⑧	Mental foramen
④	Mandibular condyle	⑨	Genial tubercles
⑤	Coronoid process		

Figure 10-8 ■ **A,** Panoramic radiograph. **B,** Panoramic anatomy of the lower face. (**A,** From Bath-Balogh M, Fehrenbach M: *Illustrated dental embryology, histology, and anatomy*, ed 3, St Louis, 2010, Saunders. **B,** Modified from Olson SS: *Dental radiography laboratory manual*, Philadelphia, 1995, Saunders; and in Fehrenbach MJ, Herring SW: *Illustrated anatomy of the head and neck*, ed 3, St Louis, 2007, Saunders.)

protuberance the bony prominence of the chin, is located deep to the roots of the mandibular incisors. In the midline on the anterior surface of the mandible is a faint ridge, an indication of the mandibular symphysis, where the bone is formed by the fusion of right and left processes.

Farther posteriorly on the lateral surface of the mandible, usually between the apices of the mandibular first and second premolars, is an opening, the mental foramen (see Figures 10-2, 10-9, 10-10, and 10-25, and Table 10-1). As mandibular growth proceeds in children, the mental foramen alters in direction from anterior to posterosuperior. The mental foramen allows the entrance of the mental nerve and blood vessels into the mandibular canal (discussed later).

The mental foramen's posterosuperior opening in adults signifies the changed direction of the emerging mental nerve. This is an important landmark to note intraorally and on a radiograph before administration of both the mental and incisive blocks (see Chapter 13 and see Table 13-6, Figure L).

The heavy horizontal part of the lower jaw is the body of the mandible, which is inferior to the mental foramen (see Figures 10-9 and 10-10). Superior to this, the part of the lower jaw that usually contains the roots of the mandibular teeth is the alveolar process of the mandible (see Table 10-2). The body of the mandible, along with the alveolar process, elongates to provide space for additional teeth as the child nears adulthood.

The mandibular alveolar process can become resorbed if a patient becomes completely edentulous in the mandibular arch (occasionally noted also in partially edentulous cases), which can change the landmarks when administering both the mental or incisive blocks as well as the inferior

alveolar block (see Chapter 13). This resorption can occur to such an extent that the mental foramen is virtually on the superior border of the mandible, instead of opening on the anterior surface, changing its relative position. The height of the mandibular foramen can also seem to be more inferior without the presence of teeth in the arch. However, the more inferior body of the mandible is not affected and remains thick and rounded.

The alveolar process of the mandibular incisors is also less dense and more porous than the body of the mandible and even less dense than the alveolar process of the mandibular posterior teeth as can be viewed on a panoramic radiograph (see Figure 10-8). This allows a supraperiosteal injection or local infiltration of the mandibular anteriors by a local anesthetic agent to have a higher degree of success

Ramus Mandibular symphysis Alveolar process

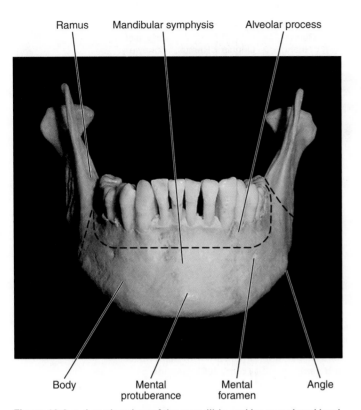

Body Mental Mental Angle
protuberance foramen

Figure 10-9 ■ Anterior view of the mandible and its associated landmarks. (From Fehrenbach MJ, Herring SW: *Illustrated anatomy of the head and neck*, ed 3, St Louis, 2007, Saunders.)

Temporomandibular Coronoid Coronoid
joint process notch

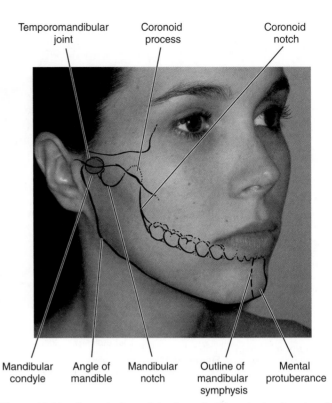

Mandibular Angle of Mandibular Outline of Mental
condyle mandible notch mandibular protuberance
symphysis

Figure 10-11 ■ Lateral view of the face showing the landmarks of the mandible. (From Fehrenbach MJ, Herring SW: *Illustrated anatomy of the head and neck*, ed 3, St Louis, 2007, Saunders.)

Coronoid Articulating
process surface of
Mandibular Alveolar Pterygoid Coronoid Mandibular condyle
teeth process fovea notch notch

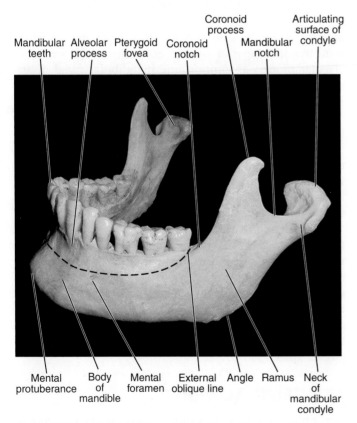

Mental Body Mental External Angle Ramus Neck
protuberance of foramen oblique line of
mandible mandibular
condyle

Figure 10-10 ■ Slightly oblique lateral view of the mandible and its associated landmarks. (From Fehrenbach MJ, Herring SW: *Illustrated anatomy of the head and neck*, ed 3, St Louis, 2007, Saunders.)

than the mandibular posterior teeth but always less success than all the maxillary teeth (see Chapters 12 and 13).

On the lateral aspect of the mandible, the stout, flat plate of the ramus extends superiorly and posteriorly from the body of the mandible on each side (see Figure 10-10). During growth of the body, the body of the mandible and alveolar process elongates posteriorly to the mental foramen, providing space for three additional permanent teeth. The ramus, which serves as the primary area for the attachment of the muscles of mastication, grows superiorly and posteriorly, displacing the mental protuberance of the chin inferiorly and anteriorly when nearing adulthood.

The anterior border of the ramus is a thin, sharp margin that terminates in the coronoid process (see Figure 10-19 and Table 10-2). The main part of the anterior border of the ramus forms a concave forward curve, the coronoid notch. The coronoid notch is a landmark for the administration of the inferior alveolar block (see Chapter 13). Inferior to the coronoid notch, the anterior border of the ramus becomes the external oblique line. The external oblique line or ridge is a crest where the ramus joins the body of the mandible. The line is noted as a radiopaque line on a radiograph superior to the mylohyoid line; clinicians may use this line intraorally to help locate the coronoid notch (see Figure 10-8).

The posterior border of the ramus is thickened and extends from the angle of the mandible to a projection, the condyle of the mandible with its neck (see Figures 10-7 to

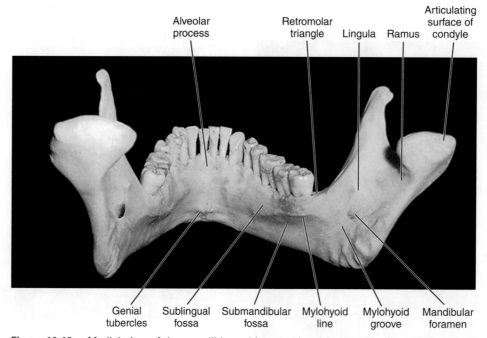

Alveolar process — Retromolar triangle — Lingula — Ramus — Articulating surface of condyle

Genial tubercles — Sublingual fossa — Submandibular fossa — Mylohyoid line — Mylohyoid groove — Mandibular foramen

Figure 10-12 ■ Medial view of the mandible and its associated landmarks. (From Fehrenbach MJ, Herring SW: *Illustrated anatomy of the head and neck*, ed 3, St Louis, 2007, Saunders.)

10-11 and Figure 10-12). The anteromedial border of the mandibular condylar neck is a landmark for the Gow-Gates mandibular block (see Chapter 13). The articulating surface of the condyle is an oval head involved in the temporomandibular joint. Between the coronoid process and the condyle is a depression, the mandibular notch.

Visible on the medial view of the mandible are the body of the mandible, alveolar process of the mandible (see Table 10-2), and ramus (see Figure 10-12). In addition, near the midline of the mandible is a cluster of small projections, the genial tubercles, which is another muscle attachment area.

At the lateral edge of each mandibular alveolar process is a rounded, roughened area, the retromolar triangle, just posterior to the most distal molar of the mandibular dentition. The retromolar triangle is a bony landmark that, when covered with soft tissue, is the retromolar pad.

Along each medial surface of the body of the mandible is the mylohyoid line or internal oblique ridge that extends posteriorly and superiorly, becoming more prominent as it moves superiorly on each body. The mylohyoid line is the point of attachment of the mylohyoid muscle that forms the floor of the mouth; the line can be noted on a radiograph as the radiopaque line inferior to the external oblique line (see Figure 10-8). The roots of the posterior mandibular teeth often extend internally inferior to the mylohyoid line.

On the medial surface of the ramus is the opening of the mandibular canal, the mandibular foramen (see Figure 10-12 and Table 10-1). The mandibular foramen is three fourths the distance from the coronoid notch to the posterior border of the ramus, which is a landmark for the

inferior alveolar block (see Chapter 13). The inferior alveolar nerve and blood vessels exit the mandible through the mandibular foramen after traveling in the mandibular canal (see discussion later). With age and tooth loss, the alveolar process is absorbed so that the mandibular canal is nearer the superior border. Sometimes with excessive alveolar process absorption, the mandibular canal disappears entirely and leaves the inferior alveolar nerve without its bony protection, although it is still covered by soft tissue.

Rarely, a patient may have a bifid inferior alveolar nerve, in which case a second mandibular foramen, more inferiorly placed, exists and can be detected by noting a doubled mandibular canal on a radiograph. Keeping this anatomic variant concerning the mandibular foramen, as well as its usual location, in mind is important when administering an inferior alveolar block (see Chapter 13).

Overhanging the mandibular foramen is a bony spine, the lingula, which serves as an attachment for the sphenomandibular ligament associated with the temporomandibular joint. A small groove, the mylohyoid groove, passes anterior to and inferior from the mandibular foramen. The mylohyoid nerve and blood vessels travel in the mylohyoid groove (discussed later), which in some cases can have an unusual pathway that complicates an inferior alveolar block (see Chapter 13).

TRIGEMINAL NERVE

The fifth cranial or trigeminal nerve provides sensory information (see Chapter 2) for the teeth and associated tissue. It is the branches of the trigeminal nerve that are anesthetized before most dental procedures (see Chapters

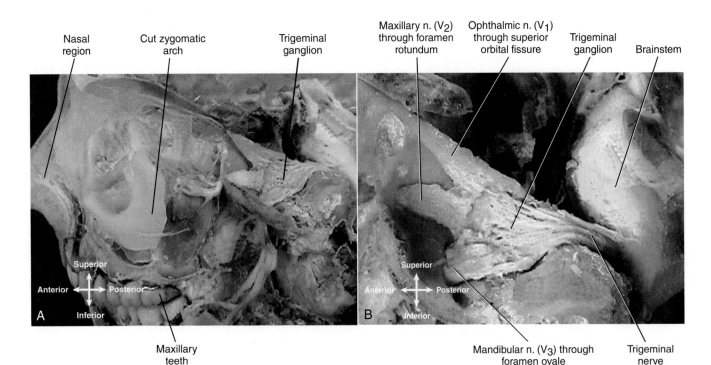

Figure 10-13 ■ Dissection of the trigeminal ganglion **(A)** and the three divisions or nerves **(B)**. (Reprinted with permission of Jeremy S, Melker, MD, 1999.) (From Fehrenbach MJ, Herring SW: *Illustrated anatomy of the head and neck,* ed 3, St Louis, 2007, Saunders.)

12 and 13). Thus the dental hygienist must have a thorough understanding of the trigeminal nerve to effectively and safely administer local anesthetics to patients.

Each trigeminal nerve is a short nerve trunk composed of two closely adapted roots (Figures 10-13 and 10-14). These roots of the nerve consist of a thicker sensory root and thinner motor root.

Within the skull, a bulge can be noted in the sensory root of the trigeminal nerve. This bulge is the trigeminal ganglion (or semilunar or gasserian ganglion), which is located on the anterior surface of the petrous part of the temporal bone. Anterior to the trigeminal ganglion, the sensory root arises from three divisions that pass into the skull by way of different fissures or foramina.

These divisions of the sensory root are the ophthalmic, maxillary, and mandibular nerves. The ophthalmic and maxillary nerves of the sensory root carry only afferent nerves (see Chapter 2). In contrast, the mandibular nerve off the sensory root runs together with the motor root and thus carries both afferent and efferent nerves. Important to note is that the commonly used terms V_1, V_2, and V_3 are simply shorthand notation for these divisions of the fifth cranial or trigeminal nerve. The "V" is the Roman numeral 5.

OPHTHALMIC NERVE

The first (V_1) division of the sensory root of the trigeminal nerve is the ophthalmic nerve (Figures 10-15 and 10-16). The smallest division serves as an afferent nerve for the conjunctiva, cornea, eyeball, orbit, forehead, ethmoidal

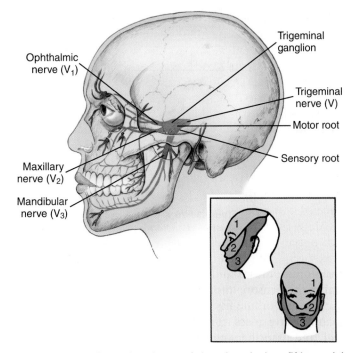

Figure 10-14 ■ General pathway of the trigeminal or fifth cranial nerve and its motor and sensory roots and three divisions or nerves (inset shows the pattern of innervations for each nerve division). (From Fehrenbach MJ, Herring SW: *Illustrated anatomy of the head and neck,* ed 3, St Louis, 2007, Saunders.)

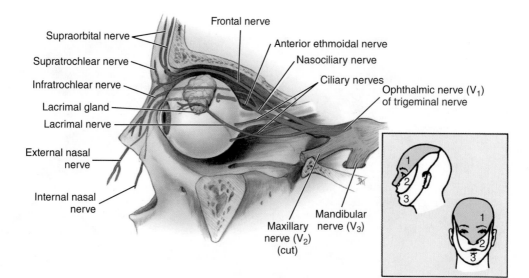

Figure 10-15 ■ Lateral view of the cut-away orbit with the pathway of the ophthalmic nerve (V₁) of the trigeminal nerve highlighted (inset shows the pattern of innervation). (From Fehrenbach MJ, Herring SW: *Illustrated anatomy of the head and neck*, ed 3, St Louis, 2007, Saunders.)

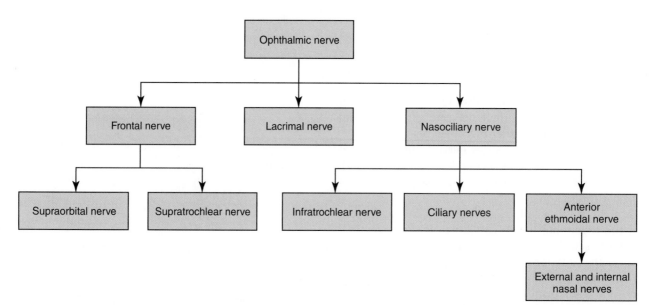

Figure 10-16 ■ Ophthalmic nerve (V₁) to the facial region. (From Fehrenbach MJ, Herring SW: *Illustrated anatomy of the head and neck*, ed 3, St Louis, 2007, Saunders.)

and frontal sinuses, and a part of the dura mater. The nerve carries this sensory information toward the brain by way of the superior orbital fissure of the sphenoid bone. The ophthalmic nerve arises from three major nerves: frontal, lacrimal, and nasociliary nerves.

MAXILLARY NERVE

The second division (V₂) from the sensory root of the trigeminal nerve is the maxillary nerve, which is set between the other two divisions both in size and location (Figures 10-17 and 10-18). The afferent nerve branches of the maxillary nerve carry sensory information (see Chapter 2) for the maxilla and overlying skin, maxillary sinuses, nasal cavity, palate, nasopharynx, and a part of the dura mater.

The maxillary nerve is a nerve trunk formed in the pterygopalatine fossa by the convergence of many nerves; the largest contributor is the infraorbital nerve. Tributaries of the infraorbital nerve or maxillary nerve trunk include the zygomatic, anterior, middle and posterior superior alveolar, greater and lesser palatine, and nasopalatine nerves.

After all these branches come together in the pterygopalatine fossa to form the maxillary nerve, the nerve enters the skull through the foramen rotundum of the sphenoid bone. Small afferent meningeal branches from parts of the

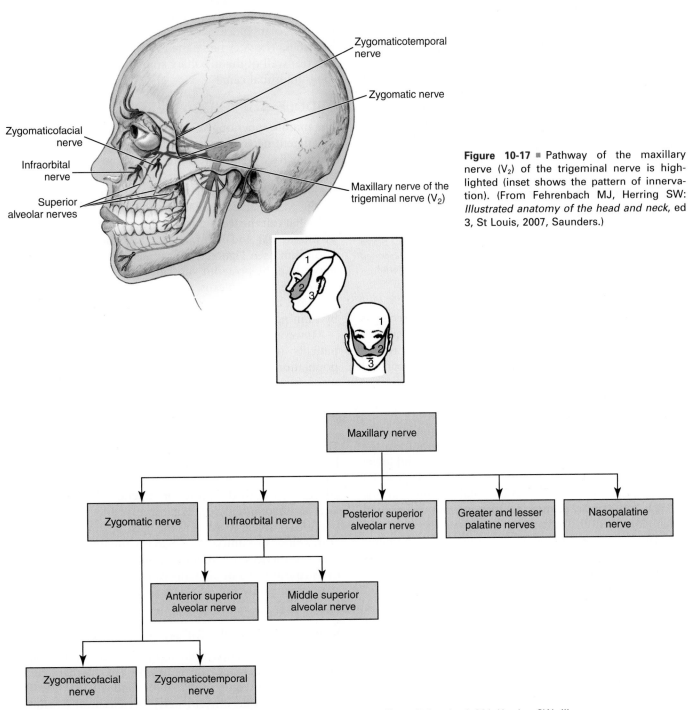

Figure 10-17 ■ Pathway of the maxillary nerve (V₂) of the trigeminal nerve is highlighted (inset shows the pattern of innervation). (From Fehrenbach MJ, Herring SW: *Illustrated anatomy of the head and neck*, ed 3, St Louis, 2007, Saunders.)

Figure 10-18 ■ Maxillary nerve (V₂) to the oral cavity. (From Fehrenbach MJ, Herring SW: *Illustrated anatomy of the head and neck*, ed 3, St Louis, 2007, Saunders.)

dura mater join the maxillary nerve as it enters the trigeminal ganglion.

ZYGOMATIC NERVE

The zygomatic nerve is an afferent nerve composed of the merger of the zygomaticofacial nerve and the zygomaticotemporal nerve in the orbit. This nerve also conveys the postganglionic parasympathetic fibers for the lacrimal gland to the lacrimal nerve. The zygomatic nerve courses posteriorly along the lateral orbit floors; enters the pterygopalatine fossa through the inferior orbital fissure, between the sphenoid bone and maxilla, and finally joins V₂.

The rather small zygomaticofacial nerve serves as an afferent nerve for the skin of the cheek. This nerve pierces the frontal process of the zygomatic bone and enters the orbit through its lateral wall. The zygomaticofacial nerve then turns posteriorly to join with the zygomaticotemporal nervesee (see Figures 10-17 and 10-18).

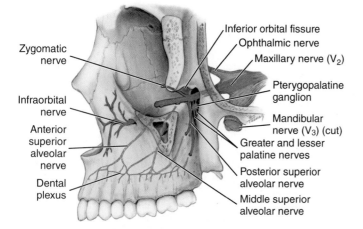

Figure 10-19 ■ Lateral view of the skull (part of lateral wall of the orbit has been removed) with the branches of the maxillary nerve (V₂) highlighted. (From Fehrenbach MJ, Herring SW: *Illustrated anatomy of the head and neck*, ed 3, St Louis, 2007, Saunders.)

The other nerve, the zygomaticotemporal nerve, serves as an afferent nerve for the skin of the temporal region, pierces the temporal surface of the zygomatic bone, and traverses the lateral wall of the orbit to join the zygomaticofacial nerve, forming the zygomatic nerve.

INFRAORBITAL NERVE

The infraorbital nerve, or IO nerve, is an afferent nerve formed from the merger of cutaneous branches from the upper lip, medial part of the cheek, side of nose, and lower eyelid (Figure 10-19; see Figures 10-1 and 10-3). The IO nerve then passes into the infraorbital foramen of the maxilla and travels posteriorly through the infraorbital canal, along with the infraorbital blood vessels, where the anterior superior alveolar nerve then joins it. The IO nerve is anesthetized by the infraorbital block, which anesthetizes both the anterior and middle superior alveolar nerves at this site (discussed next).

From the infraorbital canal and groove, the IO nerve passes into the pterygopalatine fossa through the inferior orbital fissure. After it leaves the infraorbital groove and within the pterygopalatine fossa, the IO nerve receives the posterior superior alveolar nerve.

ANTERIOR SUPERIOR ALVEOLAR NERVE

The anterior superior alveolar nerve, or ASA nerve, serves as an efferent nerve of sensation (including pain) for the maxillary central incisors, lateral incisors, and canine, as well as their associated tissue.

The ASA nerve originates from dental branches in the pulp of these teeth that exit through the apical foramina (see Figures 10-3 and 10-19). The ASA nerve also receives interdental branches from the surrounding periodontium, forming a dental plexus or nerve network in the maxilla for the region. The ASA nerve also innervates the facial gingival tissue. The ASA nerve can be anesthetized by either the anterior superior alveolar block at this site, or along with the middle superior alveolar nerve by the infraorbital block, as well as with the use of the anterior middle superior alveolar block along with other maxillary nerve branches. The ASA nerve then moves superiorly along the anterior wall of the maxillary sinus to join the IO nerve in the infraorbital canal.

MIDDLE SUPERIOR ALVEOLAR NERVE

The middle superior alveolar nerve, or MSA nerve, serves as an afferent nerve of sensation (including pain), usually for the maxillary premolar teeth and in some cases, the mesiobuccal root of the maxillary first molar, and their associated periodontium and overlying buccal soft tissue.

The MSA nerve originates from dental branches in the pulp that exit the teeth through the apical foramina, as well as interdental and interradicular branches from the periodontium (see Figures 10-2, 10-3, and 10-19). The MSA nerve, like the posterior superior alveolar and ASA nerves, forms the dental plexus or nerve network in the maxilla. The MSA nerve then moves superiorly to join the IO nerve by running in the lateral wall of the maxillary sinus.

However, the MSA nerve is not always present in all patients; it is only present in approximately 28% of the population. If this nerve is not present, the area is innervated by both the ASA and posterior superior alveolar nerves, but mainly by the ASA nerve. If the MSA nerve is present, there is communication between the MSA nerve and both the ASA and posterior superior alveolar nerves. These considerations are important when administering local anesthesia for the maxillary posterior teeth and associated tissue (see Chapter 12). Thus the clinician usually administers both the posterior superior alveolar block as well as the middle superior alveolar block in order to provide complete coverage to the maxillary premolar region at this site. The clinician can also use the infraorbital block that anesthetizes the MSA nerve along with the ASA nerve or use the anterior middle superior alveolar block that anesthetizes not only the MSA but also other maxillary nerve branches.

POSTERIOR SUPERIOR ALVEOLAR NERVE

The posterior superior alveolar, or PSA nerve, joins the IO nerve (or the maxillary nerve directly) in the pterygopalatine fossa (see Figures 10-2, 10-5, and 10-19). The PSA nerve serves as an afferent nerve of sensation (including pain) for most parts of the maxillary molar teeth and their periodontium and buccal soft tissue, as well as the maxillary sinus.

Some branches of the PSA nerve remain external to the posterior surface of the maxilla. These external branches provide afferent innervations for the buccal gingival tissue of the maxillary molars.

Other afferent nerve branches of the PSA nerve originate from dental branches in the pulp of each of the maxillary molar teeth that exit the teeth by way of the apical foramina. These dental branches are then joined by interdental branches and interradicular branches from the

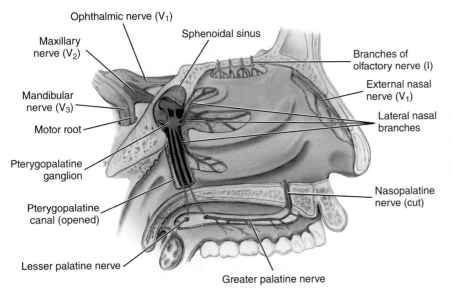

Figure 10-20 ■ Medial view of the lateral nasal wall and opened pterygopalatine canal highlighting the maxillary nerve (V₂) and its palatine branches (nasal septum has been removed, thus severing the nasopalatine nerve). (From Fehrenbach MJ, Herring SW: *Illustrated anatomy of the head and neck*, ed 3, St Louis, 2007, Saunders.)

periodontium, forming a dental plexus or a nerve network in the maxilla for the region.

All these internal branches of the PSA nerve then move superiorly together along the maxillary tuberosity, which forms the posterolateral wall of the maxillary sinus, to join either the IO nerve or maxillary nerve. The PSA nerve usually provides afferent innervations for the maxillary second and third molars and the palatal and distal buccal root of the maxillary first molar, as well as the mucous membranes of the maxillary sinus. The PSA nerve is anesthetized by the posterior superior alveolar block at this site.

GREATER PALATINE NERVES

Both palatine nerves join with the maxillary nerve from the palate (Figure 10-20; see Figure 10-6). The greater palatine nerve, or GP nerve, also called the anterior palatine nerve, is located between the mucoperiosteum and bone of the anterior hard palate. This nerve serves as an afferent nerve for the posterior hard palate and posterior lingual gingival tissue of the posterior teeth; this is the tissue that embryologically was associated with the palatal shelves. The GP nerve is anesthetized by the greater palatine block at this site as well as when giving the anterior middle superior alveolar block along with other maxillary nerve branches. Communication occurs with the terminal fibers of the nasopalatine nerve in the hard palate area, lingual to the maxillary canines, which may complicate the use of local anesthesia in the region (see Chapter 12).

Posteriorly, the GP nerve enters the greater palatine foramen in the palatine foramen in the palatine bone near the maxillary second or third molar to travel in the pterygopalatine canal, along with the greater palatine blood vessels.

NASOPALATINE NERVE

The nasopalatine nerve, or NP nerve, originates in the mucosa of the anterior hard palate, lingual to the maxillary anterior teeth (see Figures 10-4 and 10-20). Both the right

and left NP nerves enter the incisive canal by way of the incisive foramen, deep to the incisive papilla, thus exiting the oral cavity.

The nerve then travels along the nasal septum. The NP nerve serves as an afferent nerve for the anterior hard palate and the anterior lingual gingival tissue of the maxillary anterior teeth, as well as the nasal septal tissue; this is the tissue that embryologically was associated with the intermaxillary segment. The NP nerve is anesthetized by the nasopalatine block at this site, as well as the anterior middle superior alveolar block along with other maxillary nerve branches. Communication also occurs with the GP nerve in the area that is located lingual to the maxillary canines, which may complicate the use of local anesthesia in the region (see Chapter 12).

MANDIBULAR NERVE

The third division (V₃) of the trigeminal nerve is the mandibular nerve, which is the short main trunk formed by the merger of a smaller anterior trunk and a larger posterior trunk in the infratemporal fossa, before the nerve passes through the foramen ovale of the sphenoid bone (Figures 10-21 to 10-23). The mandibular nerve then joins with the ophthalmic and maxillary nerves to form the trigeminal ganglion of the trigeminal nerve. The mandibular nerve is the largest of the three divisions that form the trigeminal nerve.

Anterior and posterior trunks are branches from the undivided mandibular nerve include the meningeal branches, which are afferent nerves (see Chapter 2) for parts of the dura mater (see Figure 10-26). Also, from the undivided mandibular nerve are muscular branches, which are efferent nerves for the medial pterygoid, tensor tympani, and tensor veli palatine muscles.

The anterior trunk of the mandibular nerve is formed by the merger of the (long) buccal nerve and additional muscular nerve branches (Figure 10-24). The posterior trunk of the mandibular nerve is formed by the merger of the auriculotemporal, lingual, and inferior alveolar nerves (see Figure 10-14).

BUCCAL NERVE

The buccal nerve (or long buccal nerve) serves as an afferent nerve for the skin of the cheek, buccal mucous membranes, and buccal gingival tissue of the mandibular posterior teeth. The nerve is located on the surface of the buccinator muscle (see Figures 10-9, 10-10, 10-22, 10-23 and 10-24).

The buccal nerve then travels posteriorly in the cheek, deep to the masseter muscle.

At the level of the occlusal plane of the most distal mandibular molar, the nerve crosses anteriorly to the anterior border of the ramus and goes between the two heads of the lateral pterygoid muscle to join the anterior trunk of V₃. The buccal nerve is anesthetized by the buccal block at this site; however, this nerve must not be confused with the buccal nerve that innervates the buccinator muscle and is an efferent nerve branch from the facial nerve. The buccal nerve is

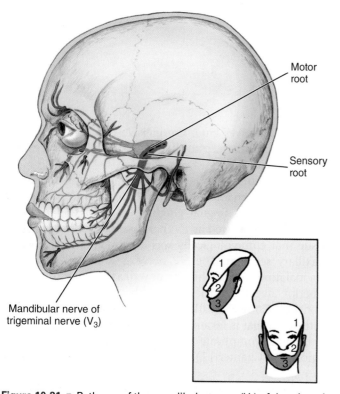

Figure 10-21 ■ Pathway of the mandibular nerve (V₃) of the trigeminal nerve is highlighted (inset shows the pattern of innervation). (From Fehrenbach MJ, Herring SW: *Illustrated anatomy of the head and neck*, ed 3, St Louis, 2007, Saunders.)

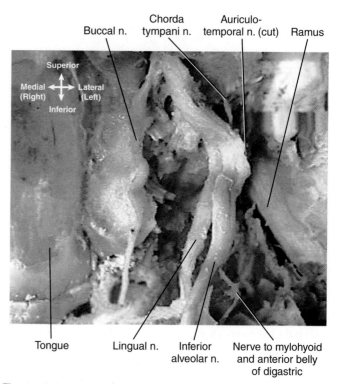

Figure 10-22 ■ Dissection of the mandibular nerve (V₃) of the trigeminal nerve. (Reprinted with permission of Jeremy S, Melker, MD, 1999.) (From Fehrenbach MJ, Herring SW: *Illustrated anatomy of the head and neck*, ed 3, St Louis, 2007, Saunders.)

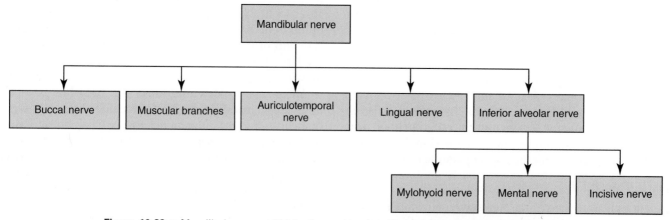

Figure 10-23 ■ Mandibular nerve (V₃) to the oral cavity. (From Fehrenbach MJ, Herring SW: *Illustrated anatomy of the head and neck*, ed 3, St Louis, 2007, Saunders.)

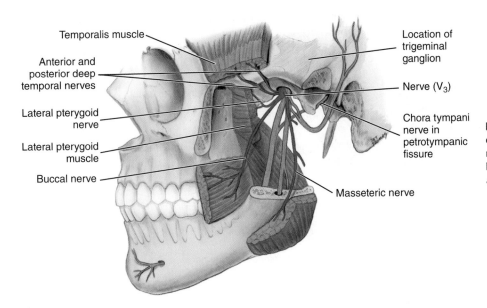

Temporalis muscle

Anterior and posterior deep temporal nerves

Lateral pterygoid nerve

Lateral pterygoid muscle

Buccal nerve

Location of trigeminal ganglion

Nerve (V₃)

Chora tympani nerve in petrotympanic fissure

Masseteric nerve

Figure 10-24 ■ Pathway of the anterior trunk of the mandibular nerve of the trigeminal nerve is highlighted. (From Fehrenbach MJ, Herring SW: *Illustrated anatomy of the head and neck*, ed 3, St Louis, 2007, Saunders.)

also anesthetized by the Gow-Gates mandibular block along with other branches of the mandibular nerve.

MUSCULAR BRANCHES

Several muscular branches are part of the anterior trunk of V_3 (see Figure 10-24). They arise from the motor root of the trigeminal nerve. The deep temporal nerves, usually two in number, anterior and posterior, are efferent nerves that pass between the sphenoid bone and the superior border of the lateral pterygoid muscle and turn around the infratemporal crest of the sphenoid bone to end in the deep surface of the temporalis muscle that they innervate. The posterior temporal nerve may arise in common with the masseteric nerve, and the anterior temporal nerve may be associated at its origin with the buccal nerve.

The masseteric nerve is also an efferent nerve that passes between the sphenoid bone and the superior border of the lateral pterygoid muscle. The nerve then accompanies the masseteric blood vessels through the mandibular notch to innervate the masseter muscle. A small sensory branch also goes to the temporomandibular joint. The lateral pterygoid nerve, after a short course, enters the deep surface of the lateral pterygoid muscle between the muscle's two heads of origin and serves as an efferent nerve for that muscle.

AURICULOTEMPORAL NERVE

The ariculotemporal nerve travels with the superficial temporal artery and vein and serves as an afferent nerve for the external ear and scalp (Figures 10-25 and 10-26 and see Figures 10-22 and 10-23). The nerve also carries postganglionic parasympathetic nerve fibers to the parotid salivary gland. Important to note is that these parasympathetic fibers arise from the lesser petrosal branch of the glossopharyngeal or ninth, cranial nerve, joining the auriculotemporal nerve only after relaying in the otic ganglion near the foramen ovale.

Communication of the auriculotemporal nerve with the facial nerve near the ear also occurs. The nerve courses deep to the lateral pterygoid muscle and neck of the mandible, then splits to encircle the middle meningeal artery, and finally joins the posterior trunk of V_3. The auriculotemporal nerve is anesthetized with the Gow-Gates mandibular block and also inadvertently in some cases with the inferior alveolar block due to its close proximity.

LINGUAL NERVE

The lingual nerve is formed from afferent branches from the body of the tongue that travel along the lateral surface of the tongue (Figure 10-27 and see Figures 10-22, 10-23, 10-25 and 10-26). The nerve then passes posteriorly, passing from the medial to the lateral side of the duct of the submandibular salivary gland by going inferior to the duct.

The lingual nerve communicates with the submandibular ganglion located superior to the deep lobe of the submandibular salivary gland (see Figure 10-27). The submandibular ganglion is a part of the parasympathetic system (see Chapter 2). Parasympathetic efferent innervations for both the sublingual and submandibular salivary gland arise from the facial nerves (specifically, a branch of the facial nerve and the chorda tympani), but travels along with the lingual nerve.

At the base of the tongue, the lingual nerve moves superiorly and runs between the medial pterygoid muscle and the mandible, anterior and slightly medial to the inferior alveolar nerve. The lingual nerve is anesthetized when administering an inferior alveolar block through localized diffusion of the local anesthetic agent through the tissue due to its close proximity to the inferior alveolar nerve (see Chapter 13). Because the lingual nerve is only a short distance posterior to the roots of the most distal mandibular molar tooth and is covered only by a thin layer of oral mucosa, its location is sometimes visible clinically. In

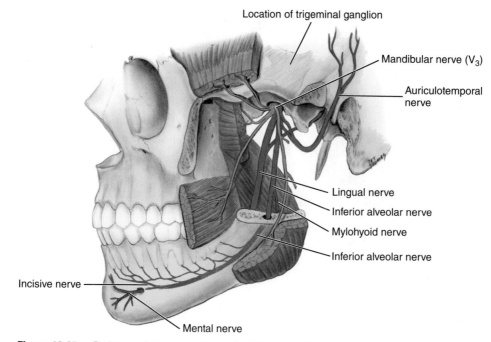

Figure 10-25 ∎ Pathway of the posterior trunk of the mandibular nerve of the trigeminal nerve is highlighted. (From Fehrenbach MJ, Herring SW: *Illustrated anatomy of the head and neck*, ed 3, St Louis, 2007, Saunders.)

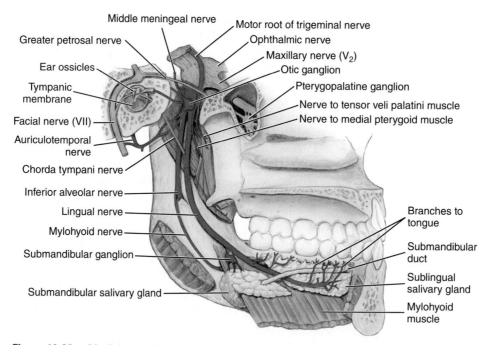

Figure 10-26 ∎ Medial view of the mandible with the motor and sensory branches of the mandibular nerve highlighted. (From Fehrenbach MJ, Herring SW: *Illustrated anatomy of the head and neck*, ed 3, St Louis, 2007, Saunders.)

addition, the Gow-Gates mandibular block can be used to anesthetize the lingual nerve along with other branches of the mandibular nerve

The lingual nerve then continues to travel superiorly to join the posterior trunk of V₃. Thus the lingual nerve serves as an afferent nerve for general sensation for the body of the tongue, floor of the mouth, and lingual gingival tissue of the mandibular teeth. Current thought has implicated most of paresthesia complications of the mandible with this nerve (see Chapters 13 and 14).

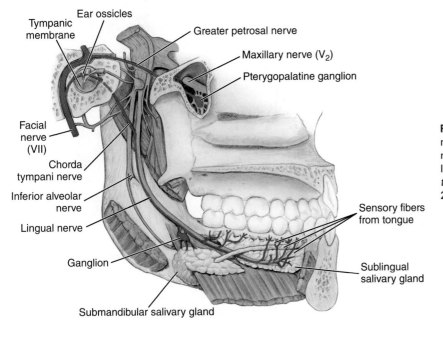

Figure 10-27 ■ Pathway of the trunk of the facial nerve, greater petrosal nerve, and chorda tympani nerve (note relationship with lingual nerve) is highlighted. (From Fehrenbach MJ, Herring SW: *Illustrated anatomy of the head and neck*, ed 3, St Louis, 2007, Saunders.)

INFERIOR ALVEOLAR NERVE

The inferior alveolar nerve, or IA nerve, is an afferent nerve formed from the merger of the mental and incisive nerves (see Figures 10-8 to 10-12 and 10-22, 10-23, 10-25 and 10-27). The mental and incisive nerves are discussed later in this section.

After forming, the IA nerve continues to travel posteriorly through the mandibular canal, along with the inferior alveolar artery and vein. The IA nerve is joined by dental branches and interdental and interradicular branches from the mandibular posterior teeth, forming a dental plexus or nerve network in the region. The IA nerve then exits the mandible from the mandibular canal through the mandibular foramen where it is joined by the mylohyoid nerve (discussed later). The mandibular foramen is an opening for the mandibular canal on the medial surface of the ramus, three fourths the distance from the coronoid notch to the posterior border of the ramus.

The IA nerve then travels laterally to the medial pterygoid muscle, between the sphenomandibular ligament and ramus of the mandible within the pterygomandibular space (or pterygomandibular triangle). This is posterior and slightly lateral to the lingual nerve. The IA nerve then joins the posterior trunk of V_3 (see Figures 10-25 and 10-26). The IA nerve carries afferent innervations for the mandibular teeth. The IA nerve, along with the lingual nerve, is anesthetized by the inferior alveolar block at this site. In addition, the Gow-Gates mandibular block can be used to anesthetize the IA nerve along with other branches of the mandibular nerve.

In some cases there are two nerves present on the same side, creating bifid IA nerves. This situation can occur unilaterally or bilaterally and can be detected on a radiograph by the presence of a double mandibular canal. Thus there

can be more than one mandibular foramen, usually inferiorly placed, either unilaterally or bilaterally, along with the presence of bifid IA nerves. These considerations must be kept in mind when administering local anesthesia for the mandibular teeth and associated tissue (see Chapter 13).

MENTAL NERVE

The mental nerve is composed of external branches that serve an afferent nerve for the chin, lower lip, and labial mucosa of the mandibular anterior teeth and premolars (see Figures 10-8 to 10-10 and Figures 10-23 and 10-25). The mental nerve then enters the mental foramen on the lateral surface of the mandible, usually between the apices of the mandibular first and second premolars, and merges with the incisive nerve to form the IA nerve in the mandibular canal before its exits the mandibular foramen. The mental nerve is anesthetized by the mental block this site, or along with the incisive nerve, with the incisive block at the same site. In addition, the inferior alveolar nerve or Gow-Gates mandibular block can be used to anesthetize the mental nerve along with other branches of the mandibular nerve.

INCISIVE NERVE

The incisive nerve is an afferent nerve composed of dental branches from the mandibular anterior teeth and premolar that originate in the pulp, exit the teeth through the apical foramina, and join with interdental branches from the surrounding periodontium, forming a dental plexus in the region (see Figures 10-8 to 10-10, Figures 10-23 and 10-25). The incisive nerve then merges with the mental nerve, just posterior to the mental foramen, to form the IA nerve in the mandibular canal before it exits the mandibular foramen. The incisive nerve serves as an afferent nerve for the mandibular anterior teeth and premolars.

The incisive nerve is anesthetized by the incisive block at this site, or with the inferior alveolar nerve or Gow-Gates mandibular block along with other branches of the mandibular nerve. Crossover from the contralateral incisive nerve sometimes occurs, which is an important consideration when administering local anesthesia for the mandibular anterior teeth and premolars and associated tissue (see Chapter 13).

MYLOHYOID NERVE

After the inferior alveolar nerve exits the mandibular foramen, a small branch occurs, the mylohyoid nerve (see Figures 10-22, 10-25 and 10-26). This nerve pierces the sphenomandibular ligament and runs inferiorly and anteriorly in the mylohyoid groove and then onto the inferior surface of the mylohyoid muscle. The nerve serves as an efferent nerve to both the mylohyoid muscle and anterior belly of the digastric muscle (posterior belly of the digastric muscle is innervated by a branch from the facial nerve).

However, this nerve may in some cases also serve as an afferent nerve (see Chapter 2) for the mandibular first molar which needs to be considered when there is failure of the inferior alveolar block (see Chapter 13). If there is a concern, the mylohyoid nerve can be additionally anesthetized by giving a supraperiosteal injection at the apex of the mesial root of the mandibular first molar on the lingual surface of the mandible (see Figure 13-12), or a periodontal ligament injection directly into the periodontium of the tooth to be anesthetized (see Table 13-12, Figure V). The mylohyoid nerve is also anesthetized by the Gow-Gates mandibular block along with other branches of the mandibular nerve.

▌FACIAL NERVE

The dental hygienist must also have an understanding of the seventh cranial (VII) or facial nerve and its importance when administering local anesthetics. The facial nerve carries both efferent and afferent nerves (see Chapter 2). The facial nerve emerges from the brain and enters the internal acoustic meatus in the petrous part of the temporal bone. Within the bone, the nerve gives off a small efferent branch to the muscle in the middle ear and two larger branches, the greater petrosal and chorda tympani nerves, both of which carry parasympathetic fibers (see Figures 10-26 and 10-27).

The main trunk of the nerve emerges from the skull through the stylomastoid foramen of the temporal bone and gives off two branches, the posterior auricular nerve and a branch to the posterior belly of the digastric and stylohyoid muscles (Figure 10-28). The facial nerve then passes into the parotid salivary gland and divides into numerous branches to supply the muscles of facial expression, but not the parotid salivary gland itself (discussed later). Avoiding anesthesia of this nerve at this location is important when administering an inferior alveolar block because it may result in transient facial paralysis if given incorrectly (see Chapters 13 and 14).

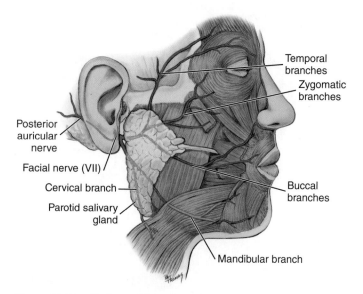

Figure 10-28 ■ Pathway of the branches of the facial nerve to the muscles of facial expression is highlighted. (From Fehrenbach MJ, Herring SW: *Illustrated anatomy of the head and neck*, ed 3, St Louis, 2007, Saunders.)

▌OVERVIEW OF ADJACENT VASCULAR AND GLANDULAR STRUCTURES

The dental hygienist must also know the location of certain adjacent soft tissue structures, such as major blood vessels and glandular tissue, so as to avoid inadvertently injecting these structures when administering local anesthesia. If these larger soft tissue structures are accidentally injected with local anesthetic agent, complications may occur. Infections may also be spread to deeper tissue by needle-tract contamination. (See Chapter 14.)

However, the dental hygienist should use the hemostatic control properties of certain components of the local anesthetic solution to reduce the bleeding from smaller blood vessels in the region instrumented so as to provide better visibility and root coverage, especially with furcations and root concavities (see Chapter 4).

The vascular system of the head and neck, as is the case in the rest of the body, consists of an arterial blood supply, a capillary network, and venous drainage. A large network of blood vessels is a plexus. The head and neck area contains certain important venous plexuses. Blood vessels also may communicate with each other by an anastomosis (plural, anastomoses), a connecting channel among the vessels.

An artery is a component of the vascular system that arises from the heart, carrying blood away from it. Each artery starts as a large vessel and branches into smaller vessels, each one a smaller artery or an arteriole. Each arteriole branches into even smaller vessels until it becomes a network of capillaries. Each capillary is smaller than an arteriole and can supply blood to a large tissue area only because there are so many of them.

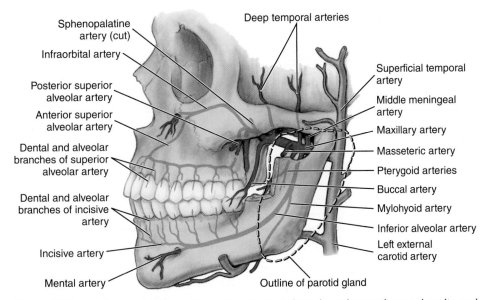

Figure 10-29 ■ Pathway of the maxillary artery (except those branches to the nasal cavity and palate). (From Fehrenbach MJ, Herring SW: *Illustrated anatomy of the head and neck*, ed 3, St Louis, 2007, Saunders.)

A **vein** is another component of the vascular system. A vein, unlike an artery, travels to the heart and carries blood. Valves in the veins are mostly absent in the head and neck area, unlike in the rest of the body. This leads to two-way flow dictated by local pressure changes, which is the reason that facial or dental infections can lead to serious complications (see Chapter 14). After each smaller vein or **venule** drains the capillaries of the tissue area, the venules coalesce to become larger veins. Veins are much larger and more numerous than arteries. Veins anastomose freely and have a greater variability in location in comparison with arteries.

There are also different kinds of venous networks found in the body. Superficial veins are found immediately deep to the skin. Deeper veins usually accompany larger arteries in a more protected location within the tissue. **Venous sinuses** are blood-filled spaces between the two layers of tissue. All these networks are connected by anastomoses.

Relating the structures supplied and the area's blood vessels is an important way of understanding the location of the various blood vessels and their relationship to the administration of local anesthesia. Remember that, unlike innervation supplied by the nerves to the muscles, which is a one-to-one relationship, blood supply is regional. Arteries supply all structures in their vicinity, and veins receive blood from all nearby structures. Associated salivary glandular tissue in the related regions will be noted during the overall discussion of the vascular system.

MAXILLARY ARTERY

The maxillary artery is the larger terminal branch of the external carotid artery (Figures 10-29 and 10-30 and Table 10-4). The maxillary artery begins at the neck of the mandibular condyle within the parotid salivary gland. The

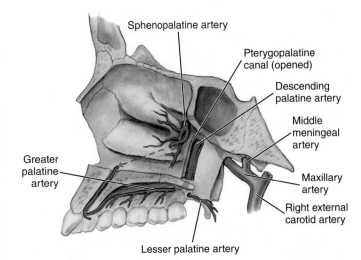

Figure 10-30 ■ Pathways of the greater palatine artery, lesser palatine artery, and sphenopalatine artery. (From Fehrenbach MJ, Herring SW: *Illustrated anatomy of the head and neck*, ed 3, St Louis, 2007, Saunders.)

maxillary artery runs between the mandible and the sphenomandibular ligament anteriorly and superiorly through the infratemporal fossa. The artery may run either superficially or deep to the lateral pterygoid muscle.

After traversing the infratemporal fossa, the maxillary artery enters the pterygopalatine fossa. The pterygopalatine fossa is deep and inferior to the eye. Within the infratemporal and pterygopalatine fossae, the maxillary artery gives off many branches. The branches within the infratemporal fossa include the middle meningeal and inferior alveolar arteries and several arteries to muscles (see Table 10-4).

The middle meningeal artery supplies the meninges of the brain by way of the foramen spinosum, located on the

TABLE 10-4	Branches of the Maxillary Artery	
MAJOR BRANCHES OF MAXILLARY ARTERY	**FURTHER BRANCHES**	**STRUCTURES SUPPLIED**
Middle meningeal		Meninges of brain and bones of skull
Inferior alveolar	Mylohyoid, mental, and incisive	Mandibular teeth, mouth floor, and mental region
Deep temporal(s)		Temporalis muscle
Pterygoid(s)		Lateral and medial pterygoid muscles
Masseteric		Masseter muscle
Buccal		Buccinator muscle and buccal region
Posterior superior alveolar		Posterior maxillary teeth and maxillary sinus
Infraorbital	Orbital and anterior superior alveolar	Orbital region, face, and anterior maxillary teeth
Greater palatine	Lesser palatine(s)	Hard and soft palates
Sphenopalatine	Lateral nasal, septal, and nasopalatine	Nasal cavity and anterior hard palate

inferior surface of the skull, as well as the skull bones (see Figure 10-29).

The inferior alveolar artery also arises from the maxillary artery in the infratemporal fossa (see Figure 10-29). The artery turns inferiorly to enter the mandibular foramen and then the mandibular canal, along with the inferior alveolar nerve; both the artery and nerve are anterior to the deeper parotid salivary gland that contains the seventh cranial nerve or facial nerve, which must be avoided when administering an inferior alveolar block (see Figures 10-29 and 13-6). The mylohyoid artery branches from the inferior alveolar artery before it enters the canal.

The mylohyoid artery arises from the inferior alveolar artery before the main artery enters the mandibular canal by way of the mandibular foramen (see Figure 10-29). The mylohyoid artery travels in the mylohyoid groove on the medial surface of the mandible and supplies the floor of the mouth and the mylohyoid muscle.

Within the mandibular canal, the inferior alveolar artery gives off the dental and alveolar branches (see Figure 10-29). The dental branches of the inferior alveolar artery supply the pulp of the mandibular posterior teeth by way of each tooth's apical foramen. The alveolar branches of the inferior alveolar artery supply the periodontium of the mandibular posterior teeth, including the lingual gingival tissue. The inferior alveolar artery then branches into two arteries within the mandibular canal: the mental and incisive arteries.

The mental artery arises from the inferior alveolar artery and exits the mandibular canal by way of the mental foramen (see Figure 10-29). The mental foramen is located on the lateral surface of the mandible, usually deep to the apices of the mandibular first and second premolar teeth. After the mental artery exits the canal, the artery supplies the tissue of the chin and anastomoses with the inferior labial artery.

The incisive artery branches off the inferior alveolar artery and remains in the mandibular canal to divide into dental and alveolar branches (see Figure 10-29). The dental branches of the incisive artery supply the pulp of the mandibular anterior teeth by way of each tooth's apical foramen.

The alveolar branches of the incisive artery supply the periodontium of the mandibular anterior teeth, including the facial gingival tissue, and anastomose with the alveolar branches of the incisive artery on the other side.

The maxillary artery also has branches that are located near the muscle they supply (see Figure 10-29 and Table 10-4). These arteries all accompany branches of the mandibular division of the fifth cranial or trigeminal nerve. The deep temporal arteries supply the anterior and posterior parts of the temporalis muscle. The pterygoid arteries supply the lateral and medial pterygoid muscles. The masseteric artery supplies the masseter muscle. The buccal artery supplies the buccinator muscle and other soft tissue of the cheek.

Just as the maxillary artery leaves the infratemporal fossa and enters the pterygopalatine fossa, it gives off the posterior superior alveolar artery (see Figure 10-29). This artery enters the posterior superior alveolar foramina on the maxillary tuberosity and then gives off dental branches and alveolar branches. The posterior alveolar superior alveolar artery also anastomoses with the anterior superior alveolar artery.

The dental branches of the posterior superior alveolar artery supply the pulp of the posterior maxillary teeth by way of each tooth's apical foramen. The alveolar branches of the posterior superior alveolar artery supply the periodontium of the maxillary posterior teeth, including the buccal gingival tissue. Some branches also supply the maxillary sinus.

The infraorbital artery branches from the maxillary artery in the pterygopalatine fossa and may share a common trunk with the posterior superior alveolar artery (see Figure 10-29). The infraorbital artery then enters the orbit through the inferior orbital fissure. While in the orbit, the artery travels in the infraorbital canal. Within the canal, the infraorbital artery provides orbital branches to the orbit and gives off the anterior superior alveolar artery.

The anterior superior alveolar artery arises from the infraorbital artery and gives off dental and alveolar branches (see Figure 10-29). The anterior superior alveolar artery also anastomoses with the posterior superior alveolar artery. The dental branches of the anterior superior alveolar artery supply the pulp of the maxillary anterior teeth by way of each tooth's apical foramen. The alveolar branches of the anterior superior alveolar artery supply the periodontium of the maxillary anterior teeth, including the facial gingival tissue.

After giving off these branches in the infraorbital canal, the infraorbital artery emerges onto the face from the infraorbital foramen (see Figure 10-29). The artery's terminal branches supply parts of the infraorbital region of the face and anastomose with the facial artery.

Also in the pterygopalatine fossa, the maxillary artery gives rise to the descending palatine artery, which travels to the palate through the pterygopalatine canal which then terminates in both the greater palatine artery and lesser palatine artery by way of the greater and lesser palatine foramina to supply the hard and soft palates, respectively (see Figure 10-30). The maxillary artery ends by becoming the sphenopalatine artery, which supplies the nasal cavity. The sphenopalatine artery gives rise to the posterior lateral nasal branches and septal branches, including a nasopalatine branch that accompanies the nasopalatine nerve through the incisive foramen on the maxilla.

PTERYGOID PLEXUS OF VEINS

The pterygoid plexus of veins is a collection of small anastomosing vessels located around the pterygoid muscles and surrounding the maxillary artery on each side of the face in the infratemporal fossa (Figures 10-31 and 10-32). This plexus anastomoses with both the facial and retromandibular veins. The pterygoid plexus protects the maxillary artery from being compressed during mastication. By either filling or emptying, the pterygoid plexus can accommodate

changes in volume of the infratemporal fossa that occur when the mandible moves.

The pterygoid plexus drains the veins from the deep parts of the face and then drains into the maxillary vein (Figure 10-32). The middle meningeal vein also drains the blood from the meninges of the brain into the pterygoid plexus.

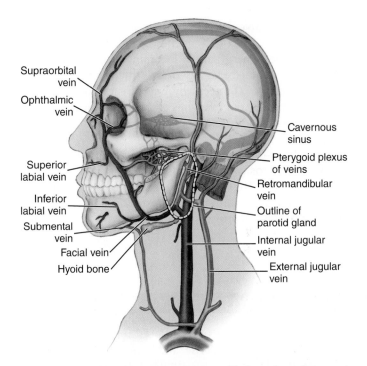

Figure 10-31 ■ Pathways of the retromandibular vein and external jugular vein including the anterior jugular vein. (From Fehrenbach MJ, Herring SW: *Illustrated anatomy of the head and neck*, ed 3, St Louis, 2007, Saunders.)

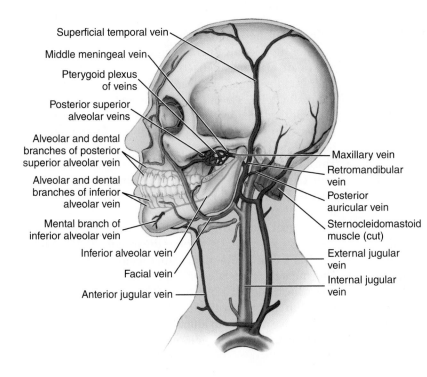

Figure 10-32 ■ Pathways of the internal jugular view and facial vein, as well as the location of the cavernous sinus. (From Fehrenbach MJ, Herring SW: *Illustrated anatomy of the head and neck*, ed 3, St Louis, 2007, Saunders.)

The pterygoid plexus of veins also drains the posterior superior alveolar vein, which is formed by the merging of its dental and alveolar branches. The dental branches of the posterior superior alveolar vein drain the pulp of the maxillary teeth by way of each tooth's apical foramen. The alveolar branches of the posterior alveolar vein drain the periodontium of the maxillary teeth, including the gingiva.

The inferior alveolar vein forms from the merging of its dental branches, alveolar branches, and mental branches in the mandible, where they also drain into the pterygoid plexus. The dental branches of the inferior alveolar vein drain the pulp of the teeth by way of each tooth's apical foramen. The alveolar branches of the inferior alveolar vein drain the periodontium of the mandibular teeth, including the gingiva.

Some parts of the pterygoid plexus of veins are near the maxillary tuberosity, reflecting the drainage of dental tissue into the plexus. Thus there is a possibility of piercing the pterygoid plexus of veins when a posterior superior alveolar block is given incorrectly (see Chapter 12). When the pterygoid plexus is pierced, a small amount of the blood escapes and enters the tissue, causing tissue tenderness, swelling, and the discoloration of a hematoma (see Chapter 14 and Figure 14-2).

A spread of infection along the needle tract deep into the tissue can also occur when the posterior superior alveolar block is incorrectly administered. This may involve a serious spread of infection into the pterygoid plexus of veins and then on to the cavernous sinus, a venous sinus within the skull (see Figure 10-32 and see Chapter 14).

MAXILLARY VEIN

The maxillary vein begins in the infratemporal fossa by collecting blood from the pterygoid plexus, accompanying the maxillary artery (see Figure 10-32). Through the pterygoid plexus, the maxillary vein receives the middle meningeal, posterior superior alveolar, inferior alveolar, and other veins such as those from the nasal cavity and palate (those areas served by maxillary artery). The maxillary vein then drains into the retromandibular vein, which forms part of the external jugular vein.

DENTAL HYGIENE CONSIDERATIONS

- The maxillary bone over the facial surface of the maxillary teeth is less dense and more porous than the mandibular bone over similar teeth, which allows a greater incidence of clinically adequate local anesthesia for the maxillary teeth when the local anesthetic agent is administered as a supraperiosteal injection or local infiltration than would occur with similar teeth on the mandibular arch.
- The median palatine raphe along with the pores in the anterior hard palate are landmarks for the administration of the anterior middle superior alveolar block.
- The incisive foramen carries both branches of the right and left nasopalatine nerve, and is the landmark for the nasopalatine block.
- The maxillary tuberosity is a landmark for the administration of the posterior superior alveolar block.
- The greater palatine foramen is a landmark for the greater palatine block.
- The mental foramen is a landmark for both the mental and incisive blocks and is located between the apices of the mandibular first and second premolars.
- The alveolar process of the mandibular incisors is less dense and more porous than the body of the mandible and even less dense than the alveolar process of the mandibular posterior teeth, which allows a supraperiosteal injection or local infiltration of the mandibular anteriors by a local anesthetic agent to have a higher degree of success than the mandibular posterior teeth but always less success than all the maxillary teeth.
- The coronoid notch is a landmark for the administration of the inferior alveolar block.
- The anteromedial border of the mandibular condylar neck is a landmark for the Gow-Gates mandibular block.
- The mandibular foramen is a landmark for the inferior alveolar block and is located three fourths the distance from the coronoid notch to the posterior border of the ramus.
- When the infraorbital nerve is anesthetized both the anterior superior alveolar and middle superior alveolar nerves are also anesthetized.
- The middle superior alveolar nerve is present in approximately 28% of the population.
- In rare cases, a patient may have a bifid inferior alveolar nerve, in which a second mandibular foramen may be seen on radiographs.
- The (long) buccal nerve is an afferent nerve for the skin of the cheek, buccal mucous membranes, and buccal gingival tissue of the mandibular posterior teeth.
- The lingual nerve is afferent for general sensation of the body of the tongue, floor of the mouth, and lingual gingival tissue of the mandibular teeth.
- The mental nerve is an afferent nerve for the chin, lower lip, and labial mucosa of the mandibular anterior teeth and premolars.
- The incisive nerve is an afferent nerve for the mandibular anterior teeth and premolars.

- The mylohyoid nerve in some cases may serve as an afferent nerve for the mandibular first molar and needs to be considered when there is failure of the inferior alveolar block.
- The facial nerve may be inadvertently anesthetized during the inferior alveolar block if given incorrectly,

causing transient facial paralysis since it travels through the parotid salivary gland.
- The pterygoid plexus of veins may be pierced during the posterior superior alveolar block if given incorrectly, causing a hematoma.

CHAPTER REVIEW QUESTIONS

1. Which of the following BEST describes the reason for greater incidence of clinically adequate local anesthesia for the maxillary teeth when the local anesthetic agent is administered as a supraperiosteal injection or local infiltration than would occur with similar teeth on the mandibular arch?
   A. More porous alveolar process
   B. Denser alveolar process
   C. Presence of adjacent nerve canals
   D. Increased pulpal lymphatic channels
2. Which foramen carries branches of BOTH the right and left nasopalatine nerves?
   A. Greater palatine foramen
   B. Lesser palatine foramen
   C. Incisive foramen
   D. Infraorbital foramen
3. Which of the following is a landmark for the posterior superior alveolar local anesthetic block?
   A. Zygomatic process
   B. Maxillary tuberosity
   C. Palatine process
   D. Retromolar pad
4. Which of the following is a landmark for the administration of the anterior middle superior alveolar local anesthetic block?
   A. Incisive foramen
   B. Greater palatine foramen
   C. Median palatine raphe
   D. Lesser palatine foramen
5. Which of the following skull bones is the ONLY freely movable bone of the skull?
   A. Maxilla
   B. Zygomatic bone
   C. Palatal bone
   D. Mandible
6. The mental foramen USUALLY located between the apices of the mandibular:
   A. first and second premolars.
   B. first and second molars.
   C. first premolar and canine.
   D. central and lateral incisors.
7. For which of the following mandibular teeth is a supraperiosteal local anesthetic injection or local infiltration MOST effective?

A. Anteriors
B. Premolars
C. Molars
D. Premolars and molars

8. Which of the following is a landmark for the inferior alveolar local anesthetic block?
   A. Mental foramen
   B. Coronoid notch
   C. Mandibular notch
   D. Incisive foramen
9. Which of the following is a landmark for the Gow-Gates mandibular local anesthetic block?
   A. Coronoid notch
   B. Mental foramen
   C. Condylar neck
   D. Mandibular canal
10. A patient may have a bifid inferior alveolar nerve, and a second mandibular canal can be detected on radiographs.
    A. Both statements are true
    B. Both statements are false
    C. First statement is true and second is false
    D. Second statement is false and second is true
11. Which of the following nerves is ONLY present in approximately 28% of the population?
    A. Anterior superior alveolar
    B. Middle superior alveolar
    C. Posterior superior alveolar
    D. Infraorbital
12. Which of the following BEST describes the (long) buccal nerve?
    A. Efferent nerve for the facial gingival tissue of the mandibular anterior teeth.
    B. Afferent nerve for the facial gingival tissue of the mandibular anterior teeth.
    D. Efferent nerve for the buccal gingival tissue of the mandibular posterior teeth.
    E. Afferent nerve for the buccal gingival tissue of the mandibular posterior teeth.
13. Which of the following is the division of the trigeminal nerve that does NOT innervate the teeth?
    A. Ophthalmic
    B. Maxillary

CHAPTER REVIEW QUESTIONS

C. Mandibular
D. Facial

14. The zygomatic nerve is a branch of which of the following nerves?
    A. Ophthalmic
    B. Maxillary
    C. Mandibular
    D. Facial

15. Which nerve when anesthetized also anesthetizes BOTH the anterior and middle superior alveolar nerves?
    A. Posterior superior alveolar
    B. Inferior alveolar
    C. Incisive
    D. Infraorbital

16. Which of the following is considered the largest division of the trigeminal nerve?
    A. Ophthalmic
    B. Maxillary
    C. Mandibular
    D. Facial

17. Which of the following nerves is formed from afferent branches from the body of the tongue?
    A. Inferior alveolar
    B. Lingual

C. Mental
D. Incisive

18. Which of the following nerves may also innervate the mandibular first molar in some cases?
    A. Mylohyoid
    B. Mental
    C. Incisive
    D. Ariculotemporal

19. The mental nerve serves as an afferent nerve for the:
    A. labial mucosa of the mandibular anterior teeth.
    B. lingual gingival tissue of the mandibular anterior teeth.
    C. buccal mucosa of the mandibular posterior teeth.
    D. lingual gingival tissue of the mandibular posterior teeth.

20. Which of the following local anesthetic block injections when given INCORRECTLY may pierce the pterygoid plexus of veins causing a hematoma?
    A. Anterior superior alveolar
    B. Middle superior alveolar
    C. Infraorbital
    D. Posterior superior alveolar

CHAPTER 11

Basic Injection Techniques

Demetra Daskalos Logothetis RDH, MS

CHAPTER OUTLINE

LEARNING OBJECTIVES

1. Describe the four anesthetic administration techniques.
2. Describe patient preparation and rapport strategies inherent in stress reduction protocol used for all anesthetic procedures.
3. Describe the steps to providing a successful injection and the importance of each.
4. Successfully complete review questions and activities for this chapter.

KEY TERMS

Aspirate on two planes The procedure of rotating the barrel of the syringe 45 degrees and aspirating following the initial aspiration test to ensure that the bevel of the needle is not abutting a blood vessel producing a false negative aspiration.

Deposit location Target area where local anesthetic will be deposited.

Depth of needle penetration Describes needle depth covered in tissue when target area is reached.

Field block Form of regional anesthesia deposited near large terminal nerve branches.

Informed consent Written agreement from the patient consenting to treatment following a discussion of the benefits and risks associated with the treatment.

Local infiltration Provides soft tissue anesthesia of the smaller terminal nerve endings only in the area of anesthetic deposition.

Needle insertion point Injection site where bevel of needle is covered with tissue.

Negative aspiration A clear air bubble entering the cartridge, or no return, after negative pressure is applied to the cartridge.

Nerve block Injection of local anesthetic in the vicinity of a major nerve trunk to anesthetize the nerve's area of innervations, usually at a distance from the area of treatment.

Positive aspiration Any blood entering the cartridge, after negative pressure is applied to the cartridge.

Supraperiosteal injection Form of regional anesthesia deposited near large terminal nerve branches providing pulpal and soft tissue anesthesia of a single tooth.

Surface anesthesia Anesthesia achieved by application of topical anesthetics to the mucosal surface by gels, creams, or sprays to block the free nerve endings.

INTRODUCTION

Successful delivery of local anesthetic agents by the dental hygienist requires careful consideration of many factors. Many of those factors have already been discussed, such as, patient assessment and selection of the appropriate anesthetic. Equally important factors are choosing the appropriate injection to be administered, safe administration of the drug, and effective patient management. The information presented in this chapter is intended to assist the dental hygienist with the skills necessary to provide safe, comfortable injections.

ADMINISTRATION TECHNIQUES

When choosing the appropriate administration technique, the dental hygienist must consider the area to be treated, the duration of anesthesia needed, and the comfort needs of the patient. Local anesthesia administration techniques are divided into four major categories: surface anesthesia, local infiltration, field block, and nerve block (Figure 11-1).

SURFACE ANESTHESIA

Surface anesthesia is used when topical anesthetics are applied to the surface by gels, creams, or sprays to block the free nerve endings supplying the mucosal surfaces. The effect is short lasting and limited to the direct area of contact. Topical anesthetics are used as a preinjection technique to obtund the pain associated with needle insertion.[1]

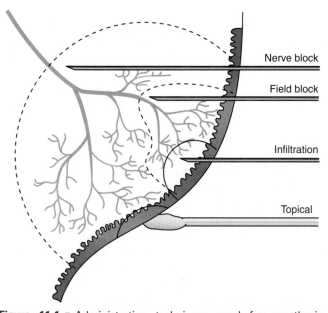

Figure 11-1 ■ Administration techniques used for anesthesia. Dashed lines and solid lines represent the areas of anesthesia produced by regional (nerve block, field block) and local (infiltration, topical application) anesthetic techniques, respectively. (Modified from Jastak T, Yagiela J, Donaldson D: *Local anesthesia of the oral cavity*, St Louis, 1995, Saunders.)

LOCAL INFILTRATION

Local infiltration techniques are used when soft tissue anesthesia is needed in a limited area. The anesthesia is deposited close to the smaller terminal nerve endings providing pain relief only in the area of anesthetic diffusion. Dental hygienists can use this technique during nonsurgical periodontal therapy when anesthesia is needed only in the immediate area of injection, and for bleeding control provided by the vasoconstrictor.[1,2]

FIELD BLOCK

Field block is a form of regional anesthesia deposited near large terminal nerve branches. It is also referred to as supraperiosteal injections. Anesthesia usually involves pulpal and soft tissue anesthesia of a single tooth in the maxilla (by depositing the solution above the apex of the tooth to be anesthetized) except in the area of the anterior superior alveolar block (ASA) and middle superior alveolar block (MSA) where anesthesia is achieved on more than one tooth using this technique (see Chapter 12). Field block injections are most effective in the maxillary arch due to the porous nature of the bone allowing the anesthetic to easily diffuse through the bone to the nerve. However, this technique can be used on the mandibular laterals and incisors, and is an excellent injection technique when crossover anesthesia is needed (see Chapters 12 and 13). In dentistry, field block injections are often referred to incorrectly as infiltration injections.

NERVE BLOCK

Nerve block anesthesia refers to the injection of local anesthetic in the vicinity of a major nerve trunk to anesthetize the nerve's area of innervations, usually at a greater distance from the area of treatment. This technique offers an advantage over the other techniques by providing profound pulpal and soft tissue anesthesia over a larger area. The disadvantage is that arteries and veins accompany major nerve trunks, and the potential for piercing the artery or vein with this technique is greatly enhanced.[1] Examples of nerve blocks are the inferior alveolar, posterior superior alveolar, mental/incisive, and infraorbital blocks.

STEPS TO PROVIDING A SUCCESSFUL INJECTION

The administration of local anesthetics will become routine to the experienced dental hygienist, but it is often a very stressful experience for the patient. For many patients, the fear and anticipation of pain from receiving a "shot" could produce an emergency situation.[3-5] Vasodepressor syncope is the most common medical emergency observed in the dental office, and it is most frequently linked to the administration of local anesthesia.[3-5]

Dental hygienists must be cognizant not to allow the administration of local anesthetics to become routine. Providing effective communication and psychological support is essential to build patient confidence and to reduce the risk of an emergency situation. Using the following steps, the dental hygienist can provide appropriate pain control during and after the treatment in a safe, effective, and comfortable manner for the patient.

STEP 1: PREANESTHETIC PATIENT ASSESSMENT AND CONSULTATION

The patient assessment should be conducted as described in Chapter 7, and vital signs should be obtained and recorded. Appropriate medical and dental consultations should be completed before administration of local anesthetics.

Selection of Anesthetic

The selection of the anesthetic should be based on the patient's medical history, taking into consideration many additional factors:

The physical status of the patient: The choice of local anesthetic agent and vasoconstrictor must be based on the patient's physical status. Absolute and relative contraindications should be carefully evaluated, and an anesthetic agent with the least adverse effects according to the patient's physical status should be selected.

Duration of treatment and postoperative pain control: Duration of effect in pulpal and soft tissue varies for each agent, and consideration should be made as to whether profound pulpal anesthesia is indicated. For nonsurgical periodontal therapy in shallow pockets with soft tissue sensitivity but no root sensitivity, a short-acting anesthetic such as 3% mepivacaine may be appropriate. For half-mouth nonsurgical periodontal therapy with deep pockets and heavy deposits, a longer-acting anesthetic may be appropriate.

Volume of anesthetic: Profound pulpal anesthesia necessary for restorative procedures, extractions, and nonsurgical periodontal therapy with heavy deposits, for example, is essential and will require more anesthetic volume than less invasive procedures.

Need for hemostasis: Limited visibility decreases the efficiency in providing thorough deposit removal. If heavy bleeding is anticipated, a vasoconstrictor should be selected to constrict the blood vessels for greater visibility. Caution should be taken when using epinephrine 1:50,000 in patients with significant cardiovascular disease. For excessive bleeding, it is recommended to infiltrate epinephrine 1:50,000 in small amounts directly into the area of bleeding for greatest visibility and hemostatic control.

Possibility of self-mutilation: Small children and patients with special needs are more prone to bite themselves while numb, causing self-mutilation. Longer acting anesthetics should be avoided.

Determining maximum recommended dose: The patient's maximum recommended dose (MRD) should be calculated based on the selected anesthetic and the

patient's medical history and documented in the patient's chart (see Chapter 8).

STEP 2: CONFIRM CARE PLAN

The care plan should be developed by the dental hygienist in collaboration with the patient, and confirmed before treatment. If the dental hygiene care plan involves nonsurgical periodontal therapy with anesthesia, the dental hygienist should carefully determine the extent of periodontal involvement, and how much of the treatment can be realistically accomplished in one visit. Local anesthesia should only be administered in the areas of treatment that can be completed in one visit. Overestimating the treatment and administering more anesthesia than necessary should be avoided.

Depending on the time available for treatment and the extent of periodontal involvement, the dental hygienist should design a care plan by dividing the mouth into quadrants or sextants for treatment. Figure 11-2 illustrates examples of nonsurgical periodontal therapy with anesthesia care plan designs. With advanced periodontal disease and heavy deposits the dental hygienist may only realistically be able to complete a few teeth in a single visit. The dental hygienist should then divide the mouth into sextants rather than quadrants for treatment. (see Figures 11-2A,B) If either sextant or quadrant dental hygiene treatment is planned on the maxillary arch, the posterior superior alveolar (PSA) block is given before any of the other maxillary facial injections as well as any maxillary palatal injections to allow the necessary time for the larger molars to become completely anesthetized, with instrumenting proceeding in the same manner. After the PSA block, the middle superior alvolar (MSA) and then the anterior superior alveolar (ASA) block (or infraorbital [IO] block instead) is then given (in that order). For patients with initial to moderate periodontal disease, the dental hygienist may complete one to two quadrants during a single visit. When two quadrants are treated in a single visit, it is recommended to treat upper and lower quadrants on either the right or left side of the patient's face. (Figure 11-2C) The dental hygienist should avoid administering local anesthetics to both the mandibular right and left quadrants during a single treatment to prevent the inability of the patient to control his or her mandible. Administering bilateral inferior alveolar nerve blocks also increases the possibility of the patient causing self-mutilation of their soft tissues (see Chapter 14). If half-mouth treatment is planned, the inferior alveolar and buccal blocks are given first, then the maxillary facial, and then palatal injections follow in order as described earlier, with instrumenting proceeding first on the maxillary arch. This allows time for the entire mandibular arch to become completely anesthetized. When designing the dental hygiene care plan, the dental hygienist must consider the amount of anesthetic needed to complete the procedure (always staying within the patient's MRD).

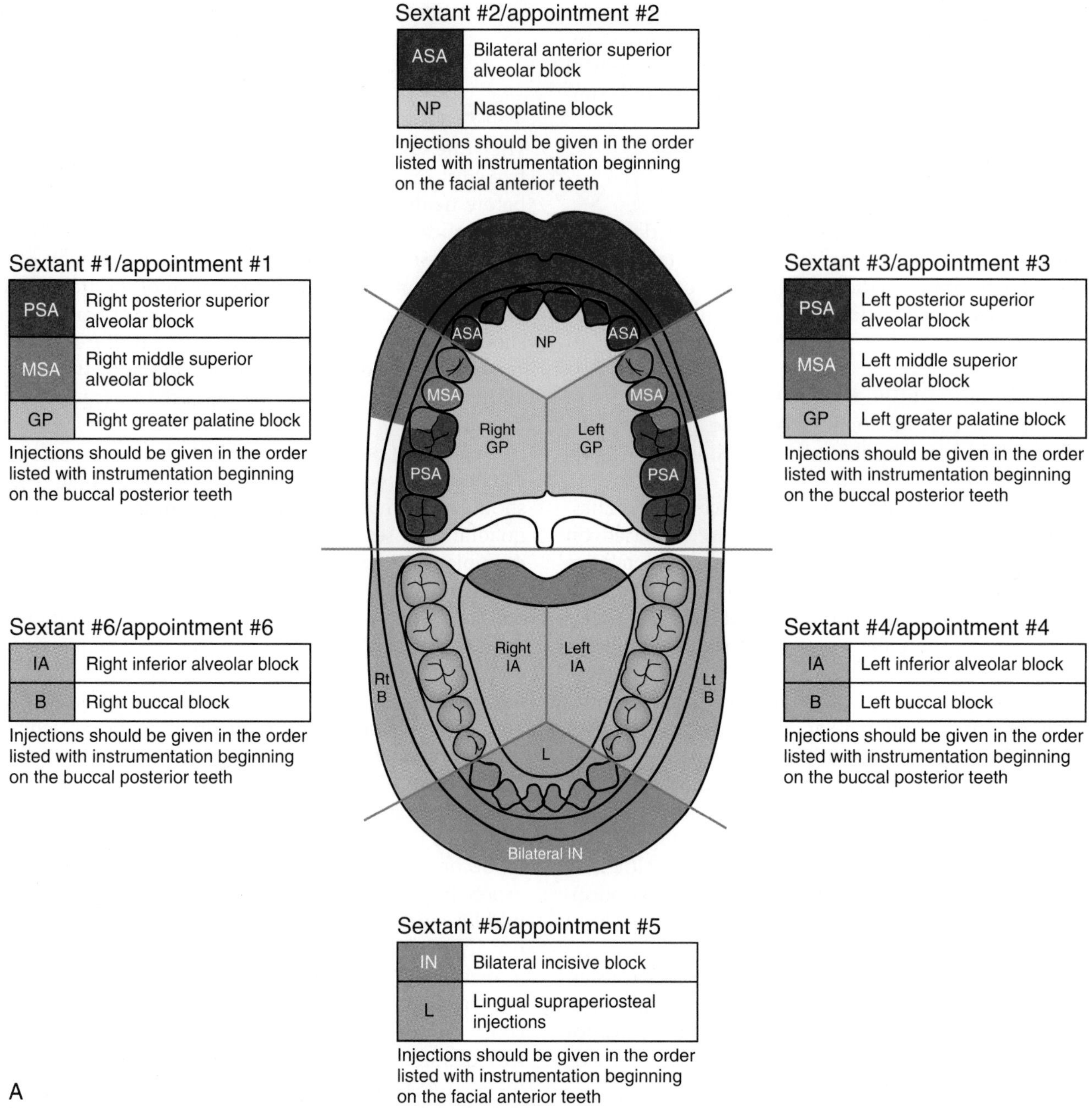
Sextant #2/appointment #2
ASA Bilateral anterior superior alveolar block
NP Nasoplatine block
Injections should be given in the order listed with instrumentation beginning on the facial anterior teeth
Sextant #1/appointment #1
PSA Right posterior superior alveolar block
MSA Right middle superior alveolar block
GP Right greater palatine block
Injections should be given in the order listed with instrumentation beginning on the buccal posterior teeth
Sextant #3/appointment #3
PSA Left posterior superior alveolar block
MSA Left middle superior alveolar block
GP Left greater palatine block
Injections should be given in the order listed with instrumentation beginning on the buccal posterior teeth
ASA
ASA
NP
MSA
MSA
Right GP
Left GP
PSA
PSA
Right IA
Left IA
Rt B
Lt B
L
Bilateral IN
Sextant #6/appointment #6
IA Right inferior alveolar block
B Right buccal block
Injections should be given in the order listed with instrumentation beginning on the buccal posterior teeth
Sextant #4/appointment #4
IA Left inferior alveolar block
B Left buccal block
Injections should be given in the order listed with instrumentation beginning on the buccal posterior teeth
Sextant #5/appointment #5
IN Bilateral incisive block
L Lingual supraperiosteal injections
Injections should be given in the order listed with instrumentation beginning on the facial anterior teeth
A

Figure 11-2 ■ Examples of nonsurgical periodontal therapy care plan with anesthesia. **A,** Sextant dental hygiene care plan for nonsurgical periodontal therapy with anesthesia. The mouth is divided into six sextants for six appointments.

STEP 3: INFORMED CONSENT

The benefits and risks associated with all treatment including the administration of local anesthetics should be discussed, as should the risks involved in not receiving treatment. The dental hygienist should discuss with the patient the type of anesthetic that will be used, and the injection procedure. The patient should be advised of the temporary numbing feeling associated with the administration of the drug, and the anticipated duration of anesthesia. Following the care plan discussion, informed consent to treatment should be received by the patient. In the case of a minor, the informed consent must be given by the parent or guardian. Figure 11-3 is a sample informed consent form that includes the consent to the administration of anesthetics. The written agreement of the care plan becomes a legal contract between the patient and the dental hygienist.[2]

STEP 4: SELECTION OF INJECTION

After the care plan has been determined, the dental hygienist should determine the appropriate injections for

Quadrant #1/appointment #1

PSA	Right posterior superior alveolar block
MSA	Right middle superior alveolar block
ASA	Right anterior superior alveolar block
GP	Right greater palatine block
NP	Nasopalatine

Injections should be given in the order listed with instrumentation beginning on the buccal posterior teeth
Note: Can substitute infraorbital (IO) block for MSA and ASA blocks

Quadrant #4/appointment #4

IA	Right inferior alveolar block
B	Right buccal block

Injections should be given in the order listed with instrumentation beginning on the buccal posterior teeth

Quadrant #2/appointment #2

PSA	Left posterior superior alveolar block
MSA	Left middle superior alveolar block
ASA	Left anterior superior alveolar block
GP	Left greater palatine block
NP	Nasopalatine

Injections should be given in the order listed with instrumentation beginning on the buccal posterior teeth
Note: Can substitute infraorbital (IO) block for MSA and ASA blocks

Quadrant #3/appointment #3

IA	Left inferior alveolar block
B	Left buccal block

Injections should be given in the order listed with instrumentation beginning on the buccal posterior teeth

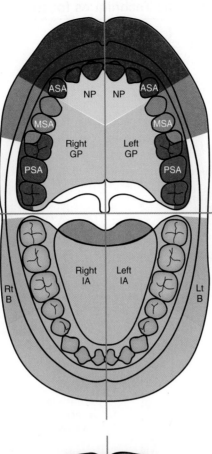

B

Half mouth #1/appointment #1

IA	Right inferior alveolar block
B	Right buccal block
PSA	Right posterior superior alveolar block
MSA	Right middle superior alveolar block
ASA	Right anterior superior alveolar block
GP	Right greater palatine block
NP	Nasopalatine block

Injections should be given in the order listed with instrumentation beginning on the buccal posterior teeth of the maxillary quadrant
Note: Can substitute infraorbital (IO) block for MSA and ASA blocks

Half mouth #2/appointment #2

IA	Left inferior alveolar block
B	Left buccal block
PSA	Left posterior superior alveolar block
MSA	Left middle superior alveolar block
ASA	Left anterior superior alveolar block
GP	Left greater palatine block
NP	Nasopalatine block

Injections should be given in the order listed with instrumentation beginning on the buccal posterior teeth of the maxillary quadrant
Note: Can substitute infraorbital (IO) block for MSA and ASA blocks

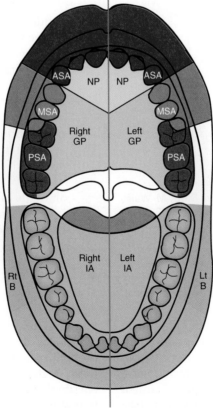

C

Figure 11-2, cont'd ■ **B,** Quadrant dental hygiene care plan for nonsurgical periodontal therapy with anesthesia. The mouth is divided into four quadrants for four appointments. **C,** Half-mouth dental hygiene care plan for nonsurgical periodontal therapy with anesthesia. The mouth is divided in half (maxillary/mandibular) for treatment of two quadrants in one appointment. (Modified from Fehrenbach MF, Herring SW: *Illustrated anatomy of the head and neck,* ed 3, St Louis, 2007, Saunders.)

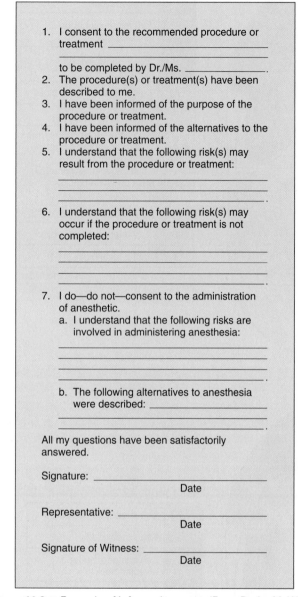

1. I consent to the recommended procedure or treatment _____

   to be completed by Dr./Ms. _____.
2. The procedure(s) or treatment(s) have been described to me.
3. I have been informed of the purpose of the procedure or treatment.
4. I have been informed of the alternatives to the procedure or treatment.
5. I understand that the following risk(s) may result from the procedure or treatment:

   _____
   _____
   _____.
6. I understand that the following risk(s) may occur if the procedure or treatment is not completed:

   _____
   _____
   _____
   _____.
7. I do—do not—consent to the administration of anesthetic.
   a. I understand that the following risks are involved in administering anesthesia:

      _____
      _____
      _____.
   b. The following alternatives to anesthesia were described: _____

      _____
      _____.

All my questions have been satisfactorily answered.

Signature: _____
                              Date

Representative: _____
                              Date

Signature of Witness: _____
                              Date

Figure 11-3 ■ Example of informed consent. (From Darby M, Walsh M: *Dental hygiene theory and practice*, ed 3, St Louis, 2010, Saunders, Elsevier.)

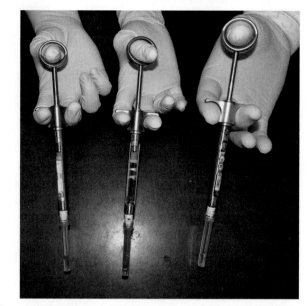

Figure 11-4 ■ Syringe selection depending upon the hand size of the dental hygienist. Small (blue) Septodont syringe should only be used for very small hands, medium (silver) Septodont syringe is typically used for average hand size, and large (gold) Septodont syringe is used for larger hands. An important factor to consider in selecting a syringe is the ability to pull back on the thumb ring in an easy manner to achieve an aspiration.

complete pulpal and/or soft tissue anesthesia. There are many factors to take into consideration for injection selection:

Areas needing to be anesthetized: For maximum patient comfort, the dental hygienist should select injections to completely anesthetize the areas needed with minimal tissue penetrations, such as choosing nerve blocks rather than field blocks for larger treatment areas. In addition, the dental hygienist should take into consideration the density of the bone in the area of treatment and the selection of injection technique. Supraperiosteal injections are much more effective on the maxilla because the bone is callous. The mandible requires nerve blocks because the cortical plate is thick. The mandibular anterior teeth are more conducive to supraperiosteal injections but to a lesser degree than the maxilla.

Presence of infection: Infection in the area of anesthetic administration will decrease the effectiveness of the anesthetic. The acidic nature of the anesthetic deposited into acidic tissue from the infection decreases the ability of the anesthetic to readily dissociate for nerve penetration. (See Chapter 3.) It is recommended to administer nerve blocks away from the infected area.

Hemostasis: If hemostasis is needed in the area for greater visibility, it is recommended to infiltrate small amounts of anesthetic with a vasoconstrictor directly into the papillary, interdental or marginal gingival. Epinephrine 1:50,000 produces the greatest hemostatic control.

STEP 5: PREPARATION OF EQUIPMENT

The preparation of equipment should be completed as described in Chapter 9. The appropriate selection of a syringe is important, taking into consideration the hand size of the dental hygienist and the hygienist's ability to properly conduct the aspiration test (Figure 11-4). The bulkiness of the anesthetic syringe and the length of dental anesthetic needles can be frightening to the patient; therefore, they should be covered or placed out of the patient's sight (Figure 11-5). The equipment may be set up before the patient's arrival if the care plan and selection of appropriate anesthetic has already been determined at a previous appointment. However, any recent changes in the patient's medical history may require a modification in anesthetic selection.

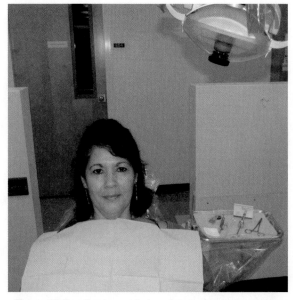

Figure 11-5 ■ Equipment placed out of patient's sight.

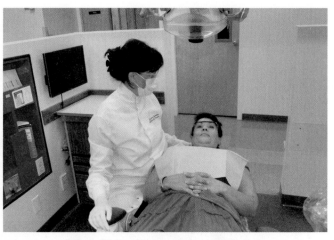

Figure 11-6 ■ Proper supine positioning.

STEP 6: CHECK THE ANESTHETIC EQUIPMENT

Before administration of the local anesthetic, the dental hygienist should check the needle bevel orientation for planned injections in close proximity to the periosteum. The bevel should be oriented toward the bone. For these injections, the bevel indicator (Figure 9-21) should be turned opposite the large window. This will ensure that when the dental hygienist is holding the syringe palm up with the large window facing him or her, the bevel will be toward the bone when the injection is commenced. Although the bevel of the needle does not affect success rates of the injection, it will provide added comfort to the patient and less trauma to the periosteum if the bone is contacted.

It is recommended to expel a few drops of anesthetic to ensure free flow of the solution. The dental hygienist should confirm that the harpoon is fully secured into the rubber stopper by gently pulling back on the thumb ring. The syringe is then ready for use. The dental hygienist should confirm that all protective equipment is in place, including re-capping devices, and personal protective equipment for the clinician and patient.

STEP 7: PATIENT POSITION

Supine positioning (head and heart parallel to the floor) (Figure 11-6) with the patient's feet slightly elevated is the most effective position to administer anesthesia. Because supine positioning is the recommended position to treat vasodepressor syncope, this adds the benefit of decreasing the risk of a patient fainting before, during, or after the administration of the anesthetic.[3,4] The dental hygienist should ask the patient to turn his or her head appropriately for the greatest visibilty of the penetration site.

STEP 8: TISSUE PREPARATION AND PATIENT COMMUNICATION

A topical antiseptic (Betadine or merthiolate) may be applied to the tissue to reduce the possibility of septic material entering the soft issues.[3] This step is optional and before application the patient must be screened for a possible allergy to iodine. The tissue should be dried with a 2×2 gauze square (Figure 11-7A) and the antiseptic should be applied to the area of needle insertion with a cotton tip applicator (see Figure 11-7B).

A topical anesthetic should be applied after the topical antiseptic; this should be applied only to the area of needle insertion (see Figure 11-7C). Topical anesthetics are commonly used before needle insertion to provide soft tissue anesthesia of the terminal nerve endings; these are most effective when applied for 1–2 minutes. Topical anesthetics do not contain vasoconstrictors and are absorbed rapidly when applied to the mucous membranes. Because of the rapid absorption and higher concentrations of surface applications, caution should be taken to avoid toxic reactions (see Chapter 6). While applying the topical anesthetic, the dental hygienist may use the cotton tip applicator to visualize and practice the angulations necessary for the injection (see Figure 11-7D).

During application of the topical anesthetic is also a good time for supportive communication with the patient to help alleviate his or her fears. Communicating in a positive manner will enhance the patient's trust in the clinician and demonstrate the clinician's desire to provide a pain-free injection. For example, the dental hygienist might say "I am applying a topical anesthetic for 2 minutes to numb the surface of the tissue, which will provide a more comfortable experience for you, and then I will make sure to administer the anesthetic slowly, which will provide additional comfort." (Do not use negative words, such as *pain*, *shot*, or *hurt*.) (See Chapter 15 for more information on effective communication prior to the administration of local anesthetics.)

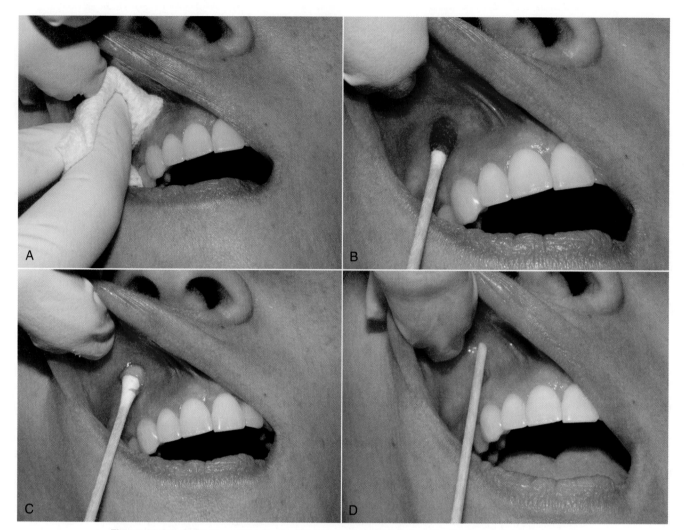

Figure 11-7 ■ **A,** Drying of the tissue. **B,** Applying topical antiseptic. **C,** Applying topical anesthetic. **D,** Using cotton tip applicator to visualize and practice injection angulations before needle insertion.

STEP 9: DRY TISSUE AND VISUALIZE OR PALPATE THE PENETRATION SITE

Following the application of topical anesthetic, re-dry the injection site to remove any excess topical anesthetic and to provide a dry area for effective visualization of the injection site. Palpate appropriate areas to determine any needle access problems associated with exostosis etc., and to determine the insertion point (such as with the IA injection). Pick up the prepared syringe, palm up, making sure the large window is facing up in clear view. See Figure 11-8 for correct hand positioning.

STEP 10: ESTABLISH A FULCRUM

The anesthetic syringe is large and can be cumbersome, so syringe stabilization is necessary. Selection of an appropriate fulcrum is determined by the finger length, personal preference, and physical abilities. A firm hand rest is essential to providing safe, comfortable injections. Of particular importance to a firm hand rest is to ensure syringe stability necessary for proper aspiration with limited needle movement. A fulcrum must always be used, and as with dental hygiene instrumentation, secure extraoral fulcrums are acceptable. The dental hygienist should never use the patient's arm to rest the syringe-holding arm. Any sudden movement of the patient's arm may cause injury to the patient or dental hygienist. Dental hygienists with small hands may not be able to achieve appropriate stabilization using only their fingers of the dominant hand. If firm finger placement cannot be achieved, the dental hygienist may maintain stability through arm-to-body support. For dental hygiene students or practicing dental hygienists administering their first local anesthetic injections on a fellow classmate, some degree of nervousness and shaking of the hands are to be expected. Syringe stabilization utilizing firm fulcrums will help alleviate the shaking. Students are encouraged to practice maintaining a solid fulcrum utilizing the syringe with a capped needle prior to administering the

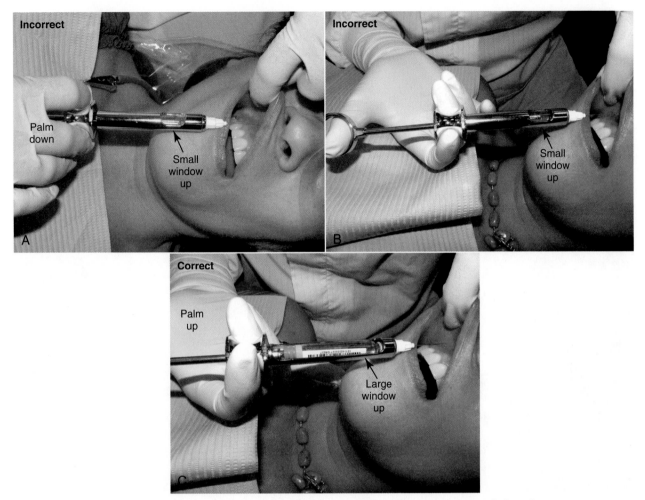

Figure 11-8 ■ **A,** Palm down, large window down, **incorrect. B,** Palm up, large window down, **incorrect. C,** Palm up, large window up, **correct.**

injection. Figures 11-9 illustrates successful fulcrums; additional fulcrums are demonstrated for each injection technique in Chapters 12 and 13.

STEP 11: MAKE TISSUE TAUT

Retracting the tissue taut at the penetration site (Figure 11-10A) will assist the dental hygienist with visibility of the injection site and allow easier, less traumatic needle insertion. A 2 × 2 piece of sterile gauze may be used if the tissues are slippery (see Figure 11-10B).

STEP 12: KEEP SYRINGE OUT OF PATIENT'S SIGHT

Keeping the syringe out of the patient's sight will help prevent any unnecessary anxiety for the patient (Figure 11-11A). The sight of the dental needle and the large anesthetic syringe could provoke excess anxiety, leading to a possible medical emergency (see Figure 11-11B). It is important, however, that the dental hygienist knows the exact location of the uncovered needle at all times. This can prevent needlestick exposure to the clinician or accidentally touching a surface outside of the patient's mouth before

insertion and thus contaminating the needle (see Figure 11-11C–D).

STEP 13: GENTLY INSERT THE NEEDLE/ WATCH/COMMUNICATE

Gently insert the needle until the bevel is covered keeping the tissue taut (Figure 11-12). This is the needle insertion point. Watch for signs of discomfort or distress. Slowly move toward the target while communicating to the patient in a positive manner. A few drops of anesthetic will be unconsciously deposited ahead of the needle due to the gentle contact by the clinician's thumb on the inner surface of the thumb ring. Proceed slowly, utilizing appropriate angulations, to the depth of needle penetration which is the target location or deposit location of the anesthetic.

STEP 14: ASPIRATION

In order to prevent the possibility of an intravascular injection, an aspiration test should be conducted before any anesthetic solution is deposited. This is one of the most important steps to reduce the incidence of injecting anesthetic solution directly into a blood vessel. Once the target

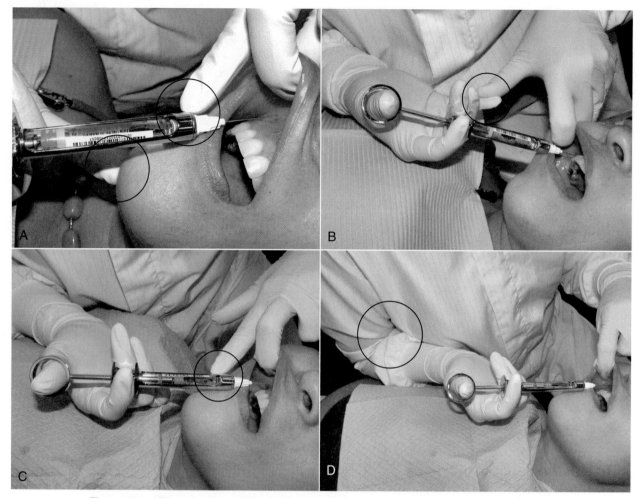

Figure 11-9 ■ Example of an appropriate fulcrum during the administration of local anesthetics. **A,** Pinky of dominant hand resting on patient's chin; index finger of non-dominant hand supporting the syringe barrel. **B,** Double-handed fulcrum. **C,** Index finger of non-dominant hand supporting the syringe barrel. **D,** Arm to body fulcrum.

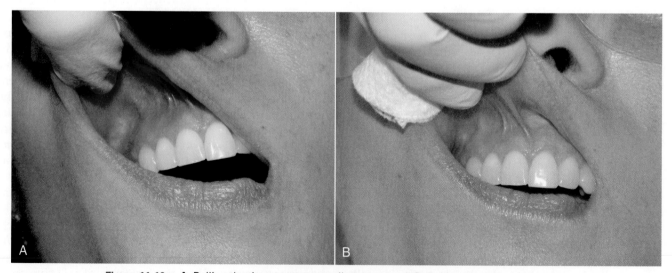

Figure 11-10 ■ **A,** Pulling the tissue taut; no sterile gauze used. **B,** Pulling the tissue taut, using sterile gauze for slippery tissue.

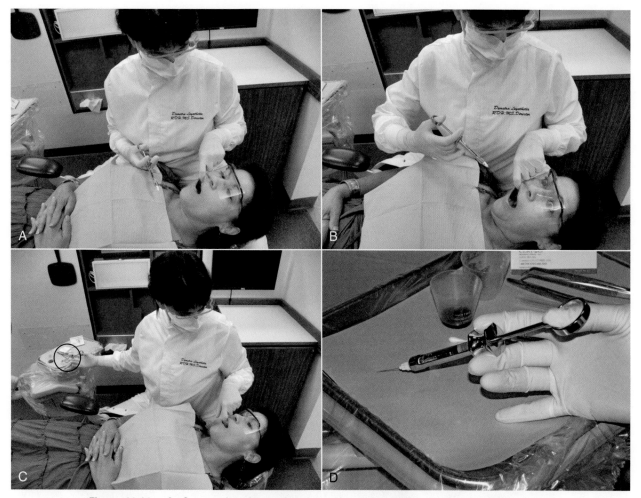

Figure 11-11 ■ **A,** Correct: keeping syringe out of patient's sight. (Keep syringe low out of patient's direct line of vision without contaminating the needle.) **B,** Incorrect: syringe in direct line of patient's sight, producing fear. **C,** Incorrect: dental hygienist not paying attention to the location of the uncovered needle, causing accidental contamination of the needle. **D,** Close-up view of dental hygienist's hand demonstrating needle contamination.

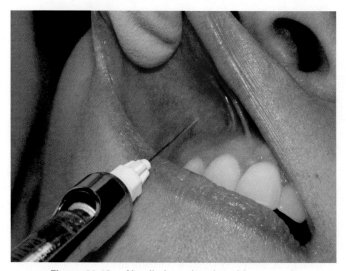

Figure 11-12 ■ Needle insertion; bevel is covered.

location is reached, aspirate by pulling back on the thumb ring (only about 1–2 mm for standard syringes) to change the pressure in the cartridge from positive to negative (Figure 11-13A). Care should be taken not to allow the thumb ring to slip down to the bottom of the thumb, making it difficult to achieve the full range of backward motion needed for a successful aspiration (see Figure 11-13B). For self-aspirating syringes, this is accomplished by applying positive pressure to either the thumb ring or thumb disk and releasing it to create the negative pressure (Figure 11-14). The needle should not move with either type of syringe. Beginners, especially those who do not have a firm fulcrum, have a tendency to overexaggerate the pulling back motion of the thumb ring, which pulls the needle away from the proper depth of penetration.

Following the initial successful negative aspiration, the dental hygienist should rotate the barrel of the syringe about 45 degrees and aspirate a second time. This is called aspirating on two planes. This ensures that the needle is

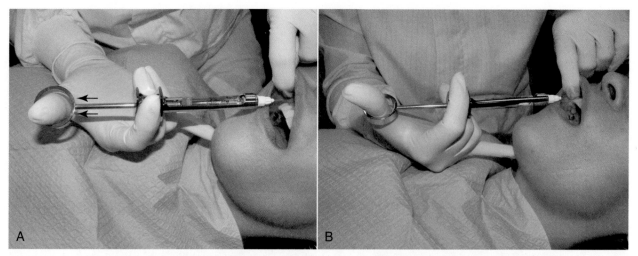

Figure 11-13 ■ Aspiration utilizing a standard syringe. **A,** Pulling back on the thumb ring for standard syringe with thumb ring in correct location for full range of backward motion. **B,** Thumb ring not in proper location, restricting full range of backward motion.

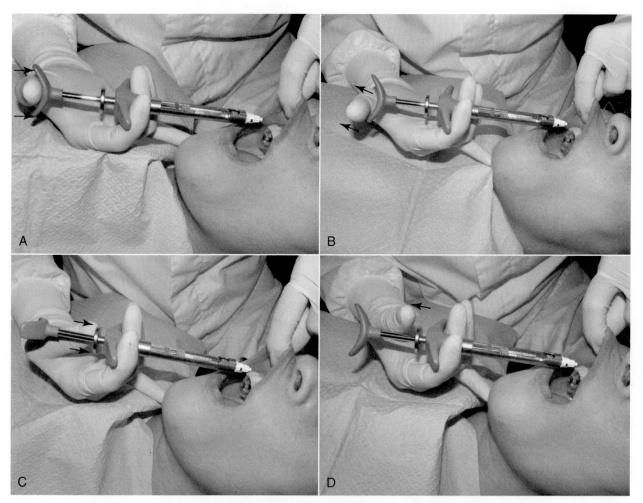

Figure 11-14 ■ Aspiration utilizing a self-aspirating syringe. **A,** Applying positive pressure to thumb ring for self-aspirating syringe. **B,** Releasing positive pressure from thumb ring to create negative pressure. **C,** Applying positive pressure to thumb disk for self-aspirating syringe. **D,** Releasing positive pressure from thumb disk to create negative pressure.

not located within a blood vessel and possibly abutting the blood vessel wall, providing a false-negative aspiration. This slight rotation will reposition the bevel away from the wall of a blood vessel. When injecting near highly vascular areas, such as near the pterygoid venous plexus with the posterior superior alveolar block, the dental hygienist should aspirate several times during the injection to ensure that any movement of the needle has not placed it within the blood vessel.

Any blood entering the cartridge is considered a positive aspiration. A clear air bubble, or no return after definite movement backward of the rubber stopper, is a negative aspiration (Figure 11-15). If a positive aspiration is observed, the dental hygienist is required to address the situation immediately. If only a small amount of blood has entered the cartridge and does not obstruct the view of successive aspirations, the dental hygienist can slightly reposition the needle a few millimeters, and the aspiration can be reattempted. If the second aspiration is negative, the anesthetic can be delivered (Figure 11-16). If blood fills and clouds the cartridge or a second aspiration cannot be clearly seen after redirection, it is necessary to remove the syringe

from the tissue, change the cartridge and needle and redo the procedure (Figure 11-17).

If repeated positive aspirations are observed at the same injection site, it may be necessary for the dental hygienist to consider postponing treatment, or treating a different section of the mouth, if possible. Repeated penetrations in the same area can cause bleeding at the target location, increase risk of hematoma, trismus, postoperative pain, and infection. Effective patient communication and education regarding these concepts is an important component to the delivery of local anesthetics so that the patient is aware that best practices are maintained at all times.[2]

Disengagement of the harpoon from the rubber stopper can occur when the dental hygienist is attempting aspiration (Figure 11-18). This is usually caused by a dull harpoon or improper engagement during setup. If the harpoon disengages, the dental hygienist cannot ensure that a negative aspiration has occurred; the syringe must be removed, the harpoon must be reembedded into the rubber stopper, and the procedure must be redone. The best practice to reembed the needle into the rubber stopper is to recap the needle (utilizing the one-handed scoop technique), remove the

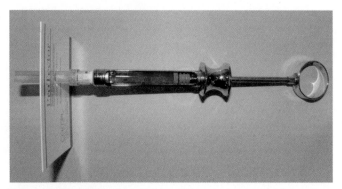

Figure 11-17 ■ Positive aspiration filling the cartridge; it is necessary to remove the syringe, change the cartridge and needle, and redo the procedure.

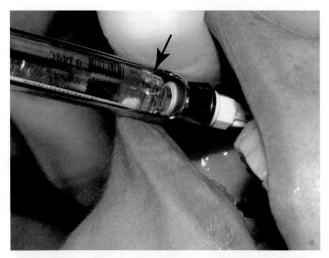

Figure 11-15 ■ Negative aspiration produces a clear bubble.

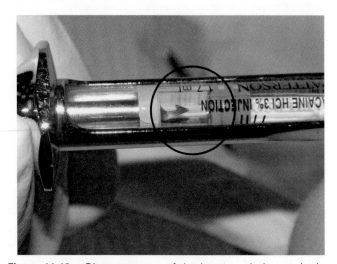

Figure 11-18 ■ Disengagement of the harpoon during aspiration: the dental hygienist must remove the needle from the tissues, reengage the harpoon, and redo the procedure.

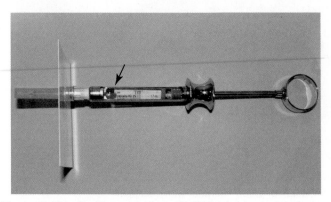

Figure 11-16 ■ Positive aspiration with little blood entering the cartridge; redirection is possible.

needle from the syringe, and apply pressure to the thumb ring. If the dental hygienist attempts to reembed the harpoon into the rubber stopper with the needle still on, anesthetic solution will be expressed without the harpoon adequately embedding into the rubber stopper.

STEP 15: SLOWLY DEPOSIT THE LOCAL ANESTHETIC SOLUTION

Once the dental hygienist has reached the target destination and has successfully aspirated on two planes, the anesthetic should be deposited slowly by gently and evenly pressing on the thumb ring. Slowly depositing the anesthetic solution is a very important safety factor for two reasons: it reduces the risk of overdose even if the anesthetic is accidentally administered intravascularly, and it prevents the tearing of tissue.[3] In addition, it improves patient comfort. The anesthetic should be deposited at a rate of 1 mL of solution per minute.[2] Local anesthetic cartridges contain 1.8 mL of solution, so an entire cartridge would be deposited in approximately 2 minutes. It is

important to continue communicating with the patient while depositing the solution. The dental hygienist should inform the patient why the solution is being deposited slowly, for example, "I am depositing the solution slowly to improve comfort." See Box 11-1 for a recommended method for slow deposition of solution while implementing the safety of re-aspiration.

BOX 11-1	Recommended Method to Ensure Slow Deposit of Solution

Following negative aspiration on two planes → deposit slowly ¼ cartridge of solution → reaspirate (negative) → continue to deposit another ¼ solution → reaspirate (negative) → continue to deposit another ¼ solution to complete the procedure.

　　This process will take approximately 2 minutes, ensuring the slow flow of solution and aspirating throughout the procedure in case of needle movement.

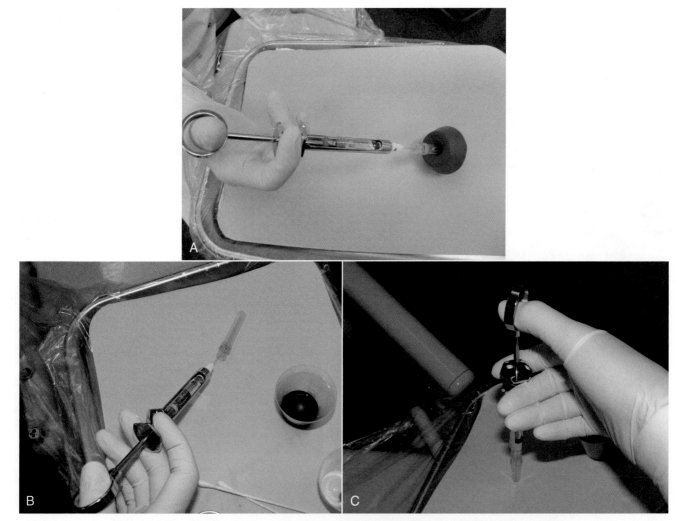

Figure 11-19 ■ Needle capping procedures. **A,** One-handed scoop method with recapping device. **B,** Basic one-handed scoop method without recapping device. **C,** Securing the cap one-handed without a recapping device.

STEP 16: SLOWLY WITHDRAW THE SYRINGE AND SAFELY CAP THE NEEDLE

Following completion of the injection, slowly withdraw the needle from the tissues. The procedure is not completed until the needle is safely capped. Once the needle leaves the tissue, it is contaminated with blood, tissue, and saliva and must be covered with its protective shield before anything else is done. This prevents inadvertent operator needle puncture. Because dental procedures require multiple injections, it is impractical to change the needle after each injection, disposing of it immediately in the sharps container after the injection as is required in other medical professions. It is therefore recommended that the needle be capped using at least the basic CDC-recommended one-handed scoop method (Figures 11-19 and Chapter 9). Safer needle recapping devices or fabricated methods are available to help the dental hygienist secure the needle shield, allowing for easy, safe capping of a contaminated needle. Figure 11-20 illustrates safe needle capping.

STEP 17: OBSERVE THE PATIENT FOR POSSIBLE REACTION TO ANESTHETIC

Following the safe covering of the contaminated needle, the dental hygienist should observe the patient to monitor any signs of a reaction to the anesthetic or from the procedure. Most reactions, or dental emergencies associated with the administration of an anesthetic, occur within 5 minutes after the procedure.[5] Therefore the dental hygienist should remain in the room while the anesthetic blood levels increase, and observe the patient for possible signs of an adverse reaction. If no adverse reactions are demonstrated, the dental hygienist should evaluate the effectiveness of the anesthetic, which should take approximately 3 to 10 minutes depending upon the selected anesthetic's pKa (see Chapter 3), and injection technique.

STEP 18: DOCUMENT PROCEDURE

Following the procedure, document the injection in the patient's permanent record. This should include (1) date of drug administration, (2) the drug used and concentration, (3) vasoconstrictor used if any, (4) the amount of drug and vasoconstrictor administered in milligrams, (5) the gauge and type of needle, (6) the injections given, (7) the time of administration, and (8) any patient reactions. The time the drug was administered is important for long procedures when additional anesthetic might be needed, especially when a patient has received anesthetic solution close to the maximum recommended dose. By noting the time, the dental hygienist may be able to administer more anesthetic once the half-life of the drug is considered. See Box 11-2 for examples of patient documentation.

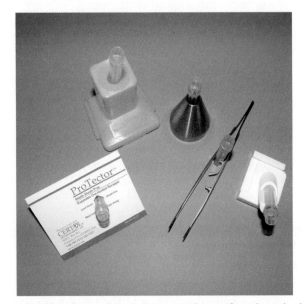

Figure 11-20 ▪ Recapping devices are the preferred method to safely cap needles.

BOX 11-2	**Examples of Treatment Notes Following the Administration of 1.6 Cartridges of Lidocaine 2%, 1:100,000 Epinephrine**

EXAMPLE 1

Date	Treatment	Signature
11/17/10	5% lidocaine topical, 57.6 mg of lidocaine 2%, 1:100,000 epinephrine (0.028 mg) was administered for the Rt. IA,B* blocks using 25-gauge long needle at 9:00 a.m.; no patient reaction or complications.	*D Logothetis*

EXAMPLE 2

Date	Treatment	Signature
11/17/10	57.6 mg of lidocaine 2%, 1:100,000 epinephrine (0.028 mg) was administered for the Rt. IA,B* blocks using 25-gauge long needle at 9:00 a.m. Hematoma developed immediately after the Rt. IA block. Applied pressure and ice to the area, and instructed the patient to continue with ice today and apply warm packs tomorrow. Patient requested treatment be postponed. Released patient after no further swelling developed. Further homecare instructions were given to the patient.	*D Logothetis*
11/17/10	Follow-up phone call at 5:00: patient is doing much better, swelling has decreased. No further complications. Informed patient to call if any problems arise.	*D Logothetis*

*IA (inferior alveolar block), B (buccal block).

DENTAL HYGIENE CONSIDERATIONS

- Dental hygienists should never allow the administration of local anesthetics to become routine. Dental hygienists should always take great care in the pre-anesthetic assessment, drug selection, and drug delivery.
- Vasodepressor syncope is the most common medical emergency observed in the dental office, and is most frequently associated with the administration of local anesthesia.
- If two quadrants are to be completed in a single visit, anesthesia should be administered to upper and lower quadrants on the same side of the patient's face, administering the mandibular anesthesia first.
- Profound pulpal anesthesia necessary for restorative procedures, nonsurgical periodontal therapy with heavy deposits, and extractions, require more anesthetic volume than less invasive procedures.
- Nerve block anesthesia provides profound anesthesia over a larger area with fewer injections needed.
- There is a greater potential for piercing an artery or vein during nerve blocks.
- Good patient communication before and during the injection will help alleviate the patient's fears.
- A firm fulcrum allows the dental hygienist to properly control the anesthetic syringe and provides ease of aspiration and a safer, more comfortable injection.

- Keeping the syringe and needle out of the patient's range of vision may prevent unnecessary anxiety.
- The dental hygienist should aspirate on two planes prior to depositing anesthetic to ensure that the needle is not abutting the blood vessel wall, providing a false-negative aspiration.
- If the blood of a positive aspiration does not completely fill the cartridge, the dental hygienist can slightly reposition the needle and attempt a second aspiration.
- If repeated positive aspirations are observed at the same injection site, it may be necessary for the dental hygienist to consider postponing treatment.
- If the harpoon disengages after an aspiration, the dental hygienist must remove the needle from the tissue and the harpoon must be reembedded into the rubber stopper. The procedure will need to be redone.
- To provide safe and comfortable injections, the dental hygienist should administer the anesthetic solution slowly at a rate of 1.8 mL over approximately 2 minutes.
- The dental hygienist should always cap the contaminated needle using the one-handed scoop method utilizing a needle shield prop.
- The dental hygienist should observe the patient for possible adverse reactions to the anesthetic and should never leave the patient unattended after providing anesthesia.

CASE STUDY 11-1

Christine is feeling anxious following administration of a local anesthetic

Christine, a 130-lb patient, is in the office for a routine class I amalgam on tooth #19. Christine's medical history reveals that she is nervous about the dental appointment, has a history of hypertension, and is taking Tenormin. The dental hygienist, Diana, calculates Christine's MRD and determines that Christine can have 2.2 cartridges of lidocaine 2% 1:100,000 epinephrine. Diana begins the administration of the inferior alveolar block. Once the needle is at the penetration site, Diana aspirates and hears a popping noise, which startles the patient. Diana is concerned about the patient's nervousness and quickly injects the cartridge of anesthetic. Shortly following the

completion of the injection, Christine is experiencing increased heart rate and blood pressure, and a throbbing headache. Christine leaves the patient in a supine position to make her more comfortable.

Critical Thinking Questions
- Why can Christine only receive 2.2 cartridges of the selected anesthetic?
- What reaction is Christine experiencing?
- What is the likely cause of the reaction?
- What could Diana have done to prevent the reaction?
- How should Diana properly treat the reaction?

CHAPTER REVIEW QUESTIONS

1. Surface anesthesia can be achieved by all of the following EXCEPT:
   A. Gels
   B. Creams
   C. Sprays
   D. Injections

2. When soft tissue anesthesia is needed in a limited area, it is best to perform a:
   A. Field block
   B. Local infiltration
   C. Nerve block
   D. Surface anesthesia

CHAPTER REVIEW QUESTIONS

3. The dental hygienist will provide nonsurgical periodontal therapy of teeth #18–24. Which injection administration technique should the dental hygienist use?
   A. Field block
   B. Local infiltration
   C. Nerve block
   D. Surface anesthesia

4. If the dental hygienist wants to anesthetize tooth #12, which injection administration technique should the clinician use?
   A. Field block
   B. Local infiltration
   C. Nerve block
   D. Surface anesthesia

5. What type of injection administration technique is the ASA?
   A. Field block
   B. Local infiltration
   C. Nerve block
   D. Surface anesthesia

6. What is the most common medical emergency observed in the dental office?
   A. Cardiac arrest
   B. Vasodepressor syncope
   C. Seizures
   D. Respiratory failure

7. During the preanesthetic assessment, what are appropriate clinical considerations?
   A. Vitals signs
   B. Length of appointment
   C. Anticipated postoperative pain control
   D. All are important considerations

8. When checking the armamentarium, why is it important to expel a few drops of solution?
   A. To decrease the amount of anesthetic that would be administered to the patient
   B. To ensure the harpoon is fully engaged into the rubber stopper
   C. To ensure the rubber stopper is not sticky
   D. To ensure a free flow of anesthetic through the needle

9. What is the recommended patient position when administering anesthesia?
   A. Supine
   B. Semisupine
   C. Upright
   D. Head below heart level

10. Following a positive aspiration, the dental hygienist must always change the cartridge and redo the procedure.
    A. True
    B. False

11. Topical anesthetic should be applied after the application of a topical antiseptic. Topical antiseptic can be used to decrease infection.
    A. Both statements are true
    B. Both statements are false
    C. First statement is true, second statement is false
    D. First statement is false, second statement is true

12. After the patient has consented to treatment, when is a good time to communicate with the patient to alleviate fears of needle injection?
    A. After the procedure is over so as to not distract the clinician from the procedure
    B. When preparing the equipment
    C. When inserting the needle
    D. When preparing the tissue for injection

13. What are the benefits of establishing a fulcrum during the administration of a local anesthetic?
    A. To ensure safe, comfortable injections
    B. To ensure proper aspiration without needle movement
    C. To provide more stability
    D. All of the above

14. Pulling the tissue taut before needle insertion helps all of the following EXCEPT:
    A. Visibility
    B. Ease of needle insertion
    C. Ease of needle penetration through the tissue
    D. Burning sensation felt by the patient

15. What is the main goal of aspirating on two planes?
    A. To determine if the bevel of the needle is abutting against a blood vessel providing a false negative aspiration on the first aspiration test.
    B. To determine definite backward movement of the rubber stopper.
    C. To determine if disengagement of the harpoon occurred.
    D. To provide the clinician a second chance to see if a clear bubble entered the cartridge.

16. What is the minimum number of times a clinician should aspirate before administering the anesthetic solution?
    A. Once
    B. Twice
    C. Zero, only during nerve blocks
    D. Four

17. Depositing anesthetic solution should be done quickly to promote patient comfort.
    A. True
    B. False

18. After removing the needle, what is the immediate next step?
    A. Rinsing the patient's mouth
    B. Documenting the procedure

CHAPTER REVIEW QUESTIONS

C. Recapping the needle

D. Monitor the patient for reactions

19. When do most reactions or dental emergencies associated with the administration of local anesthetics happen?

A. Before the procedure

B. When the patient gets home

C. Within 5 minutes of the procedure

D. Within 1 hour of the procedure

20. Following the local anesthetic procedure, what information is important to document?

A. Time the anesthetic was administered

B. Anesthetic used and amount

C. Vasoconstrictor used

D. B and C only

E. All of the above

REFERENCES

1. Jastak T, Yagiela J, Donaldson D: *Local anesthesia of the oral cavity*, St Louis, 1995, Saunders.

2. Darby M, Walsh M: *Dental hygiene theory and practice*, ed 3, St Louis, 2010, Saunders.

3. Malamed S: *Handbook of local anesthesia*, ed 5, St Louis, 2004, Mosby.

4. Malamed SF: *Medical emergencies in the dental office*, ed 6, St Louis, 2007, Mosby.

5. Matsuura H: Analysis of systemic complications and deaths during dental treatment in Japan, *Anesth Prog* 36: 219-228, 1989.

Sharps Management: Center for Disease Control (CDC) Guidelines for Infection Control in the Dental Health Care Setting

EXPOSURE PREVENTION FACTS

Preventing occupational exposures in dentistry can significantly preclude the transmission of HBV, HCV, and HIV, to Dental Health Care Personnel (DHCP). (19,96,97)

Occupational exposures occur through percutaneous injury (e.g., a needlestick or cut with a sharp object), through contact between potentially infectious blood, tissues, body fluids, and mucous membranes of the eye, nose, mouth, or nonintact skin).

The incidence of occupational exposures is not reduced for the experienced clinician. (100,104,107)

Occupational exposures in dentistry are preventable when standard precautions are consistently utilized and devices engineered to alleviate sharps injuries are employed. (98–100,103)

STANDARD PRECAUTIONS

Engineering controls incorporate safer designs of instruments to reduce the exposures to blood and other potentially infectious material (OPIM) from sharp instruments and needles. These include self-sheathing anesthetic needles to reduce percutaneous injuries. (101,103,108)

Needles are a substantial source of percutaneous injury in dental practice, and engineering of safe devices and work-practice controls for needle handling are paramount. The 2001 OSHA bloodborne pathogens standards as mandated by the Needlestick Safety and Prevention Act of 2000 emphasizes the need for employers to consider available safer needle devices and to involve clinicians (e.g., dentists, hygienists, and dental assistants) in identifying and choosing such devices. (109)

Safety controls for needles and other sharps are mandatory, which include placing used disposable syringes and needles, scalpel blades, and other sharp items in appropriate puncture-resistant containers located as close as feasible to the area of use. (2,7,13,113–115)

Contaminated needles should never be recapped or otherwise manipulated by using both hands, or directed toward any part of the body. (2,7,13,97,113,114)

A one-handed scoop technique, a recapping device designed for holding the needle cap to facilitate one-handed recapping, or an engineered sharps injury protection device (e.g., needles with resheathing mechanisms) should be employed for recapping needles between uses and before disposal. (2,7,13,113,114)

DHCP should never bend or break needles before disposal because this practice requires unnecessary manipulation and a greater chance for needlestick injury.

To prevent injuries, the DHCP should safely recap contaminated needles utilizing the one-handed scoop technique before attempting to remove needles from nondisposable aspirating syringes. For procedures involving multiple injections with a single needle, the practitioner should recap the needle between injections by using a one-handed scoop technique or use a device with a needle-resheathing mechanism.

Avoid passing a syringe with an unsheathed needle between clinicians to avoid risk for injury.

Strategic steps for needlestick prevention programs are:

Form a sharps injury prevention team that includes workers to (1) develop, implement, and evaluate a plan to reduce needlestick injuries and (2) evaluate needle devices with safety features.

Identify priorities based on assessments of how needlestick injuries are occurring, patterns of device use in the institution, and local and national data on injury and disease transmission trends. Give the highest priority to needle devices with safety features that will have the greatest impact on preventing occupational infection.

When selecting a safer device, identify its intended scope of use in the dental care facility and any special technique or design factors that will influence its safety, efficiency, and user acceptability. Seek published, Internet, or other sources of data on the safety and overall performance of the device.

Conduct a product evaluation, making sure that the participants represent the scope of eventual product users. The following steps will contribute to a successful product evaluation:

- Train DHCP in the correct use of the new device.
- Establish clear criteria and measures to evaluate the device. (Safety feature evaluation forms are available.)

- Conduct onsite follow-up to obtain informal feedback, identify problems, and provide additional guidance.
- Monitor the use of a new device after it is implemented to determine the need for additional training, solicit informal feedback on health care worker experience with the device (e.g., using a suggestion box), and identify possible adverse effects of the device on patient care.

Additional information for developing a safety program and for identifying and evaluating safer dental devices is available at http://www.cdc.gov/OralHealth/infectioncontrol/forms.htm and http://www.cdc.gov/niosh/topics/bbp (state legislation on needlestick safety).

Source: http://www.cdc.gov/mmwr/preview/mmwrhtml/rr5217a1.htm.

Safe and Unsafe Needle Recapping Techniques

Exposures to bloodborne pathogens can happen by getting stuck with a used needle or getting cut by a sharp instrument that has blood on it. Job-related needlesticks can lead to serious or potentially fatal infections from bloodborne pathogens such as hepatitis B virus, hepatitis C virus, or human immunodeficiency virus (HIV). Even when a serious infection is not transmitted, the emotional impact of a needlestick injury can be severe and long-lasting. It is essential that dental health care providers consistently employ safe needle handling, recapping, and disposal of contaminated needles based upon the CDC and OSHA guidelines for infection control in the dental health care setting. A one-handed scoop technique is crucial to safe and effective needle recapping in the dental setting. The use of recapping devices with the one-handed scoop method provides safer engineering controls for recapping procedures. The following examples demonstrate "safe" and "unsafe" needle recapping techniques.

"Safe" basic one-handed scoop method without recapping device.

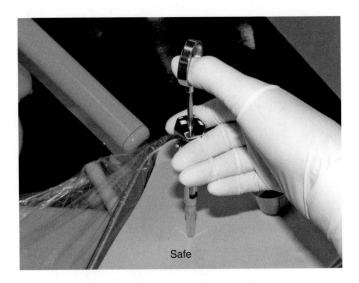

Safe

"Safe" one-handed scoop method utilizing weighted needle cap holder.

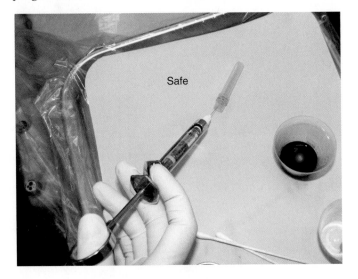

Safe

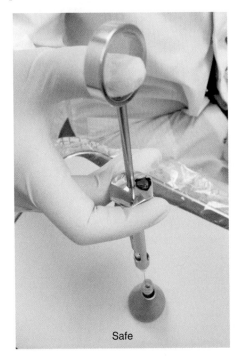

Safe

"Safe" one-handed scoop method utilizing plastic recapping devices.

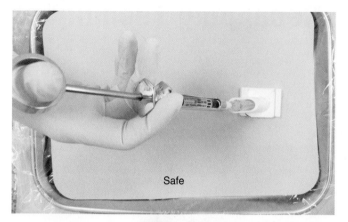

Safe

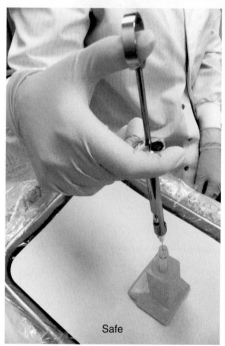

Safe

"Unsafe" two-handed technique holding the needle cap should never be performed.

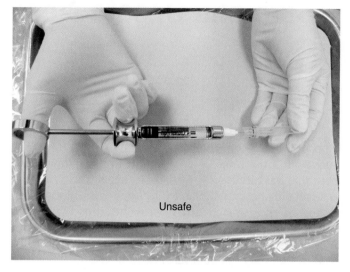

Unsafe

"Unsafe" two-handed techniques holding the rubber recapping device should never be performed.

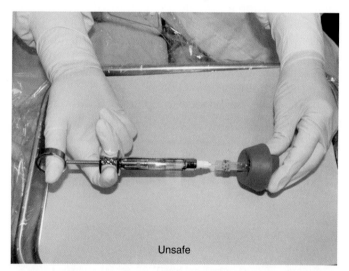

Unsafe

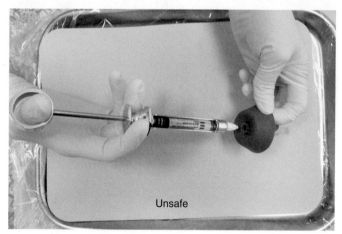

Unsafe

"Safe" one-handed technique utilizing assisted rubber recapping device.

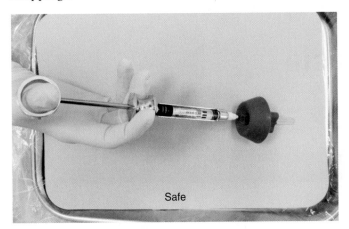

Safe

"Unsafe" two-handed technique utilizing the needle sheath prop. Note that it is unsafe to hold the card at the corner as well as in the back of the card as the needle can easily penetrate the card injuring the clinician, and should never be utilized in this manner.

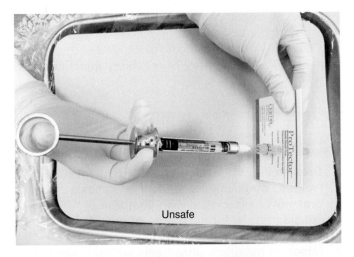

Unsafe

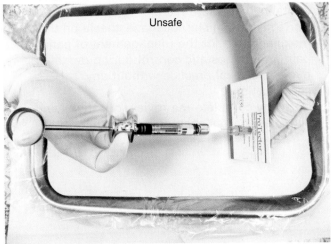

Unsafe

"Safe" one-handed scoop technique with a needle sheath prop to aid in covering and securing the contaminated needle. This device is disposable after use and is the preferred recapping device.

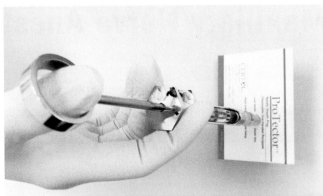

Safe

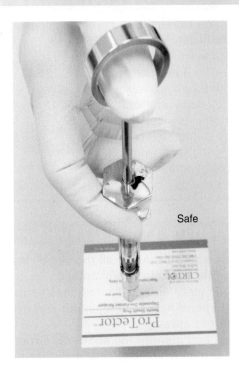

Safe

"Safe" one-handed shielding of safety syringe.

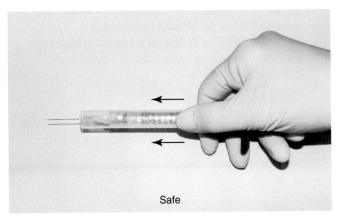

Safe

CHAPTER 12

Maxillary Nerve Anesthesia

Margaret Fehrenbach RDH, MS and Demetra Daskalos Logothetis RDH, MS

CHAPTER OUTLINE

LEARNING OBJECTIVES

1. Define and pronounce all the key terms and anatomic terms in this chapter.
2. List the teeth and structures anesthetized by each type of maxillary injection and describe the target areas.
3. Locate and identify the anatomic structures used to determine the local anesthetic needle's injection site for each type of maxillary injection on a skull and a patient.
4. Demonstrate the correct placement of the local anesthetic needle for each type of maxillary injection on a skull and a patient.
5. Identify the correct tissue penetrated by the local anesthetic needle for each type of maxillary injection.
6. Discuss the indications of successful injections as well as complications of local anesthesia of the oral cavity associated with anatomic considerations for each type of maxillary injection.
7. Integrate maxillary anesthesia with the needs of a dental hygiene care plan.
8. Correctly administer local anesthesia on the maxillary arch for the management of patient pain and hemostatic control during dental hygiene clinical practice without any complications.
9. Correctly complete the review questions and activities for this chapter.

KEY TERMS

Anterior middle superior alveolar (AMSA) block Type of injection that anesthetizes .most of the maxillary teeth and their associated periodontium as well as most of the facial and lingual gingival tissue in one quadrant

Anterior superior alveolar (ASA) block Type of injection that anesthetizes the maxillary anterior teeth and associated structures when the local anesthetic agent is deposited superior to the apex of the maxillary canine.

Crossover-innervation Overlap of terminal nerve fibers from the contralateral side.

Deposit location Target area where local anesthetic will be deposited.

Depth of needle penetration Describes needle depth covered in tissue when target area is reached.

Greater palatine (GP) block Type of injection that anesthetizes the lingual soft tissue distal to the maxillary canine in one quadrant.

Hematoma Swelling that develops when a blood vessel, particularly an artery, is punctured or lacerated by the needle.

Infraorbital (IO) block Type of injection that anesthetizes the maxillary anterior and premolar teeth and associated structures when the local anesthetic agent is deposited at the infraorbital foramen.

Middle superior alveolar (MSA) block Type of injection that anesthetizes the maxillary

premolars, and the mesial buccal root of the maxillary first molar and associated structures when the local anesthetic agent is deposited superior to the apex of the maxillary second premolar.

Nasopalatine (NP) block Type of injection that anesthetizes the lingual soft tissue between the maxillary right and left canines.

Needle insertion point Injection site where bevel of needle is covered with tissue.

Nerve block Type of injection that anesthetizes a larger area than the local infiltration because the local anesthetic agent is deposited near large nerve trunks.

Posterior superior alveolar (PSA) block Type of injection that anesthetizes the maxillary molars and associated structures when the local anesthetic solution is deposited superior to the apex of the maxillary second molar and posterior and superior to posterior border of maxilla at posterior superior alveolar foramina.

Supraperiosteal injection Type of injection that anesthetizes a small area—one or two teeth and associated structures—when the local anesthetic agent is deposited near terminal nerve endings.

Visual analog scale (VAS) An instrument used to measure pain.

INTRODUCTION TO MAXILLARY NERVE ANESTHESIA

The maxillary nerve and its branches can be anesthetized in a number of ways by the dental hygienist for patient pain management with hemostatic control depending upon the extent of procedure anticipated and the structures needing to be anesthetized (Figure 12-1 and Table 12-1).[1] But the dental hygienist must understand that giving maxillary anesthesia has its own considerations compared with giving mandibular anesthesia.

First, most local anesthesia of the maxilla is more successful than that of the mandible because the facial plate of the maxillary bone over the maxillary teeth is less dense than that of the mandible over similar teeth and even lingual anesthesia from the palatal surface is easily accomplished (see Chapters 10 and 13). This can be easily noted with a panoramic radiograph (see Figures 10-2 and 10-8).

Second, there is less anatomic variation of the maxillary and palatine bones and associated nerves with respect to local anesthetic landmarks than there is in similar mandibular structures, making the maxillary injections more

routine and usually without the need for troubleshooting failures (see Chapter 10).[2]

MAXILLARY FACIAL INJECTIONS

All the maxillary facial injections have a Visual Analog Scale (VAS) of 0–2 using the correct technique by the clinician.[3] (See Chapter 1.) To achieve this level of comfort, there is no bony contact of the overlying sensitive periosteum of the maxilla with the needle during the injection except at the final deposition point of the infraorbital (IO) block. In all cases, the solution is placed in the vestibule at the height of the mucobuccal fold of the soft tissue of the redder superior alveolar mucosa, avoiding the firmer and pinker inferior attached gingiva (Figure 12-2). To locate this general target area, the cotton tip applicator is used to gently palpate the injection site to ensure soft tissue entry before the needle is inserted and to provide topical anesthesia. It is important to advise the patient that a slight prick of the needle may be felt before proceeding.

To increase patient comfort during maxillary facial injections, the needle should not be moved within the tissue,

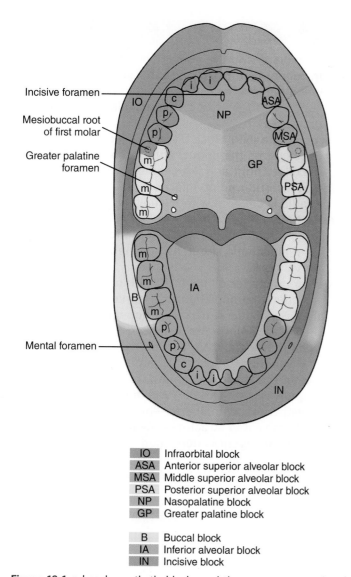

IO	Infraorbital block
ASA	Anterior superior alveolar block
MSA	Middle superior alveolar block
PSA	Posterior superior alveolar block
NP	Nasopalatine block
GP	Greater palatine block

B	Buccal block
IA	Inferior alveolar block
IN	Incisive block

Figure 12-1 ■ Local anesthetic blocks and the structures anesthetized (anterior middle superior alveolar block is not included; see associated figures for clarification of this block). (From Fehrenbach MJ, Herring SW: *Illustrated anatomy of the head and neck*, ed 3, St Louis, 2007, Saunders.)

nor should the patient's upper lip be shaken, which was mistakenly done in the past. In this distractor technique, the clinician used the retraction finger to shake the patient's upper lip to distract the patient during the injection; however, this movement may increase discomfort when the needle bevel is moved and the anesthetic may not be placed at the target area. To reduce patient discomfort, the local anesthetic agent should be deposited slowly and topical anesthesia used.

Any pulpal anesthesia for the maxillary blocks is achieved through anesthesia of each tooth's dental branches as they extend into the pulp by way of the apical foramen. Both the hard and soft tissue of the periodontium are anesthetized by way of the interdental and interradicular branches for each tooth.

The supraperiosteal injection is recommended when pulpal anesthesia is needed on a limited number of teeth or when anesthesia of the periodontium is needed in a localized area.

The posterior superior alveolar (PSA) block is generally recommended for anesthesia of the maxillary molar teeth and associated periodontium as well as buccal soft tissue in one quadrant. The middle superior alveolar (MSA) block is generally recommended for anesthesia of the maxillary premolars and associated periodontium as well as buccal soft tissue in one quadrant.

The anterior superior alveolar (ASA) block is recommended for anesthesia of the maxillary canine and incisors and their associated periodontium as well as facial soft tissue in one quadrant. The infraorbital (IO) block is generally recommended for anesthesia of the maxillary anterior and premolar teeth and associated periodontium as well as facial soft tissue in one quadrant.

If either sextant or quadrant dental hygiene treatment is planned on the maxillary arch, the PSA block is given before any of the other maxillary facial injections as well as any maxillary palatal injections to allow the necessary time for the larger molars to become completely anesthetized, with instrumenting proceeding in the same manner. After the

Figure 12-2 ■ For maxillary facial injections, the solution is placed in the height of the mucobuccal fold of the soft tissue of the redder superior alveolar mucosa, avoiding the firmer and pinker inferior attached gingiva. Note that for certain mandibular injections, such as the mental block and incisive block, a similar method is used in the depth of the mucobuccal fold. (From Bath-Balogh M, Fehrenbach MJ: *Illustrated dental embryology, histology, and anatomy*, ed 3, St Louis, 2011, Saunders.)

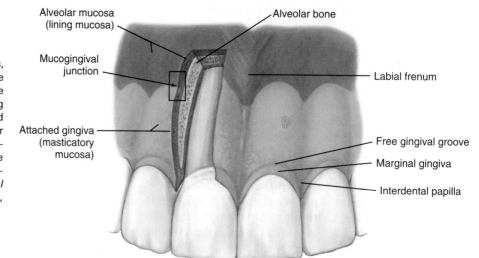

TABLE 12-1	Summary of Maxillary Local Anesthesia of the Teeth and Associated Structure						
MAXILLARY TOOTH AND STRUCTURE	**ASA BLOCK**	**PSA BLOCK**	**MSA BLOCK**	**IO BLOCK**	**NP BLOCK**	**GP BLOCK**	**AMSA BLOCK**
Central incisor							
Pulp/ periodontium/facial soft tissue	X			X			X
Lingual soft tissue					X		X
Lateral incisor							
Pulp/periodontium/facial soft tissue	X			X			X
Lingual soft tissue					X		X
Canine							
Pulp/Periodontium/facial soft tissue	X			X			X
Lingual soft tissue					X		X
First premolar							
Pulp/periodontium/buccal soft tissue			X	X			X
Lingual soft tissue						X	X
Second premolar							
Pulp/periodontium/buccal soft tissue			X	X			X
Lingual soft tissue						X	X
First molar							
Pulp/periodontium/buccal soft tissue		X					
Lingual soft tissue						X	
Second molar							
Pulp/periodontium/buccal soft tissue		X					
Lingual soft tissue						X	
Third molar							
Pulp/periodontium/buccal soft tissue		X					
Lingual soft tissue						X	

The anesthesia is not included for the mesiobuccal root of the first molar nor for anatomical variants.
AMSA, Anterior middle superior alveolar; *ASA,* anterior superior alveolar; *GP,* greater palatine; *IO,* infraorbital; *MSA,* middle superior alveolar; *NP,* nasopalatine; *PSA,* posterior superior alveolar.
From Fehrenbach MJ, Herring SW: *Illustrated anatomy of the head and neck,* ed 3, St Louis, 2007, Saunders.

PSA block, the MSA and then ASA blocks (or IO block instead) is then given (in that order). If half-mouth treatment is planned, the inferior alveolar and buccal blocks are given first, then the maxillary facial and then palatal injections follow in order, with instrumenting proceeding first on the maxillary arch. This allows time for the entire mandibular arch to become completely anesthetized. See Figure 11-2 for examples of nonsurgical periodontal therapy care plan with anesthesia. Local anesthesia should only be administered in the areas of treatment that can be completed in one visit. Overestimating the treatment to be completed on patients with heavy deposits and thus administering more anesthesia than necessary should be avoided. In some cases, there can be access difficulties for the clinician on getting the needle to the target site. The patient may have exostoses present on the facial surface of the maxillary arch, especially in the posterior sextants, forcing the clinician to work around these bony growths in order to maintain needed angulations. Similarly, a bulky facial alveolar ridge may hinder ideal angulation of the needle; increasing retraction and moving the needle injection site more superior usually helps the clinician adapt to this anatomic variation. Palpating the injection site with a cotton tip applicator before the injection helps determine these needle access problems.

SUPRAPERIOSTEAL INJECTION

The supraperiosteal injection, commonly referred to as *local infiltration* or *field block*, is generally recommended for anesthesia of individual teeth and associated periodontium as well as facial or lingual soft tissue (Table 12-2A–C and Procedure 12-1). The supraperiosteal injection can be accomplished on any tooth of either dental arch by depositing the anesthetic solution adjacent to the periosteum overlying the apex of the tooth to be anesthetized. In the case of the maxillary arch with its relatively porous bone, the anesthetic solution readily diffuses through its thinner facial plates of the maxillary bone to anesthetize the terminal fibers of the dental plexus (see Chapter 10).

This injection technique is especially useful for dental hygiene care during limited nonsurgical periodontal therapy when the anesthetic is used in combination with a vasoconstrictor to provide hemostasis in the smaller circumscribed area, such as during a maintenance or recare appointment.

Text continued on p. 230

TABLE 12-2   Supraperiosteal Injection Review

Indications

One or two teeth

Figure A ■ Supraperiosteal injection of maxillary central incisor.

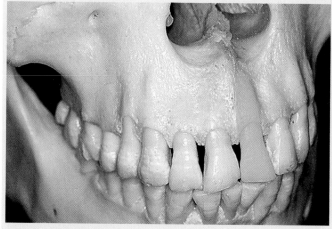

1. Areas anesthetized.

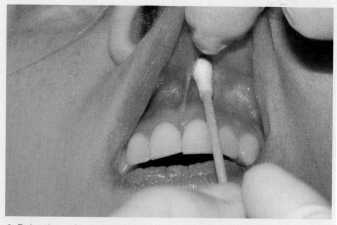

2. Palpation of height of mucobuccal fold at tooth apex to ensure soft tissue deposition. (Modified from Darby M, Walsh M: *Dental hygiene theory and practice*, ed 3, St Louis, 2010, Saunders.)

Nerves anesthetized	Terminal branches of dental plexus
Teeth anesthetized	Selected tooth (or teeth)
Other structures anesthetized	Periodontium of anesthetized tooth (or teeth) and either facial or lingual soft tissue in area
Administration technique	See Procedure 12-1
Needle gauge and length	27-gauge short

Figure B ■ Syringe stabilization for supraperiosteal injection

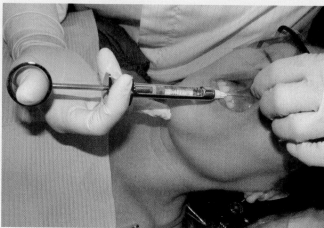

1. Rest pinky finger of dominant hand on patient's chin.

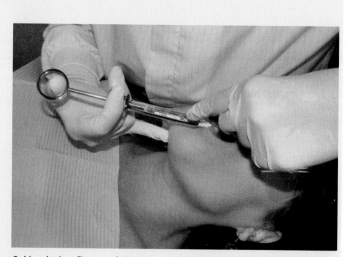

2. Use index finger of the retraction hand to support the syringe barrel.

TABLE 12-2	**Supraperiosteal Injection Review—cont'd**
Landmarks	Mucobuccal fold or lingual surface Selected tooth or teeth
Needle insertion point (see Figure A2)	Apex of selected tooth or teeth at the height or depth of mucobuccal fold or lingual surface
Depth of needle penetration	Approximately 5 mm or one-fourth the depth of short needle

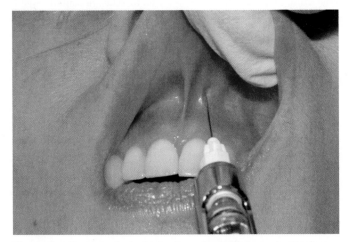

Figure C ■ Supraperiosteal injection of maxillary central incisor.

Deposit location	Superior or inferior to apex of selected tooth or teeth
Amount of anesthetic*	Approximately 0.6 mL or one-third of cartridge
Length of time to deposit	Approximately 30–60 seconds

*Approximate recommended amounts given are for 2% solutions of local anesthetic agents for adults; if using 4% solutions of local anesthetic agents, the approximate recommended amounts would be at least one-half of the amount of 2% solutions.

PROCEDURE 12-1   Supraperiosteal Injection Procedure

STEP 1 Assume the correct operator position depending on area anesthetized.

STEP 2 Ask the supine patient to open his or her mouth and then retract the patient's upper lip pulling the tissue taut using the thumb and index finger of the nondominant hand (one inside and one outside); a piece of sterile gauze may be used to help retract slippery tissue.

STEP 3 Prepare the alveolar mucosal tissue in the vestibule at the height (or depth) of the mucobuccal fold at the apex of the selected tooth (as discussed in Chapter 11), and palpate the injection site to ensure that only soft tissue is injected (see Table 12-2, Figure A2).

STEP 4 Using a 27-gauge short needle in the syringe in the dominant hand, orient the bevel of the needle away from the large window of the syringe to ensure bevel orientation toward the bone.

STEP 5 Establish a fulcrum (see Table 12-2, Figure B for fulcrum recommendations).

STEP 6 Place the syringe parallel with the long axis of the tooth with the large window facing the operator.

STEP 7 Insert the needle at the height (or depth) of the mucobuccal fold, parallel to the long axis of the tooth, and approximately one-fourth of the depth of the short needle (approximately 5 mm), or until the bevel is slightly superior (or inferior) to the apex of the tooth (see Table 12-2, Figure C). There should be no resistance or bony contact.

STEP 8 Aspirate within two planes.

STEP 9 If negative aspiration, slowly deposit approximately 0.6 mL of solution (one-third of cartridge) over approximately 30–60 seconds; if the tissue balloons, the clinician is injecting too rapidly.

STEP 10 Carefully withdraw the syringe and immediately recap the needle using the one-handed scoop method utilizing a needle sheath prop (see Chapter 11).

STEP 11 Wait approximately 3–5 minutes until anesthesia takes effect before starting treatment.

TABLE 12-3	**Average Size and Root Length of Selected Maxillary Teeth**	
TOOTH	**TOTAL LENGTH (mm)**	**ROOT LENGTH (mm)**
Central incisor	24.0	12.4
Lateral incisor	22.5	13.5
Canine	27.0	17.0
First premolar	22.5	13.8
Second premolar	21.5	13.0
First molar	20.5	12.8
Second molar	19.5	12.0

From Jastak T, Yagiela J, Donaldson D: *Local anesthesia of the oral cavity,* St Louis, 1995, Saunders.

However, because the anesthetic is deposited in close proximity to the area of treatment, any severe inflammation or infection in the area may inhibit achieving profound anesthesia. In this situation, it is recommended to instead administer the anesthetic at a distance from the infection using a nerve block where normal healthy tissue is located, thus allowing for more profound anesthesia (see Chapter 3).

Finally, supraperiosteal injections are not recommended when several teeth in the quadrant need to be anesthetized. Using supraperiosteal injections for nonsurgical periodontal therapy of several teeth in the quadrant would require several supraperiosteal injections and thus larger volumes of anesthetic solution to achieve anesthesia of the entire quadrant. Therefore using nerve block anesthesia techniques would be a more appropriate choice for this situation (see Chapter 11 and Figure 11-2).

Target Area and Injection Site for Supraperiosteal Injection

The deposit location or target area for the supraperiosteal injection is the apex of the selected tooth. Because the root lengths of teeth vary among patients, the depth of needle penetration will vary among teeth and among patients. For the maxillary arch, the clinician should review the average root lengths of maxillary teeth to help make this adjustment of needle depth more accurate (Table 12-3).[4]

The needle insertion point or injection site for the supraperiosteal injection is the height (maxillary arch) or depth (mandibular arch) of the mucobuccal fold or lingual (or palatal) surface, with the needle inserted toward the apex of the tooth to be anesthetized (see Table 12-2, Figure A). The bevel orientation of the needle should be toward the bone, and the needle should be inserted parallel to the long axis of the tooth. The needle tip is then placed superior or inferior to the apex (deposit location) of the selected tooth depending on the dental arch, without resistance or contacting bone in order to reduce trauma, and then the injection is administered (see Table 12-2, Figure C).

TABLE 12-4	**Supraperiosteal Injection Complications**
COMPLICATION	**TECHNIQUE ADJUSTMENT**
Pain on insertion with needle against the periosteum	Withdraw needle and reinsert farther away (or lateral) from periosteum
Pain during injection from injecting too rapidly	Due to acidic anesthetic agent, care should be taken to inject slowly so as to not exceed recommended deposit time
Possibly inadequate anesthesia from injecting into area of infection and also risking needle-track infection	Instead administer appropriate nerve block (see Tables 12-5 to 12-18)
Possibly inadequate anesthesia from dense bone covering apex or apices	Instead administer appropriate nerve block (see Tables 12-5 to 12-18)

Indications of Successful Supraperiosteal Injection and Possible Complications

Indications of a successful supraperiosteal injection include numbness of any associated soft tissue and absence of discomfort during dental procedures. However, the patient may feel pain if the needle makes bony contacts against the periosteum; in this case, the needle should be withdrawn and reinserted farther away (or lateral) from the periosteum (Table 12-4). Inadequate anesthesia may result when solution is deposited inferior to the apex of the tooth or when dense bone covers the apices, as is seen in children or around the maxillary central incisors where the apex of the tooth lies beneath the nasal cavity. Positive aspiration occurs in less than 1% of cases; thus overinsertion with complications of hematoma are rare with supraperiosteal injections.

POSTERIOR SUPERIOR ALVEOLAR BLOCK

The posterior superior alveolar block or PSA block is used to achieve pulpal anesthesia in the maxillary third, second, and first molars in most patients (Table 12-5, Figures D through H, and Procedure 12-2). Thus the PSA block is indicated when the dental procedure involves two or more maxillary molars or their associated periodontium and buccal gingival tissue. Most times this occurs during quadrant nonsurgical periodontal therapy, but the dental hygienist should consider using this injection also during maintenance or recare appointments. Many times the maxillary molars, even unilaterally, are the first teeth involved in periodontal disease.

However, in some patients the mesiobuccal root of the maxillary first molar is not innervated by the posterior

Text continued on p. 234

TABLE 12-5	**Posterior Superior Alveolar Block Review**

Indications	Maxillary molars in one quadrant

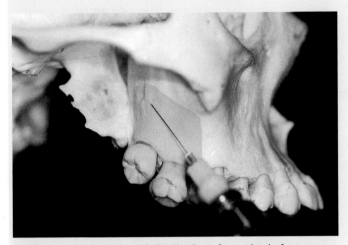

Figure D ■ Target area and distribution of anesthesia for posterior superior alveolar block. (From Fehrenbach MJ, Herring SW: *Illustrated anatomy of the head and neck*, ed 3, St Louis, 2007, Saunders.)

Nerves anesthetized	Posterior superior alveolar nerve
Teeth anesthetized	Third, second, maxillary first molars completely in 72% of population; mesiobuccal root of maxillary first molar not anesthetized in 28% of population
Other structures anesthetized	Periodontium of anesthetized teeth and buccal soft tissue of maxillary molar region
Administration technique	See Procedure 12-2
Needle gauge and length	Using 25-gauge short is preferred; a 27-gauge needle is also acceptable and may be more readily available (long needle may not be as safe)
Operator position	Right-handed: 8, 9, or 10 o'clock Left-handed: 4 or 2 o'clock

Figure E ■ Operator position of right-handed clinician for posterior superior alveolar block.

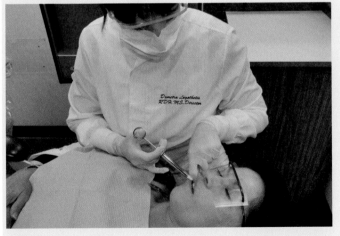

1. Right: 8 or 9 o'clock.

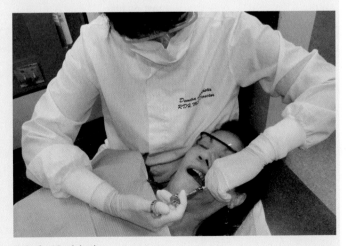

2. Left: 10 o'clock.

continued next page

TABLE 12-5	**Posterior Superior Alveolar Block Review—cont'd**

Figure F ■ Syringe stabilization for posterior superior alveolar block

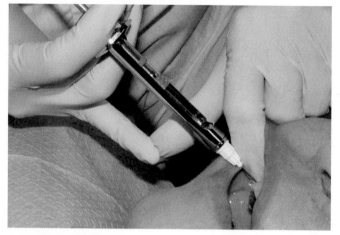

1, Double finger support.

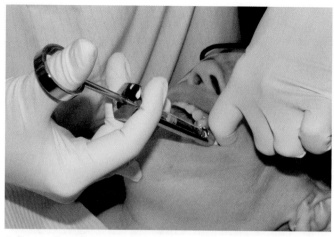

2, Rest syringe barrel on index finger or thumb of retraction hand for left side, and if possible use pinky finger of dominant hand to rest on chin.

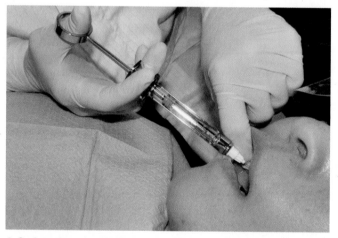

3, Syringe barrel resting on index finger of retraction hand for right side, and if possible use pinky finger of dominant hand to rest on chin.

Landmarks	Maxillary tuberosity
	Maxillary mucobuccal fold
	Maxillary second molar
	Maxillary occlusal plane
	Midsagittal plane

TABLE 12-5   Posterior Superior Alveolar Block Review—cont'd

Needle insertion point	Height of mucobuccal fold superior to apex of maxillary second molar

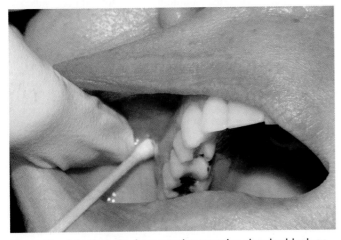

Figure G ■ Injection site for posterior superior alveolar block on right side.

Depth of needle penetration	Using short needle at 16 mm or three-fourths the depth of short needle

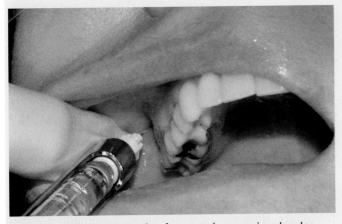

Figure H ■ Needle penetration for posterior superior alveolar block demonstrated on right side. Note: needle depth is three-fourths the depth of a short needle.

Deposit location	Superior to apex of maxillary second molar and posterior and superior to posterior border of maxilla at posterior superior alveolar foramina
Amount of anesthetic*	Approximately 0.9–1.7 (1.8) mL or one-half to full cartridge
Length of time to deposit	Approximately 60–120 seconds

*Approximate recommended amounts given are for 2% solutions of local anesthetic agents for adults; if using 4% solutions of local anesthetic agents, the approximate recommended amounts would be at least one-half of the amount of 2% solutions.

PROCEDURE 12-2 | Posterior Superior Alveolar (PSA) Block Procedure

STEP 1 Assume the correct operator position for right-handed at 8 o'clock (right side) or 10 o'clock (left side); left-handed at 4 o'clock (right side) or 2 o'clock (left side) (see Table 12-5 Figure E).

STEP 2 Ask the supine patient to partially open his or her mouth and to slide the mandible toward the injection side, opening the area for greater visibility. Retract the cheek vertically and not horizontally, pulling the tissue taut using the index finger for intraoral retraction and thumb for extraoral retraction on the dominant side (and vice versa on nondominant side) for visibility and to help with a fulcrum. A piece of sterile gauze may be used to help retract slippery tissue.

STEP 3 Prepare the alveolar mucosal tissue in the vestibule at the height of the mucobuccal fold superior to the apex of the maxillary second molar (as discussed in Chapter 11) and palpate the injection site to ensure that only soft tissue is injected (see Table 12-5, Figure G).

STEP 4 Using a 25- or 27-gauge short or long needle in the syringe in the dominant hand (see Step 6), orient the bevel of the needle away from the large window of the syringe to ensure bevel orientation toward the bone in case of accidental bone contact.

STEP 5 Establish a fulcrum by resting the syringe on the index finger or thumb that is retracting the cheek to ensure that the syringe is backward at a 45° angle from the midsagittal plane, while the index finger or thumb rests on the zygomatic arch while retracting (see Table 12-5, Figure F for fulcrum recommendations). The syringe should be extended from the ipsilateral corner of the mouth, possibly pressing downward on the lower lip to maintain the angulations.

STEP 6 Insert the needle at the height of the mucobuccal fold superior to the apex of the maxillary second molar and gently advance the needle in an upward, inward, and backward direction until desired depth of the needle is achieved (using short needle at 16 mm or three-fourths the depth is recommended for most situations) (Table 12-5, Figure H). Angulation may need adjusting once the syringe is in the mouth but before tissue is entered; do not move the needle in the tissue to establish correct angulation. There should be no resistance or bony contact.

STEP 7 Aspirate within three planes: due to the high vascularity in the area of anesthetic deposition, it is recommended to aspirate three times within different planes to ensure that the bevel of the needle is not abutted against the interior of a blood vessel, providing a false aspiration. To accomplish this, first aspirate as usual at the depth of penetration. If aspiration is negative, rotate the syringe barrel gently toward the operator and reaspirate; if aspiration is negative, rotate the syringe barrel gently back to the original position and aspirate again.

STEP 8 If a negative aspiration is achieved after each of three aspirations, slowly deposit approximately 0.9–1.7 (1.8) mL of solution (one-half to one cartridge) over approximately 60–120 seconds and aspirate in the same plane after each one-fourth of the cartridge is administered.

STEP 9 Carefully withdraw the syringe, possibly stepping it up to avoid nicking the lower lip with the tip of the needle, and immediately recap the needle using the one-handed scoop method utilizing a needle sheath prop (see Chapter 11).

STEP 10 Wait approximately 3–5 minutes until anesthesia takes effect before starting treatment.

---

superior alveolar nerve but rather by the middle superior alveolar nerve. Therefore a second injection to anesthetize the middle superior alveolar nerve is recommended after the PSA block (see next section on MSA block) to ensure pulpal anesthesia of all the roots of the maxillary first molar even during recare appointments.

The PSA block also anesthetizes the periodontium and buccal soft tissue overlying the maxillary third, second, and first molars, including the buccal gingival tissue. With many patients now retaining their third molars, this injection when done correctly can ensure the pulpal anesthesia of the sometimes elusive third molars, unlike supraperiosteal injections of the maxillary second molar.

If anesthesia of the lingual (or palatal) soft tissue is desired, the greater palatine block also may be necessary; this is an important consideration with any palatal molar furcation and root concavity involvement.

Target Area and Injection Site for Posterior Superior Alveolar Block

The deposit location or target area for the PSA block is the posterior superior alveolar nerve as it enters the maxilla through the posterior superior alveolar foramina on the maxilla's infratemporal surface (see Table 12-5, Figure D). This area is posterosuperior and medial on the maxillary tuberosity. However, intraoral surface landmarks are used to ensure close proximity to the target area.

The depth of needle penetration is 16 mm or three-fourths the depth of a short needle, and should not vary much from patient to patient with an average skull size. This average depth for the average skull may be too deep for patients with smaller than average skull size, increasing the risk for hematoma (discussed later). In contrast, using the average depth of needle penetration in a patient with a larger than average skull size may not provide adequate anesthesia and a long needle may need to be used. However, to decrease the risk for hematoma, a short 25-gauge needle is recommended except in a very large patient. This is the current educational method taught in most dental hygiene and dental school programs,[5,6] and will be the method specifically described in Table 12-5 and Procedure 12-2. Dental hygiene students are tested on clinical and written board examinations using this method.

However, a more conservative insertion technique may be considered that is being used by clinicians with proven success so as to reduce possible complications (discussed later). This includes never using a long needle and going to less depth of the mucobuccal fold (only one-fourth the depth, or 5–10 mm) with a short needle.

To achieve visibility of the intraoral surface landmarks for maximum success, the alveolar mucosa is retracted vertically about 1 cm distal to the zygomatic process so that the distal part of the maxillary tuberosity is exposed. If this is done correctly, a concavity in the mucobuccal fold distal to the maxillary tuberosity will be present. If horizontal retraction is used, the overlying upper lip will prevent needle access using the correct angulation.

The needle insertion point or injection site for the PSA block is the height of the mucobuccal fold superior to the apex of the maxillary second molar, as well as distal to the zygomatic process of the maxilla (Figures 12-3 and 12-4; see Table 12-5, Figure G). Thus, to reduce trauma, the needle is inserted into the mucobuccal fold in a distal and

medial direction to the tooth and maxilla without resistance or bony contact, then the injection is administered (see Table 12-5, Figure H). It is important to make sure that the needle will be at the apex of the maxillary second molar before entering the tissue, especially on the nondominant side, where visualization may be difficult. Otherwise, not all of the three maxillary molars or their associated tissue will be anesthetized if the anesthetic is incorrectly administered at the apex of the maxillary first molar.

In addition, a certain overall angulation of the needle to the injection site must be maintained throughout the injection. The angulation of the needle should be upward (or superiorly) at a 45° angle to the occlusal plane, inward (or medially) at a 45° angle to the occlusal plane, and backward (or posteriorly from the midsagittal plane) at a 45° angle to the long axis of the maxillary second molar.

To accomplish this injection in these three planes within one pass, the syringe should be extended from the ipsilateral corner of the mouth, possibly pressing downward on the lower lip to maintain the angulations (Figure 12-5). Resting the index finger or thumb on the inside of the zygomatic arch when retracting can make the clinician feel more confident.

When attempting the nondominant side, the correct angulation may be harder again to ascertain from across the patient's face; however, the needle should follow the same pathway as the nondominant arm, always toward the surface of the maxilla and the operator's body.

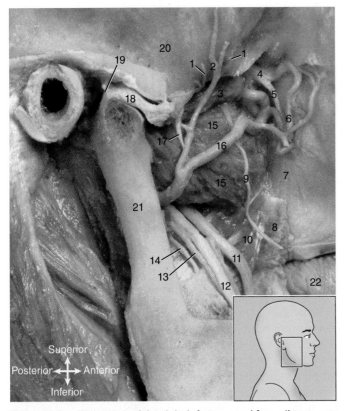

Figure 12-3 ■ Dissection of the right infratemporal fossa (inset, note zygomatic arch and mandible removed) in target area for the posterior superior alveolar block (as well as the inferior alveolar block discussed in Chapter 13). *1,* Deep temporal nerve; *2,* deep temporal artery; *3,* lateral pterygoid muscle; *4,* maxillary nerve; *5,* PSA nerve; *6,* PSA artery; *7,* infratemporal surface of maxilla; *8,* buccinator muscle; *9,* buccal nerve; *10,* medial pterygoid muscle; *11,* lingual nerve; *12,* IA nerve; *13,* IA artery; *14,* nerve to mylohyoid muscle; *15,* lateral pterygoid muscle; *16,* maxillary artery; *17,* masseteric nerve; *18,* disc of the joint and mandibular condyle; *19,* joint capsule; *20,* temporal bone; *21,* mandibular ramus; *22,* tongue. (From Logan BM, Reynold PA, Hutching RT: *McMinn's color atlas of head and neck anatomy,* ed 3, London, 2004, Mosby. In: Fehrenbach MJ, Herring SW: *Illustrated anatomy of the head and neck,* ed 3, St Louis, 2007, Saunders.)

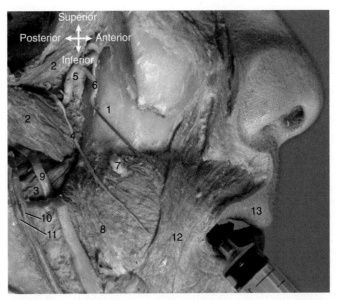

Figure 12-4 ■ Dissection showing the needle at the injection site for a posterior superior alveolar block. *1,* Posterior surface of maxilla; *2,* lateral pterygoid muscle; *3,* medial pterygoid muscle; *4,* buccal nerve; *5,* maxillary artery; *6,* PSA nerve and vessels; *7,* parotid salivary duct; *8,* buccinator muscle; *9,* lingual nerve; *10,* IA nerve; *11,* IA artery; *12,* corner of lip; *13,* upper lip. (From Logan BM, Reynold PA, Hutching RT: *McMinn's color atlas of head and neck anatomy,* ed 3, London, 2004, Mosby. In: Fehrenbach MJ, Herring SW: *Illustrated anatomy of the head and neck,* ed 3, St Louis, 2007, Saunders.)

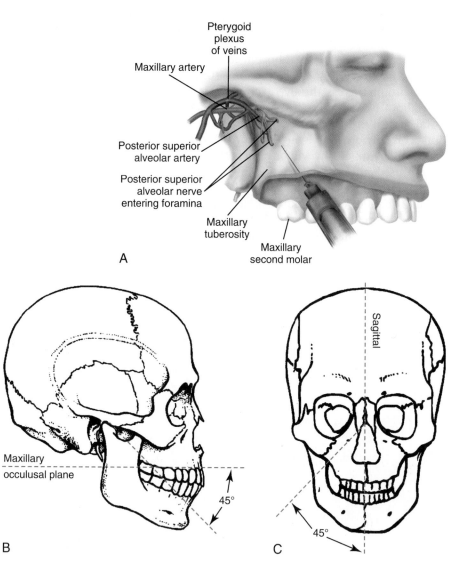

A

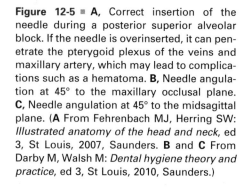

B

C

Figure 12-5 ■ **A,** Correct insertion of the needle during a posterior superior alveolar block. If the needle is overinserted, it can penetrate the pterygoid plexus of the veins and maxillary artery, which may lead to complications such as a hematoma. **B,** Needle angulation at 45° to the maxillary occlusal plane. **C,** Needle angulation at 45° to the midsagittal plane. (**A** From Fehrenbach MJ, Herring SW: *Illustrated anatomy of the head and neck*, ed 3, St Louis, 2007, Saunders. **B** and **C** From Darby M, Walsh M: *Dental hygiene theory and practice*, ed 3, St Louis, 2010, Saunders.)

With this injection there should be no bending of the needle shank in order to accomplish the necessary needle angulations. The needle can break when bent and there is little control over the direction of needle, angulation of needle, and bevel. Nor should there be movement of the needle within the tissue to obtain correct angulation; angulations should be correct before entering the soft tissue.

Indications of Successful Posterior Superior Alveolar Block and Possible Complications

Usually there are no indications of a successful PSA block. Thus the patient frequently has difficulty determining the extent of anesthesia because the lip or the tongue does not feel numb (e.g., with the more commonly used inferior alveolar or mandibular block). Instead, the patient will state that the teeth in the area feel dull when gently tapped, and there will be an absence of discomfort during dental procedures. It may be necessary to inform the patient of this situation before starting the procedure so as to reduce fears that the local anesthetic has not worked.

Bone should not be contacted at any time during the PSA injection. If bone is contacted or resistance is felt, the angle of the needle toward the midline is too great at more than a 45° angle and the syringe needs to be closer to the occlusal plane, thereby reducing the angle to less than 45°.

Complications can occur if the needle is advanced too far distally into the tissue during a PSA block (Table 12-6; see Figures 12-4 and 12-5). The needle may penetrate the pterygoid plexus of veins and the maxillary artery if overinserted, possibly causing a hematoma in the infratemporal fossa. This results in a bluish-reddish extraoral swelling of hemorrhaging blood in the tissue on the affected side of the face in the infratemporal fossa a few minutes after the injection, progressing over time inferiorly and anteriorly toward the lower anterior region of the cheek, causing an extraoral hematoma. This is a basic risk of local anesthesia; however, care must be taken to avoid this situation. If the needle is additionally contaminated, there may be a spread of infection to the cavernous sinus (see Chapter 14). The clinician should always assess the infection level of the

TABLE 12-6 — Posterior Superior Alveolar Block Complications

COMPLICATION	TECHNIQUE ADJUSTMENT/ RECOMMENDATION
Bone is contacted because angle of needle toward midline is too great at more than 45° angle	Withdraw syringe and reinsert it closer to occlusal plane, thereby reducing angle to less than 45°
Hematoma caused by overinsertion into pterygoid plexus of veins and/or maxillary artery	Use more conservative method with only short needle; advance to one-fourth the depth of short needle and/or modify depth of needle for children and small adults as well as avoiding use in children; use extraoral pressure over region with sterile gauze square and reassure
Mandibular anesthesia from branches of mandibular division of trigeminal nerve located lateral to posterior superior alveolar nerve	Avoid depositing lateral to posterior superior alveolar nerve

patient before proceeding with dental care and use strict standard infection control.

Positive aspiration is 3.1%; it is the third highest rate of all the block injections. Thus clinicians recommend aspiration several times within different planes before administration to reduce risk and to further reaspirate if there is any movement of the needle within the tissue. In addition, clinicians believe that the PSA block should not be used in children because of its inherant risks and have found success with using supraperiosteal injections instead for the maxillary posterior sextant.

Inadvertent and harmless anesthesia of branches of the mandibular nerve may also occur with a PSA block because they may be located lateral to the PSA nerve. This may result in differing levels of lingual anesthesia and numbness of the lower lip in some patients.

MIDDLE SUPERIOR ALVEOLAR BLOCK

The middle superior alveolar block or MSA block may be indicated for dental procedures in the maxillary premolars and mesiobuccal root of the maxillary first molar (Table 12-7, Figures I through M, and Procedure 12-3). To ensure complete anesthesia to the entire quadrant, most clinicians give this block even though the middle superior alveolar

TABLE 12-7 — Middle Superior Alveolar Block Review

Indications	Maxillary premolar teeth in one quadrant

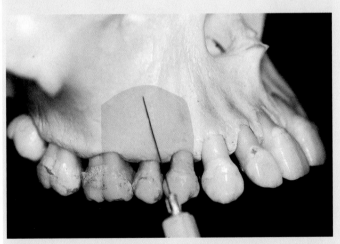

Figure I ■ Target area and distribution of anesthesia for middle superior alveolar block. (From Fehrenbach MJ, Herring SW: *Illustrated anatomy of the head and neck*, ed 3, St Louis, 2007, Saunders.)

Nerves anesthetized	Middle superior alveolar nerve
Teeth anesthetized	Maxillary first and second premolars and mesiobuccal root of maxillary first molar in 28% of population
Other structures anesthetized	Periodontium of anesthetized teeth and buccal soft tissue of premolar region
Administration technique	See Procedure 12-3
Needle gauge and length	27-gauge short

continued next page

TABLE 12-7   **Middle Superior Alveolar Block Review—cont'd**

Operator position	Right-handed: 8 or 9 o'clock.
	Left-handed: 4 or 3 o'clock.

Figure J ■ Operator position of right-handed clinician for middle superior alveolar block (same as for anterior superior alveolar block).

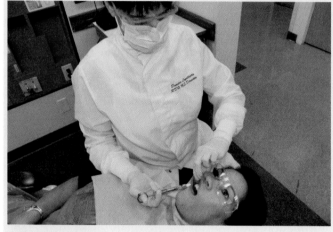

1, Right: 8 o'clock.

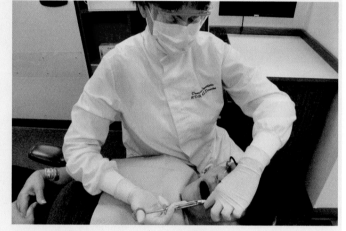

2, Left: 9 o'clock.

Figure K ■ Syringe stabilization for middle superior alveolar block

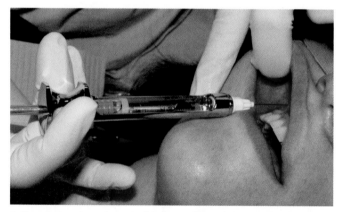

1, Support syringe barrel with finger from the retraction hand.

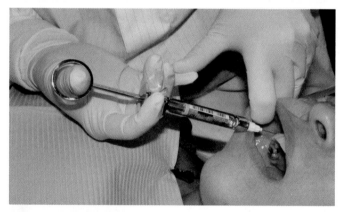

2, Double finger support.

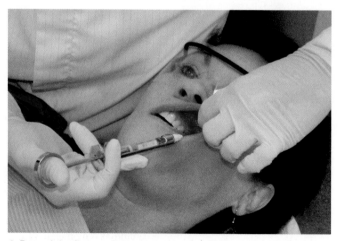

3, Rest pinky finger of dominant hand on patient's chin.

TABLE 12-7	Middle Superior Alveolar Block Review—cont'd
Landmarks	Maxillary mucobuccal fold Maxillary second premolar
Needle insertion point	Height of mucobuccal fold at apex of maxillary second premolar

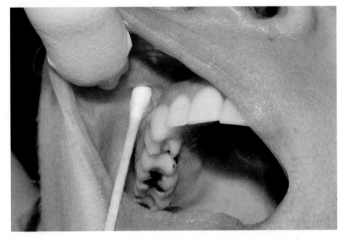

Figure L ■ Injection site for middle superior alveolar block.

Depth of needle penetration	Approximately 5 mm or one-fourth the depth of short needle

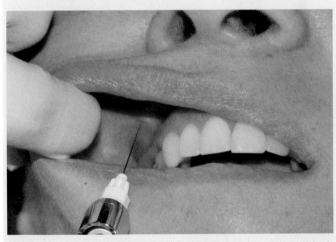

Figure M ■ Needle penetration for middle superior alveolar block demonstrated on right side.

Deposit location	Superior to apex of maxillary second premolar
Amount of anesthetic*	Approximately 0.9–1.2 mL or one-half to two-thirds of cartridge
Length of time to deposit	Approximately 60–90 seconds

*Approximate recommended amounts given are for 2% solutions of local anesthetic agents for adults; if using 4% solutions of local anesthetic agents, the approximate recommended amounts would be at least one-half of the amount of 2% solutions.

nerve may not be present or when only instrumenting the maxillary premolars. Where the middle superior alveolar nerve is absent (in approximately 68% of the population), the area is innervated by both the posterior superior alveolar and anterior superior alveolar nerves.

Thus the MSA block anesthetizes the pulp of the maxillary first and second premolars and possibly the mesiobuccal root of the maxillary first molar and the associated periodontium and buccal soft tissue, including the buccal gingival tissue if the middle superior alveolar nerve is present. Using this block will ensure complete comfort when the dental hygienist is instrumenting the mesial root of the first premolar with its root depression that is prone to heavier deposits. If anesthesia of the palatal (or lingual) soft tissue of these teeth is desired, the greater palatine block may also be necessary.

PROCEDURE 12-3   Middle Superior Alveolar (MSA) Block Procedure

STEP 1   Assume the correct operator position for right-handed at 8 o'clock (right side) or 9 o'clock (left side); left-handed at 4 o'clock (right side) or 3 o'clock (left side) (see Table 12-7 Figure J).

STEP 2   Ask the supine patient to open his or her mouth and then retract the upper lip, pulling the tissue taut; a piece of sterile gauze may be used to help retract slippery tissue. Pull the upper lip more anteriorly to avoid having to go through any large frena.

STEP 3   Prepare the alveolar mucosal tissue in the vestibule at the height of the mucobuccal fold superior to the apex of the maxillary second premolar (see Chapter 11) and palpate the injection site to ensure only soft tissue is injected (see Table 12-7, Figure L).

STEP 4   Using a 27-gauge short needle in the syringe in the dominant hand, orient the bevel of the needle away from the large window of the syringe to ensure the bevel orientation is toward the bone.

STEP 5   Establish a fulcrum (see Table 12-7, Figure K for fulcrum recommendations).

STEP 6   Place the syringe parallel with the long axis of the tooth with the large window facing the operator.

STEP 7   Insert the needle at the height of the mucobuccal fold at the apex of the maxillary second premolar, approximately one-fourth of the depth of the short needle (approximately 5 mm), or until the bevel is slightly superior to the apex of the tooth. There should be no resistance or bony contact; move to a more posterior site to avoid going through any large frena (see Table 12-7, Figure M).

STEP 8   Aspirate within two planes.

STEP 9   If a negative aspiration is achieved, slowly deposit approximately 0.9–1.2 mL of solution (one-half to two-thirds of cartridge over approximately 60–90 seconds; if the tissue balloons, injection is too rapid.

STEP 10 Carefully withdraw the syringe and immediately recap the needle using the one-handed scoop method utilizing a needle sheath prop (see Chapter 11).

STEP 11 Wait approximately 3–5 minutes until anesthesia takes effect before starting treatment.

Target Area and Injection Site for Middle Superior Alveolar Block

The deposit location or target area for the MSA block is the middle superior alveolar nerve at the apex of the maxillary second premolar (see Table 12-7, Figure I). Thus the needle insertion point or injection site is the height of the mucobuccal fold at the apex of the maxillary second premolar (Figure 12-6; see Table 12-7, Figure L). Thus the needle is inserted into the mucobuccal fold until its tip is located superior to the apex of the maxillary second premolar without resistance or bony contact in order to reduce trauma, and then the injection is administered (see Table 12-7, Figure M).

Because the root length varies among patients, the depth of needle penetration will vary among the maxillary second premolar among patients. For the MSA block, the clinician should review the average root length of the maxillary second premolar to help make this adjustment of needle depth more accurate to achieve a more successful injection (see Table 12-3)[2]. If one of the maxillary premolars has been removed for orthodontic therapy, thereby moving the existing premolars from their original place in the dental arch, the target area can be estimated by having the injection site halfway in the dental arch to provide the best anesthetic coverage to the maxillary premolars. Finally, pulling the upper lip more anteriorly helps to avoid having to go through any large frena; if not able to avoid them, give the injection slightly posterior than anterior to the recomended site for more complete coverage.

Indications of Successful Middle Superior Alveolar Block and Possible Complications

Indications of a successful MSA block include harmless tingling and numbness of the upper lip and absence of

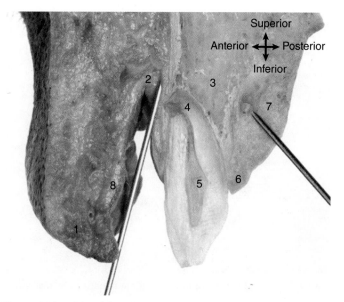

Figure 12-6 ■ Dissection showing a coronal section of maxilla and buccal mucosa through the permanent maxillary first premolar tooth. With one needle (left) at the injection site for middle superior alveolar block and the other needle (right) at the injection site for the anterior middle superior alveolar block. *1,* Upper lip; *2,* height of mucobuccal fold; *3,* alveolar process of maxilla; *4,* apex of tooth; *5,* pulp cavity; *6,* gingival margin; *7,* mucoperiosteum of hard palate; *8,* labial mucosa. (From Logan BM, Reynold PA, Hutching RT: *McMinn's color atlas of head and neck anatomy,* ed 3, London, 2004, Mosby. In: Fehrenbach MJ, Herring SW: *Illustrated anatomy of the head and neck,* ed 3, St Louis, 2007, Saunders.)

discomfort during dental procedures. Positive aspiration less than 3.1%; thus overinsertion with complications such as a hematoma is rare with the MSA block (Table 12-8).

ANTERIOR SUPERIOR ALVEOLAR BLOCK

The anterior superior alveolar block, or ASA block, is commonly used in conjunction with a MSA block instead of using an infraorbital block (Table 12-9, Figures N–R and Procedure 12-4). Communication occurs between the anterior superior alveolar, the middle superior alveolar and posterior superior alveolar nerves. In addition, many times crossover-innervation may occur when the anterior superior alveolar nerve crosses over the midline to the contralateral side in a patient; this may need to be taken into account when using local anesthesia in this area. Bilateral injections of the ASA block or supraperiosteal injections over the contralateral maxillary central incisor may be indicated if the patient still reports discomfort during treatment. Some clinicians consider the ASA block an infiltration injection.

The ASA block anesthetizes the pulp of the maxillary canine and incisor teeth, as well as the associated periodontium and facial soft tissue including the gingival tissue. If palatal (or lingual) anesthesia of the soft tissue of these teeth is desired, a nasopalatine block may also be necessary.

Target Area and Injection Site for Anterior Superior Alveolar Block

The deposit location or target area for the ASA block is the anterior superior alveolar nerve at the apex of the maxillary

TABLE 12-8	Middle Superior Alveolar Block Complications
COMPLICATION	**TECHNIQUE ADJUSTMENT**
Presence of large buccal frenum (frena) at site of needle insertion	Insert needle more posterior to injection site and retract lip and frenum more anteriorly to avoid going through large frenum; however, avoid moving injection site too anterior to lose maxillary premolar coverage
Pain on insertion with needle against the periosteum	Withdraw needle and reinsert farther away (or lateral) from periosteum
Pain during injection from injecting too rapidly	Due to acidic anesthetic agent, care should be taken to inject slowly so as to not exceed recommended deposit time
Inadequate anesthesia from injecting inferior to apex of maxillary second premolar	Increase depth of penetration upon reinsertion to ensure placement of solution just superior to apical region of maxillary second premolar
Possible inadequate anesthesia from dense bone covering apices	Instead administer infraorbital block (see Table 12-11)
Possible inadequate anesthesia from injecting into an area of infection or risk of needle tract infection	Instead administer infraorbital block (see Table 12-11)

TABLE 12-9	Anterior Superior Alveolar Block Review

Indications   Maxillary anterior teeth in one quadrant

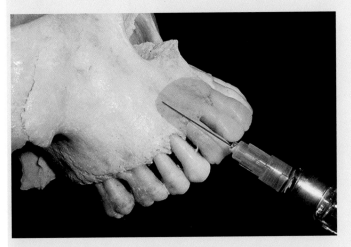

Figure N ■ Target area and distribution of anesthesia for anterior superior alveolar block. (From Fehrenbach MJ, Herring SW: *Illustrated anatomy of the head and neck,* ed 3, St Louis, 2007, Saunders.)

Text continued on p. 244

TABLE 12-9	**Anterior Superior Alveolar Block Review—cont'd**
Nerves anesthetized	Anterior superior alveolar nerve
Teeth anesthetized	Maxillary central and lateral incisors and canine
Other structures anesthetized	Periodontium of anesthetized teeth and facial soft tissue of maxillary anterior region in one quadrant
Administration technique	See Procedure 12-4
Needle gauge and length	27-gauge short
Operator position	Right-handed: 8 or 9 o'clock Left-handed: 4 or 3 o'clock

Figure O ▪ Operator position of right-handed clinician for anterior superior alveolar block (same as for middle superior alveolar block).

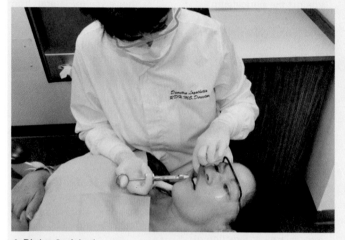

1, Right: 8 o'clock.

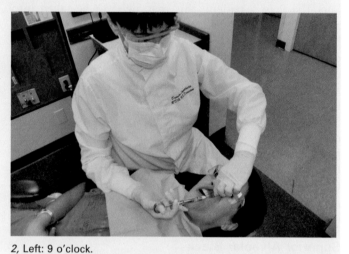

2, Left: 9 o'clock.

Figure P ▪ Syringe stabilization for anterior superior alveolar block

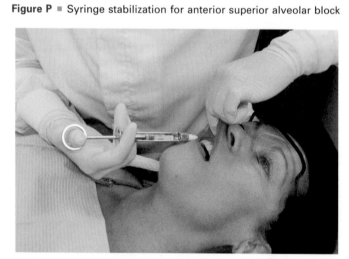

1. Rest pinky finger of dominant hand on patient's chin.

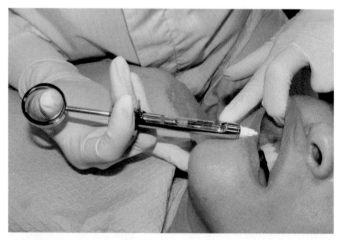

2. Support syringe barrel with finger from the retraction hand.

TABLE 12-9	**Anterior Superior Alveolar Block Review—cont'd**

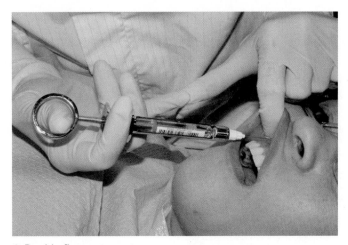

3. Double finger support.

Landmarks	Canine eminence
	Canine fossa
	Maxillary mucobuccal fold
	Maxillary canine

Needle insertion point	Height of mucobuccal fold at apex of maxillary canine

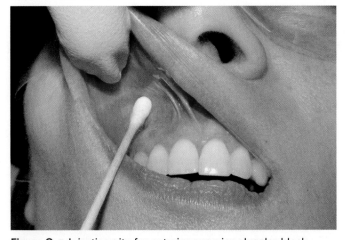

Figure Q ■ Injection site for anterior superior alveolar block.

TABLE 12-9	Anterior Superior Alveolar Block Review—cont'd
Depth of needle penetration	Approximately 5 mm or one-fourth the depth of short needle

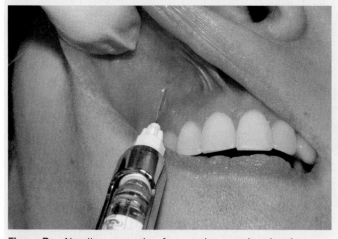

Figure R ■ Needle penetration for anterior superior alveolar block demonstrated on right side.

Deposit location	Superior to apex of maxillary canine
Amount of anesthetic*	Approximately 0.6–0.9 mL or one-third to one-half of cartridge
Length of time to deposit	Approximately 30–60 seconds

*Approximate recommended amounts given are for 2% solutions of local anesthetic agents for adults; if using 4% solutions of local anesthetic agents, the approximate recommended amounts would be at least one-half of the amount of 2% solutions.

PROCEDURE 12-4	Anterior Superior Alveolar (ASA) Block Procedure

STEP 1 Assume the correct operator position for right-handed at 8 o'clock (right side) or 9 o'clock (left side); left-handed at 4 o'clock (right side) or 3 o'clock (left side) (see Table 12-9, Figure O).

STEP 2 Ask the supine patient to open his or her mouth, and then retract the upper lip by pulling the tissue taut only at the tip using the index finger and thumb of the non-dominant hand (one inside and one outside); a piece of sterile gauze may be used to help retract slippery tissue.

STEP 3 Prepare the alveolar mucosal tissue in the vestibule at the height of the mucobuccal fold superior to the apex of the maxillary canine, just anterior to and parallel with the canine eminence (see Chapter 11) and palpate the injection site to ensure only soft tissue is injected (see Table 12-9, Figure Q).

STEP 4 Using a 27-gauge short needle in the syringe, orient the bevel of the needle away from the large window of the syringe to ensure the bevel orientation is toward the bone.

STEP 5 Establish a fulcrum (see Table 12-9, Figure P for fulcrum recommendations).

STEP 6 Place the syringe parallel with the long axis of the tooth with the large window facing the operator.

STEP 7 Insert the needle at the height of the mucobuccal fold at the apex of the maxillary canine, just anterior to and parallel with the canine eminence and approximately 10° angle off an imaginary line drawn to the long axis of the tooth, and approximately one-fourth the depth of the short needle (approximately 5 mm) or until the bevel is slightly superior to the apex of the tooth (see Table 12-9, Figure R). There should be no resistance or bony contact.

STEP 8 Aspirate within two planes.

STEP 9 If a negative aspiration is achieved, slowly deposit approximately 0.6–0.9 mL of solution (one-third to one-half of cartridge) over approximately 30–60 seconds; if the tissue balloons, injection is too rapid.

STEP 10 Carefully withdraw the syringe and immediately recap the needle using the one-handed scoop method utilizing a needle sheath prop (see Chapter 11).

STEP 11 Wait approximately 3–5 minutes until anesthesia takes effect before starting treatment.

canine (see Table 12-9, Figure N). The injection site is the height of the mucobuccal fold at the apex of the maxillary canine, just anterior to and parallel with the canine eminence and approximately 10° angle off an imaginary line drawn parallel to the long axis of the tooth. Note that this is slightly over the slight depression or canine fossa located anterior to the canine eminence (see Table 12-9, Figure Q).

The needle tip is placed superior to the apex of the maxillary canine without resistance or bony contact in order to reduce trauma, and then the injection is administered (see Table 12-9, Figure R). This is approximately 10° off an imaginary line drawn parallel to the long axis of the canine tooth. Because the root length varies among patients, the depth of needle penetration will vary among the maxillary canine and among patients. For the ASA block, the clinician should review the average root length of the maxillary canine to help make this adjustment of needle depth more accurate to achieve a more successful injection (see Table 12-3).

If the patient needs extensive nonsurgical periodontal therapy of the maxillary arch, treatment planning using a sextant approach instead of quadrant should be considered (along with the use of a nasopalatine block) (see Figure 11-2, A)

Indications of Successful Anterior Superior Alveolar Block and Possible Complications

Indications of a successful ASA block include harmless tingling and numbness of the upper lip and an absence of discomfort during dental procedures. Positive aspiration is less than 1%; thus overinsertion with complications such as a hematoma is rare with ASA block (Table 12-10).

INFRAORBITAL BLOCK

The infraorbital block, or IO block, is a useful block because it anesthetizes both the anterior superior alveolar and middle superior alveolar nerves with one injection (Table 12-11, Figures S through V, and Procedure 12-5). The IO block is used for anesthesia of the maxillary incisors, maxillary canine, and premolars. The IO block is indicated when the dental procedures involve more than two anterior teeth or maxillary premolars and the periodontium and facial soft tissue including the gingival tissue. Some clinicians believe that this block should be referred to as the *anterior superior block* to reflect the anesthetized tissue, but the correct name comes from the foramen where the injection is administered. If anesthesia of palatal (or lingual) soft tissue is necessary, both a nasopalatine block and greater palatine block may also be necessary; this is an important consideration with any palatal molar furcation and root concavity involvement.

In many patients the anterior superior alveolar nerve crosses over the midline from the contralateral side, so bilateral injections of the infraorbital block (or ASA block, depending on extent of procedures) or even supraperiosteal injection over the contralateral maxillary central incisor may be indicated if the patient still feels discomfort.

Target Area and Injection Site for Infraorbital Block

The deposit location or target area for the IO block is the anterior superior alveolar and middle superior alveolar nerves as they move superiorly to join the infraorbital nerve after it enters the infraorbital foramen (see Table 12-11, Figure S). Branches of the infraorbital nerve to the upper lip, side of the nose, and lower eyelid are also inadvertently anesthetized (see Table 12-11, Figure S2).

To locate the infraorbital foramen, palpate extraorally the patient's infraorbital rim and then move slightly downward about 10 mm, applying gentle pressure until the

TABLE 12-10	Anterior Superior Alveolar Block Complications
COMPLICATION	**TECHNIQUE ADJUSTMENT**
Pain on insertion with needle against the periosteum	Withdraw needle and reinsert farther away (or lateral) from periosteum
Pain during injection from injecting too rapidly	Due to acidic anesthetic agent, care should be taken to inject slowly so as to not exceed recommended deposit time
Inadequate anesthesia from injecting inferior to apex of maxillary canine	Increase depth of penetration upon reinsertion to assure placement of solution just superior to apical region of maxillary canine
Possibly inadequate anesthesia from crossover of contralateral anterior superior alveolar nerve	Bilateral injections of anterior superior alveolar block or supraperiosteal injection over contralateral maxillary central incisor (Table 12-2 Figure C)
Possibly inadequate anesthesia from dense bone covering apices	Instead administer infraorbital nerve (see Table 12-11)
Possibly inadequate anesthesia from injecting into area of infection or risking needle-tract infection	Instead administer infraorbital block (see Table 12-11)

depression created by the infraorbital foramen is located (Figure 12-7). The patient may feel a dull aching sensation when pressure is applied to the nerves in the region. The infraorbital foramen is about 1–4 mm medial to the pupil of the eye if the patient looks straight forward. There is a linear relationship between the pupil of the eye, the infraorbital notch, and the ipsilateral corner of the mouth (Figure 12-8).

The needle insertion point or injection site for the IO block is the height of the mucobuccal fold at the apex of the maxillary first premolar (see Table 12-11, Figure U). A preinjection approximation of the depth of needle penetration for the IO block can be made by placing one finger on the infraorbital foramen and the other one on the injection site and estimating the distance between them. The approximate depth of needle penetration for the IO block may vary, but typically is one-half the depth of a long needle and three-fourths the depth of a short needle. In a patient with a higher or deeper mucobuccal fold or more inferior infraorbital foramen, less tissue penetration will be required than in a patient with a much lower or shallower mucobuccal fold or more superior infraorbital foramen.

The needle is inserted for the IO block into the height of the mucobuccal fold while keeping the finger of the other hand on the infraorbital foramen during the injection to help keep the syringe toward the foramen (see Table 12-11,

Text continued on p. 249

TABLE 12-11	**Infraorbital Block Review**

Indications	Maxillary anterior teeth and premolars in one quadrant or if other injections considered would not be as effective due to dense bone or local infection, such as a supraperiosteal injection, MSA block, or ASA block

Figure S ■ Target area and distribution of anesthesia for infraorbital block.

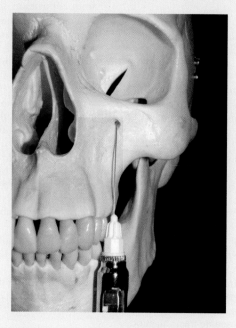

1, Target area and distribution of anesthesia for infraorbital block.

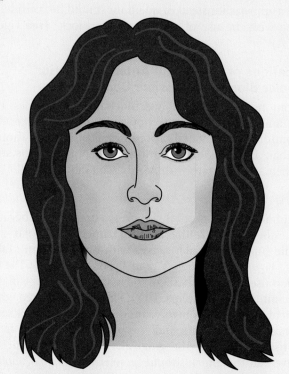

2, Facial view of anesthetic distribution after an infraorbital nerve block.

Nerves anesthetized	Infraorbital nerve Anterior superior alveolar nerve Middle superior alveolar nerve Inferior palpebral nerve Lateral nasal nerve Superior labial nerve
Teeth anesthetized	Maxillary central and lateral incisors and canine, first and second premolars, and mesiobuccal root of maxillary first molar in 28% of population
Other structures anesthetized	Periodontium of anesthetized teeth and facial soft tissue of maxillary arch, except for maxillary molar region Upper lip to midline, medial part of the cheek, side of nose, and lower eyelid
Administration technique	See Procedure 12-5
Needle gauge and length	Either 27-gauge long or short (for children or small adults)
Operator position	Right-handed: 8 or 9 o'clock Left-handed: 4 or 3 o'clock

TABLE 12-11 **Infraorbital Block Review—cont'd**

Figure T ■ Syringe stabilization for infraorbital block

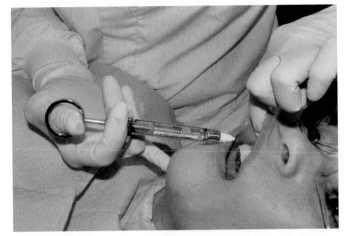

1, Pinky finger of dominant hand resting on patient's chin for right side.

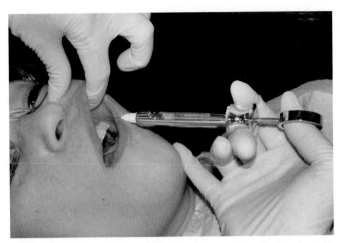

2, Pinky finger of dominant hand resting on patient's chin for left side.

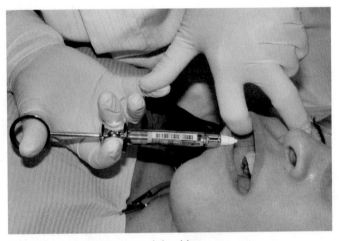

3, Double finger support on right side.

Landmarks	Infraorbital notch
	Infraorbital ridge
	Infraorbital depression
	Infraorbital foramen
	Maxillary first premolar
	Maxillary mucobuccal fold

continued next page

TABLE 12-11	Infraorbital Block Review—cont'd

Needle insertion point	Height of mucobuccal fold superior to maxillary first premolar

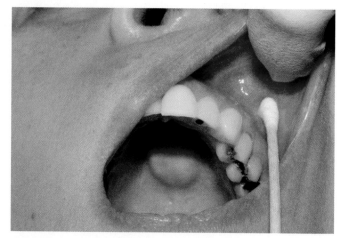

Figure U ■ Injection site for infraorbital block.

Depth of needle penetration	Approximately 16 mm or one-half the depth of long needle or three fourths of short needle

Figure V ■ Needle penetration for infraorbital block.

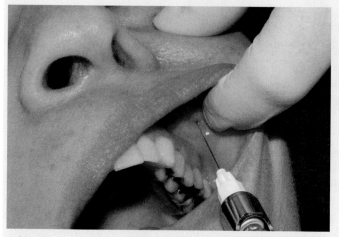

1, Needle penetration showing finger pressure over IO foramen.

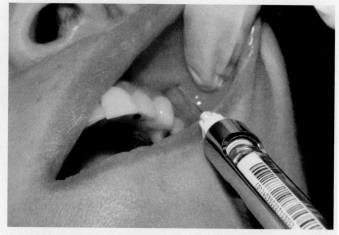

2, Needle depth of long needle approximately half its length.

Deposit location	Upper rim of infraorbital foramen until bone is gently contacted
Amount of anesthetic*	Approximately 0.9–1.2 mL or one-half to two-thirds of cartridge
Length of time to deposit	Approximately 60–90 seconds

*Approximate recommended amounts given are for 2% solutions of local anesthetic agents for adults; if using 4% solutions of local anesthetic agents, the approximate recommended amounts would be at least one-half of the amount of 2% solutions.

PROCEDURE 12-5 | Infraorbital Block (IO) Procedure

STEP 1 Assume the correct operator position for right-handed at 8 o'clock (right side) or 9 o'clock (left side); left-handed at 4 o'clock (right side) or 3 o'clock (left side).

STEP 2 Ask the supine patient to open his or her mouth, and then retract the upper lip, pulling the tissue taut with the index finger or thumb of the nondominant hand (one inside and one outside); a piece of sterile gauze may be used to help retract slippery tissue.

STEP 3 Prepare the alveolar mucosal tissue in the vestibule at the height of the mucobuccal fold superior to the apex of the maxillary first premolar (see Chapter 11) and palpate the injection site to ensure soft tissue is injected (see Table 12-11, Figure U).

STEP 4 Using a 27-gauge short or long needle in the syringe in the dominant hand, orient the bevel of the needle away from the large window of the syringe to ensure the bevel orientation is toward the bone.

STEP 5 Locate the infraorbital foramen (see Figures 12-7 and 12-8) by palpating extraorally for the infraorbital notch which is the inferior outer bulge of the inferior border of the orbit with the index finger or thumb of the non-dominant hand; maintain finger pressure in this area before, during, and after the injection. Advise patient that he or she may feel some slight discomfort with this slight pressure.

STEP 6 Establish a fulcrum (see Table 12-11, Figure T for fulcrum recommendations).

STEP 7 Place the syringe parallel with the long axis of the maxillary first premolar orienting the needle in line with the infraorbital foramen using the finger over the foramen as a guide, with the large window facing the operator.

STEP 8 Insert the needle at the height of the mucobuccal fold at the apex and parallel to the long axis of the maxillary first premolar, and approximately one-half of the depth of the long needle and three-fourths of the depth of the short needle (approximately 16 mm), until the needle gently contacts bone at the superior rim of the infraorbital foramen (see Table 12-11, Figure V).

STEP 9 Aspirate within two planes.

STEP 10 If negative aspiration is achieved, slowly deposit approximately 0.9–1.2 mL of solution (one-half to two-thirds of cartridge) over approximately 60–90 seconds. The operator will be able to feel the anesthetic solution being deposited beneath the finger over the infraorbital foramen.

STEP 11 Carefully withdraw the syringe and immediately recap the needle using the one-handed scoop method utilizing a needle sheath prop (see Chapter 11).

STEP 12 Maintain pressure and massage the solution into the infraorbital foramen for approximately 2 minutes after the injection.

STEP 13 Wait approximately 3–5 minutes until anesthesia takes effect before starting treatment.

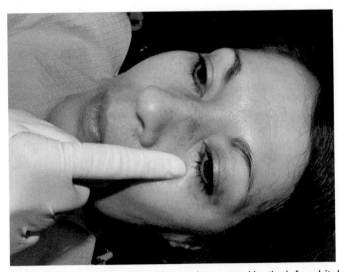

Figure 12-7 ■ Palpation of the depression created by the infraorbital foramen by moving slightly downward on the face from the infraorbital rim for the infraorbital block.

Figure V1). The needle is advanced while keeping it parallel with the long axis of the tooth to avoid premature contact with the maxillary bone. The point of contact of the needle with the maxillary bone should be the upper rim of the infraorbital foramen and then the injection is administered (see Table 12-11, Figure V2). Keeping the needle in contact with the bone at the roof of the infraorbital foramen prevents overinsertion and possible puncture of the orbit. Once the needle is carefully withdrawn and capped, an

important postinjection procedure is to maintain pressure and massage the solution into the infraorbital foramen for approximately 2 minutes to enhance anesthetic diffusion.

Indications of Successful Infraorbital Block and Possible Complications

Indications of a successful IO block include harmless tingling and numbness of the upper lip, medial part of the cheek, side of the nose, and lower eyelid because there is inadvertent anesthesia of the branches of the infraorbital nerve. Additionally, there is numbness of the teeth and associated tissue along the distribution of the anterior superior alveolar and middle superior alveolar nerves and absence of discomfort during dental procedures. Rarely, the complication of a hematoma may develop across the lower eyelid and the tissue between it and the infraorbital foramen (Table 12-12).

■ MAXILLARY PALATAL INJECTIONS

All the palatal maxillary injections have a somewhat higher VAS of 2–4 even when using correct technique by the clinician because there is bony contact, including initially the sensitive periosteum overlying maxillary and palatal bones; most maxillary facial injections have a lower VAS of 0–2 and are given through soft tissue and have no bony contact (except the IO block) (see Chapter 1).[3]

However, there is no need to avoid these successful injections because of their somewhat greater level of discomfort; the clinician and the rest of the dental team should be

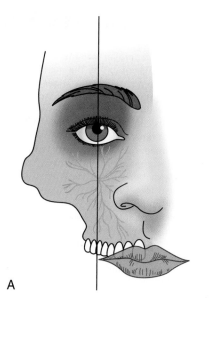 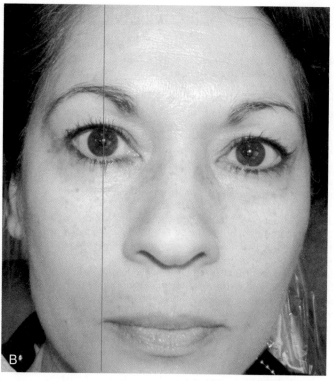

Figure 12-8 ■ **A,** Linear relationship between the pupil of the eye, zygomaticomaxillary suture, infraorbital foramen, and corner of the mouth. **B,** Facial view of linear relationship. (**A** Modified from Jastak T, Yagiela J, Donaldson D: *Local anesthesia of the oral cavity*, St Louis, 1995, Saunders.)

TABLE 12-12	Infraorbital Block Complications
COMPLICATION	**TECHNIQUE ADJUSTMENT**
Pain on insertion with needle against the periosteum	Withdraw needle and reinsert farther away (or lateral) from periosteum
Inadequate anesthesia from needle contacting bone inferior to infraorbital foramen	Direct needle toward finger over foramen to help line up needle with infraorbital foramen, making sure to contact bone
Possibly inadequate anesthesia from crossover of contralateral anterior superior alveolar nerve	Contralateral anterior superior alveolar block (Table 12-9, Figure R) or supraperiosteal injection over contralateral maxillary central incisor (Table 12-12, Figure C)

careful in their discussion of this injection in front of the patient. The goal is overall pain management as well as hemostatic control during the sometimes longer appointment time needed for nonsurgical periodontal therapy and instrumenting of exposed roots with possible dentinal hypersensitivity.

Because the overlying palatal tissue is dense and adheres firmly to the underlying palatal bone, the use of pressure anesthesia with a cotton tip applicator (always along with topical anesthesia) to the injection site before, during, and after the injection to blanch the tissue will reduce patient discomfort. This pressure anesthesia of the tissue produces a dull ache that blocks pain impulses that arise from needle penetration. It is important to advise patients that they may feel some slight discomfort from the gentle pressure and that there may still be an initial slight prick of the needle. It is important to keep the cotton tip applicator firmly engaged with the hard palatal tissue surface; this reassures the patient that the applicator, which feels like it is near the soft palate, will not be moving down the throat to be choked on.

A cotton tip applicator is the best tool to use to accomplish pressure anesthesia because its roundness results in less damaging pressure. After topical anesthetic has been placed, a new cotton tip applicator without topical anesthesia should be used to ensure minimal slippage while still being able to bear down on the tissue with the pressure anesthesia during the injection.

The needle will naturally withdraw from the periosteum when bony contact is made, so there is no need to withdraw further upon bony contact and possibly miss the target area. Use of a topical anesthetic as well as the slow deposition of the local anesthetic agent will also reduce patient discomfort.

Because the palatal tissue adheres so tightly to the bone and the injection is quite shallow, the solution may leak out of the injection site and run down the patient's throat. Quickly rinsing the patient's mouth immediately following safe capping of the needle will help reduce any bad taste of the solution. Even though positive aspiration is less than 1% for all palatal injections, because of increased vascularity and density of the palatal tissue, the tissue may continue to bleed even after the removal of the needle and rinsing. Pressure against the palatal tissue with folded sterile gauze, avoiding the soft palate, will stem the bleeding and prevent the patient from becoming alarmed.

Palatal anesthesia usually involves anesthesia of both the soft and hard tissue of the palate including the lingual gingival tissue. However, palatal anesthesia usually does not provide any pulpal anesthesia to the maxillary teeth or associated periodontium and facial soft tissue so that maxillary facial injections would need to be given for complete coverage of either a sextant or quadrant when planning treatment. The greater palatine (GP) block is generally recommended for anesthesia of the lingual soft tissue distal to the maxillary canine in one quadrant. The nasopalatine (NP) block is generally recommended for anesthesia of the lingual soft tissue between the maxillary right and left canines.

Separate from these palatal blocks that only provide anesthesia of the lingual soft tissue and not any pulpal anesthesia is another block administered on the palate, the anterior middle superior alveolar (AMSA) block. This block is generally recommended for anesthesia of most of the maxillary teeth and their associated periodontium as well as most of the facial and lingual gingival tissue in one quadrant, except for those structures innervated by the posterior superior alveolar nerve. Thus the maxillary molars and associated periodontium as well as the buccal gingival tissue are not involved in the anesthesia provided by this block. However, if using this block, the PSA block is additionally given first in most cases to complete the coverage of the quadrant so as to include the maxillary molars.

If quadrant dental hygiene treatment is planned for the maxillary arch, the greater palatine block is given after any maxillary facial injections but before the nasopalatine block, with instrumenting proceeding in the same manner to have complete anesthesia coverage. Because of its regional coverage of the palatal region of the maxillary molars, the greater palatine block easily covers any sextant dental hygiene care. (see Figure 11-2 A) Discussion of the nasopalatine block and its use with sextants or even quadrants is discussed in detail later.

GREATER PALATINE BLOCK

The greater palatine block, or GP block, is used during dental procedures that involve more than two maxillary posterior teeth distal to the maxillary canine (Table 12-13, Figures W through AA, and Procedure 12-6). This maxillary block anesthetizes the posterior hard palate, anteriorly as far as the maxillary first premolar and medially to the midline as well as the lingual gingival tissue in the area.

Because the GP block does not provide pulpal anesthesia of the area teeth, the use of the ASA, PSA, and MSA blocks or the IO block may also be indicated, especially during nonsurgical periodontal therapy because dentinal hypersensitivity is possible when instrumenting exposed root surfaces. In addition, anesthesia in the palatal area of the maxillary first premolar may prove inadequate because of overlapping nerve fibers from the nasopalatine nerve if only instrumenting the patient within the posterior sextant. This

TABLE 12-13	Greater Palatine Block Review
Indications	Lingual gingival tissues of maxillary premolars and molars in one quadrant

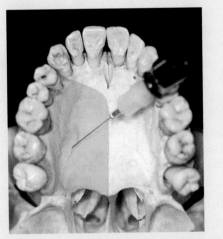

Figure W ■ Target area and distribution of anesthesia for greater palatine block. (From Fehrenbach MJ, Herring SW: *Illustrated anatomy of the head and neck*, ed 3, St Louis, 2007, Saunders.)

continued next page

TABLE 12-13	Greater Palatine Block Review—cont'd
Nerves anesthetized	Greater palatine nerve
Teeth anesthetized	None
Other structures anesthetized	Lingual gingival tissue of maxillary premolars and molars as well as posterior hard palate in one quadrant
Administration technique	See Procedure 12-6
Needle gauge and length	27-gauge short
Operator position	Right-handed: 8–9 or 11 o'clock Left-handed: 4–3 or 1 o'clock

Figure X ■ Operator position of right-handed clinician for greater palatine block.

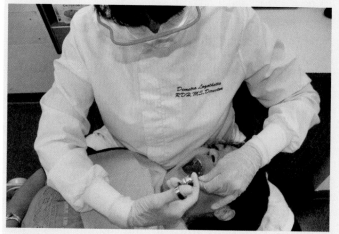

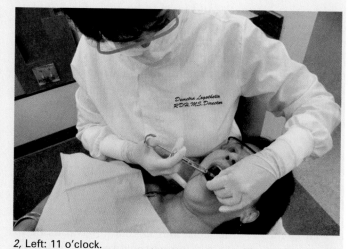

1, Right: 8 to 9 o'clock.

2, Left: 11 o'clock.

Figure Y ■ Syringe stabilization for greater palatine block

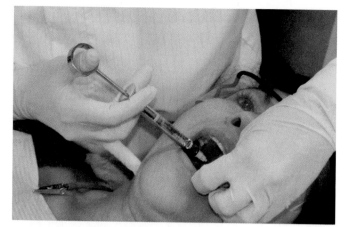

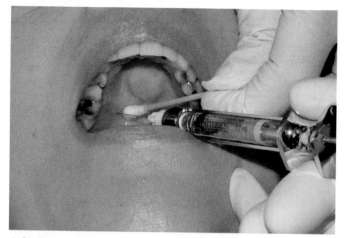

1, Pinky finger resting on patient's chin for left side.

2, Syringe barrel resting on index finger of nondominant hand and pinky finger of dominant hand on chin for right side.

Landmarks	Maxillary third molar Junction of maxillary alveolar process and posterior hard palate Greater palatine foramen

| **TABLE 12-13** | **Greater Palatine Block Review—cont'd** |

| Needle insertion point | Anterior to greater palatine foramen |

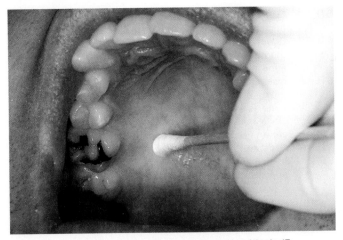

Figure Z ▪ Injection site for the greater palatine block. (From Fehrenbach MJ, Herring SW: *Illustrated anatomy of the head and neck*, ed 3, St Louis, 2007, Saunders.)

| Depth of needle penetration | Approximately 3–6 mm or until contact with palatine bone |

Figure AA ▪ Needle penetration for the greater palatine block demonstrated on right side. (From Fehrenbach MJ, Herring SW: *Illustrated anatomy of the head and neck*, ed 3, St Louis, 2007, Saunders.)

Deposit location	At greater palatine foramen
Amount of anesthetic*	Approximately 0.45 mL or one-fourth of cartridge until blanching of tissue
Length of time to deposit	Approximately 20–30 seconds

*Approximate recommended amounts given are for 2% solutions of local anesthetic agents for adults; if using 4% solutions of local anesthetic agents, the approximate recommended amounts would be at least one-half of the amount of 2% solutions.

PROCEDURE 12-6 Greater Palatine Block (GP) Procedure

STEP 1 Assume the correct operator position for right-handed at 8–9 o'clock (right side) or 11 o'clock (left side); left-handed at 4–3 o'clock (right side) or 1 o'clock (left side) (see Table 12-13, Figure X).

STEP 2 Ask the patient to open his or her mouth and extend the neck either to the right or left. Locate the greater palatine foramen by gently sliding a cotton tip applicator along the hard palate surface, starting at the junction of the maxillary alveolar process and the posterior hard palate foramen near the maxillary first molar, and moving distally until the cotton tip applicator falls into the depression of the greater palatine foramen. Usually the foramen is located near the maxillary third molar, although it can be located anterior or distal to this area (see Table 12-13 Figure Z). Be careful to not cross the more yellow-tinged soft palate with the applicator or else gagging will occur.

STEP 3 Prepare the tissue slightly anterior to the greater palatine foramen (see Chapter 11).

STEP 4 Using a 27-gauge short needle in the syringe in the dominant hand, orient the bevel of the needle toward the hard palate.

STEP 5 Using a new cotton tip applicator in the nondominant hand, apply firm pressure with the cotton tip applicator directly over the depression created by the greater palatine foramen until blanching is seen. Continue the pressure for 30 seconds before inserting the needle. Advise

patient that some slight discomfort from the pressure may be felt.

STEP 6 Establish a fulcrum (see Table 12-13, Figure Y for fulcrum recommendations).

STEP 7 Direct the syringe from the contralateral side of the mouth at a 90° angle to the palate toward the cotton tip applicator, with the large window facing the operator.

STEP 8 Insert the needle at approximately slightly anterior to the greater palatine foramen 3–6 mm until the palatine bone is contacted, with the needle bowing slightly, while maintaining pressure on the foramen with the cotton tip applicator (see Table 12-13, Figure AA).

STEP 9 Aspirate.

STEP 10 If negative aspiration is achieved, slowly deposit approximately 0.45 mL of solution (one-fourth of cartridge) over approximately 20–30 seconds; tissue in area will blanch even further when the anesthetic is administered. Continue to maintain pressure anesthesia for a short time with cotton tip applicator after solution is deposited.

STEP 11 Carefully withdraw the syringe and immediately recap the needle using the one-handed scoop method utilizing a needle sheath prop (see Chapter 11).

STEP 12 Rinse the patient's mouth and wait approximately 3–5 minutes until anesthesia takes effect before starting treatment.

---

lack of anesthesia may be corrected by additional administration of the nasopalatine block if the patient is still feeling discomfort, especially with the considerations of palatal molar furcation and palatal root concavity involvement of the maxillary molars or premolars.

Target Area and Injection Site for Greater Palatine Block

The deposit location or target area for the GP block is anterior to where the greater palatine nerve enters the greater palatine foramen from its location between the mucoperiosteum and palatine bone of the posterior hard palate (see Table 12-13, Figure W).

The greater palatine foramen is usually seen as a depression on palatal surface at the junction of the maxillary alveolar process and posterior hard palate, at the apex of the maxillary second (in children) or third molar, about 10 mm medial and directly superior to the lingual gingival margin (Figure 12-9). In patients who have a vaulted palate, the foramen appears closer to the dentition. Conversely, in patients with a more shallow palate, the foramen appears closer to the midline. Some patients do not have a visible depression so the landmarks listed will be useful to the clinician or palpation of the area will emphasize the depression of the foramen.

Thus, this depression created by the foramen can be palpated about midway between the median palatine raphe and lingual gingival margin of the maxillary molar tooth; this is where pressure anesthesia is applied throughout the

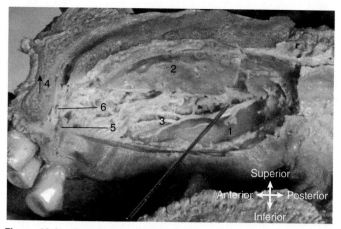

Figure 12-9 ■ Dissection of the hard palate showing a needle at the injection site for the greater palatine block (also showing landmarks for the nasopalatine block). *1,* GP foramen; *2,* mucoperiosteum of the hard palate; *3,* GP nerve traveling horizontally; *4,* incisive canal (and arrow), *5,* incisive foramen; *6,* nasopalatine nerve. (From Logan BM, Reynold PA, Hutching RT: *McMinn's color atlas of head and neck anatomy,* ed 3, London, 2004, Mosby. In: Fehrenbach MJ, Herring SW: *Illustrated anatomy of the head and neck,* ed 3, St Louis, 2007, Saunders.)

injection. The actual site of injection is in palatal tissue slightly anterior to the depression created by the greater palatine foramen (see Table 12-13, Figure Z). The needle for the GP block is inserted into the previously blanched anterior palatal tissue at a 90° angle to the palate, with the needle bowing slightly (see Table 12-13, Figure AA). The needle is advanced during the GP block until the palatine bone is contacted and then the injection is administered.

There is no need to enter the greater palatine canal and it would be difficult with the angulation of the needle as recommended. Although such an entrance is not potentially hazardous, it is not necessary for this block.

Indications of Successful Greater Palatine Block and Possible Complications

Indications of a successful GP block are numbness in the posterior palate and absence of discomfort during dental procedures. However, some patients may become uncomfortable and may gag if the soft palate becomes inadvertently and harmlessly anesthetized, which is possible given the proximity of the lesser palatine nerve and its foramen (Table 12-14). It may also be necessary to work around a midline palatal torus if present or a high vaulted palate when giving the injection; the clinician must try to maintain the perpendicular angle to the palatal tissue as much as possible.

NASOPALATINE BLOCK

The nasopalatine block, or NP block, is useful for anesthesia of the bilateral anterior palate or maxillary anterior sextant, from the mesial of the maxillary right first premolar to the mesial of the maxillary left first premolar or from maxillary canine to canine, including the maxillary bone as well as the lingual gingival tissue (Table 12-15, Figures BB through FF, and Procedure 12-7). The injection is useful on the more difficult nonsurgical periodontal therapy cases that are treated in sextants as well as in patients who have extensive lingual deposits in the region.

Both the right nasopalatine nerve and the left nasopalatine nerve are anesthetized by this block so only one injection is needed for both sides of the anterior palate. The NP block is used when anesthesia of the lingual gingival tissue is required for two or more maxillary anterior teeth. In the past, more than one injection may have been used by clinicians, such as entering the gingival tissue from the facial initially for a first injection and then following up with a second injection from the lingual or palatal with the thought of reducing soft tissue discomfort. However, if given correctly, one injection can be used comfortably for the patient. Creative dental hygiene treatment planning using sextants and administering only one NP block may be helpful in more sensitive patients with heavier deposits (see Figure 11-2A).

The NP block does not provide pulpal anesthesia of these teeth, so additional anesthesia such as the ASA block or the IO block may be indicated and is usually given before this block. In addition, anesthesia in the palatal area of the maxillary canine may prove inadequate because of overlapping nerve fibers from the posteriorly placed greater palatine nerve. This lack of anesthesia may be corrected by additional administration of the ipsilateral GP block if the patient is still feeling discomfort during treatment.

TABLE 12-14	Greater Palatine Block Complications
COMPLICATION	**TECHNIQUE ADJUSTMENT**
Inadequate anesthesia from injecting too far anterior to greater palatine foramen	Direct needle more posteriorly toward greater palatine foramen upon reinsertion
Inadequate anesthesia of maxillary first premolar due to crossover innervations from nasopalatine nerve	Additionally administer nasopalatine block (see Table 12-15, Figure FF)
Patient gags slightly due to soft palate anesthesia	Inadvertently anesthetized the lesser palatine nerve because its foramen is in close proximity; reassure patient and have the patient avoid swallowing until anesthesia wears off

Target Area and Injection Site for Nasopalatine Block

Both the right and left nasopalatine nerves enter the incisive foramen from the mucosa of the anterior hard palate (Figure 12-10). The deposit location or target area for the NP block is the incisive foramen beneath the incisive papilla (see Table 12-15, Figure BB).

However, the needle insertion point or injection site is the palatal tissue lateral to the incisive papilla, which is located at the midline (see Table 12-15, Figure EE). This is also 10 mm lingual to the maxillary central incisor teeth in case there is no telltale bulge of the structure of the incisive papilla. Never insert the needle directly into the incisive papilla because this can be extremely painful. Pressure anesthesia is performed utilizing a cotton tip applicator on palatal tissue on the contralateral side of the incisive papilla.

The needle is inserted for this block into the previously blanched palatal tissue at a 45° angle to the palate (see Table 12-15, Figure FF). The needle is advanced into the tissue until the maxillary bone is contacted and then the injection is administered. There is no need to enter the incisive canal via the foramen; however, the needle cannot enter foramen with the recommended position of the needle.

Indications of Successful Nasopalatine Block and Possible Complications

Indications of a successful NP block include numbness in the anterior palate and absence of discomfort during dental procedures. Complications such as hematoma are extremely rare (Table 12-16). However, this site on the anterior hard palate surrounding the incisive papilla is prone to previous trauma from food products, for example, hot coffee, tea, or pizza cheese, or rough nacho chips, so care needs to be taken to work around any trauma that may be present.

Text continued on p. 258

TABLE 12-15   **Nasopalatine Block Review**

Indications	Tissues lingual to maxillary anterior teeth in maxillary anterior sextant (from maxillary canine to canine)

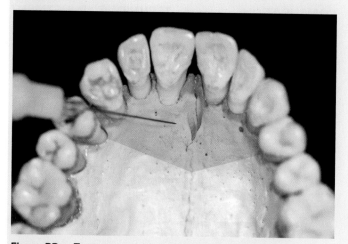

Figure BB ■ Target area and distribution of anesthesia for nasopalatine block. (From Fehrenbach MJ, Herring SW: *Illustrated anatomy of the head and neck,* ed 3, St Louis, 2007, Saunders.)

Nerves anesthetized	Nasopalatine nerve
Teeth anesthetized	None
Other structures anesthetized	Lingual gingival tissue of maxillary anterior teeth from maxillary canine to canine as well as anterior hard palate
Administration technique	See Procedure 12-7
Needle gauge and length	27-gauge short

Operator position	Right-handed: 11 o'clock Left-handed: 1 o'clock

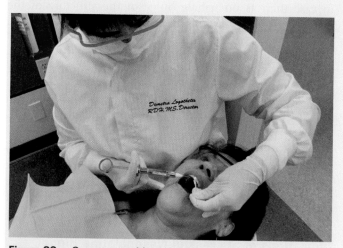

Figure CC ■ Operator position of right-handed clinician for nasopalatine block for both right and left block.

TABLE 12-15	Nasopalatine Block Review—cont'd

Syringe stabilization for nasopalatine block

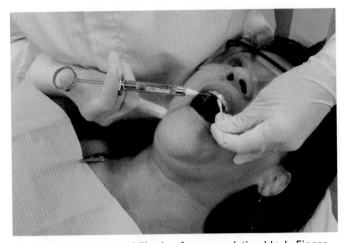

Figure DD ■ Syringe stabilization for nasopalatine block. Finger of dominant hand resting on patient's chin.

Landmarks	Maxillary central incisors Incisive papilla
Needle insertion point	Lateral to incisive papilla

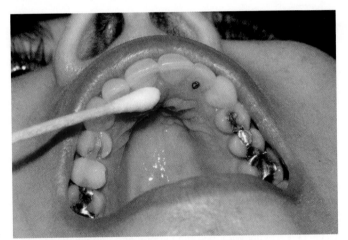

Figure EE ■ Injection site for nasopalatine block.

TABLE 12-15	Nasopalatine Block Review—cont'd
Depth of needle penetration	Approximately 3–6 mm or until contact with maxillary bone

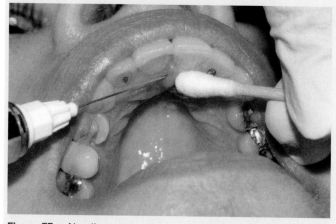

Figure FF ∎ Needle penetration for nasopalatine block.

Deposit location	At incisive foramen
Amount of anesthetic*	Approximately 0.45 mL or one-fourth of cartridge until blanching of tissue
Length of time to deposit	Approximately 20–30 seconds

*Approximate recommended amounts given are for 2% solutions of local anesthetic agents for adults; if using 4% solutions of local anesthetic agents, the approximate recommended amounts would be at least one-half of the amount of 2% solutions.

PROCEDURE 12-7	Nasopalatine (NP) Block Procedure

STEP 1 Assume the correct operator position for right-handed at 11 o'clock; left-handed at 1 o'clock (see Table 12-15, Figure CC).

STEP 2 Ask the patient to open his or her mouth and extend the neck comfortably backward.

STEP 3 Prepare the tissue on the lateral side of the incisive papilla toward the operator (see Chapter 11 and see Table 12-15, Figure EE).

STEP 4 Using a 27-gauge short needle in the syringe in the dominant hand, orient the bevel of the needle toward the hard palate.

STEP 5 Using a new cotton tip applicator in the nondominant hand, apply firm pressure to the cotton tip applicator directly to contralateral side of the incisive papilla away from the operator until tissue is blanched, and maintain pressure with the cotton tip applicator throughout the injection. Advise patient that he or she may feel some slight discomfort from the pressure.

STEP 6 Establish a fulcrum (see Table 12-15, Figure DD).

STEP 7 Direct the syringe at a 45° angle toward the base of the incisive papilla with the large window facing the operator.

STEP 8 Insert the needle approximately 3–6 mm into the tissue on the lateral side of the incisive papilla toward the operator until the maxillary bone is contacted, while maintaining pressure on the contralateral side with the cotton tip applicator (see Table 12-15, Figure FF).

STEP 9 Aspirate.

STEP 10 If negative aspiration is achieved, slowly deposit approximately 0.45 mL of solution (one-fourth of cartridge) over approximately 20–30 seconds; tissue in area will blanch even further when the anesthetic is administered. Continue to maintain pressure anesthesia for a short time with cotton tip applicator after solution is deposited.

STEP 11 Carefully withdraw the syringe and immediately recap the needle using the one-handed scoop method utilizing a needle sheath prop (see Chapter 11).

STEP 12 Rinse the patient's mouth and wait approximately 3–5 minutes until anesthesia takes effect before starting treatment.

ANTERIOR MIDDLE SUPERIOR ALVEOLAR BLOCK

The anterior middle superior alveolar block, or AMSA block, is useful for pulpal anesthesia and anesthesia of the periodontium and gingival tissue covering a large area that is normally innervated by the ASA, MSA, GP, and NP blocks in the maxillary arch (Table 12-17, Figures GG through II, and Procedure 12-8). Thus, the single-site palatal injection with the AMSA block can anesthetize multiple teeth (from the maxillary second premolar through the maxillary central incisor) and associated periodontium without causing the usual collateral anesthesia to the soft tissue of the patient's upper lip and face.

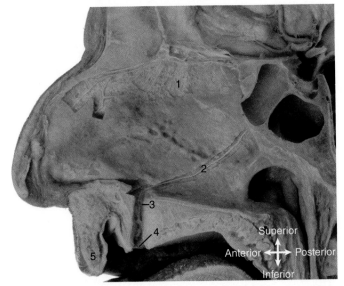

Figure 12-10 ■ Dissection showing a sagittal section of the right side of the hard palate at the target area for the nasopalatine block. *1*, Olfactory nerve; *2*, NP nerve; *3*, incisive canal; *4*, anterior ethmoidal nerve; *5*, incisive foramen; *6*, upper. (From Logan BM, Reynold PA, Hutching RT: *McMinn's color atlas of head and neck anatomy*, ed 3, London, 2004, Mosby. In: Fehrenbach MJ, Herring SW: *Illustrated anatomy of the head and neck*, ed 3, St Louis, 2007, Saunders.)

This injection is commonly used when performing cosmetic dentistry procedures because after the procedures are completed, the clinician can immediately and accurately assesses the patient's smile line. The AMSA, together with a traditional PSA block, will anesthetize a maxillary quadrant for dental procedures. Studies show that this injection is best accomplished with a computer-controlled delivery device (CCDD) (see Chapter 9) because it regulates the pressure and volume ratio of solution delivered, which is not readily attained with a manual syringe.

TABLE 12-16	Nasopalatine Block Complications
COMPLICATION	**TECHNIQUE ADJUSTMENT**
Inadequate anesthesia of maxillary first premolar or canine due to crossover innervations from greater palatine nerve	Additionally administer greater palatine injection (see Table 12-13)
Density of the tissue and constricted area for anesthetic deposition may cause the anesthetic solution to appear around the needle penetration site during administration	Inject slowly and rinse patient's mouth following safe capping of needle

TABLE 12-17	Anterior Middle Superior Alveolar Block
Indications	Maxillary teeth in one quadrant, except for those innervated by posterior superior alveolar nerve

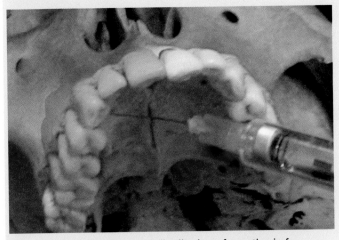

Figure GG ■ Target area and distribution of anesthesia for anterior middle superior alveolar block. (From Fehrenbach MJ, Herring SW: *Illustrated anatomy of the head and neck*, ed 3, St Louis, 2007, Saunders.)

Nerves anesthetized	Anterior superior alveolar nerve Middle superior alveolar nerve Greater palatine nerve Nasopalatine nerve
Teeth anesthetized	Most maxillary teeth in one quadrant, except for maxillary molars

continued next page

TABLE 12-17   **Anterior Middle Superior Alveolar Block—cont'd**

Other structures anesthetized	Periodontium of anesthetized teeth as well as facial and lingual gingival tissue of maxillary arch in one quadrant, except for the buccal soft tissue of maxillary molars (no regional soft tissue anesthesia of upper lip and face)
Administration technique	See Procedure 12-8
Needle gauge and length	Using computer-controlled delivery device with short needle
Operator position	Right-handed: 8–9 or 11 o'clock Left-handed: 4–3 or 1 o'clock
Landmarks	Maxillary premolars Lingual gingival margin Median palatine raphe

Needle insertion point	Apices of maxillary premolars on hard palate, midway between median palatal raphe and lingual gingival margin

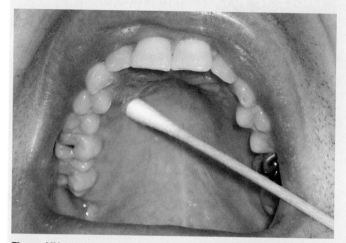

Figure HH ■ Injection site for anterior middle superior alveolar block. (From Fehrenbach MJ, Herring SW: *Illustrated anatomy of the head and neck*, ed 3, St Louis, 2007, Saunders.)

Depth of needle penetration	Approximately 3–6 mm until until contact with maxillary bone

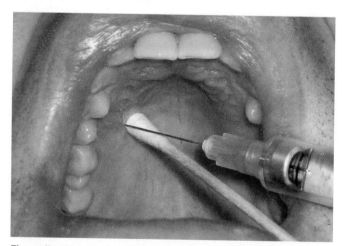

Figure II ■ Needle penetration for anterior middle superior alveolar block demonstrated on right side. (From Fehrenbach MJ, Herring SW: *Illustrated anatomy of the head and neck*, ed 3, St Louis, 2007, Saunders.)

Deposit location	Pores on maxillary bone on one side of hard palate
Amount of anesthetic*	Approximately 0.45 mL or one-fourth of cartridge until blanching of tissue
Length of time to deposit	Approximately 20–30 seconds

*Approximate recommended amounts given are for 2% solutions of local anesthetic agents for adults; if using 4% solutions of local anesthetic agents, the approximate recommended amounts would be at least one-half of the amount of 2% solutions.

PROCEDURE 12-8	Anterior Middle Superior Alveolar (AMSA) Block Procedure

STEP 1 Assume the correct operator position for right-handed at 8–9 o'clock (right side) or 11 o'clock (left side); left-handed at 4–3 o'clock (right side) or 1 o'clock (left side).

STEP 2 Prepare the tissue on the surface of the hard palate at the apices of the maxillary premolars, midway between the median palatal raphe and the lingual gingival margin (see Chapter 11 and Table 12-17, Figure HH).

STEP 4 Using a computer-controlled delivery device and short needle in the dominant hand, orient the bevel of the needle toward the hard palate. Have the patient extend the neck either to the right or left for visibility.

STEP 5 Using a new cotton tip applicator in the dominant hand, apply firm pressure with the applicator nearby the apices of the maxillary premolars on the surface of the hard palate until tissue is blanched. Maintain pressure with the cotton tip applicator throughout the injection (see Table 12-17, Figure II). Advise patient that he or she may feel some slight discomfort from the pressure.

STEP 6 Establish a fulcrum and direct the handpiece of the syringe from the contralateral premolars at a 45° angle to the apices of the maxillary premolars on the hard

palate, with the large window facing the operator (see Table 12-17, Figure II).

STEP 7 Insert the needle approximately 3–6 mm into the tissues over the hard palate at the apices of the maxillary premolars until the maxillary bone is contacted, while maintaining pressure nearby with the applicator (see Table 12-17, Figure II).

STEP 8 Aspirate.

STEP 9 If negative aspiration is achieved, slowly deposit approximately 0.45 mL of solution (one-fourth of cartridge) over approximately 20–30 seconds; tissue in area will blanch even further when the anesthetic is administered. Continue to maintain pressure anesthesia for a short time with cotton tip applicator after solution is deposited.

STEP 10 Carefully withdraw the syringe and immediately recap the needle using the one-handed scoop method utilizing a needle sheath prop (see Chapter 11).

STEP 11 Rinse the patient's mouth and wait approximately 3–5 minutes until anesthesia takes effect before starting treatment.

However, even more recent studies show that due to the extensive anatomy involved, this block may be variable in depth and duration of anesthesia, which may compromise its use for nonsurgical periodontal therapy by the dental hygienist that usually needs full depth and long duration of anesthesia to complete the treatment. Instead, reliance on the traditional blocks may allow the dental hygienist to treatment plan instrumentation in either quadrants or sextants with more confidence of pain and hemostatic control.

Target Area and Injection Site for Anterior Middle Superior Alveolar Block

The deposit location or target area for the AMSA block is the tissue of the hard palate (see Table 12-17, Figure GG). This block takes advantage of a number of small pores in the maxillary bone in the region as well as the tight attachment of the palatal tissue. As the solution penetrates through the pores, it has access to the anterior to middle part of the dental plexus, which then anesthetizes the teeth and associated facial tissue as well as the lingual tissue of the surrounding palate (see Figure 12-6).

The injection site for the AMSA block is at the apices of the maxillary premolars on the hard palate, midway between the median palatal raphe and the lingual gingival margin (see Table 12-17, Figure HH). Orientation of the handpiece of the syringe should be from the contralateral premolars. The previously blanched tissue is approached with the needle at a 45° angle until the maxillary bone is contacted, and then the injection is administered (see Table 12-17, Figure II).

Indications of Successful Anterior Middle Superior Alveolar Block and Possible Complications

Indications of a successful AMSA block include variable numbness of the large area that is normally innervated by

TABLE 12-18	Anterior Middle Superior Alveolar Block Complication

COMPLICATION	TECHNIQUE ADJUSTMENT
Excessive blanching on palatal tissue that may lead to postoperative tissue ischemia and sloughing	Slowing or stopping device to let solution dissipate as well as controlling overall amount used

the ASA, MSA, GP, and NP blocks. Blanching also occurs on the palatal tissue after the AMSA block. However, if excessive, it may cause postoperative tissue ischemia and sloughing (Table 12-18). Thus if excessive blanching is noted, slowing or stopping the device for a few seconds to let the solution dissipate will diminish the chance of this postoperative event as well as controlling the overall amount used. Other complications are extremely rare.

COMMON TECHNIQUE ERRORS ASSOCIATED WITH MAXILLARY INJECTIONS

Most technique errors associated with maxillary injections are due to the angulation of the needle and syringe, and are typically associated with the maxillary facial injections. To ensure safe and effective pain control, the dental hygienist should follow all recommended injection technique guidelines addressed in this chapter. This section describes common technique errors associated with maxillary facial injections.

COMMON ERRORS: SUPRAPERIOSTEAL INJECTIONS OR ANTERIOR SUPERIOR ALVEOLAR, AND MIDDLE SUPERIOR ALVEOLAR BLOCKS

The most common technique error associated with supra-periosteal injections or ASA and MSA blocks is the angle of the syringe barrel and needle. The angle of the syringe barrel should be parallel to the long access of the tooth following the normal contour of the tooth. If the syringe barrel angle is too steep, the needle will be inserted too shallow into the mucobuccal fold. The needle would

possibly be into the attached gingiva so the maxillary bone will be contacted causing discomfort to the patient, and the target location will be missed, causing a decreased level of anesthesia. Figure 12-11 demonstrates *incorrect syringe/needle angulation* for supraperiosteal injections, ASA and MSA blocks, and Figure 12-12 demonstrates *correct syringe/needle angulation*.

COMMON ERRORS: POSTERIOR SUPERIOR ALVEOLAR BLOCK

The most common technique error associated with the PSA block is not obtaining the correct syringe angulation of the

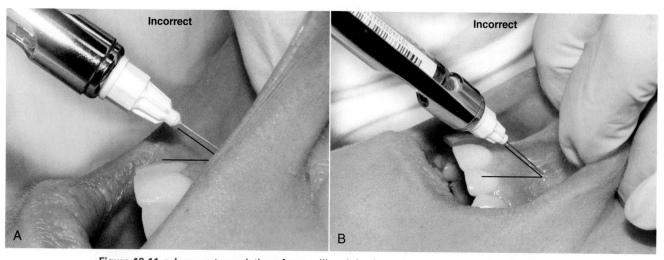

Figure 12-11 ■ **Incorrect** angulations for maxillary injections. Incorrect: syringe/needle angulation for supraperiosteal injections, ASA and MSA blocks. **A,** Incorrect: syringe angle is too steep and not parallel with the long axis of the tooth. **B,** Incorrect: the needle insertion point is too shallow. Bone will be contacted causing discomfort to the patient and inferior deposition of solution below the apex of the tooth.

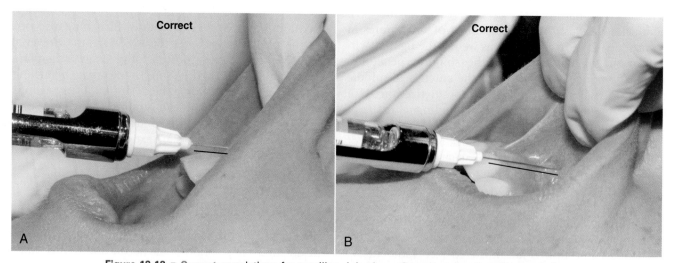

Figure 12-12 ■ **Correct** angulations for maxillary injections. Correct syringe/needle angulation for supraperiosteal injections, ASA and MSA blocks: syringe angulation is parallel with the long axis of the tooth, allowing the needle to be inserted at the proper height within the mucobuccal fold. This allows the needle to be inserted superior to the apex of the tooth for correct placement of anesthetic solution. Note stable fulcrum of clinician's pinky finger resting on the patient's chin.

needle in an upward (or superiorly) 45° angle to the occlusal plane, inward (or medially) at a 45° angle to the occlusal plane, and backward (or posteriorly) at a 45° angle to the long axis of the maxillary second molar. To achieve these angulations it is important for the barrel of the syringe to be at the corner of the patient's mouth, and resting on the clinician's retraction finger. It is also important for the clinician to retract the tissue upward and outward rather than horizontally. Figures 12-13 demonstrates *incorrect syringe angulation*, and Figure 12-14 demonstrates *correct syringe angulation*.

COMMON ERRORS: INFRAORBITAL BLOCK

The most common technique error associated with the IO block is not aligning the syringe barrel toward the infraorbital foramen in the same plane as the pupil of the eye. Inserting the needle too shallow into the mucobuccal fold will cause premature bone contact and an inferior deposit of anesthetic solution to the infraorbital foramen. This will cause a decreased level of anestheisa. Figure 12-15 demonstrates *incorrect syringe/needle angulation* for the IO block. Figure 12-16 demonstrates *correct syringe/needle angulation* for the IO block.

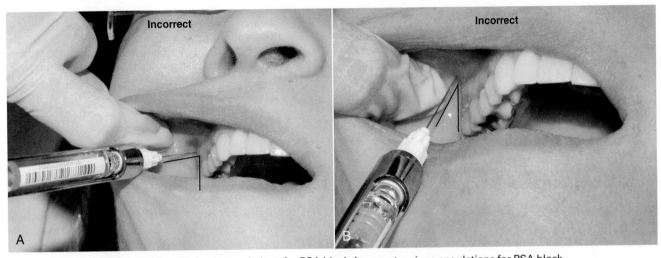

Figure 12-13 ■ **Incorrect** angulations for PSA block. Incorrect syringe angulations for PSA block. **A,** Syringe angulation is greater than 45° backward from the apex of the maxillary second molar, causing needle tip to be too medial and bone will be contacted. Need to decrease angulation to 45°. **B,** Syringe angulation is not 45° backward from the apex of the maxillary second molar. Syringe barrel needs to be resting on the clinician's retraction finger and at the corner of the patient's mouth.

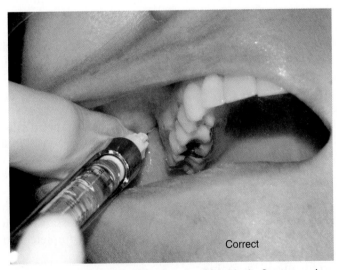

Figure 12-14 ■ **Correct** angulation for PSA block. Correct syringe angulation for PSA block: syringe angle is 45° backward, inward, and upward from the occlusal plane. Note stable fulcrum of syringe resting on clinician's retraction finger and at the corner of the patient's mouth.

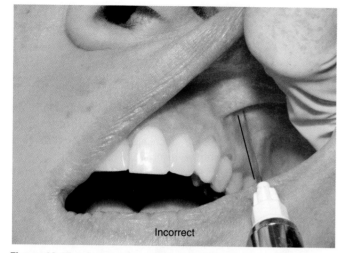

Figure 12-15 ■ **Incorrect** angulation for IO block. Incorrect syringe alignment for IO block: the syringe barrel is not aligned toward the infraorbital foramen in the same plane as the pupil of the eye, and is angled toward the bone. This will cause premature bone contact with the needle and an inferior deposition of anesthetic solution. Needle insertion point is too shallow within the mucobuccal fold.

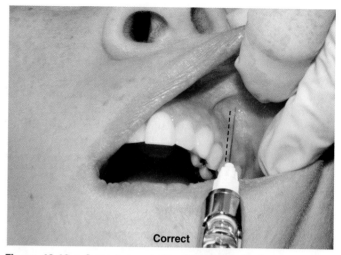

Figure 12-16 ■ **Correct** angulation for IO block. Correct syringe alignment for IO block: the syringe barrel is correctly aligned toward the infraorbital foramen along a plane parallel to the pupil of the eye.

DENTAL HYGIENE CONSIDERATIONS

- Local anesthesia of the maxillae is more successful than that of the mandible because the facial plates of bone over the teeth are less dense than that of the mandible over similar teeth.
- Certain distractor techniques involving lip movement can actually increase patient discomfort as the needle bevel can be moved, and anesthetic solution may be deposited away from the target site.
- Supraperiosteal injections can usually be successfully administered on every tooth in the maxillary quadrant.
- Supraperiosteal injections are recommended when pulpal anesthesia is needed on a limited number of teeth.
- The PSA block is recommended for pulpal anesthesia of the maxillary molar teeth and associated periodontium.
- The MSA block may be useful for pulpal anesthesia of the maxillary premolar teeth and associated periodontium.
- The ASA block is recommended for pulpal anesthesia of the maxillary anterior teeth and associated periodontium.
- The IO block is recommended for pulpal anesthesia of the maxillary anterior teeth and premolars and associated periodontium in one quadrant.
- The GP block is recommended when lingual soft tissue anesthesia is needed distal to the maxillary canine.

- The NP block is recommended when lingual soft tissue anesthesia is needed from maxillary canine to canine.
- The anterior middle superior alveolar block, or AMSA block, is recommended for pulpal anesthesia and anesthesia of the periodontium and gingival tissue covering the area that is normally innervated by the ASA, MSA, GP, and NP blocks.
- In order to maximize patient comfort during a palatal injection, pressure anesthesia utilizing a cotton tip applicator is recommended in the area of needle insertion during the injection.
- To decrease the risk of hematoma associated with the PSA block, a short needle should be used for most patients at three-fourths its depth, and less for children and small adults.
- To decrease the risk of intravascular injection with the PSA block, it is recommended to aspirate within three planes before anesthetic deposition and then to reaspirate every one fourth of anesthetic deposition.
- If sextant or quadrant dental hygiene treatment is planned, it is recommended that the PSA block be given before any of the other maxillary facial injections, as well as any maxillary palatal injections, to allow the necessary time for the larger maxillary molars to become completely anesthetized.

CASE STUDY 12-1

Patient with abscess formation

A new patient has come into the dental office today due to pain on her maxillary right canine. Following a complete examination, the supervising dentist determines that the tooth needs an extraction due to a chronic periapical abscess formation noted on the radiographs, even though there are no intraoral signs. The dentist asks the dental hygienist to administer the anesthesia since the schedule is running behind and there is not even time to enter the patient history into the patient record. The newly-hired dental hygienist hurridly selects both the right ASA and NP blocks necessary for the surgical procedure, and administers the usual volume of anesthetic without further discussing the case with the supervising dentist. When the dentist begins the procedure, the patient informs him that she is still in pain.

Critical Thinking Questions
- Why is the patient still feeling pain?
- How should the dental team have proceeded for a more successful outcome in pain control for the patient?
- What serious complications could have occurred for this patient?

CHAPTER REVIEW QUESTIONS

1. Anesthesia of the maxillary teeth is MORE successful than the mandibular teeth BECAUSE the maxillary bone overlying the teeth is more dense.
   A. Both the statement and the reason are correct and related.
   B. Both the statement and the reason are correct but NOT related.
   C. The statement is correct, but the reason is NOT.
   D. The statement is NOT correct, but the reason is correct.
   E. NEITHER the statement NOR the reason is correct.

2. When performing maxillary nerve anesthesia, which is the ONLY local anesthetic block that requires the clinician to contact bone with the needle to ensure success?
   A. Infraorbital block
   B. Anterior superior alveolar block
   C. Middle superior alveolar block
   D. Posterior superior alveolar block

3. Which block is MOST appropriate to successfully anesthetize the buccal tissue of the maxillary premolars?
   A. Greater palatine block
   B. Nasopalatine block
   C. Anterior superior alveolar block
   D. Middle superior alveolar block

4. Where is the target area for local anesthetic deposition of the agent located when administering a supraperiosteal injection?
   A. Cervix of the tooth
   B. Height or depth of the mucobuccal fold
   C. Between the mucoperiosteum and bone
   D. Between the gingival tissue and bone

5. It is ALWAYS important for the clinician to orient the needle as close as possible to the periosteum. This is to ensure the needle glides along the periosteum allowing for more stability.
   A. Both the statement and the reason are correct and related.
   B. Both the statement and the reason are correct but NOT related.
   C. The statement is correct, but the reason is NOT.
   D. The statement is NOT correct, but the reason is correct.
   E. NEITHER the statement NOR the reason is correct.

6. Which of the following local anesthetic blocks anesthetizes the mesial buccal root of tooth #3 in ONLY 28% of the population?
   A. Greater palatine block
   B. Nasopalatine block
   C. Anterior superior alveolar block
   D. Middle superior alveolar block

7. Which of the following structures does the infraorbital local anesthetic block anesthetize?
   A. The teeth and periodontium in either the upper left or upper right quadrant
   B. The teeth and peridontium in the entire maxillary arch
   C. The anterior and middle superior alveolar nerves in one maxillary quadrant
   D. The anterior and middle superior alveolar nerves in both maxillary quadrants

8. Where is the target area located for the posterior superior alveolar local anesthetic block?
   A. The posterior superior alveolar nerve as it enters infratemporal fossa
   B. The posterior superior alveolar nerve as it exits the ptergopalatine fossa
   C. The posterior superior alveolar nerve as it exits the parotid salivary gland near the facial nerve

D. The posterior superior alveolar nerve as it enters the maxilla through the posterior superior alveolar foramina

9. Which local anesthetic block listed below requires the needle insertion point to be at the height of the mucobuccal fold, superior to the apex of the maxillary second molar?
   A. Infraorbital block
   B. Anterior superior alveolar block
   C. Middle superior alveolar block
   D. Posterior superior alveolar block

10. If the clinician wanted to anesthetize teeth #9-11, and associated buccal and lingual gingival tissue, it would be BEST to administer which of the following local anesthetic blocks?
    A. Infraorbital block only
    B. Infraorbital and nasopalatine blocks
    C. Infraorbital and greater palatine blocks
    D. Anterior superior alveolar and middle superior alveolar blocks

11. BECAUSE the greater palatine block local anesthetic does NOT provide pulpal anesthesia, the use of the middle superior alveolar block and/or posterior superior alveolar block is also indicated when instrumenting on the maxillary premolars.
    A. Both the statement and the reason are correct and related.
    B. Both the statement and the reason are correct but NOT related.
    C. The statement is correct, but the reason is NOT.
    D. The statement is NOT correct, but the reason is correct.
    E. NEITHER the statement NOR the reason is correct.

12. Which of the following local anesthetic blocks require the needle angulation to be at 45 degrees within three separate planes during administration?
    A. Infraorbital block
    B. Anterior superior alveolar block
    C. Middle superior alveolar block
    D. Posterior superior alveolar block

13. Where is the needle insertion point recommended for the nasopalatine local anesthetic block?
    A. Lateral to the incisive papilla
    B. Anterior to the greater palatine foramen
    C. Posterior to the incisive foramen
    D. Near the maxillary labial frenum

14. Where is the target area located for the middle superior alveolar local anesthetic block?
    A. Apex of the maxillary canine
    B. Apex of the maxillary first premolar
    C. Apex of the maxillary second premolar
    D. Mesial buccal root of the maxillary first molar

15. Where is the needle insertion point for the anterior superior alveolar local anesthetic block?
    A. Mucobuccal fold at the apex of the maxillary canine
    B. Mucobuccal fold at the apex of the maxillary first premolar
    C. Mucobuccal fold at the apex of the maxillary second premolar
    D. Mucobuccal fold at the apex of the maxillary first molar

16. What is the usual depth of needle penetration for the anterior superior alveolar local anesthetic block?
    A. 5 mm
    B. 10 mm
    C. 16 mm
    D. 20 mm

17. What is the needle insertion point for the infraorbital local anesthetic block?
    A. Mucobuccal fold at the apex of the maxillary canine
    B. Mucobuccal fold at the apex of the maxillary first premolar
    C. Mucobuccal fold at the apex of the maxillary second premolar
    D. Mucobuccal fold at the apex of the maxillary first molar

18. After receiving an infraorbital local anesthetic block, the patient reports slight numbness of the lower eyelid. What should the clinician do?
    A. Stop treatment and explain facial nerve paralysis to the patient
    B. Nothing since this is normal for this block
    C. Place a cold compress to prevent hematoma
    D. Immediately administer an oral antihistamine

19. Where is the greater palatine foramen usually located?
    A. About 10 mm medial and directly superior to the lingual gingival margin
    B. About 10 mm medial and directly inferior to the lingual gingival margin
    C. Lateral to the incisive papilla and lingual to the maxillary central incisors
    D. Lateral to the lesser palatine foramen and posterior to the hard plate

20. Pressure anesthesia to control patient discomfort upon injection with the needle can be used during which of the following local anesthetic blocks?
    A. Posterior alevolar and greater palatine local anesthetic blocks
    B. Greater palatine and nasopalatine local anesthetic blocks
    C. Nasopalatine and infraorbital local anesthetic blocks
    D. Nasopalatine local anesthetic block only

REFERENCES

1. Fehrenbach MJ, Herring SW: *Illustrated anatomy of the head and neck*, ed 3, St Louis, 2007, Saunders.
2. Logan BM, Reynold PA, Hutching RT: *McMinn's color atlas of head and neck anatomy*, ed 3, London, 2004, Mosby.
3. Kaufman E, Epstein JB, Naveh E, Gorsky M, Gross A, Cohen G: A survey of pain, pressure, and discomfort induced by commonly used oral anesthesia injections, *Anesth Prog* 54(4): 122-127, 2005 Winter.
4. Jastak T, Yagiela J, Donaldson D: *Local anesthesia of the oral cavity*, St Louis, 1995, Saunders.
5. Malamed S: *Handbook of local anesthesia*, ed 5, St Louis, 2004, Mosby.
6. Darby M, Walsh M: *Dental hygiene theory and practice*, ed 3, St Louis, 2010, Saunders.

Summary of Maxillary Injections

SUPRAPERIOSTEAL INJECTION

AREAS ANESTHETIZED	LANDMARKS	ADMINISTRATION SITES	TECHNIQUE	ADVERSE EFFECTS
Teeth Single tooth (or teeth) **Other Structures** Periodontium of anesthetized tooth (or teeth) and either facial or lingual soft tissue in area	Muccobuccal fold or lingual surface of selected tooth or teeth	**Penetration Site** Height of muccobuccal fold or lingual surface of selected tooth or teeth **Deposit Location** Superior or inferior to apex of selected tooth or teeth	Parallel to long axis of the tooth (teeth) superior or inferior to the apex; Aspirate **Depth of Penetration** Short needle approximately 5 mm or one-fourth the needle length; 27 gauge **Anesthetic Solution** 0.6 mL, or one-third cartridge	Pain from scraping periosteum; pain from injecting too rapidly; inadequate anesthesia from infection in area; inadequate anesthesia from dense bone

POSTERIOR SUPERIOR ALVEOLAR (PSA) BLOCK

AREAS ANESTHETIZED	LANDMARKS	ADMINISTRATION SITES	TECHNIQUE	ADVERSE EFFECTS
Teeth Pulpal anesthesia of the third, second, and first maxillary molars entirely in 72% of population, mesiobuccal root not anesthetized in 28% of population **Other Structures** Periodontium of anesthetized teeth and buccal soft tissue of maxillary molar region	Maxillary mucobuccal fold; maxillary second molar; maxillary tuberosity; maxillary occlusal plane; midsagittal plane	**Penetration site** Height of mucobuccal fold superior to the apex of the maxillary second molar **Deposit Location** Superior to apex of maxillary second molar and posterior and superior to posterior border of maxilla at posterior superior alveolar foramina	Upward 45° to occlusal plane, inward and backward 45° to midsagittal plane; Aspirate **Depth of Penetration** Short needle three-fourths of needle length; 25 or 27 gauge **Anesthetic Solution** 0.9–1.7 (1.8) mL, or half to a full cartridge 60–120 seconds	Needle inserted too far posterior and superior may tear maxillary artery or pterygoid plexus of veins resulting in hematoma; mandibular anesthesia

MIDDLE SUPERIOR ALVEOLAR (MSA) BLOCK

AREAS ANESTHETIZED	LANDMARKS	ADMINISTRATION SITES	TECHNIQUE	ADVERSE REACTIONS
Teeth Pulpal anesthesia of maxillary first and second premolars and mesiobuccal root of maxillary first molar in 28% of population **Other Structures** Periodontium of anesthetized teeth and buccal soft tissue of premolar region	Mucobuccal fold; maxillary second premolar	**Penetration Site** Height of mucobuccal fold of maxillary second premolar **Deposit Location** Superior to the apex of the maxillary second premolar	Parallel to long axis of the maxillary second premolar superior to the apex; Aspirate **Depth of Penetration** Short needle approximately 5 mm or one-fourth of needle length; 27 gauge **Anesthetic Solution** 0.9–1.2 mL, or one-half to two-thirds the cartridge 60–90 seconds to deposit seconds	Pain from scraping periosteum; pain from injecting too rapidly; inadequate anesthesia from infection in area; inadequate anesthesia from dense bone; inadequate anesthesia from injecting inferior to apex

ANTERIOR SUPERIOR ALVEOLAR (ASA) BLOCK

AREAS ANESTHETIZED	LANDMARKS	ADMINISTRATION SITES	TECHNIQUE	ADVERSE REACTIONS
Teeth Pulpal anesthesia of maxillary central, lateral and canine **Other Structures** Periodontium of anesthetized teeth and facial soft tissue of anterior area	Mucobuccal fold; canine eminence; canine fossa; maxillary canine	**Penetration Site** Height of mucobuccal fold slightly mesial to the canine eminence **Deposit Location** Superior to apex of the maxillary canine	Parallel to the long axis of the canine superior to the apex; Aspirate **Depth of Penetration** Short needle approximately 5 mm or one-fourth of needle length; 27 gauge **Anesthetic Solution** 0.6–0.9 mL, or one third to one half of a cartridge 30–60 seconds	Pain from scraping periosteum; pain from injecting too rapidly; inadequate anesthesia from infection in area; inadequate anesthesia from dense bone over apecies; inadequate anesthesia from injecting inferior to apex; inadequate anesthesia from crossover-innervation from contralateral ASA nerve

INFRAORBITAL (IO) BLOCK

AREAS ANESTHETIZED	LANDMARKS	ADMINISTRATION SITES	TECHNIQUE	ADVERSE EFFECTS
Teeth Pulpal anesthesia of the maxillary central incisor, lateral incisor, canine, premolars, mesiobuccal root of the first molar in 28% of population **Other Structures** Periodontium of anesthetized teeth and facial soft tissue of maxillary arch, except for maxillary molar region; upper lip to midline; medial part of the cheek; side of nose; lower eyelid	Maxillary mucobuccal fold; infraorbital notch; infraorbital ridge; infraorbital depression; infraorbital foramen; maxillary first premolar	**Penetration Site** Height of mucobuccal fold superior to the maxillary first premolar **Deposit Location** Height of mucobuccal fold above the maxillary first premolar	Locate infraorbital foramen; Maintain pressure with finger over the foramen during injection; bevel toward bone; direct needle toward the foramen Aspirate Massage solution into foramen for 2 minutes **Depth of Penetration** Long or short needle, one half length of long needle and three-fourths the length of short needle; 25 or 27 gauge **Anesthetic Solution** 0.9–1.2 ml, or one half to two thirds of a cartridge 60–90 seconds	Pain from scraping periosteum; pain from injecting too rapidly; inadequate anesthesia from needle contacting bone inferior to infraorbital foramen; inadequate anesthesia from crossover-innervation from contralateral ASA nerve

GREATER PALATINE (GP) BLOCK

AREAS ANESTHETIZED	LANDMARKS	ADMINISTRATION SITES	TECHNIQUE	ADVERSE REACTIONS
Teeth None **Other Structures** Lingual gingival tissue of maxillary premolars and molars and posterior hard palate in one quadrant	Maxillary third molar Junction of maxillary alveolar process and posterior hard palate Greater palatine foramen	**Penetration Site** Slightly anterior to the greater palatine foramen **Deposit Location** At greater palatine foramen	Advance syringe from opposite side of mouth at right angle to target area; use pressure anesthesia utilizing cotton tip applicator Aspirate **Depth of Penetration** Short needle approximately 3–6 mm or until palate is lightly contacted; 27 gauge **Anesthetic Solution** 0.45 mL, or one fourth of a cartridge until blanching of tissue is observed 20–30 seconds	Gagging from touching the soft palate; inadequate anesthesia from injecting too far anterior; inadequate anesthesia of maxillary first premolar due to crossover-innervation of NP nerve

continued next page

NASOPALATINE (NP) BLOCK

AREAS ANESTHETIZED	LANDMARKS	ADMINISTRATION SITES	TECHNIQUE	ADVERSE REACTIONS
Teeth None **Other Structures** Anterior hard palate and overlying soft tissue of the maxillary anterior teeth bilaterally (canine to canine)	Maxillary central incisors Incisive papilla	**Penetration Site** Lateral to the incisive papilla **Deposit Location** At incisive foramen	45°–90° to tissue at the edge of incisive papilla; watch for blanching of the tissue; pressure anesthesia utilizing cotton tip applicator Aspirate **Depth of Penetration** Short needle approximately 3–6 mm or until bone is lightly contacted; 27 gauge **Anesthetic Solution** 0.45 mL, or one fourth of a cartridge until blanching of tissue is observed 20–30 seconds	Because of the density of the tissues, the anesthetic solution may appear around the needle penetration site during administration; inadequate anesthesia of maxillary first canine due to crossover-innervations from the GP nerve

ANTERIOR MIDDLE SUPERIOR ALVEOLAR (AMSA) BLOCK

AREAS ANESTHETIZED	LANDMARKS	ADMINISTRATION SITES	TECHNIQUE	ADVERSE REACTIONS
Teeth Most maxillary teeth in one quadrant, except for the maxillary molars **Other Structures** Periodontium of anesthetized teeth; facial and lingual gingival tissue of maxillary arch over same teeth	Maxillary premolars Lingual gingival margin Median palatine raphe	**Penetration Site** Apices of maxillary premolars on hard palate, midway between median palatal raphe and lingual gingival margin **Deposit Location** Pores on maxillary bone on one side of hard palate	Direct handpiece 45° angle to the apices of maxillary premolars on hard palate until the maxillary bone is contacted **Depth of Penetration** 3–6 mm until contact of maxillary bone **Anesthetic Solution** 0.45 mL, or one fourth of a cartridge	Excessive blanching of palatal tissue leading to possible ischemia and sloughing

CHAPTER 13

Mandibular Nerve Anesthesia

Margaret Fehrenbach RDH, MS and Demetra Daskalos Logothetis RDH, MS

CHAPTER OUTLINE

LEARNING OBJECTIVES

1. Define and pronounce all the key terms and anatomic terms in this chapter.
2. List the teeth and structures anesthetized by each type of mandibular injection and describe the target areas.
3. Locate and identify the anatomic structures used to determine the local anesthetic needle's injection site for each type of mandibular injection on a skull and a patient.
4. Demonstrate the correct placement of the local anesthetic needle for each type of mandibular injection on a skull and a patient.
5. Identify the correct tissue penetrated by the local anesthetic needle for each type of mandibular injection.
6. Discuss the indications of a successful injections as well as complications of local anesthesia of the oral cavity associated with anatomic considerations for each type of mandibular injection.
7. Integrate mandibular anesthesia with the needs of a dental hygiene care plan.
8. Correctly administer local anesthesia on the mandibular arch for the management of patient pain with hemostatic control during clinical dental hygiene practice without any complications.
9. Correctly complete the review questions and activities for this chapter.

KEY TERMS

Buccal block Type of injection that anesthetizes the buccal soft tissue of the mandibular molars.

Crossover-innervation Overlap of terminal nerve fibers from the contralateral side.

Deposit location Target area where local anesthetic will be deposited.

Depth of needle penetration Describes needle depth covered in tissue when target area is reached.

Gow-Gates mandibular block (GG Block) Type of injection that anesthetizes most of the mandibular nerve.

Incisive block Type of injection that anesthetizes the teeth and associated periodontium as well as facial soft tissue anterior to the mental foramen.

Inferior alveolar (IA) block Type of injection that anesthetizes the mandibular teeth and their associated periodontium and lingual soft tissue to the midline.

Mental block Type of injection that anesthetizes the facial soft tissue anterior to the mental foramen.

Needle insertion point Injection site where bevel of needle is covered with tissue.

Nerve block Type of injection that anesthetizes a larger area than the local infiltration due to the local anesthetic agent deposited near large nerve trunks.

Paresthesia Persistent anesthesia beyond the expected duration, or altered sensation such as tingling or itching that is beyond a normal level.

Periodontal ligament (PDL) injection Supplemental injection used when pulpal anesthesia is indicated on a single tooth, is administered directly into the periodontium of the tooth to be anesthetized.

Supraperiosteal injection Type of injection that anesthetizes a small area—one or two teeth and associated structures—due to the local anesthetic agent deposited near terminal nerve endings.

Visual analog scale (VAS) An instrument used to measure pain.

INTRODUCTION TO MANDIBULAR NERVE ANESTHESIA

The mandibular nerve and its branches can be anesthetized in a number of ways by the dental hygienist for patient pain management with hemostatic control depending on the extent of procedure anticipated and the structures needing to be anesthetized (Figure 13-1 and Table 13-1).[1] But the dental hygienist must understand that, compared with maxillary anesthesia, mandibular anesthesia has its own considerations.

First, supraperiosteal injection (an anesthetic option discussed in Chapter 12) of the mandible is not as successful as that of the maxillae because overall the mandible is denser than the maxillae over similar teeth, especially in the area of the posterior teeth. This can be easily noted using a panoramic radiograph (see Figures 10-2 and 10-8). For this reason, a nerve block is preferred to supraperiosteal injection in most parts of the mandible, unlike the maxillae.

Second, substantial variation exists in the anatomy of local anesthetic landmarks of the mandibular bone and nerves compared with similar structures in the maxilla, complicating mandibular anesthesia for the clinician, and possibly with the need for troubleshooting of failure cases (see Chapter 10).[2] This chapter covers some of the most common mandibular variations; variation in the anatomy of the mandible gives individuals facial "character."

The inferior alveolar (IA) block is generally recommended for anesthesia of the mandibular teeth and their associated periodontium and lingual soft tissue to the midline, as well as the facial soft tissue anterior to

the mandibular first molar. The buccal block is generally recommended for anesthesia of the buccal soft tissue of the mandibular molars to complete the anesthesia of a mandibular quadrant for nonsurgical periodontal therapy by the dental hygienist.

The mental block is generally recommended for anesthesia of the facial soft tissue anterior to the mental foramen, usually the mandibular anterior teeth and premolars. More commonly used than the mental block but with similar technique, the incisive block is generally recommended for anesthesia of the teeth and associated periodontium as well as facial soft tissue anterior to the mental foramen, usually the mandibular anterior teeth and premolars.

Finally, the more encompassing Gow-Gates mandibular block or GG block anesthetizes most of the mandibular nerve and is useful for extensive procedures during quadrant dentistry or with failure of the IA block.

Any pulpal anesthesia for these blocks is achieved through anesthesia of each nerve's dental branches as they extend into the pulp by way of each tooth's apical foramen (see Chapter 10). The hard and soft tissue of the periodontium are anesthetized by way of the interdental and interradicular branches for each tooth.

If quadrant dental hygiene treatment is planned on the mandible after anesthesia, the clinician must proceed with instrumentation first of the mandibular molars (third, second, and then first) and then premolars (second and then first), and finally the anterior teeth to allow for complete anesthesia of the core bundles of the last teeth in the anterior sextant of the dental arch (see Chapter 3). If half-mouth treatment is planned, the IA and buccal blocks

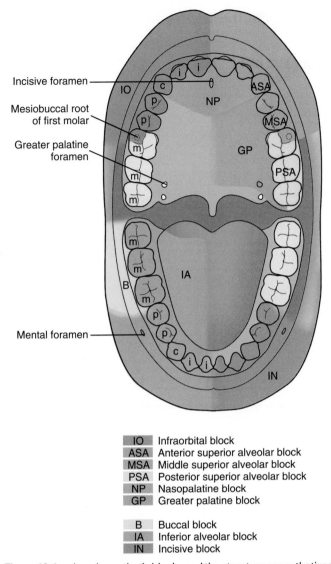

Incisive foramen

Mesiobuccal root of first molar

Greater palatine foramen

Mental foramen

IO	Infraorbital block
ASA	Anterior superior alveolar block
MSA	Middle superior alveolar block
PSA	Posterior superior alveolar block
NP	Nasopalatine block
GP	Greater palatine block

B	Buccal block
IA	Inferior alveolar block
IN	Incisive block

Figure 13-1 ■ Local anesthetic blocks and the structures anesthetized (note that the mental block and Gow-Gates mandibular block are not included; see associated figures for more clarification of these blocks). (From Fehrenbach MJ, Herring SW: *Illustrated anatomy of the head and neck*, ed 3, St Louis, 2007, Saunders.)

are given first, then the maxillary facial injections, and then palatal injections follow in order, as discussed in Chapter 12. Instrumentation, however, proceeds first on the maxillary arch, followed by the mandibular arch, allowing time for the entire mandibular arch to become completely anesthetized due to the larger length and breadth of the mandible. (See Figure 11-2.)

■ INFERIOR ALVEOLAR BLOCK

The IA block, also known as the *mandibular block*, is the most commonly used injection in dentistry, especially during restorative care but also during nonsurgical periodontal therapy (Table 13-2 and Procedure 13-1). The IA block is used when dental procedures are performed on the mandibular teeth and pulpal anesthesia is necessary. This

block also gives anesthesia of the lingual soft tissue of all the mandibular teeth, as well as anesthesia of the facial soft tissue of the mandibular anterior teeth and premolars. Because not all of the mandibular nerve is anesthetized, calling it a mandibular block is incorrect; the Gow-Gates mandibular block is a mandibular block (discussed later).

The Visual Analog Scale (VAS) of the IA block is 0–5 when the correct technique is used by the clinician; the discomfort is mainly due to the reaction of the needle near the lingual nerve (discussed later) (see Chapter 1).[3] In addition, patients may feel uncomfortable after this injection because the proprioceptor fibers that innervate the tongue and lower lip are blocked, thus numbing these structures (see Table 13-2, Figure A). Both the tongue and lower lip then feel swollen or "fat" because the neurosensory feedback is temporarily absent; patients who look in the patient mirror directly after the injection is completed will be assured that this is not the case.

Additional use of the buccal block may be considered when anesthesia of the buccal soft tissue of the mandibular molars is also necessary, which is usually the case with nonsurgical periodontal therapy by the dental hygienist. In some cases, there is overlap of the left and right incisive nerves, known as crossover-innervation. The incisive nerve is a branch of the mandibular nerve that serves the pulp of the mandibular anterior teeth. If this is the case, a bilateral IA block can be used, but it is not recommended.

Thus, bilateral IA blocks are usually avoided unless absolutely necessary. This is because bilateral mandibular injections produce complete anesthesia of the body of the tongue and floor of the mouth, which can cause difficulty with swallowing and speech, especially in patients with full or partial removable mandibular dentures, until the effects of the local anesthetic agent wear off, which may take several hours. Comprehensive dental hygiene treatment planning can usually prevent the need for bilateral IA blocks by treating the mandible in quadrants or even sextants (see Figure 11-2).

More often, the use of an incisive block or supraperiosteal injection at the apices of the mandibular anterior teeth that fail to achieve initial pulpal anesthesia may be indicated (see earlier discussion). Supraperiosteal injections on the facial surface of the anterior mandible are more successful than more posterior injections but less successful than injections over the maxillae in similar locations (see Chapter 12). Again, these differences in success rates are due to differences in the density of the facial plates of the mandible compared with those of the maxillae.

TARGET AREA AND INJECTION SITE FOR INFERIOR ALVEOLAR BLOCK

The deposit location or target area for the IA block is at the entry point of the IA nerve as it moves inferiorly to enter into the mandibular foramen, overhung anteriorly by the lingula (see Figure 13-2 and Table 13-2, Figures A and B). The adjacent anteriorly placed lingual nerve will also be

Text continued on p. 277

TABLE 13-1		Summary of Mandibular Local Anesthesia of the Teeth and Associated Structures			
MANDIBULAR TOOTH AND STRUCTURES		**IA BLOCK**	**BUCCAL BLOCK**	**MENTAL BLOCK**	**INCISIVE BLOCK**
Central incisor pulp/periodontium		X			X
Facial soft tissue		X		X	X
Lingual soft tissue		X			
Lateral incisor pulp/periodontium		X			X
Facial soft tissue		X		X	X
Lingual soft tissue		X			
Canine pulp/periodontium		X			X
Facial soft tissue		X		X	X
Lingual soft tissue		X			
First premolar pulp/periodontium		X			X
Facial soft tissue		X		X	X
Lingual soft tissue		X			
Second premolar pulp/periodontium		X			X
Facial soft tissue		X		X	X
Lingual soft tissue		X			
First molar pulp/periodontium/lingual soft tissue		X			
Buccal soft tissue			X		
Second molar pulp/periodontium/lingual soft tissue		X			
Buccal soft tissue			X		
Third molar pulp/periodontium/lingual soft tissue		X			
Buccal soft tissue			X		

IA, Inferior alveolar.
The anesthesia for anatomic variants is not included.
From Fehrenbach MJ, Herring SW: *Illustrated anatomy of the head and neck*, ed 3, St Louis, 2007, Saunders.

TABLE 13-2	Inferior Alveolar Block Review

Indications — Mandibular teeth in one quadrant

Figure A ■ Area anesthetized by inferior alveolar block.

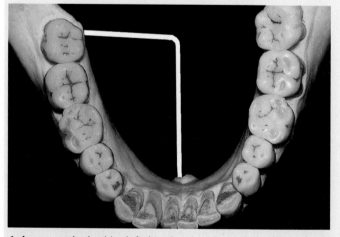

1, Area anesthetized by inferior alveolar block. (From Fehrenbach MJ, Herring SW: *Illustrated anatomy of the head and neck*, ed 3, St Louis, 2007, Saunders.)

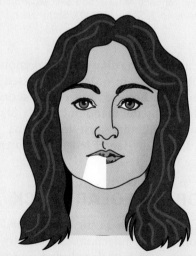

2, Facial view of anesthetic distribution after an inferior alveolar nerve block. (*2,* Modified from Jastak T, Yagiela J, Donaldson D: *Local anesthesia of the oral cavity.* St Louis, 1995, Saunders.)

TABLE 13-2	Inferior Alveolar Block Review—cont'd

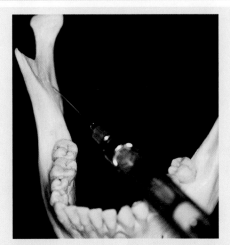

Figure B ■ Target area for inferior alveolar block. (From Fehrenbach MJ, Herring SW: *Illustrated anatomy of the head and neck*, ed 3, St Louis, 2007, Saunders.)

Nerves anesthetized	Inferior alveolar nerve Lingual nerve Mental nerve Incisive nerve
Teeth anesthetized	Mandibular teeth to midline
Other structures anesthetized	Periodontium anterior to mental foramen as well as facial gingival tissue Lingual soft tissue to midline Lower lip to midline, anterior two-thirds of tongue, and floor of the mouth
Administration technique	See Procedure 13-1
Needle gauge and length	Using 25-gauge long (smaller diameter gauge would not provide reliable aspiration and short needle would be dangerously inserted to its hub)
Operator position	Right-handed: 8–9 or 10 o'clock Left-handed: 4–3 or 2 o'clock

Figure C ■ Operator position of right-handed clinician for inferior alveolar block.

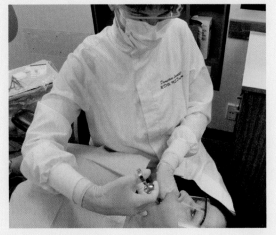

1, Right: 8–9 or 10 o'clock.

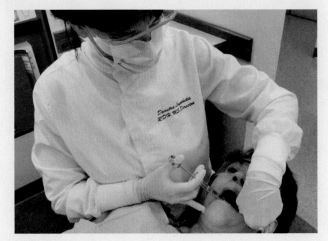

2, Left: 10 o'clock.

continued next page

TABLE 13-2   Inferior Alveolar Block Review—cont'd

Figure D ■ Syringe stabilization for inferior alveolar block

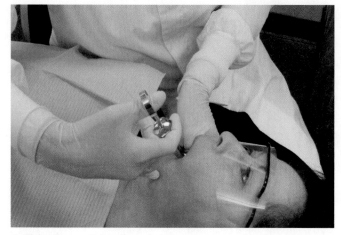

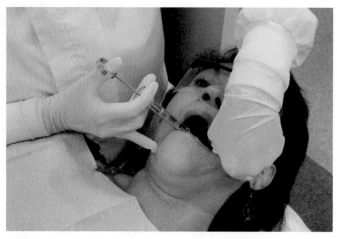

1, Pinky finger of dominant hand resting on patient's chin for right side.

2, Pinky finger of dominant hand resting on patient's chin for left side.

Landmarks	Medial surface of ramus Coronoid notch Pterygomandibular fold (raphe) Pterygomandibular space Mandibular occlusal plane Internal oblique ridge
Needle insertion point	At intersection of horizontal imaginary line and imaginary vertical line using coronoid notch and pterygomandibular fold; middle of pterygomandibular space at 6–10 mm superior to occlusal plane of mandibular molars

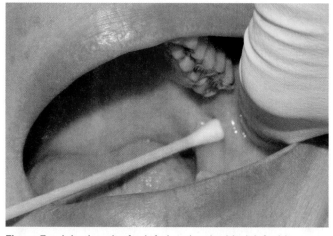

Figure E ■ Injection site for inferior alveolar block left side.

TABLE 13-2	Inferior Alveolar Block Review—cont'd
Depth of penetration	Approximately 20–25 mm or two-thirds to three-fourths the depth of long needle until bone is contacted

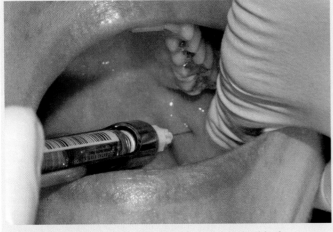

Figure F ▪ Needle penetration for inferior alveolar block demonstrated on left side. Note the three-fourths depth of long needle to reach the target location.

Deposit location	At mandibular foramen with inferior alveolar nerve
Amount of anesthetic*	Approximately 1.7 (1.8)–3.4 (3.6) mL cartridges (save some for buccal block, if needed; see Table 13-4)
Length of time to deposit	Approximately 60–120 seconds

*Approximate recommended amounts given are for 2% solutions of local anesthetic agents for adults; if using 4% solutions of local anesthetic agents, the approximate recommended amounts would be at least one-half of the amount of 2% solutions.

anesthetized as the local anesthetic agent diffuses so there is no need for a separate injection for this nerve. However, the agent must be accurately deposited within 1 mm of the target area to achieve anesthesia, which may be difficult because most of the deeper anatomy is not visible to the clinician, so surface landmarks must be relied upon. The technique discussed is also known as the *Halstead technique,* named after a medical doctor who first gave an intraoral injection of local anesthesia (1886); it is also called the *direct approach* of anesthesia for the IA nerve.

The injection site for the IA block is the mandibular tissue on the medial surface of the mandibular ramus at the height and anteroposterior direction determined for the injection (Figure 13-3; see Table 13-2, Figure E). Mainly hard tissue is used for landmarks to locate the injection site, such as the coronoid notch and the occlusal plane of the mandibular molars, to reduce errors caused by patient soft tissue variance.

The height of the injection for the IA block is determined by palpating the coronoid notch, the greatest depression on the anterior border of the ramus, which can be demonstrated using a finger or cotton tip applicator (see Figure 10-11). To determine the injection height, it helps to visualize an imaginary horizontal line that extends posteriorly from the coronoid notch to the pterygomandibular fold

as it turns upward toward the soft palate, demarcating the posterior border of the ramus (see Figure 13-4). Clinicians can palpate extraorally the posterior border of the ramus but with this intraoral technique that is not necessary.

The pterygomandibular fold extends behind the most distal mandibular molar and retromolar pad and runs horizontally to the posterior border of the mandible and then turns superior to the junction of hard and soft palates, separating the buccal mucosa from the pharynx. The pterygomandibular fold covers the deeper pterygomandibular raphe, which is located between the buccinator and superior pharyngeal constrictor muscles. This fold stretches, becoming accentuated when the patient opens the mouth wider, which is an important instruction to give to the patient when performing this block.

This imaginary horizontal line showing the height of IA block injection site is also parallel to and 6–10 mm superior to the occlusal plane of the mandibular molars in most adults. The clinician's retracting finger can be kept at this height to help maintain this level throughout the injection because being too low is the most commonly cited cause of missed IA blocks. This will also help keep the needle and syringe barrel parallel to the occlusal plane at all times to ensure correct placement of the needle tip and the agent near the mandibular foramen. Thus, it is important not to

PROCEDURE 13-1   Inferior Alveolar Block Procedure

STEP 1 Assume the correct operator position at 8 to 9 o'clock (right side) or 10 o'clock (left side) for right-handed clinician or 4 to 3 o'clock (right side) or 2 o'clock (left side) for left-handed clinician (see Table 13-2, Figure C).

STEP 2 Ask the supine patient to open his or her mouth comfortably wide. Use the index finger for intraoral retraction and thumb for extraoral retraction on dominant side and vice versa on nondominant side.

STEP 3 Prepare the alveolar mucosal tissue at the location of the pterygomandibular space, lateral to the pterygomandibular fold and the sphenomandibular ligament (see Chapter 11).

STEP 4 Using a new cotton tip applicator, palpate the coronoid notch on the anterior border of the mandible from the contralateral side, which is the greatest concavity on the anterior border of the ramus, usually superior to the mandibular second premolar, practicing the actual injection pathway (see Table 13-2, Figure E).

STEP 5 Palpate the pterygomandibular fold, the tissue that extends from behind the most distal mandibular molar and retromolar pad and horizontally to the posterior border of the mandible.

STEP 6 For the height of the injection, imagine a horizontal line that extends posteriorly from the coronoid notch to the pterygomandibular fold, as it turns upward toward the palate, marking the posterior border of the ramus. It is usually 6–10 mm superior to the occlusal plane of the mandibular molars in most adults; the inside retracting finger can be kept at this height to help maintain it throughout the injection. For anteroposterior direction, imagine a vertical line, three-fourths the distance between the coronoid notch and the posterior border of the ramus or where the pterygomandibular fold turns superior to the palate and marks the posterior border of the ramus (see Figures 13-4 and 13-5). Palpate the depression created by the pterygomandibular space and at the intersection of these two imaginary lines; note any access problems created by the pterygomandibular fold, buccal fat pad, or tongue.

STEP 7 Using a 25-gauge long needle with the bevel toward the bone and with the large window of the syringe toward the operator, direct the syringe from over the contralateral mandibular second premolar, with the syringe barrel resting on the corner of the mouth, superior and parallel to the occlusal plane.

STEP 8 Establish a fulcrum (see Table 13-2, Figure D for fulcrum recommendations).

STEP 9 Insert the needle in the deepest part of the depression created by the pterygomandibular space and at the intersection of these two imaginary lines, using any means needed if there are access problems (see Table 13-2, Figure F). Use the needle tip to depress the space further to ensure its location.

STEP 10 Advance the needle into the soft tissue until gently contacting bone of the medial surface of the ramus over the mandibular foramen; do not move the needle except in a forward pathway. This is approximately two-thirds to three-fourths the depth of the long needle (approximately 20–25 mm). Continue advancement even when the patient experiences a reaction by the lingual nerve ("lingual shock").

STEP 11 Aspirate within three planes. Due to the high vascularity in the area of anesthetic deposition, it is recommended to aspirate three times within different planes to ensure that the bevel of the needle is not abutted against the interior of a blood vessel, providing a false aspiration. To accomplish this, first aspirate as usual at the depth of penetration. If aspiration is negative, rotate the syringe barrel gently toward the operator and reaspirate; if aspiration is negative, rotate the syringe barrel gently back to the original position and aspirate again.

STEP 12 If a negative aspiration is achieved after each aspiration, slowly deposit approximately 1.7 (1.8)–3.4 (3.6) mL of solution (one to one-and-half to two cartridges) over 60–90 seconds. Aspirate in one plane after each one-fourth of the cartridge is administered. If administering a buccal block immediately following the inferior alveolar block, a small amount of solution should be saved for the buccal block (give 1.5 mL or most of the second cartridge but save the remaining approximately 0.3 mL or one-eighth of the cartridge). Maintain the height and direction of the syringe barrel throughout the injection.

STEP 13 Carefully withdraw the syringe in the same pathway as penetration, and immediately administer the buccal block (see Procedure 13-2) or carefully recap the needle using the one-handed scoop method utilizing needle sheath prop (see Chapter 11).

STEP 14 Place the patient upright or semi-upright and wait approximately 3–5 minutes until anesthesia takes effect before starting treatment. If unsuccessful or the patient feels uncomfortable during treatment, proceed with the troubleshooting injection paradigm (see Figures 13-9 and 13-10).

move the syringe barrel side to side or up and down within the tissue when dispensing the agent, nor should the syringe barrel rest on the masticatory surfaces of the mandibular teeth at any time since they can also move.

With a patient having an Angle's classification of malocclusion class II with a prognathic mandible, the clinician should insert the needle at least 1 cm more superior than the usual height of the injection. However, in children and small adults, this imaginary horizontal line for the height of the injection should be more inferior than the usual given height (around 6–10 mm) of the injection, to just at the occlusal plane of the mandibular molars. For children,

this is because the mandible has not reached its full mature size.

In contrast, are partially edentulous patients with only their mandibular anterior teeth and premolars present; the mandibular foramen may appear to be more superior than when the posterior dentition is present because the occlusal plane of molars is not present as a guide, when indeed it is at the usual height.

The anteroposterior direction of the IA block injection is achieved at the same time as the determination of the correct height of the injection. To determine this anteroposterior direction, it helps to visualize an imaginary

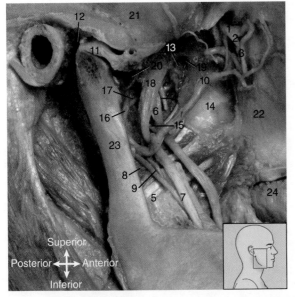

Figure 13-2 ■ Dissection of the right infratemporal fossa (after removal of the lateral pterygoid muscle, zygomatic arch, and part of mandible) to show the injection site of the inferior alveolar block (also posterior superior alveolar block as discussed in Chapter 12). *1,* Maxillary nerve; *2,* PSA nerve; *3,* PSA artery; *4,* (long) buccal nerve; *5,* medial pterygoid muscle; *6,,* lingual nerve; *7,* IA nerve; *8,* IA artery; *9,* nerve to mylohyoid muscle; *10,* maxillary artery; *11,* disc of joint and mandibular condyle; *12,* joint capsule; *13,* nerve to medial pterygoid muscle; *14,* lateral pterygoid plate; *15,* chorda tympani nerve; *16,* middle meningeal artery; *17,* accessory meningeal artery; *18,* mandibular nerve; *19,* nerve to lateral pterygoid muscle; *20,* auriculotemporal nerve; *21,* temporal bone; *22,* maxilla; *23,* mandibular ramus; *24,* tongue. (From Logan BM, Reynold PA, Hutching RT: *McMinn's color atlas of head and neck anatomy,* ed 3, London, 2004, Mosby. In Fehrenbach MJ, Herring SW: *Illustrated anatomy of the head and neck,* ed 3, St Louis, 2007, Saunders.)

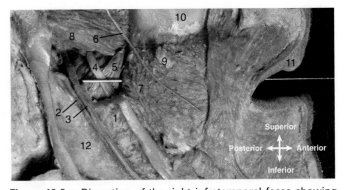

Figure 13-3 ■ Dissection of the right infratemporal fossa showing the injection site for the inferior alveolar block. *1,* Lingula; *2,* IA artery; *3,* IA nerve; *4,* lingual nerve; *5,* medial pterygoid muscle; *6,* long buccal nerve; *7,* buccinator muscle; *8,* lateral pterygoid muscle; *9,* parotid duct; *10,* maxilla; *11,* upper lip; *12,* mandibular ramus. (From Logan BM, Reynold PA, Hutching RT: *McMinn's color atlas of head and neck anatomy,* ed 3, London, 2004, Mosby. In Fehrenbach MJ, Herring SW: *Illustrated anatomy of the head and neck,* ed 3, St Louis, 2007, Saunders.)

vertical line, three-fourths of the distance between the coronoid notch and the posterior border of the ramus, demarcated by the pterygomandibular fold as it turns upward toward the soft palate (see Figure 13-4).

Thus, the injection site of the IA block is determined by the intersection of these two imaginary lines, one horizontal and one vertical, which is located at the deepest or most posterior part of the pterygomandibular space (also known as the *pterygomandibular triangle*), lateral to the pterygomandibular fold and the sphenomandibular ligament (see Table 13-2, Figure E and Figure 13-4). To accomplish this, the syringe barrel is usually superior to the contralateral mandibular second premolar, with the syringe barrel at the corner of mouth. There is a tendency for the clinician to place the syringe barrel too far forward (anterior), possibly superior to the mandibular canine, when giving the injection on the clinician's nondominant side due to poor visibility. Using a pathway directly from the corner of mouth to the injection site for both the right and left injection can help avoid this possible blind sight situation.

The needle is inserted into the soft tissue of the pterygomandibular space until the mandible is gently contacted

approximately two-thirds to three-fourths the depth of the long needle (or 20–25 mm). This may seem extra deep in comparison to injections for other blocks with less depth such as the maxillary injections, but the extra depth is necessary to gain access to the target area (Figures 13-4, 13-5, 13-6, 13-7; see Table 13-2, Figure F).

The pterygomandibular space mimics an inverted tear drop in its outer shape: the injection is given in the superior basin-like part (Figure 13-8A,B). However, the overall shape and size of the space can vary and in some cases may not be readily visible to the clinician unless it is palpated with a cotton tip applicator. Additionally, using the tip of the needle to initially depress the pterygomandibular space before fully entering the tissue may reassure the clinician that he or she has correctly located where the injection should be made (see Figure 13-8C).

The needle will naturally withdraw from the periosteum when gentle bony contact is made, so there is no need to withdraw the needle farther and possibly miss the target area. It is also usually not necessary to deposit small amounts of the local anesthetic agent as the needle enters the tissue for the IA block to anesthetize the adjacent anteriorly placed lingual nerve because anesthesia of the lingual nerve will occur through diffusion of the local anesthetic agent placed near the IA nerve. These small amounts injected early will not reduce any tissue discomfort for the patient. Administering the solution only after gentle bony contact and at the target area will provide the most anesthetic power.

Often scar tissue is present in the pterygomandibular space when there has been extensive local anesthesia procedures and/or complicated extraction of the adjacent mandibular third molar. This tissue feels firm ("tough") instead of bony hard like the medial surface of the mandible to the clinician as the needle goes through it but may still prove difficult to penetrate on the way to the injection site of the

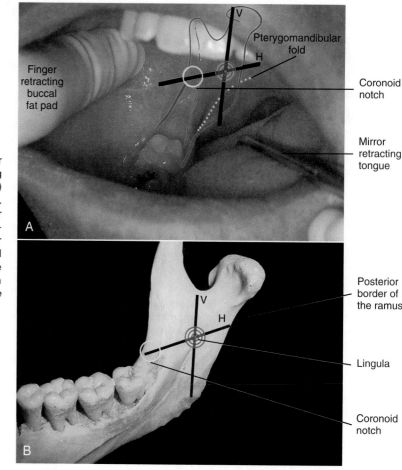

Figure 13-4 ■ A, Oral view of the pterygomandibular space showing imaginary horizontal solid line (H) showing the correct height and imaginary vertical solid line (V) showing the anteroposterior direction for the injection. The intersection of these two lines is the injection site for this block (*bull's-eye*), which is at the depth of the ptery-gomandibular space, lateral to the pterygomandibular fold (*dashed line*) and at the same height as the coronoid notch (*yellow circle*). B, Medial surface of the mandible showing the bony landmarks and imaginary lines (From Fehrenbach MJ, Herring SW: *Illustrated anatomy of the head and neck*, ed 3, St Louis, 2007, Saunders.)

mandibular foramen. It is important, therefore, to always use a sharp needle to accomplish all injections and change needles as the situation demands.

In addition, the needle may need to be used to gently deflect the laterally placed pterygomandibular fold even farther laterally if it prevents the needle from entering into the superior basin-like part of the pterygomandibular space from across the mouth. Additionally, an extensive buccal fat pad superior to the site may need to be gently deflected. Strong retraction of the tongue that lies over the space can be accomplished by assistance using a mirror (never using fingers).

Palpation with a cotton tip applicator of the pterygo-mandibular space before the injection will allow the clini-cian to note these needle access problems and be able to accommodate them in order to get to the target area. Similar to maxillary facial injections, there is no need for the clinician to shake or vibrate the tissue of the cheek to distract the patient; this action would move the needle and its bevel out of the correct pathway to the target area causing less effective administration and possible pain to the patient.

TROUBLESHOOTING INFERIOR ALVEOLAR BLOCK

Even though the IA block is the most commonly used dental injection, it is not always initially successful; failure rates are approximately 15%–20%. This may mean that the patient must be reinjected to achieve the necessary anesthe-sia of the tissue. However, the careful clinician will use a troubleshooting injection paradigm in order to achieve success. The clinician should re-assess the area visually and by palpation of the landmarks. In addition, consideration should be made to the height of the insertion point, syringe angulations, and depth of penetration. Lack of consistent success is due in part to anatomic variation in the height of the mandibular foramen on the medial side of the ramus and the great depth of soft tissue penetration required to achieve pulpal anesthesia.

To further complicate matters, not many patients are sym-metric in their anatomic positioning of structures so each paradigm for the IA block is different on each side of the patient's oral cavity. Documenting these anatomic variations as well as any technique adjustments that were implemented

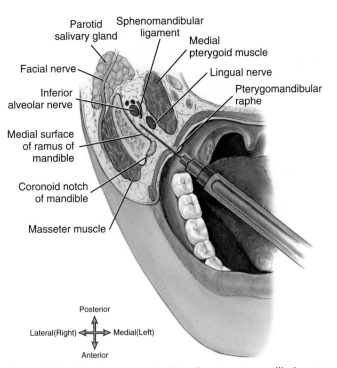

Figure 13-5 ■ Needle penetration into the pterygomandibular space (dashed line) for an inferior alveolar block. If the needle is inserted too far posteriorly, it may enter the parotid salivary gland containing the facial nerve, causing the complication of transient facial paralysis due to temporary anesthesia of the facial nerve. (From Fehrenbach MJ, Herring SW: *Illustrated anatomy of the head and neck*, ed 3, St Louis, 2007, Saunders.)

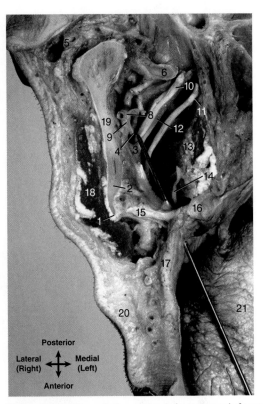

Figure 13-7 ■ Dissection of the right infratemporal fossa on a horizontal section showing the needle at the injection site for the inferior alveolar block. *1,* Coronoid notch (superior to external oblique ridge); *2,* mylohyoid line; *3,* lingula; *4,* mandibular foramen; *5,* parotid salivary gland; *6,* styloid process; *7,* maxillary artery; *8,* IA vein; *9,* IA artery; *10,* IA nerve; *11,* lingual nerve; *12,* sphenomandibular ligament; *13,* medial pterygoid muscle; *14,* long buccal nerve; *15,* temporalis muscle; *16,* pterygomandibular raphe; *17,* buccinator muscle; *18,* masseter muscle; *19,* mandibular ramus; *20,* buccal fat pad; *21,* tongue. (From Logan BM, Reynold PA, Hutching RT: *McMinn's color atlas of head and neck anatomy*, ed 3, London, 2004, Mosby. In Fehrenbach MJ, Herring SW: *Illustrated anatomy of the head and neck*, ed 3, St Louis, 2007, Saunders.)

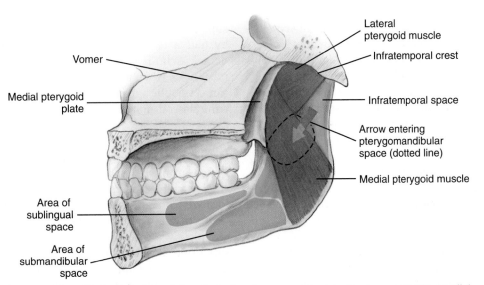

Figure 13-6 ■ Median section of the skull showing an arrow (similar to anesthetic needle) entering the pterygomandibular space (dotted line). (From Fehrenbach MJ, Herring SW: *Illustrated anatomy of the head and neck*, ed 3, St Louis, 2007, Saunders.)

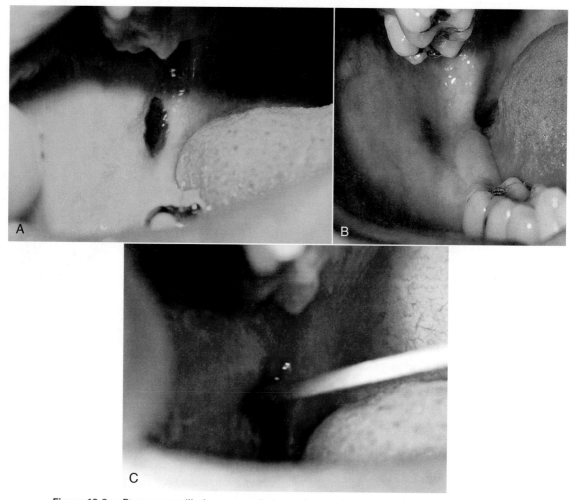

Figure 13-8 ■ Pterygomandibular space mimics an inverted tear drop; the injection site for the inferior alveolar block is in its superior basin-like part. **A,** Space has been dyed to show its depth and shape. **B,** Hematoma within the space, a possible risk of local anesthesia, again shows its most common depth and shape. **C,** Pressure with the opposite end of the cotton applicator mimics the correct needle insertion point in the pterygomandibular space. (Courtesy Margaret J. Fehrenbach, RDH, MS.)

in the patient's chart will assist the clinician in subsequent appointments. Other techniques to achieve mandibular anesthesia, such as the Gow-Gates mandibular block, may also be used when the IA block fails (discussed later). Putting the patient upright or semiupright after the injection helps the solution diffuse by gravity into the region.

If bone is contacted immediately after the needle penetrates the soft tissue, it is possible that the insertion point was too low and/or too far lateral from the pterygomandibular raphe. The clinician should remove the needle completely and re-palpate to assess the anatomical landmarks. Adjustments should be made accordingly, and the needle re-inserted.

When bone is contacted early (at half the length to less than half the depth of the long needle, or less than 16 mm) during administration of an IA block, the needle tip is located too far anterior on the ramus (Figure 13-9). Correction is made by withdrawing the needle partially or completely and bringing the syringe barrel more closely

superior to the mandibular anterior teeth; the correction is by half a tooth at a time, moving anteriorly across the dental arch. This correction moves the needle tip more posteriorly when it is newly directed or reinserted. Injections can even be given with the syringe barrel over the contralateral mandibular lateral incisor or canine in some cases.

In contrast, when the bone is not contacted even with the usual depth of penetration by the needle (two-thirds to three-fourths the length of the long needle, or 20–25 mm) when trying to administer an IA block, the needle tip is located too far posterior on the ramus (Figure 13-10). Correction is made by withdrawing the needle partially or completely and bringing the syringe barrel more closely superior to the mandibular molars; the correction is by half a tooth at a time, moving posteriorly across the dental arch. This correction moves the needle tip more anteriorly when it is newly directed or reinserted. The syringe barrel may have to press down even more on the contralateral labial

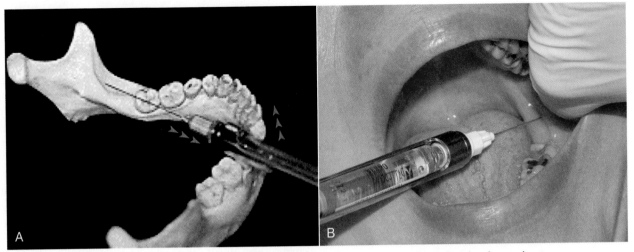

Figure 13-9 ▪ Troubleshooting inferior alveolar block. If bone is contacted early when trying to administer an inferior alveolar block, the needle tip is located too far anterior on the ramus. **A,** Correction is made by withdrawing the needle and bringing the syringe barrel more closely superior to the mandibular anterior teeth. This correction moves the needle tip more posteriorly. **B,** Intraoral view of long needle contacting bone early at approximately one-half the depth of the long needle. (**A,** Courtesy Margaret J. Fehrenbach, RDH, MS.)

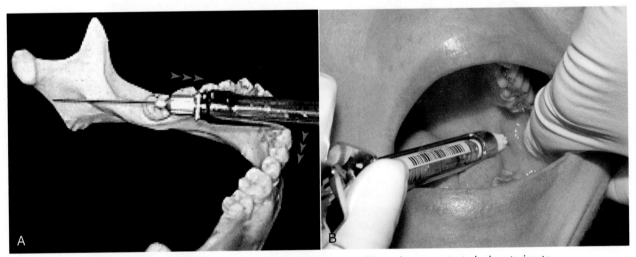

Figure 13-10 ▪ Troubleshooting inferior alveolar block. If bone is not contacted when trying to administer an inferior alveolar block, the needle tip is located too far posterior on the ramus. **A,** Correction is made by withdrawing the needle and bringing the syringe barrel more closely superior to the mandibular molars. This correction moves the needle tip more anteriorly. **B,** Intraoral view of long needle not contacting bone and needle inserted to hub. (**A,** Courtesy Margaret J. Fehrenbach, RDH, MS.)

corner of mouth when directed over the mandibular second molar so there may be some slight temporary discomfort for the patient.

At all times, it is important not to deposit the local anesthetic agent in haste if bone is not contacted on initial insertion of the needle for an IA block. The needle tip may be too posterior and thus resting within the parotid salivary gland near the seventh cranial or facial nerve, resulting in complications (see Figure 13-5).

If the insertion and deposition are too shallow and bone is not contacted but the anesthetic is given in haste, the medially located sphenomandibular ligament can become a physical barrier. The ligament can stop the important

diffusion of the local anesthetic agent to the deeper mandibular foramen and IA nerve, thus preventing the needed deeper and more profound pulpal anesthesia, allowing only the lingual nerve to be anesthetized.

If there is failure of anesthesia, mainly on the mandibular first molar, even using the troubleshooting injection paradigm, there may be accessory innervation of the mandibular teeth. Current thinking supports the mylohyoid nerve as the nerve that may be involved in this accessory mandibular innervation (see Chapter 10). To correct this problem, local anesthesia of the mylohyoid nerve using a supraperiosteal injection on the lingual border of the mandible is indicated. This reinjection technique using a supraperiosteal injection is at the apex of the mesial root of the mandibular first molar, near the mylohyoid line on the medial surface of the body of the mandible (Figure 13-11). The clinician may also want to attempt an additional block that has a higher success rate than the IA block and provides anesthesia for the mylohyoid nerve, the Gow-Gates mandibular block (discussed later).

Another reason for incomplete anesthesia following an IA block is a bifid IA nerve, which can be detected by noting a doubled mandibular canal on intraoral radiograph. In many such cases, a second mandibular foramen, more inferiorly placed, exists; studies show that it occurs in less than 1% of the population (see Chapter 10). To correct this, the local anesthetic agent is deposited more inferior to the usual anatomic landmarks for the IA block.

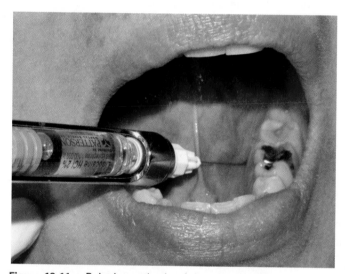

Figure 13-11 ■ Pulpal anesthesia of the mandibular first molar as well as lingual soft tissue using a supraperiosteal injection.

INDICATIONS OF SUCCESSFUL INFERIOR ALVEOLAR BLOCK AND POSSIBLE COMPLICATIONS

Indications of a successful IA block include harmless numbness and tingling of the lower lip because the mental nerve, a branch of the IA nerve, is anesthetized. This is a good indication that the IA nerve has been initially anesthetized, but it is not a reliable indicator of the depth of anesthesia, especially concerning pulpal anesthesia.

Another indication of anesthesia is harmless numbness and tingling of the body of the tongue and floor of the mouth, which indicates that the lingual nerve, a branch of the mandibular nerve, is anesthetized. Important to note is that this anesthesia of the tongue may occur without concurrent anesthesia of the IA nerve due to the barrier presented by the sphenomandibular ligament (see previous discussion of this ligament). Possibly the needle was not advanced deeply enough into the tissue to anesthetize the deeper IA nerve. It is important to remember that the most reliable indicator of a successful IA block is the absence of discomfort during dental procedures.

In addition, "lingual shock" as the needle passes by the lingual nerve (Table 13-3) may occur. The patient may make an involuntary movement, varying from a slight opening of the eyes to jumping in the chair. This reaction is only momentary, and anesthesia will quickly occur. Informing the patient that this reaction may occur before the injection can help alleviate any alarm the patient may experience. Moreover, good preanesthetic communication can help the patient understand that reactions like this are common occurrences of the anesthesia process of the mandible. The "lingual shock" occurs frequently when giving the IA block, and the clinician must be prepared to maintain control of the injection even as the patient responds to this "shock." Stable fulcrums, and slowly continuing on the intended

TABLE 13-3	Complications with Inferior Alveolar Block
COMPLICATION	**TECHNIQUE ADJUSTMENT**
Lingual shock when moving needle through tissue	Symptom is only momentary and unavoidable
Inadequate anesthesia possibly caused by depositing solution inferior to mandibular foramen	Reinject at a more superior injection site
Incomplete anesthesia of the mandibular central or lateral incisors due to crossover innervation from contralateral incisive nerve	Additionally administer supraperiosteal injection on contralateral central incisor (see Figure 13-17 and Chapter 12) or additionally administer contralateral incisive block (see Table 13-8)
Incomplete anesthesia of the mandibular first molar possibly caused by accessory innervation by the mylohyoid nerve that is not anesthetized by the inferior alveolar block	Additionally administer supraperiosteal injection with a 27-guage short needle at the apex of mandibular first molar at 3–5 mm or one-fourth the depth of needle, aspirate and deposit one fourth of cartridge over 20 seconds (see Figure 13-17 and Box 12-1)
Transient facial paralysis when facial nerve is mistakenly anesthetized due to incorrect administration of anesthetic agent into the parotid salivary gland containing the facial nerve because bone was not contacted	To prevent, always contact bone of the mandible before depositing anesthetic agent or initiating troubleshooting injection (see Figures 13-15 and 13-16)
Hematoma	Apply pressure with sterile gauze to the area if needed; reassure patient after treatment is completed

path to the target location will provide the necessary control. Trying to pull the needle out or moving the needle will not avoid the sensitive lingual nerve. In addition, trying to deposit small amounts of solution as the needle advances through the tissue to the mandibular foramen will not prevent "lingual shock" and may end up reducing the amount of agent available for anesthesia at the target area.

One serious short term complication with an IA block is transient facial paralysis if the facial nerve is mistakenly anesthetized. This can occur because of incorrect administration of anesthetic into the deeper parotid salivary gland (containing the seventh cranial or facial nerve) when the mandibular bone was not contacted. This causes temporary unilateral loss of motor function to the facial expression muscles. The patient will experience the inability to close the eyelid and drooping of the corner of lips on the affected side. The loss of motor function is temporary and fades within a few hours once the action of the anesthetic resolves. (see Chapter 14).

Because aspiration is positive in 10%–15% of cases, which is the highest positive aspiration rate of all block injections, hematoma may occur. If hematoma occurs in the area of the pterygomandibular space, it is important to let the patient see the bruising when the treatment is finished, telling him or her that it is a basic risk of anesthesia and is temporary (see Figure 13-8B, and Chapter 14).

Muscle soreness or limited movement of the mandible is rarely seen with this block. Self-inflicted trauma such as lower lip biting and resultant swelling can also occur, so notify the patient not to eat until the anesthesia wears off.

Finally, damage can occur after administration of the IA block, causing paresthesia, usually from trauma to the lingual nerve. Paresthesia is persistent anesthesia beyond the expected duration, or an altered sensation such as tingling or itching, that is beyond a normal level. Recent studies demonstrate that this paresthesia may be due to lack of adequate fascia around the lingual nerve or possibly neurotoxicity from the local anesthetic agent (see Chapter 14). Paresthesia can also occur with the spread of dental infection from a contaminated needle, but in most cases, it occurs due to problematic surgical extraction of impacted mandibular molars.

■ BUCCAL BLOCK

The buccal block or *long buccal block* is useful for anesthesia of buccal gingival tissue of the mandibular molars (Table 13-4, Figures G through K, and Procedure 13-2). Many times this block is not necessary, such as when the buccal tissue is not impacted by the dental procedures performed (such as restoration of occlusal caries). However, for nonsurgical periodontal therapy of the mandibular molars

TABLE 13-4	Buccal Block Review
Indications	Usually given immediately after inferior alveolar block to complete quadrant anesthesia

Figure G ■ Target area and distribution of anesthesia for buccal block. (From Fehrenbach MJ, Herring SW: *Illustrated anatomy of the head and neck*, ed 3, St Louis, 2007, Saunders.)

Nerves anesthetized	Long buccal nerve
Teeth anesthetized	None
Other structures anesthetized	Buccal gingival tissue of mandibular molars
Administration technique	See Procedure 13-2
Needle gauge and length	Using 25-gauge long (uses same needle since immediately after inferior alveolar block) or 27-gauge short (if given alone)

continued next page

TABLE 13-4   Buccal Block Review—cont'd

Operator position

Right-handed: 8–9 or 10 o'clock
Left-handed: 4–3 or 2 o'clock

Figure H ■ Operator position of right-handed clinician for buccal block (same as inferior alveolar block).

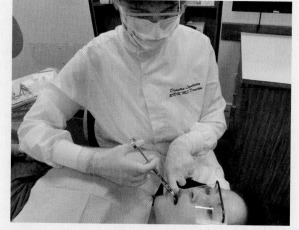

1, Right: 8 or 9 o'clock.

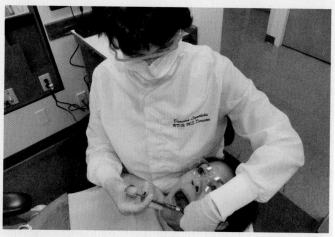

2, Left: 10 o'clock.

Figure I ■ Syringe stabilization for buccal block

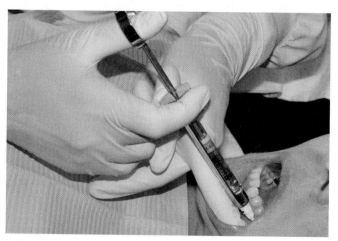

1, Retracting with index finger of nondominant hand and resting syringe barrel on top of finger.

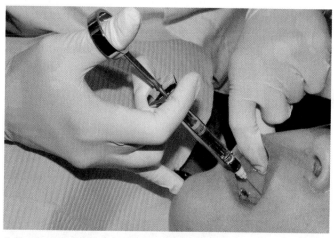

2, Resting pinky finger of dominant hand on patient's chin right side.

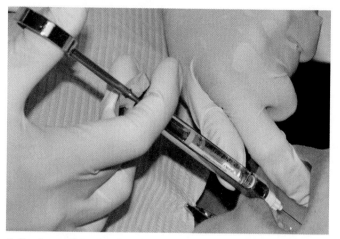

3, Resting syringe barrel on thumb of nondominant hand.

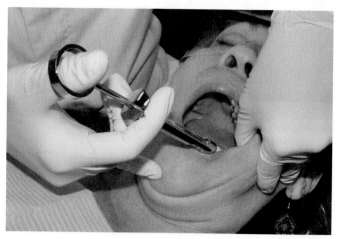

4, Resting pinky finger of dominant hand on patient's chin left side.

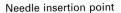 **TABLE 13-4**	**Buccal Block Review—cont'd**
Landmarks	Most distal mandibular molar Anterior border of the ramus of the mandible Occlusal plane of mandibular molars
Needle insertion point	In vestibule, distal and buccal to most distal molar in the quadrant at height of the occlusal plane

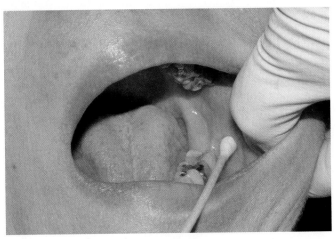

Figure J ■ Injection site for buccal block.

Depth of penetration	Approximately 1–4 mm

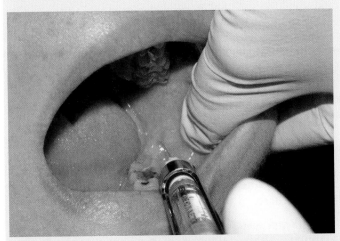

Figure K ■ Needle penetration for buccal block demonstrated on left side.

Deposit location	Long buccal nerve as it passes over the anterior border of the ramus
Amount of anesthetic *	Approximately 0.3–0.45 mL or one-eighth to one-fourth of cartridge
Length of time to deposit	Approximately 10–20 seconds

*Approximate recommended amounts given are for 2% solutions of local anesthetic agents for adults; if using 4% solutions of local anesthetic agents, the approximate recommended amounts would be at least one-half of the amount of 2% solutions.

PROCEDURE 13-2 **Buccal Block Procedure**

STEP 1 Administer the buccal block immediately following the administration of the inferior alveolar block if both are needed and keep the same operator position as the IA block (see Table 13-4, Figure H).

STEP 2 Ask supine patient to again open the mouth but not as wide as for the previous IA block. Retract the buccal soft tissue laterally, pinching it between both the index finger and thumb (as when giving the inferior alveolar block; one inner and one outer), pulling the tissue taut.

STEP 3 Prepare the alveolar mucosal tissue in the vestibule, distal and buccal to the most distal molar in the quadrant at the height of the occlusal plane because the previous inferior alveolar block will not anesthetize the buccal soft tissue (see Chapter 11).

STEP 4 Using 25-gauge long (same needle set up as the inferior alveolar block if given together) or using a 27-gauge short needle (if given alone), orient the bevel toward the bone and large window toward the operator.

STEP 5 Push the buccal fat pad into the injection site so that the bony injection will be somewhat padded, being careful to keep the retracting index finger or thumb out of the pathway of the needle.

STEP 6 Establish a fulcrum (see Table 13-4, Figures I for fulcrum recommendations).

STEP 7 Direct the syringe barrel parallel to the occlusal plane but directly superior to the mandibular molars.

STEP 8 Insert the needle into alveolar mucosal tissue distal and buccal to the most distal mandibular molar in the quadrant until gently contacting bone at a depth of 1–4 mm (see Table 13-4, Figure K).

STEP 9 Aspirate.

STEP 10 If negative aspiration is achieved, slowly deposit 0.3–0.45 mL of solution (one-third to one-fourth of cartridge) over 10–20 seconds; if the tissue balloons this is due to injecting too rapidly. The dental hygienist should stop the deposition and remove the needle or slow down the procedure.

STEP 11 Carefully withdraw the syringe and immediately recap the needle using the one-handed scoop method utilizing a needle sheath prop. (See Chapter 11.)

STEP 12 Rinse the patient's mouth and wait until anesthesia takes effect before starting treatment: approximately 3–5 minutes if given with the inferior alveolar block or 1 minute if given alone.

TABLE 13-5 **Complications with Buccal Block**

COMPLICATION	TECHNIQUE ADJUSTMENT
Leakage of solution at injection site due to bevel of needle only partially in the tissue, with bitter taste of anesthetic agent	Correct by deeper depth of penetration upon reinsertion; rinse the patient's mouth afterward
Ballooning of the tissue caused by rapid deposit of solution	Correct by slowing down injection procedure

by a dental hygienist, especially with furcation involvement and root concavities when visibility is necessary, this block is often necessary and should be administered immediately following the IA block.

This is a very successful dental block because the (long) buccal nerve is readily located on the surface of the tissue and not within bone. However, because there is bony contact with the mandible, the VAS is 2–4 if the clinician uses the correct technique, which is somewhat higher overall than the IA block, but the injection itself does not take as long (see Chapter 1).[3]

TARGET AREA AND INJECTION SITE FOR BUCCAL BLOCK

The target area for the buccal block is the (long) buccal nerve as it passes anteriorly to the anterior border of the ramus and through the buccinator muscle before it enters the buccal region (see Table 13-4, Figure G). Thus the injection site is the alveolar mucosal tissue distal and buccal to the most distal molar tooth in the arch, on the anterior border of the ramus (see Table 13-4, Figure J).

The needle is advanced until it contacts the bone of mandible, and then the injection is administered (see Table 13-4, Figure K). However, pushing or "scrunching" the softer tissue of the buccal fat pad over the injection site after initially retracting the outer cheek may make the needle

entry more comfortable to the patient. Careful placement of retraction finger or thumb away from the injection pathway will ensure safety when giving the injection.

Because the buccal tissue is so tightly adhered to the bone and the injection is quite shallow, the solution may leak out of the injection site, but rinsing the patient's mouth immediately after safely capping the needle will help reduce the bitter taste of the anesthetic agent.

INDICATIONS OF SUCCESSFUL BUCCAL BLOCK AND POSSIBLE COMPLICATIONS

Even with a successful buccal block, the patient rarely feels any symptoms because of the location and small size of the anesthetized area. There is usually only absence of discomfort with dental procedures. Self-inflicted trauma can occur as cheek bites, so it is important to notify the patient not to eat until the anesthesia wears off (Table 13-5). The complication of a hematoma rarely occurs because the rate of positive aspiration is approximately 0.7%.

❚ MENTAL BLOCK

The mental block is used to anesthetize the gingival tissue of the mandibular anterior teeth and premolars on one side (Table 13-6, Figures L through P, and Procedure 13-3). If

Text continued on p. 292

TABLE 13-6	Mental Block Review

Indications	Usually mandibular anterior teeth and premolars

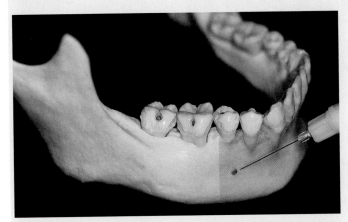

Figure L ■ Target area and distribution of anesthesia for mental block. (From Fehrenbach MJ, Herring SW: *Illustrated anatomy of the head and neck*, ed 3, St Louis, 2007, Saunders.)

Nerves anesthetized	Mental nerve
Teeth anesthetized	None
Other structures anesthetized	Facial gingival tissue from mental foramen to midline
	Lower lip and skin of chin to midline
Administration technique	See Procedure 13-3
Needle gauge and length	Using 27-gauge short

Figure M ■ Operator position for either mental or incisive block Horizontal approach	Right-handed: 8 or 9 o'clock
	Left-handed: 4 or 3 o'clock
	Vertical approach
	Right- or left-handed: 12 or 1 o'clock

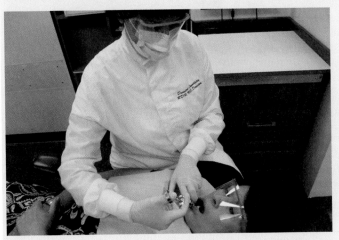

1, Horizontal approach right-handed 8 or 9 o'clock, right side.

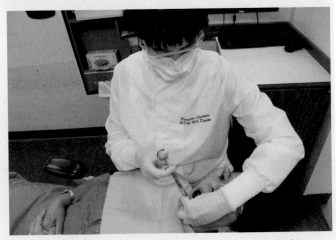

2, Horizontal approach: right-handed, 8 or 9 o'clock, left side.

continued next page

TABLE 13-6	Mental Block Review—cont'd

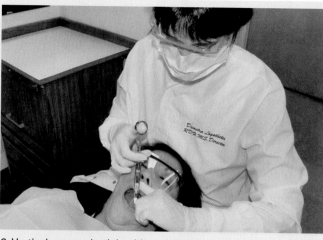

3, Vertical approach: right side or left side, 12 o'clock.

Figure N ■ Syringe stabilization for either mental or incisive block

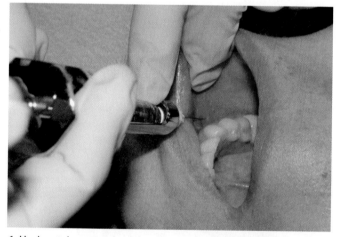

1, Horizontal approach: right side syringe barrel resting on the index finger of nondominant hand.

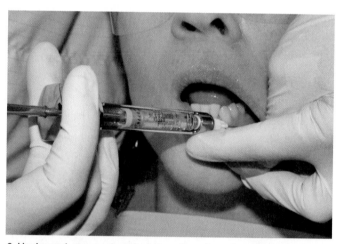

2, Horizontal approach: left side syringe barrel resting on the index finger of nondominant hand.

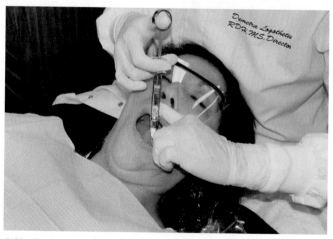

3, Vertical approach: syringe barrel resting on thumb of nondominant finger.

TABLE 13-6	**Mental Block Review—cont'd**

Landmarks	Mandibular premolars Mental foramen Mandibular mucobuccal fold

Figure O ■ Needle insertion point

Depth of mucobuccal fold anterior to mental foramen

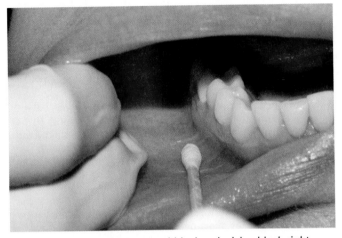

1, Injection site for either mental block or incisive block right side, horizontal approach.

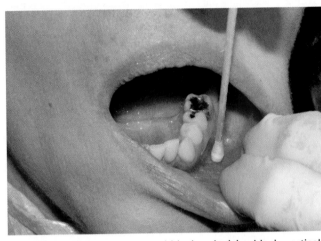

2, Injection site for either mental block or incisive block, vertical approach left side.

Figure P ■ Depth of penetration

Approximately 5–6 mm or one-fourth the depth of short needle

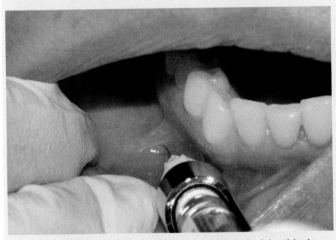

1, Needle penetration for either mental block or incisive block, horizontal approach demonstrated on right side.

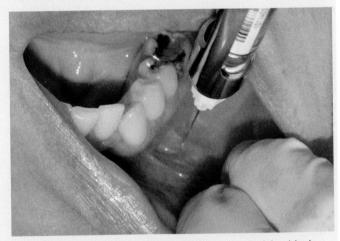

2, Needle penetration for either mental block or incisive block, vertical approach demonstrated on left side.

Deposit location	At mental foramen, between apices of mandibular premolars or location determined by radiographs and/or palpation
Amount of anesthetic*	Approximately 0.6 mL or one-third of cartridge
Length of time to deposit	Approximately 30–60 seconds

*Approximate recommended amounts given are for 2% solutions of local anesthetic agents for adults; if using 4% solutions of local anesthetic agents, the approximate recommended amounts would be at least one-half of the amount of 2% solutions.

PROCEDURE 13-3   Mental Block Procedure

STEP 1 Determine syringe approach, and assume the correct operator positioning: 8 o'clock (right side) or 9 o'clock (left side) for right-handed clinician or 4 o'clock (right side) or 3 o'clock (left side) for left-handed clinician for horizontal approach 12 or 1 o'clock for vertical approach. (See Table 13-6, Figure M.)

STEP 2 Ask supine patient to open his or her mouth and retract the lower lip outward, pulling the tissue taut; a piece of sterile gauze may be used to help retract slippery tissue.

STEP 3 Locate the mental foramen by placing cotton tip applicator in the depth of the mucobuccal fold in the area of the mandibular first molar and then palpating anteriorly until a depression is felt, usually between the apices of the mandibular premolars; radiographs may be used to assist in locating the mental foramen before palpation (see Figures 13-13 and Table 13-6, Figure O). Too much pressure on the site before the injection may be uncomfortable for the patient.

STEP 4 Prepare the alveolar mucosal tissue in the vestibule anterior to the mental foramen in the depth of the mucobuccal fold (see Chapter 11).

STEP 5 Using a 27-gauge short needle, orient the bevel toward the bone and large window toward the operator.

STEP 6 For horizontal approach, establish a fulcrum, then direct the syringe from the anterior of the mouth to the posterior in a horizontal manner, with the syringe barrel resting on the lower lip and index finger of the retraction hand (see Table 13-6, Figure N1,2). Insert the needle to the depth of the mucobuccal fold, directing the needle anterior to the mental foramen, approximately one-fourth the depth of the short needle (approximately 5–6 mm) (see Table 13-6, Figure P1). For vertical approach, establish a fulcrum using the thumb of the retraction hand (Table 13-6, Figure N3), then direct the syringe vertically with the patient's cheek toward the needle penetration site anterior to the mental foramen, approximately one-fourth the depth of the short needle (approximately 5–6 mm) (see Table 13-6, Figure P2).

STEP 7 Aspirate within two planes.

STEP 8 If negative aspiration is achieved, slowly deposit 0.6 mL or one-third of cartridge over 30–60 seconds; if the tissue balloons, the clinician is injecting too rapidly and should stop the deposition and remove the needle.

STEP 9 Carefully withdraw the syringe and immediately recap the needle using the one-handed scoop method utilizing a needle sheath prop (see Chapter 11).

STEP 10 Place the patient upright or semi-upright, rinse the mouth, and wait approximately 2–3 minutes until anesthesia takes effect before starting treatment.

---

pulpal anesthesia is necessary for the mandibular anterior teeth or premolars, administration of an incisive block (discussed later) or IA block (discussed earlier) may be considered instead.

This block also does not provide any anesthesia of the lingual gingival tissue of the involved teeth so the incisive block is more commonly used for nonsurgical periodontal therapy by the dental hygienist. However, this block may be used for maintenance or recare appointments involving the mandibular anterior teeth when neither pulpal nor lingual gingival tissue is needed, such as when dealing with Stillman's clefts that do not involve any dentinal hypersensitivity.

TARGET AREA AND INJECTION SITE FOR MENTAL BLOCK

The deposit location or target area for the mental block is anterior to where the mental nerve enters the mental foramen to merge with the incisive nerve and form the IA nerve (see Table 13-6, Figure L). The mental foramen is usually located on the surface of the mandible between the apices of the mandibular first and second premolars (Figure 13-12). The mental foramen in adults faces posterosuperiorly.

The mental foramen can be located on a radiograph before performing the block to allow for a better determination of its position during palpation (Figure 13-13). To locate the mental foramen for the mental block, palpate intraorally the depth of the mucobuccal fold between the apices of the mandibular premolars with a cotton tip applicator or at a site indicated by a radiograph

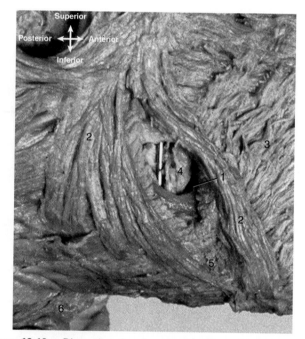

Figure 13-12 ■ Dissection showing a probe deep at the injection site for either the mental block or incisive block. *1,* Mental foramen; *2,* depressor anguli oris muscle; *3,* depressor labii inferioris muscle; *4,* mental nerve and vessels; *5,* lower chin; *6,* neck. (From Logan BM, Reynold PA, Hutching RT: *McMinn's color atlas of head and neck anatomy,* ed 3, London, 2004, Mosby. In: Fehrenbach MJ, Herring SW: *Illustrated anatomy of the head and neck,* ed 3, St Louis, 2007, Saunders.)

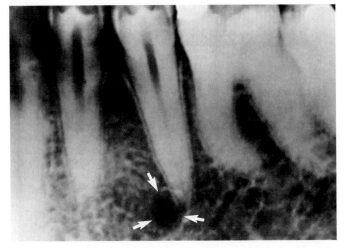

Figure 13-13 ■ Radiographs can be used to assist in locating the mental foramen. (From Darby M, Walsh M: *Dental hygiene theory and practice*, ed 3, St Louis, 2010, Saunders.)

until a depression is felt on the surface of the mandible, surrounded by smoother bone (see Table 13-6, Figure O).

However, studies show that the mental foramen can be as far posterior as the mandibular first molar or as far anterior as the distal surface of the mandibular canine, so palpation should begin as far posterior as the mandibular first molar. The patient will comment that pressure in this area produces soreness because the mental nerve is compressed against the mandible near the foramen; care must be taken not to apply too much pressure directly to the site before administration of the agent.

Currently there are two pathways or methods of anesthetizing this nerve.[4-6] The syringe barrel can either be directed from the anterior of the mouth to the posterior in a horizontal manner, with the syringe barrel resting on the lower lip, or vertically aligned with the patient's cheek with needle being inserted parallel with the long axis of the tooth. Both techniques provide the necessary anesthesia. However, the horizontal pathway is the preferred method because it keeps the syringe out of the patient's line of sight and offers a psychological advantage over the vertical approach. In addition, it offers a direct view of the large window during aspiration.

The needle insertion point for a mental block is anterior to the depression created by the mental foramen at the depth of the mucobuccal fold (see Figures 12-2 and Table 13-6, Figure O). The needle is advanced without contacting mandibular bone, and then the injection is administered (see Table 13-6, Figure P).

There is no need to enter the mental foramen to achieve anesthesia, in fact, the needle cannot enter the mandibular canal using the recommended positions of the needle. Using the horizontal angulation approach, the clinician sits more along the side of the patient, where visibility is better and the patient does not see the needle. The vertical angulation approach recommends that the clinician sit behind the patient, which may alarm the patient if he or she sees the

TABLE 13-7	Complication with Mental Block
PROBLEM	**TECHNIQUE ADJUSTMENT**
Hematoma	Apply pressure with gauze to the area

syringe; however, asking patients to close their eyes may alleviate this problem. Studies show that putting the patient upright or semi-upright after the injection helps with the diffusion of the solution by gravity into the region.

INDICATIONS OF SUCCESSFUL MENTAL BLOCK AND POSSIBLE COMPLICATIONS

The indications of a successful mental block are harmless numbness and tingling of the lower lip and absence of discomfort during dental procedures. The complication of a hematoma rarely occurs even though positive aspiration is approximately 5.7%, the second highest rate of all the block injections (Table 13-7).

■ INCISIVE BLOCK

The incisive block anesthetizes the pulp and periodontium of the mandibular teeth anterior to the mental foramen, usually the mandibular premolars and anterior teeth, as well as the facial gingival tissue (Table 13-8, Figure Q, and Procedure 13-4). If anesthesia of the lingual gingival tissue is necessary, an IA block would be administered instead because the incisive block does not provide any lingual tissue anesthesia. An additional supraperiosteal injection of the lingual tissue may also be considered (see Figure 13-11).

The incisive block has a high success rate because the incisive nerve is readily accessible. This block is useful when there is crossover innervation of the contralateral incisive nerve and there is still discomfort on the mandibular anterior teeth after giving an IA block, as well as when performing nonsurgical periodontal therapy on a maintenance case with sensitive mandibular anterior teeth from previous care or if the patient does not have any posterior teeth. The injection is also very useful on the more difficult nonsurgical periodontal therapy cases that are treated by the dental hygienist in sextants (see Figure 11-2A).

TARGET AREA AND INJECTION SITE FOR INCISIVE BLOCK

The target area for the incisive block is the same as the mental block: anterior to where the mental nerve enters the mental foramen to merge with the incisive nerve and form the IA nerve (see Table 13-8, Figure Q).

The mental foramen is usually located on the surface of the mandible between the apices of the mandibular first and second premolars. The mental foramen in adults faces posterosuperiorly. The mental foramen can be located on a radiograph before performing the block to allow for a better determination of its position during palpation. To locate

TABLE 13-8	Incisive Block Review

Indications

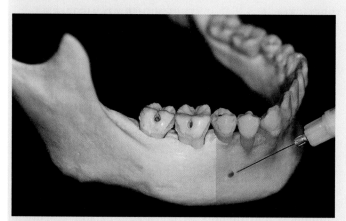

Figure Q ▪ Target area and distribution of anesthesia for incisive block. (From Fehrenbach MJ, Herring SW: *Illustrated anatomy of the head and neck*, ed 3, St Louis, 2007, Saunders.)

	Usually mandibular anterior teeth and premolars; when the anesthesia provided for inferior alveolar block is not needed (no scheduled mandibular molars instrumentation)
Nerves anesthetized	Mental nerve Incisive nerve
Teeth anesthetized	Mandibular teeth anterior to mental foramen
Other structure anesthetized	Periodontium of anesthetized teeth and facial gingival tissue from mental foramen to midline Lower lip and skin of chin to midline
Administration technique	See Procedure 13-3
Needle gauge and length	Using 27-gauge short
Operator position (see Table 13-6, Figure M)	Horizontal approach: Right-handed: 8 or 9 o'clock Left-handed: 4 or 3 o'clock Vertical approach: 12 or 1 o'clock
Syringe stabilization (see Table 13-6, Figures N)	1, Horizontal approach: right side of syringe barrel resting on index finger of retraction hand 2, Horizontal approach: left side of syringe barrel resting on index finger of retraction hand 3, Vertical approach: syringe barrel resting on thumb of retraction finger
Landmarks	Mandibular premolars Mental foramen Mandibular mucobuccal fold
Needle insertion point (see Table 13-6, Figure O)	Depth of mucobuccal fold anterior to mental foramen
Depth of penetration (see Table 13-6, Figure P)	Approximately 5–6 mm or one-fourth the depth of short needle
Deposit location	At mental foramen, between apices of mandibular premolars or location determined by radiographs and/or palpation
Amount of anesthetic*	Approximately 0.6–0.9 mL or one-third to one-half of cartridge
Length of time to deposit	Approximately 30–60 seconds

*Approximate recommended amounts given are for 2% solutions of local anesthetic agents for adults; if using 4% solutions of local anesthetic agents, the approximate recommended amounts would be at least one-half of the amount of 2% solutions.

the mental foramen for the mental block, palpate with a cotton tip applicator intraorally the depth of the mucobuccal fold between the apices of the mandibular premolars or at a site indicated by a radiograph until a depression is felt on the surface of the mandible, surrounded by smoother bone (see Figure 13-13 and Table 13-6, Figure O).

However, studies show that the mental foramen can be as far posterior as the mandibular first molar or as far anterior as the distal surface of the mandibular canine, so it is wise to start palpating for it as far posterior as the first molar. The patient will comment that pressure in this area produces soreness as the mental nerve is compressed against

PROCEDURE 13-4   Incisive Block Procedure

STEP 1 Determine syringe approach, and assume the correct operator positioning at 8 o'clock (right side) or 9 o'clock (left side) for right-handed clinician or 4 o'clock (right side) or 3 o'clock (left side) for left-handed clinician for horizontal approach or 12 or 1 o'clock for vertical approach (see Table 13-6, Figure M).

STEP 2 Ask supine patient to open their mouth and retract the lower lip outward, pulling the tissue taut; a piece of sterile gauze may be used to help retract slippery tissue.

STEP 3 Locate the mental foramen by placing cotton applicator tip in the depth of the mucobuccal fold in the area of the mandibular first molar and palpating anteriorly until a depression is felt, usually between the apices of the mandibular premolars. Radiographs may be used to assist in locating the mental foramen before palpation (see Figures 13-13 and Table 13-6, Figure O). Too much pressure on the site before the injection may be uncomfortable for the patient.

STEP 4 Prepare the alveolar mucosal tissue anterior to the mental foramen in the depth of the mucobuccal fold (see Chapter 11).

STEP 5 Using a 27-gauge short needle, orient the bevel toward the bone and large window toward the operator.

STEP 6 For horizontal approach, establish a fulcrum, then direct syringe from the anterior of the mouth to the posterior in a horizontal manner, with the syringe barrel resting on the lower lip and index finger of the retraction hand (see Table 13-6, Figure N1,2). Insert the needle to the depth of the mucobuccal fold, directing the needle anterior to the mental foramen, approximately one-fourth the depth of the short needle (approximately 5–6 mm) (see Table 13-6, Figure P1). For vertical approach, establish a fulcrum using the thumb (Table 13-6, Figure N3) of the retraction hand, then direct the syringe vertically with the patient's cheek toward the needle penetration site anterior to the mental foramen, approximately one-fourth the depth of the short needle (approximately 5–6 mm) (see Table 13-6, Figure P2).

STEP 7 Aspirate within two planes.

STEP 8 If negative aspiration is achieved, slowly deposit 0.6–0.9 mL or one-third to one-half of the cartridge over 30–60 seconds; if the tissue balloons, the clinician is injecting too rapidly and should stop the deposition and remove the needle.

STEP 9 Carefully withdraw the syringe and immediately recap the needle using the one-handed scoop method utilizing a needle sheath prop (see Chapter 11).

STEP 10 Place the patient upright or semi-upright and apply firm pressure intraorally to the injection site for a minimum of 2 minutes to assist the solution into the mental foramen and then rinse the patient's mouth.

STEP 11 (Optional) If anesthesia of the lingual periodontium is necessary in the area of the incisive block, an additional supraperiosteal injection can be administered by inserting a 27-gauge short needle at the apex of the selected tooth or teeth and slowly depositing 0.6–0.9 mL or one-third to one-half of a cartridge over 30–60 seconds (see Figure 13-11 and Procedure 12-1).

STEP 12 Wait approximately 2–3 minutes until anesthesia takes effect before starting treatment.

the mandible near the foramen, so care must be taken not to apply too much pressure to the site before administering the agent.

The syringe barrel can either be directed from the anterior of the mouth to the posterior in a horizontal manner, with the syringe barrel resting on the lower lip, or vertically aligned with the patient's cheek, in the same manner as the mental block. As with the mental block, the horizontal approach is the preferred method. The injection site for an incisive block is anterior to the depression created by the mental foramen in the depth of the mucobuccal fold (see Figure 12-2 and Table 13-6, Figure O). The needle is advanced without contacting the mandible, and then the injection is administered (see Table 13-6, Figure P).

It is not necessary to have the needle enter the mental foramen to achieve anesthesia, in fact, the needle cannot enter the mandibular canal using the recommended positions of the needle. However, more local anesthetic agent is deposited within the tissue for the incisive block than for the mental block, and gentle pressure to the site is applied intraorally after the injection. This pressure given by soothing massage of the area for at least 2 minutes forces more local anesthetic agent into the mental foramen, thus anesthetizing first the shallow mental nerve and then the deeper incisive nerve.

Anesthesia of the tissue innervated by the mental nerve will precede that of the deeper incisive nerve's tissue; thus the soft tissue anesthesia precedes pulpal anesthesia so the careful clinician needs to wait for the latter when instrumenting sensitive root surfaces. Also putting the patient upright or semi-upright after the injection and then gently applying recommended pressure to the mental foramen has shown in studies to help with further diffusion of the solution by gravity into the region.

INDICATIONS OF SUCCESSFUL INCISIVE BLOCK AND POSSIBLE COMPLICATIONS

The indications of a successful incisive block are the same as those for a mental block, except that there is pulpal anesthesia of the involved teeth. Thus, there is no discomfort during dental procedures. As with a mental block, it has the same percentage of positive aspiration, approximately 5.7%, the second highest rate of all the block injections, but still a hematoma rarely occurs (Table 13-9).

■ GOW-GATES MANDIBULAR BLOCK

The Gow-Gates mandibular block or GG block is a mandibular block because it anesthetizes almost the entire V_3 or mandibular nerve. Thus, the nerves anesthetized with a

TABLE 13-9	**Complications with Incisive Block**
COMPLICATION	**TECHNIQUE ADJUSTMENT**
Inadequate anesthesia due to inadequate volume of anesthetic into mental foramen or inadequate duration of pressure over the mental foramen after injection	Correct by reinjecting in correct location with additional anesthetic agent and applying firm pressure to deposition site for a minimum of 2 minutes
Hematoma	Apply pressure with gauze to the area, if needed

GG block are the IA, mental, incisive, lingual, mylohyoid, auriculotemporal, and (long) buccal nerves in most patients (Table 13-10, Figures R through U, and Procedure 13-5).

The GG block is indicated for use in quadrant dentistry in which the buccal soft tissue anesthesia from most distal molar to midline and anesthesia of both the pulp and periodontium is necessary, and in some cases in which a conventional IA block is unsuccessful. Thus, one of the major advantages of the block is that its success rate is higher than that of an IA block, even taking into account a slightly more complicated procedure. Studies show that its success may be related to the block providing anesthesia to the mylohyoid nerve that has been shown to be involved in failure of the IA block (see earlier discussion).

TARGET AREA AND INJECTION SITE FOR GOW-GATES MANDIBULAR BLOCK

The target area for the GG block is the anteromedial border of the neck of the mandibular condyle, just inferior to the insertion of the lateral pterygoid muscle (see Table 13-10, Figure S). The injection site is located intraorally on the oral mucosa on the medial surface of the mandibular ramus, just distal to the height of the mesiolingual cusp of the maxillary second molar, following an imaginary line extraorally from the ipsilateral intertragic notch of the ear (lower border of the tragus) to the ipsilateral corner of mouth (Figure 13-14).

The extraoral landmarks of the intertragic notch and corner of the mouth are first located (see Table 13-10, Figure T). The condyle assumes a more frontal position with the mouth open, and the injection site is closer to the mandibular nerve trunk, which is preferred for this injection. In contrast, with a more closed mouth, the condyle will move out of the injection site and the soft tissue will become thicker thus preventing effective anesthesia. Later after the injection, leaving the mouth open until inferior nerve anesthesia occurs is important until the diffusion of the agent occurs, since the open mouth allows the IA nerve to be closer to the injection site at the neck of the mandibular condyle.

Initially the needle is used to determine the height for the injection by placing the needle just inferior to the mesiolingual cusp of the maxillary second molar site. The needle is then placed distal to the maxillary second molar, maintaining the established height (Figure 13-15). The syringe barrel is maintained over the contralateral mandibular canine-to-premolar region, such that the direction of the syringe barrel parallels an imaginary line connecting the ipsilateral corner of the mouth (labial commissure) and the ipsilateral intertragic notch (Figure 13-14).

The needle is then inserted parallel to the determined imaginary line until bony contact is made with the neck of the mandibular condyle, and the injection is administered (see Table 13-10, Figure U). The needle naturally withdraws from the periosteum when bony contact is made, so there is no need to withdraw further as recommended by some clinicians and miss the target area.

The height of insertion is more superior to the mandibular occlusal plane than that of an IA block, around 10–25 mm, depending on the patient's size. When a maxillary third molar is present, the site of injection is just distal to that tooth.

INDICATIONS OF SUCCESSFUL GOW-GATES MANDIBULAR BLOCK AND POSSIBLE COMPLICATIONS

With a successful GG block, the mandibular teeth to midline, and the buccal and lingual periodontium will be numb. In addition, the anterior two-thirds of the tongue, floor of mouth, and body of the mandible and inferior ramus, as well as the facial skin over the zygomatic bone and the posterior buccal and temporal regions, are also numb.

The two main disadvantages of the GG block are the numbness of the lower lip, as well as the temporal and buccal regions, and the longer time necessary for the anesthetic to take effect (see earlier discussion). Thus this block may be contraindicated in a patient who may not be willing to undergo increased soft tissue anesthesia or wait time. The increased time of onset is due to the larger size of the nerve trunk being anesthetized and the distance of the trunk from the site of deposition, which is 5–10 mm.

However, another advantage is that the injection also lasts longer than the IA block, because the area of the injection is less vascular and a larger volume of anesthetic may be used; thus this block may be contraindicated for certain patients who do not like the feeling of numbness to last too long. However, in more advanced cases of periodontal disease with its increased levels of dentinal hypersensitivity and postinstrumentation bleeding, this longer anesthesia may be useful.

This block is also contraindicated in patients with limited ability to open the mouth, but trismus is rarely a complication (Table 13-11 and see Chapter 14). With less than 2% positive aspiration, hematoma is also rare.

TABLE 13-10	Gow-Gates Mandibular Block Review

Indications

When inferior alveolar block is unsuccessful or extensive quadrant coverage is needed for procedures since anesthetizes almost all of mandibular nerve

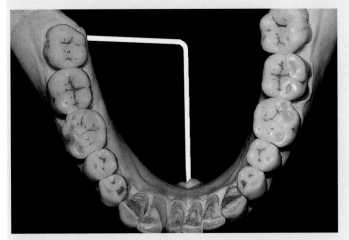

Figure R ■ Area anesthetized by Gow-Gates mandibular block. (From Fehrenbach MJ, Herring SW: *Illustrated anatomy of the head and neck*, ed 3, St Louis, 2007, Saunders.)

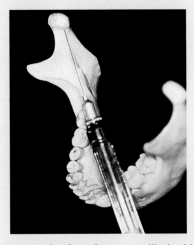

Figure S ■ Target area for Gow-Gates mandibular block. (From Fehrenbach MJ, Herring SW: *Illustrated anatomy of the head and neck*, ed 3, St Louis, 2007, Saunders.)

Nerves anesthetized	Auriculotemporal nerve
	Inferior alveolar nerve
	Mylohyoid nerve
	Lingual nerve
	Long buccal nerve
	Mental nerve
	Incisive nerve
Teeth anesthetized	Mandibular teeth to midline
Other structures anesthetized	Periodontium of anesthetized teeth as well as both buccal and lingual gingival tissue to midline overlying teeth
	Lower lip to midline, anterior two thirds of tongue and floor of the mouth
	Skin over zygomatic bone and posterior part of buccal and temporal regions
Administration technique	See Procedure 13-5
Needle gauge and length	Using 25-gauge long
Operator position	Right-handed: 8 o'clock
	Left-handed: 4 o'clock

continued next page

TABLE 13-10	Gow-Gates Mandibular Block Review—cont'd
Syringe stabilization	Resting the dominant hand on patient's chin
Landmarks	Extraoral: Intertragic notch (lower border of the tragus) Corner of mouth (labial commissure) Intraoral: Mesiolingual cusp of maxillary second molar Soft tissue just distal to maxillary second molar
Needle insertion point	Oral mucosa on medial surface of mandibular ramus, just distal to height of mesiolingual cusp of maxillary second molar

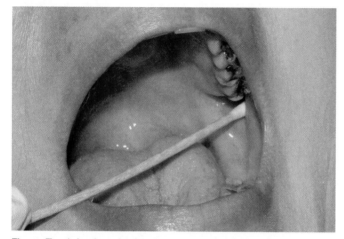

Figure T ▪ Injection site for Gow-Gates mandibular block.

Depth of penetration	Approximately 25 mm or three-fourths the depth of long needle until bone is contacted

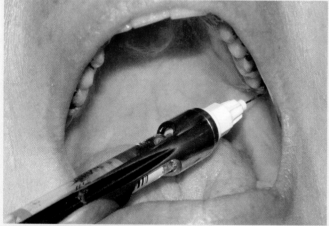

Figure U ▪ Needle penetration for Gow-Gates mandibular block demonstrated on left side.

Deposit location	Anteromedial border of neck of mandibular condyle, just inferior to insertion of lateral pterygoid muscle
Amount of anesthetic*	Approximately 1.7 (1.8) mL or full cartridge
Length of time to deposit	Approximately 60–120 seconds

*Approximate recommended amounts given are for 2% solutions of local anesthetic agents for adults; if using 4% solutions of local anesthetic agents, the approximate recommended amounts would be at least one-half of the amount of 2% solutions.

PROCEDURE 13-5   Gow-Gates Mandibular Block Procedure

STEP 1 Assume the correct operator positioning at 8 o'clock for right-handed clinician or 4 o'clock for left-handed clinician.

STEP 2 Locate the extraoral landmarks: intertragic notch (lower border of the tragus) and corner of mouth. Ask the supine patient to open his or her mouth. Visualize the intraoral landmarks: mesiolingual cusp of maxillary second molar and soft tissue just distal to the maxillary second molar (see Table 13-10, Figure S).

STEP 3 Prepare the alveolar mucosal tissue at the injection site. (See Chapter 11.)

STEP 4 Using a 25-gauge long needle, orient the bevel of the needle toward the bone and large window toward the operator and then direct the syringe over the contralateral mandibular canine-to-premolar region, such that the angulation of the syringe parallels an imaginary line connecting the ipsilateral corner of mouth and the lower border of the tragus (intertragic notch). Initially the needle is placed just inferior to the mesiolingual cusp of the maxillary second molar to determine the height for the injection (see Figures 13-14 and Table 13-10, Figure T).

STEP 5 The needle is next placed distal to the maxillary second molar, maintaining the established height (see Figure 13-15).

STEP 6 Establish a fulcrum by resting the syringe barrel on the patient's chin.

STEP 7 The height of insertion is superior to the mandibular occlusal plane, which more superior than that of an IA block, around 10–25 mm, depending on the patient's size. When a maxillary third molar is present, the site of injection is just distal to that tooth. The needle is inserted parallel to the determined imaginary line until gentle bony contact is made with the neck of the condyle (see Table 13-10, Figure U).

STEP 8 Aspirate within two planes.

STEP 9 If negative aspiration is achieved, slowly deposit 1.8 mL or one cartridge over 60–120 seconds.

STEP 10 Carefully withdraw the syringe and immediately recap the needle using the one-handed scoop method utilizing a needle sheath prop (see Chapter 11).

STEP 11 The patient should continue to keep his or her mouth open for 2 minutes until indications of inferior alveolar nerve anesthesia are present.

STEP 12 Wait approximately 5 minutes or more until anesthesia takes effect before starting treatment.

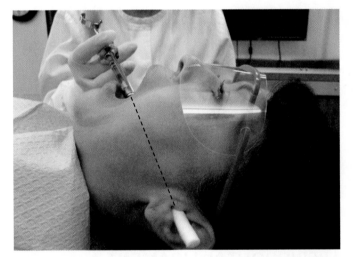

Figure 13-14 ▪ Extraoral line that is used to estimate the pathway for the Gow-Gates mandibular block. The line extends from the intertragic notch of the ear to the ipsilateral corner of the mouth.

MANDIBULAR SUPRAPERIOSTEAL INJECTION

Incomplete anesthesia of the central or lateral incisors following an IA, mental, or incisive block may be due to crossover-innervation or overlap of terminal fibers of the contralateral inferior incisive nerve (nonanesthetized incisive nerve) (Figure 13-16). This is similar to the crossover-innervation of the anterior superior alveolar (ASA) nerve on the maxillary arch. Sensory innervation from the contralateral nerve may cause pain on the mandibular anterior teeth. Because the bone is less dense on the

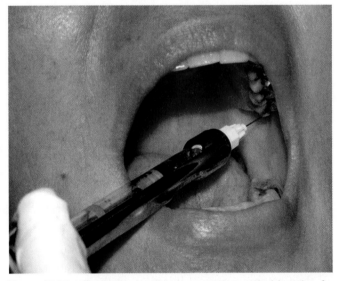

Figure 13-15 ▪ Using the needle to assess the vertical location for the Gow-Gates mandibular block by placing the needle just inferior to the mesiolingual cusp of the maxillary second molar. Note that the syringe barrel is over the contralateral mandibular canine-to-premolar region. (From Fehrenbach MJ, Herring SW: *Illustrated anatomy of the head and neck,* ed 3, St Louis, 2007, Saunders.)

TABLE 13-11	Complications with Gow-Gates Mandibular Block
COMPLICATION	**TECHNIQUE ADJUSTMENT**
Hematoma	Apply pressure with gauze to the area, if needed; reassure patient after treatment is completed

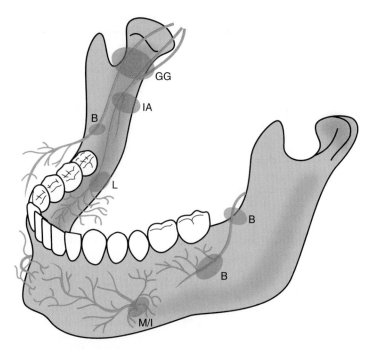

Figure 13-16 ■ An example of crossover-innervation of the mandibular arch at midline and anesthetic deposition sites for mandibular anesthesia demonstrated by circles. (GG = Gow-Gates, IA = inferior alveloar, B = buccal, L = lingual, M/I = mental/incisive.)

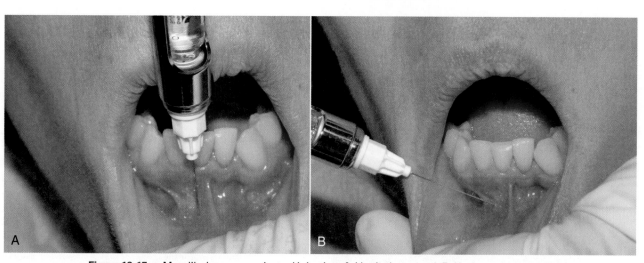

Figure 13-17 ■ Mandibular supraperiosteal injection: **A,** Vertical approach **B,** Horizontal approach

mandibular anterior teeth than on the mandibular posterior teeth, a supraperiosteal injection may be more successful than a supraperiosteal injection on the posterior teeth (see earlier discussion).

To correct this, a supraperiosteal injection for the mandibular central incisor is administered in this situation. The injection site is in the depth of the mucobuccal fold inferior to the apex of the mandibular central incisor in the contralateral quadrant than the administered IA block. This will anesthetize the terminal nerve fibers crossing over from the other side. This can be accomplished using a horizontal or vertical or approach similar to that used for the mental or incisive nerve blocks with the horizontal approach being preferred (Figure 13-17). For more information on a supraperiosteal injection, see Chapter 12. Administering an incisive block will also accomplish the same effect (see earlier discussion).

PERIODONTAL LIGAMENT INJECTION

Periodontal ligament (PDL) injection is considered a supplemental injection used when pulpal anesthesia is indicated on a single tooth mainly in the mandibular arch; the injection can also be used on the maxillary arch but is rarely used. Because of the density of the facial plate of the mandible, supraperiosteal injections are usually unsuccessful predominantly in the posterior region. As an anesthetic option, this injection is administered directly into the periodontium of the tooth to be anesthetized, providing pulpal anesthesia along with the lingual and buccal mucosa without causing numbness of the tongue or lower lip (Table 13-12, Figure V).

Use of a computer-controlled delivery device (CCDD) may be warranted since it slowly delivers the anesthetic

TABLE 13-12   Periodontal Ligament Injection Review

Indications	Pulpal anesthesia of one or two teeth in the quadrant
Nerves anesthetized	Terminal nerve endings at site of injection
Teeth anesthetized	Individual tooth at site of deposition
Other structures anesthetized	Associated periodontium
Administration technique	See Procedure 13-6
Needle gauge and length	27 gauge short or extra-short (may need to bend the needle for better access especially for posterior teeth)
Operator position	Varies with different teeth, clinician should position self with greatest visibility
Syringe stabilization	Against the patient's teeth, lips, or face
Landmarks	Root(s) of the tooth Periodontal tissues
Needle insertion point	Long axis of tooth either mesial or distal with one rooted tooth, and mesial and distal for multirooted tooth
Depth of penetration	Until reach the depth of gingival sulcus

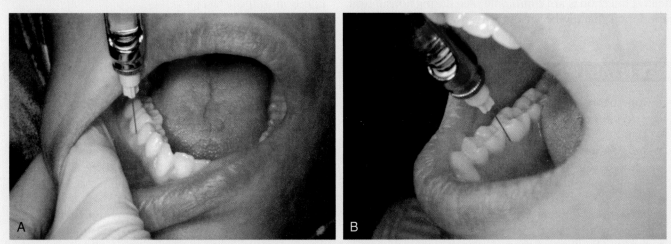

Figure V ■ Periodontal ligament injection. **A,** Buccal. **B,** Lingual. (From Malamed S: *Handbook of local anesthesia*, ed 5, St Louis, 2004, Mosby.)

Deposit location	Depth of gingival sulcus until resistance is met
Amount of anesthetic	0.2 m, one stopper full

TABLE 13-13   Advantages and Disadvantages of PDL Injection

ADVANTAGES	DISADVANTAGES
• Single dose and minimal volume of anesthetic and hemostatic agent, which is a consideration with medically compromised patients since there is a decreased risk of toxicity (0.2 mL) • Minimizes bleeding in the localized area of treatment • Alternative when other methods are ineffective • Postoperative complications are unlikely such as paresthesia since the lingual nerve is not anesthetized in most cases • Absence of lower lip or tongue numbness, which is particularly beneficial to children and mentally challenged patients so as to decrease risk of self-inflicted trauma • No postinjection discomfort due to absence of numbness of the lower lip and tongue	• Contraindicated in areas with localized infection or severe inflammation such as with periodontal disease or severe caries * • Short duration of pulpal anesthesia when patient may need it due to dentinal hypersensitivity • Excessive pressure needed for the injection may cause tissue damage and posttreatment soreness or may cause breakage of cartridge in standard syringe • Needle placement may be difficult without experience and with certain crowded dentitions or if patient has lost interdental bone • Anesthetic agent may leak into the patient's mouth causing a bitter taste, especially without adequate levels of interdental bone

*Most common reason cited for not using during nonsurgical periodontal therapy unless outweighed by the advantages such as medical history of the patient

| **PROCEDURE 13-6** | **Periodontal Ligament Injection Procedure** |

STEP 1 Assemble the standard syringe with a 27- gauge short or extra-short needle or use computer-controlled delivery device with a short needle after careful consideration of the situation.

STEP 2 Patient operator position varies from tooth to tooth.

STEP 3 Needle insertion point is the long axis of the tooth on the mesial or distal surface at a 30° angle.

STEP 4 Target location is the depth of the gingival sulcus

STEP 5 Direct syringe using appropriate fulcrum along the long axis of the tooth to be anesthetized until the depth of the sulcus is reached and resistance is felt. (see Table 13-12, Figure V)

STEP 6 Exert pressure on the syringe and administer 0.2 mL (one stopper of anesthetic agent).

STEP 7 Carefully withdraw the syringe and immediately recap the needle, using the one-handed scoop method utilizing a needle sheath prop (see Chapter 11).

STEP 8 Rinse the patient's mouth.

STEP 9 Onset of action is immediate and treatment may commence.

Note that multirooted teeth require a PDL injection for each root present.

agent, but standard local anesthetic syringes may also be used, typically with short needles. Table 13-13 lists the advantages and disadvantages of the PDL injection, and see Procedure 13-6 for administration technique. In most cases, the PDL injection is not commonly used during nonsurgical periodontal therapy because it is contraindicated in areas of infection or inflammation at the injection site such as with periodontal disease. Instead nerve blocks or supraperiosteal injections are used since the advantages of these two methods outweigh any advantages of the PDL injection in most cases.

DENTAL HYGIENE CONSIDERATIONS

- Supraperiosteal injections of the mandible are not as successful as that of the maxillae because overall the mandible is denser than the maxillae.

- Supraperiosteal injections are more effective on the mandible on the anterior teeth, and can be administered for crossover-innervation if needed.

- Substantial variation exists in the anatomy of local anesthetic landmarks of the mandibular bone and nerves complicating mandibular anesthesia.

- For quadrant dental hygiene treatment on the mandible, the clinician must proceed with instrumentation first of the mandibular molars (third, second, and then first) and then premolars (second and then first), and finally the anterior teeth to allow for complete anesthesia of the core bundles of the last teeth in the anterior sextant of the dental arch.

- If half-mouth treatment is planned, the IA and buccal blocks are given first, then the maxillary facial injections, followed by the palatal injections. Instrumentation should proceed first on the maxillary arch, to be followed by the mandibular arch.

- IA block is generally recommended for anesthesia of the mandibular teeth and their associated periodontium and lingual soft tissue to the midline, as well as the facial soft tissue anterior to the mandibular first molar.

- The deposit location of the IA block is slightly superior to the entry point of the IA nerve as it moves inferiorly to enter the mandibular foramen, overhung anteriorly by the lingula. If anesthesia fails after the first attempt of a seemingly correct injection, the dental hygienist should reattempt the injection at a slightly superior level than the first injection.

- If bone is contacted early during the IA block (half the length to less than half the depth of the long needle), the needle tip is located too far anterior to the ramus. Correction is made by withdrawing the needle partially or completely and bringing the syringe barrel more closely superior to the mandibular anterior teeth.

- If bone is not contacted with usual depths of penetration of two-thirds to three-fourths the length of the long needle, the needle tip is located too far posterior on the ramus. Correction is made by withdrawing the needle partially or completely and bringing the syringe barrel more closely superior to the mandibular molars.

- If bone is not contacted during the IA block, the anesthetic may be inadvertently deposited in the parotid salivary gland causing temporary anesthesia of the facial nerve. Symptoms of transient facial paralysis include the inability to close the eyelid and the drooping of the corner of the lips on the affected side for a couple of hours.

- Failure of anesthesia during the IA block of the mandibular first molar may be due to the innervation of the mylohyoid nerve. Local anesthesia of the mylohyoid nerve using a supraperiosteal injection on the lingual border of the mandible may be indicated.

- Incomplete anesthesia following an IA block may be because a bifid IA nerve, which can be detected by noting a doubled mandibular canal on intraoral radiograph, more inferiorly placed, exists. To correct this, the local anesthetic agent is deposited more inferior to the usual anatomic landmarks for the IA block.

DENTAL HYGIENE CONSIDERATIONS—cont'd

- "Lingual shock" may occur as the needle passes by the lingual nerve during the IA block. Communication to the patient that this may occur may alleviate the patient's fear if it happens during injection.
- IA block has the highest positive aspiration rate of all the block injections. Aspirating within three planes and reaspiration after every one-fourth of a cartridge deposited is recommended.
- Paresthesia may occur following IA block, usually from trauma to the lingual nerve and with the spread of dental infection from a contaminated needle, but in most cases, it occurs due to problematic surgical extraction of impacted mandibular molars.
- The buccal block is recommended for anesthesia of the buccal soft tissue of the mandibular molars.
- The mental block is recommended for anesthesia of the facial soft tissue anterior to the mental foramen, usually the mandibular anterior teeth and premolars.

- The incisive block is generally recommended for anesthesia of the teeth and associated periodontium as well as facial soft tissue anterior to the mental foramen, usually the mandibular anterior teeth and premolars.
- Bilateral incisive or mental blocks may be useful for sextant nonsurgical periodontal therapy from canine to canine.
- The Gow-Gates mandibular block is recommended for extensive procedures during quadrant dentistry or with failure of the IA block.
- The periodontal ligament injection can be used on the mandibular posterior teeth for single tooth anesthesia but is not usually used prior to nonsurgical periodontal therapy.

CASE STUDY 13-1

Considerations following inferior alveolar block

A patient of record has come into the dental office for scheduled nonsurgical periodontal therapy of the mandibular right quadrant. The dental hygienist prepares to administer both an inferior alveolar block and buccal block. However, when giving the inferior alveolar block, the dental hygienist has a difficult time contacting bone regardless of properly readjusting the syringe barrel more posteriorly so the needle will be at the correct injection site. The patient has had extensive past dental work in the area and there is resultant scar tissue at the injection site. Following the third attempt of readjustment, the dental hygienist feels frustration and is concerned about the

schedule getting behind, but is still unsure if the mandibular bone has been contacted. In light of this and hoping for the best, a full cartridge of anesthetic agent is deposited, and the corner of the patient's lips on the same side begins to droop.

Critical Thinking Questions:

- What is the reason why the corner of the patient's lips on the same side begins to droop?
- What should now be done to treat the patient?
- How could the dental hygienist have prevented this occurrence?

CHAPTER REVIEW QUESTIONS

1. What is the approximate needle penetration depth into soft tissue for the inferior alveolar local anesthetic block in most cases?
   - A. 10 mm
   - B. 15 mm
   - C. 16 mm
   - D. 20 mm
2. The mandibular nerve or division is a branch of which cranial nerve?
   - A. X
   - B. V
   - C. VII
   - D. IV

3. The posterior part of the mandible is MORE dense than the anterior part, which allows for MORE successful molar anesthesia.
   - A. Both the statement and the reason are correct and related.
   - B. Both the statement and the reason are correct but NOT related.
   - C. The statement is correct, but the reason is NOT.
   - D. The statement is NOT correct, but the reason is correct.
   - E. NEITHER the statement NOR the reason is correct.

CHAPTER REVIEW QUESTIONS

4. Which injection is usually recommended to be administered along with the inferior alveolar local anesthetic block to provide complete anesthesia of a mandibular quadrant on a patient before nonsurgical periodontal therapy WITHOUT any overlapping coverage?
   A. Buccal block
   B. Lingual injection
   C. Gow-Gates mandibular block
   D. Mental block
   E. Supraperiosteal injection

5. Which of the following local anesthesia blocks will NOT provide pulpal anesthesia to tooth #23 before restorative dental procedures?
   A. Inferior alveolar block
   B. Incisive block
   C. Gow-Gates mandibular block
   D. Buccal block

6. After administering a mental local anesthetic block, the patient reports slight numbness of the chin. What should the clinician do?
   A. Stop treatment and explain facial nerve paralysis to the patient
   B. Explain to the patient this is normal and continue with treatment
   C. Place a cold compress to prevent hematoma
   D. Immediately administer an oral antihistamine

7. After a few minutes following the administration of a mental local anesthetic block, a patient reports that some of her contralateral mandibular anterior teeth feel numb. What caused the patient's anterior teeth to become anesthetized?
   A. Diffusion of the anesthetic into the incisive nerve
   B. Cross innervation of the anterior part of the mandible
   C. Constriction of the incisive nerve in the area
   D. Constriction of the mental nerve in the area

8. What injection uses the mesiolingual cusp of the maxillary second molar as a landmark during administration?
   A. Gow-Gates mandibular block
   B. Inferior alveolar block
   C. Mental block
   D. Buccal block

9. When administering the inferior alveolar local anesthetic block, the barrel of the syringe should be in what relation the mandibular occlusal plane?
   A. Perpendicular
   B. Parallel
   C. At a 45° angle
   D. At a 90° angle

10. When administering the inferior alveolar local anesthetic block, the barrel of the syringe should usually be over which mandibular tooth?

A. Premolar on the injection side
B. Premolar on the contralateral side
C. First molar on the contralateral side
D. First molar on the injection side

11. If lingual gingival anesthesia is required for #25–27, an incisive block is adequate BECAUSE it anesthetizes both the facial and lingual soft tissue of the mandibular anterior teeth.
    A. Both the statement and the reason are correct and related.
    B. Both the statement and the reason are correct but NOT related.
    C. The statement is correct, but the reason is NOT.
    D. The statement is NOT correct, but the reason is correct.
    E. NEITHER the statement NOR the reason is correct.

12. Which of the following local anesthetic blocks has the HIGHEST risk of hematoma for the patient after administration?
    A. Posterior superior alveolar block
    B. Inferior alveolar block
    C. Gow-Gates mandibular block
    D. Mental or incisive blocks

13. While administering the inferior alveolar local anesthetic block, the clinician contacts bone at a depth of 10 mm on an adult patient. What should the clinician do?
    A. Aspirate correctly and then deposit anesthetic agent at the site
    B. Withdraw the needle almost completely and redirect the syringe barrel more anteriorly
    C. Withdraw the needle partially or completely and redirect the syringe barrel more posteriorly
    D. Withdraw the needle partially and redirect the syringe barrel more perpendicular to the occlusal plane

14. While administering the inferior alveolar local anesthetic block, the clinician does not contact bone. What should the clinician do?
    A. Aspirate correctly and then deposit anesthetic agent at the site
    B. Withdraw the needle almost completely and redirect the syringe barrel more anteriorly
    C. Withdraw the needle partially or completely and redirect the syringe barrel more posteriorly
    D. Withdraw the needle partially and redirect the syringe barrel more perpendicular to the occlusal plane

15. The target area for the incisive local anesthetic block is the same as the mental block, but during the mental local anesthetic block the clinician must place pressure to the injection site following the injection.
    A. Both statements are true.
    B. Both statements are false.

CHAPTER REVIEW QUESTIONS

C. First statement is true and the second is false.

D. First statement is false and the second is true.

16. There is no need to palpate for the mental foramen prior to performing the mental local anesthetic block BECAUSE the mental foramen is commonly in the same place on all patients.
    A. Both the statement and the reason are correct and related.
    B. Both the statement and the reason are correct but NOT related.
    C. The statement is correct, but the reason is NOT.
    D. The statement is NOT correct, but the reason is correct.
    E. NEITHER the statement NOR the reason is correct.

17. Which of the following local anesthetic blocks anesthetizes the mylohyoid, mental, and the auriculotemporal nerves?
    A. Gow-Gates mandibular block
    B. Inferior alveolar block
    C. Mental block
    D. Buccal block

18. Which mandibular local anesthetic blocks require the clinician to contact the mandibular bone with the anesthetic needle?

A. Inferior alveolar block, infraorbital block

B. Inferior alveolar block, Gow-Gates mandibular block

C. Buccal block, mental block

D. Gow-Gates mandibular block, mental block

19. Which of the following situations is NOT related to incomplete anesthesia on the usual areas of the mandible on an adult patient after performing an inferior alveolar local anesthetic block?
    A. Bifid inferior alveolar nerve
    B. Accessory innervation by the mylohyoid nerve
    C. Crossover local anesthetic innervation from the incisive nerve
    D. Angle's classification of malocclusion Class II case
    E. Patient experiencing lingual shock during the injection

20. Which of the following local anesthetic blocks uses BOTH the maxillary and mandibular occlusal planes as well as the pterygomandibular raphe as landmarks for administration?
    A. Gow-Gates mandibular block
    B. Inferior alveolar block
    C. Mental block
    D. Incisive block

REFERENCES

1. Fehrenbach MJ, Herring SW: *Illustrated anatomy of the head and neck*, ed 3, St Louis, 2007, Saunders.
2. Logan BM, Reynold PA, Hutching RT: *McMinn's color atlas of head and neck anatomy*, ed 3, London, 2004, Mosby.
3. Kaufman E, Epstein JB, Naveh E, Gorsky M, Gross A, Cohen G: A survey of pain, pressure, and discomfort induced by commonly used oral anesthesia injections. *Anesth Prog* 54(4): 122-127, 2005 Winter.
4. Jastak T, Yagiela J, Donaldson D: *Local anesthesia of the oral cavity*, St Louis, 1995, Saunders.
5. Darby M, Walsh M: *Dental hygiene theory and practice*, ed 3, St Louis, 2010, Saunders.
6. Malamed S: *Handbook of local anesthesia*, ed 5, St Louis, 2004, Mosby.

Summary of Mandibular Injections

INFERIOR ALVEOLAR BLOCK

AREAS ANESTHETIZED	LANDMARKS	ADMINISTRATION SITES	TECHNIQUE	ADVERSE EFFECTS
Teeth Mandibular teeth to midline **Other Structures** Periodontium anterior to mental foramen as well as facial gingival tissue; lingual soft tissue to midline; lower lip to midline; anterior two-thirds of tongue, and floor of the mouth	Medial surface of ramus; coronoid notch Pterygomandibular fold (raphe) Pterygomandibular space Mandibular occlusal plane; internal oblique ridge	**Penetration Site** At intersection of horizontal imaginary line and imaginary vertical line using coronoid notch and pterygomandibular fold; middle of pterygomandibular space at 6–10 mm superior to occlusal plane of mandibular molars **Deposit Location** At mandibular foramen with inferior alveolar nerve	Insert the needle in the deepest part of the depression created by the pterygomandibular space and at the intersection of these two imaginary lines moving through soft tissue until bone is gently contacted; aspirate **Depth of Penetration** Approximately 20–25 mm or two-thirds to three-fourths the depth of long needle until bone is contacted **Anesthetic Solution** Approximately 1.7 (1.8)–3.4 (3.6) mL cartridges; 60–120 seconds	Transient facial paralysis from deposition in parotid salivary gland Hematoma; lingual shock when moving needle through tissue; inadequate anesthesia possibly caused by depositing solution inferior to mandibular foramen; incomplete anesthesia of first molar due to mylohyoid nerve; incomplete anesthesia from crossover-innervation of incisive nerve

BUCCAL BLOCK

AREAS ANESTHETIZED	LANDMARKS	ADMINISTRATION SITES	TECHNIQUE	ADVERSE EFFECTS
Teeth None **Other Structures** Buccal gingival tissue of mandibular molars	Most distal mandibular molar Anterior border of the ramus of the mandible; occlusal plane of mandibular molars	**Penetration site** In vestibule, distal and buccal to most distal molar in the quadrant at height of the occlusal plane **Deposit Location** Long buccal nerve as it passes over the anterior border of the ramus	Direct the syringe barrel parallel to the occlusal plane but directly superior to the mandibular molars; aspirate **Depth of Penetration** Approximately 1–4 mm using same needle from the IA block; or short needle if no IA block **Anesthetic Solution** Approximately 0.3–0.45 mL or one-eighth to one-fourth of cartridge; 10–20 seconds	Leakage of solution at injection site due to bevel of needle only partially in the tissue with bitter taste of anesthetic agent Ballooning of the tissue caused by rapid deposit of solution

MENTAL BLOCK

AREAS ANESTHETIZED	LANDMARKS	ADMINISTRATION SITES	TECHNIQUE	ADVERSE REACTIONS
Teeth None **Other Structures** Facial gingival tissue from mental foramen to midline; lower lip and skin of chin to midline	Mandibular premolars Mental foramen Mandibular mucobuccal fold	**Penetration Site** Depth of mucobuccal fold anterior to mental foramen **Deposit Location** At mental foramen, between apices of mandibular premolars or location determined by radiographs and/or palpation	Horizontal approach: insert the needle to the depth of the mucobuccal fold, directing the needle anterior to the mental foramen; vertical approach: direct the syringe vertically with the patient's cheek anterior to the mental foramen Aspirate **Depth of Penetration** Short needle approximately 5 mm or one-fourth of needle length; 27 gauge **Anesthetic Solution** Approximately 0.6 mL or one third of cartridge; 30–60 seconds	Hematoma

INCISIVE BLOCK

AREAS ANESTHETIZED	LANDMARKS	ADMINISTRATION SITES	TECHNIQUE	ADVERSE REACTIONS
Teeth Mandibular teeth anterior to mental foramen **Other Structures** Periodontium of anesthetized teeth and facial gingival tissue from mental foramen to midline; lower lip and skin of chin to midline	Mandibular premolars Mental foramen Mandibular mucobuccal fold	**Penetration Site** Depth of mucobuccal fold anterior to mental foramen **Deposit Location** At mental foramen, between apices of mandibular premolars or location determined by radiographs and/or palpation	Horizontal approach: insert the needle to the depth of the mucobuccal fold, directing the needle anterior to the mental foramen; vertical approach: direct the syringe vertically with the patient's cheek anterior to the mental foramen Aspirate; deposit solution then massage solution into foramen for 2 minutes **Depth of Penetration** Short needle approximately 5 mm or one-fourth of needle length; 27 gauge **Anesthetic Solution** Approximately 0.6–0.9 mL or one-third of cartridge; 30–60 seconds	Hematoma; inadequate anesthesia due to inadequate volume of anesthetic into mental foramen or inadequate duration of pressure over the mental foramen after injection

GOW-GATES MANDIBULAR BLOCK

AREAS ANESTHETIZED	LANDMARKS	ADMINISTRATION SITES	TECHNIQUE	ADVERSE EFFECTS
Teeth Mandibular teeth to midline **Other Structures** Periodontium of anesthetized teeth as well as both buccal and lingual gingival tissue to midline overlying teeth; lower lip to midline, anterior two thirds of tongue and floor of the mouth; skin over zygomatic bone and posterior part of buccal and temporal regions	Extraoral: Intertragic notch (lower border of the tragus) Corner of mouth (labial commissure) Intraoral: Mesiolingual cusp of maxillary second molar; soft tissue just distal to maxillary second molar	**Penetration Site** Oral mucosa on medial surface of mandibular ramus, just distal to height of mesiolingual cusp of maxillary second molar **Deposit Location** Anteromedial border of neck of mandibular condyle, just inferior to insertion of lateral pterygoid muscle	Insert needle parallel to the determined imaginary line until gentle bony contact is made with the neck of the condyle **Depth of Penetration** Long needle, approximately 25 mm or three-fourths the needle depth until bone is contacted; 25 gauge **Anesthetic solution** Approximately 1.7 (1.8) mL or full cartridge 60–120 seconds	Hematoma

PERIODONTAL LIGAMENT INJECTION

AREAS ANESTHETIZED	LANDMARKS	ADMINISTRATION SITES	TECHNIQUE	ADVERSE REACTIONS
Teeth Single tooth **Other Structures** Associated periodontium	Root(s) of the tooth; Periodontal tissues	**Penetration Site** Long axis of the tooth on the mesial or distal surface at a 30° angle. **Deposit Location** The depth of the gingival sulcus when resistance is felt	Advance needle parallel to the root surface and exert pressure on the syringe **Depth of Penetration** Variable **Anesthetic Solution** 0.2 mL, one stopper of anesthetic	Postoperative soreness; may cause tissue damage

PART V

Complications, Legal Considerations, and Risk Management

CHAPTER 14

Local Anesthetic Complications

Demetra Daskalos Logothetis RDH, MS

CHAPTER OUTLINE

LEARNING OBJECTIVES

1. Define local and systemic anesthetic complications.
2. Differentiate between anesthetic overdose, vasoconstrictor overdose and allergic response, and discuss the various causes, treatments, and preventive precautions.
3. Discuss the possible complications of local anesthetic administration, such as needle breakage, hematoma, infection, sloughing of tissue; know management and prevention of same.
4. List complications related to anesthetic needle or administration technique.
5. List complications related to the anesthetic solution.
6. List the symptoms and treatment of the following emergency situation:
   a. Syncope/psychogenic shock
   b. Hyperventilation
   c. Mild/severe allergic reactions
   d. True overdose/drug reactions
   e. Asthma
   f. Angina
   g. Myocardial infarct/cardiac arrest
   h. Diabetic coma/insulin shock
   i. Epileptic seizures
   j. Cardiovascular accident
   k. Respiration arrest
7. Discuss the guidelines for emergency preparedness in the dental office.
8. Discuss the signs, symptoms, prevention, and treatment of medical emergencies in the dental office.
9. Describe how to properly document emergency reactions, treatment, and referral notations.
10. Correctly complete review questions and activities for this chapter.

KEY TERMS

Allergens or antigens Noninfectious foreign substance that trigger hypersensitivity.

Diaphoresis Excessive sweating.

Edema Abnormal accumulation of fluid beneath the skin causing swelling of the tissues, and describes a clinical complication.

Hematoma Swelling that develops when a blood vessel, particularly an artery, is punctured or lacerated by the needle.

Localized complication Occurs in the region of the injection.

Mild complication Minor complication that resolves without treatment.

Paresthesia Persistent anesthesia beyond the expected duration, or altered sensation tingling or itching beyond a normal level.

Permanent complication Has a residual effect.

Primary complication Experienced by the patient at the time of the injection.

Secondary complication Apparent after the injection is completed.

Severe complication Requires a plan of treatment to resolve the complication.

Soft tissue sloughing The loss of surface layers of epithelium due to the administration of topical anesthetics for extended periods, or anesthetic sterile abscesses developed by prolonged ischemia due to the inclusion of a vasoconstrictor in the anesthetic solution.

Syncope Fainting

Systemic complication Attributed to the drug administered.

Transient complication May appear severe at the time of its observance but eventually resolves without any residual effect.

Trismus Spasms of the muscles of mastication resulting in soreness and difficulty opening the mouth.

INTRODUCTION

Local anesthetics allow dentistry to be practiced without patient discomfort. Serious complications associated with the use of these drugs are rare. However, regardless of appropriate preanesthetic patient assessment, good patient communication, and use of proper technique according to all the recommended guidelines and procedures prior to the administration of the local anesthetic agent, localized and systemic responses to anesthetic injections are uncommon but may occur. Localized complications occur in the region of the injection and can be attributed to the anesthetic needle, administration technique, and/or to the anesthetic drug administered. Systemic complications are attributed to the drug administered (Table 14-1). According to Bennett, there are three primary categories for local anesthetic complications.[1]

1. Primary or secondary
   - Primary complication, such as burning during the injection, is experienced by the patient at the time of the injection. The patient experiences the burning sensation at the time of drug administration.
   - Secondary complication is apparent after the injection is completed. It is caused by the injection of the local anesthetic drug, but experienced by the patient later. This could occur shortly after the injection or later.
2. Mild or severe
   - Mild complications resolve without requiring treatment. For example, burning during injection is temporary and resolves shortly after the deposition of the solution.
   - Severe complications require a plan of treatment to resolve the complication. For example, anaphylaxis requires immediate treatment and drug intervention.
3. Transient or permanent
   - Transient complications may appear severe at the time of their observance but will eventually resolve without any residual effect. For example, a hematoma may cause severe swelling and bruising, but will resolve over time without leaving any residual effects.
   - Permanent complications leave a residual effect. For example, nerve damage associated with the inferior alveolar (IA) local anesthetic block may last a few weeks, months, or indefinitely.

LOCAL COMPLICATIONS

See Table 14-2 for a summary of local complications, prevention, and management.

NEEDLE BREAKAGE

Reported incidences of accidental breakage of disposable stainless steel needles are uncommon and are usually reported when thinner 30-gauge needles are used.[2,3] The most common cause of needle breakage is due to sudden unexpected movement of the patient during the injection, or poor technique by applying excessive lateral pressure on the needle. A needle that is deeply embedded into tissue increases the risk, and when it is broken, the needle fragment is more difficult to retrieve. If the end of the needle fragment remains outside the mucosa, it is readily

TABLE 14-1   Local Anesthetic Complications

COMPLICATIONS ASSOCIATED WITH THE ANESTHETIC NEEDLE OR ADMINISTRATION TECHNIQUE	COMPLICATIONS ASSOCIATED WITH THE ANESTHETIC SOLUTION
Syncopy	Burning during injection
Broken needle	Toxicity
Pain during injection	Allergic reaction
Burning during injection	Anaphylactic reaction
Hematoma	Idiosyncrasy (reactions not classified as toxic or allergic)
Facial paralysis	Edema
Paresthesia	Infection
Trismus	Soft tissue injuries
Infection	Tissue sloughing
Edema	
Postanesthetic intraoral lesions	

TABLE 14-2   Local Complications Associated with the Administration of Local Anesthetics

COMPLICATION	CAUSES	PREVENTION	MANAGEMENT
Needle breakage	Sudden, unexpected movement Poor technique	Patient communication Long, large-gauge needle Do not bend needle Advance slowly Never force needle No sudden direction changes Never insert to hub	Remain calm Keep hands in patient's mouth Remove needle fragment if visible Refer to oral surgeon Document incident
Pain during injection	Careless technique Dull needle Barbed needle Rapid deposit	Proper technique Sharp needles Topical anesthetic Sterile anesthetics Inject slowly Room temperature solutions	Good communication Reassure patient that pain is only temporary
Burning during injection	Contamination of local anesthetics Heated anesthetic Expired solution Rapid deposit	Never store in disinfecting solution Store at room temperature Check expiration date Do not use cartridge warmers Inject slowly	Reassure patient that burning will last only a few seconds
Hematoma	Inadvertent puncturing of a blood vessel Overinsertion of needle during posterior superior alveolar (PSA) block Improper technique Multiple needle penetrations	Short 25-gauge needle for PSA Know your anatomy Modify injection technique for patient size Minimize the number of needle insertions Maintain good technique	Swelling; apply direct pressure Apply ice to the region; warm packs the next day Discuss possibility of soreness and limited movement to patient Instruct patient that swelling and discoloration will disappear after 7–14 days Dismiss patient when bleeding has stopped
Facial paralysis	Bone is not contacted and local anesthetic is deposited in parotid gland during inferior alveolar (IA) block Parotid gland is located on the posterior border of the ramus where the facial nerve passes into Temporary loss of function of facial expression muscles	Proper technique for IA block Contact bone before depositing solution for the IA block Redirect barrel of syringe more posteriorly if bone is not contacted	Reassure patient that paralysis will last only a few hours Ask patient to remove contact lenses if applicable Close eyelid manually Document
Paresthesia	Irritation to nerve following injection of contaminated solution Edema places pressure on nerve Trauma to nerve sheath; electrical shock Hemorrhage around nerve sheath Higher concentrations of solutions may increase risk for paresthesia	Store dental cartridges properly Avoid placing cartridges in disinfectant Proper technique (do not move needle around in deep tissue, change needle directions when needle is almost completely withdrawn from tissue)	Reassure patient Arrange exam with dentist Consultation with oral surgeon Record incident Inform insurance carrier of incident

continued next page

TABLE 14-2	Local Complications Associated with the Administration of Local Anesthetics—cont'd		
COMPLICATION	**CAUSES**	**PREVENTION**	**MANAGEMENT**
Trismus	Trauma to muscles in infratemporal space Multiple insertions Contaminated needles Depositing contaminated solution Depositing large amounts of solution in restricted areas Hemorrhage Low-grade infection	Store anesthetic properly Sharp, sterile, needles Appropriate injection technique Minimal amount of solution Deposit anesthetic slowly	Arrange for exam from dentist Heat therapy Jaw exercises Infection; antibiotic treatment Severe pain; refer to oral surgeon Record incident
Infection	Contamination of the anesthetic needle before injection Improper handling of local anesthetic Administration of contaminated solution Improper tissue preparation Administering local anesthetics through areas of dental infection	Sterile needle Sheath needle before and immediately after injection Be aware of the location of the uncovered needle at all times Use appropriate infection protocols Store anesthetic properly Wipe off diaphragm Topical antiseptic Do not administer local anesthetics through areas of dental infection	Treat initially as trismus; if patient does not respond in 3 days, antibiotic therapy should be prescribed by the dentist or physician
Edema	Trauma during injection Administration of contaminated solution Hemorrhage Infection Allergic response; may produce airway obstruction	Appropriate infection control Appropriate technique Adequate preanesthetic assessment	Usually resolves within several days without any required treatment Edema due to infection may require antibiotic therapy
Soft tissue injuries	Lips, tongue, cheeks traumatized by patient while numb Typically seen in children and in special needs patients	Select anesthetic with appropriate duration for treatment Warn patient not to eat, drink hot fluids, or test anesthesia by biting Instruct parent or guardian of danger Place cotton rolls between teeth and soft tissues Warning stickers can be used to remind patient and guardian of dangers associated with being numb	Analgesics for pain Antibiotics should be prescribed for infections Recommend warm saline rinses to decrease swelling and discomfort Petrolatum can be used to coat the lips to minimize discomfort
Tissue sloughing	Prolonged use of topical anesthetics Sterile abscess may develop after prolonged ischemia, usually on palate due to vasoconstrictor	Topical 1–2 minutes Avoid high concentrations of vasoconstrictors	Usually requires no treatment
Postanesthetic intraoral lesions	Trauma to area of injection	Use appropriate administration techniques	Topical anesthetic solutions or pastes for discomfort

retrievable, and no emergency exists. However, if the needle fragment is embedded in the tissue, it is extremely difficult to remove and will most likely require specialized radiographic and surgical procedures to locate and remove, usually by an oral maxillofacial surgeon (Figure 14-1). Needle fragments that remain encased in scar tissue may be better left untouched because difficult surgical procedure is required for removal.

Prevention of Needle Breakage

Patient communication

Effective communication by the dental hygienist to the patient before administration of the local anesthetic drug may help alleviate the patient's fear of the unknown and could significantly reduce the possibility of sudden unexpected movements by the patient. The dental hygienist should thoroughly explain the procedure before the injection is administered, and continue the communication throughout the procedure, helping the patient anticipate the dental hygienist's actions.

Long, large-gauge needle

Long, 25-gauge needles should be used when penetrating significant soft tissue because they are less likely to break than thinner, smaller-gauge needles. Documented incidences of needle breakage have been reported predominantly when 30-gauge, and occasionally 27-gauge, needles are used.[1,2]

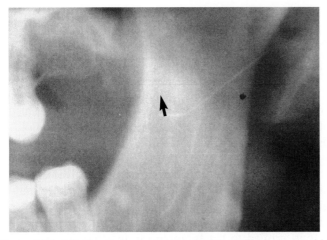

Figure 14-1 ■ Radiograph of a broken dental needle (note bend in needle: arrow). (From Malamed S: *Handbook of local anesthesia*, ed 5, St Louis, 2004, Mosby.)

Do not bend needle

Bending the needle weakens its integrity, increasing the possibility of breakage. All intraoral injections can be performed successfully without bending the needle. Bending the needle also prevents the proper recapping of the needle (see Chapters 9 and 11), increasing the likelihood of postexposure.

Advance needle slowly

Slow advancement of the needle results in gentle contact of the bone, decreasing the possibility of needle breakage. In addition, sudden forceful bone contact may startle the patient, causing sudden unexpected movement.

Never force needle

The needle should never be forced against significant resistance such as bone.

No sudden direction changes

Direction changes of the needle may be indicated during certain injections such as the IA block. Changes in needle direction should never be initiated when the needle is inserted deeply in soft tissue. The needle should be withdrawn almost completely and then redirected.

Never insert needle to hub

The most vulnerable part of the needle is at the hub, and is the location where most needle breakages are likely to occur. Inserting the needle to the hub increases the risk for breakage in this area and makes it virtually impossible to retrieve the needle. To increase the chances of retrieving a needle fragment, a portion of the needle's shaft in front of the hub should always be visible during the injection.

If needle breakage occurs and the needle fragment is visible, the following are recommendations for the dental hygienist to follow:

1. Remain calm. If the patient senses panic, he or she will close the mouth, causing the needle fragment to embed into the tissue.
2. Keep your hands in the patient's mouth, and ask the patient to open widely.
3. If the needle fragment is visible, attempt to remove it with the hemostat or cotton pliers.

If the needle fragment is not visible and cannot be retrieved, the following are recommendations for the dental hygienist to follow:

1. Remain calm, and inform the patient of the incident in a manner that will alleviate his or her fear and apprehension.
2. The dental hygienist, in consultation with the dentist, should refer the patient to an oral maxillofacial surgeon for consultation and possible further treatment.
3. Document the incident and sequence of events in the patient's permanent record. It is important to include the patient's reaction to the situation.
4. Keep the remaining needle fragment for structural evaluation.
5. Surgical procedures are indicated if the needle fragment is not deeply embedded in tissue and easily located by radiographic or clinical examination.
6. If the needle is deeply embedded in tissue, the oral maxillofacial surgeon may recommend that the needle remain in the tissue without further attempt for removal.

PAIN DURING INJECTION

As discussed in Chapter 1, patients' reactions to pain may vary according to their pain reaction thresholds. Therefore, it is impossible for the dental hygienist to ensure that every injection will be pain-free. However, it is the dental hygienist's responsibility to make every effort to take the necessary precautions to prevent pain during injection. Pain during administration of local anesthetics may be due to several reasons: careless technique, a barbed needle caused during manufacturing, hitting bone, and rapid deposition of the anesthetic solution. The following recommendations will help alleviate pain during injection.

Proper Technique

The dental hygienist should adhere to the proper techniques discussed in Chapters 11, 12, and 13. Carefully following the recommended guidelines will decrease patient discomfort and strengthen the patient's confidence in the practitioner. This allows future dental appointments requiring anesthesia to be less stressful on the patient and the practitioner.

Sharp Needles

Dull needles cause pain on insertion, and are usually due to repeated injections using the same needle. For most dental hygiene procedures requiring anesthesia, several injections are administered to achieve the necessary anesthesia. Therefore it is essential that the needle be changed after three to four needle penetrations.

Topical Anesthetic

Applying topical anesthetic for 1–2 minutes before the injection will block the free nerve endings supplying the mucosal surfaces. This procedure will significantly reduce the pain caused by needle insertion.

Anesthetics Placed in Disinfecting Solution

Anesthetics that have been placed in disinfecting solution, or have been frozen will cause burning and pain during the injection. Anesthetic cartridges should never be placed in disinfecting solution. The dental hygienist should carefully evaluate every cartridge before the syringe is set up to ensure that no large bubbles are present and that the rubber stopper is intact and does not show any signs of contamination. If the cartridge contains large bubbles or the rubber stopper is extruded, the cartridge should not be used and should be discarded. (See Chapter 9.)

Inject Slowly

Injecting the anesthetic slowly during the injection is one of the most valuable methods to reduce pain. It prevents the tissue from tearing and improves patient comfort. Because the anesthetic solutions is more acidic than the patient's tissues, the patient will feel stinging when the anesthetic is administered. To decrease or avoid this sensation, the anesthetic solution should be deposited slowly at a rate of 1 mL of solution per minute.

Room Temperature Solutions

Anesthetic cartridges should be stored in a dark place at room temperature in their original containers. Cartridge warmers should not be used.

BURNING DURING INJECTION

The patient may experience a normal burning sensation during the deposition of the anesthetic solution, usually due to the local anesthetic agent and the vasoconstrictor being more acidic than the patient's tissues. The burning sensation only lasts a few seconds until anesthesia manifests, and does not last after the anesthetic wears off. However, more severe buring sensations may be caused by other factors not related to the normal response of the anesthetic being deposited into the tissue. These factors include contaminated solutions, heated cartridges, expired solutions, and too rapid deposition of the solution into tissue. Responses to these factors may result in postanesthetic trismus, edema, and possibly paresthesia. To prevent these conditions, as well as abnormal burning sensation during the injection, the dental hygienist should follow the following guidelines:

- Never store cartridges in disinfecting solution; always store in a dark place at room temperature.
- Check expiration date; discard outdated solutions.
- Do not use cartridge warmers.

- Inject slowly at a rate of 1 mL of solution per minute, taking approximately 2 minutes for an entire cartridge.

HEMATOMA

A hematoma develops when a blood vessel, particularly an artery, is punctured or lacerated by the needle. This is observed as asymmetrical swelling and discoloration of the tissue resulting from the effusion of blood into extravascular spaces (Figure 14-2). Hematomas particularly result after administration of a posterior superior alveolar (PSA) block. However, the inferior alveolar and mental nerve blocks also commonly cause hematomas. Hematomas less often occur after an infraorbital (IO) block, because pressure is applied to the foramen immediately following the injection.[3] Hematomas are least likely to develop following palatal blocks.

Although hematomas may appear serious, they are more a cosmetic nuisance. Trismus and mild pain may also occur. A hematoma resulting from a PSA block is usually the largest due to the infratemporal fossa being able to accommodate large volumes of blood, and clinically appears as extraoral bruising. Hematomas resulting from an IA block appear as intraoral bruising. Hematomas can occur without a positive aspiration, and by nicking a blood vessel with the needle during the pathway to the target loction, or while removing the needle after the anesthetic has been deposited. In most cases positive aspirations do not produce hematomas and result in unnoticable slight leakage of blood in the tissue.[3-5]

Although hematomas can occur even when proper technique is used, to decrease the risk the dental hygienist should follow these guidelines:

1. Know your anatomy.
2. Use a short needle and modify the needle penetration depth for the PSA block for children, petite adults, and patients with small facial characteristics.
3. Minimize the number of needle insertions.
4. Follow all recommended injection techniques for all local anesthetic injections.

Management of Hematoma

1. At the first sign of swelling, apply pressure directly to the area for a minimum of 2 minutes. This involves the medial aspect of the mandibular ramus for the IA block, the mental foramen for the mental/incisive block, and because it is difficult to locate the blood vessels for the PSA block, pressure should be applied as far distally as possible without producing a gag reflex.
2. Apply ice to the region of the developing hematoma to reduce the swelling. Ice will constrict the blood vessels, decreasing the effusion of blood into the extravascular spaces, and also provide some analgesic effects for the patient.
3. Communicate to the patient that soreness and limited movement of their jaw may occur. Instruct the patient

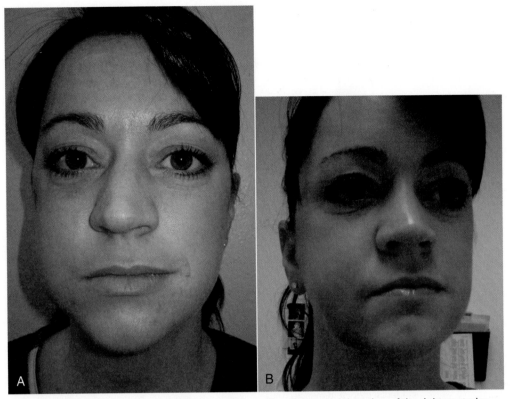

Figure 14-2 ■ **A,** Hematoma producing initial swelling from administration of the right posterior superior alveolar block. **B,** Progression of hematoma one week following initial swelling.

to use warm moist towels applied to the region the next day for 20 minutes every hour to assist in the resorption of blood. This will also provide comfort to the patient should soreness occur.

4. Inform the patient that there are no serious complications associated with hematomas, and that swelling and discoloration should disappear after 7–14 days.

5. Do not dismiss the patient until bleeding has stopped. Document the incident in the patient's record including instructions presented to the patient, and the patient's response. Dental hygiene treatment should resume after the swelling and discoloration have disappeared.

6. Follow up as indicated.

FACIAL NERVE PARALYSIS

Facial nerve paralysis is caused by the inadvertent deposition of local anesthetic solution during the inferior alveolar (IA) block into the parotid gland, located at the posterior border of the ramus anesthetizing the facial nerve that runs through the parotid gland (Figure 14-3). This is due to overinsertion of the needle penetrating the parotid gland. This produces a unilateral loss of motor function to the facial expression muscles.

The loss of motor function is temporary and fades within a few hours once the action of the anesthetic resolves.

During this time, the patient will be unable to use these muscles and will have a lopsided appearance (Figure 14-4); the corneal reflex remains functional and continues to produces tears to lubricate the eye.

To prevent inadvertent deposition of anesthetic solution into the parotid gland and prevent temporary facial paralysis, the dental hygienist should follow these guidelines:

1. Adhere to the guidelines for administering the IA block at all times as described in Chapter 13.

2. The needle must always contact bone at the medial aspect of the ramus before the dental hygienist deposits any anesthetic solution. Facial paralysis is always preventable if bone is contacted because this prevents the solution from being deposited into the parotid gland.

3. If bone is not contacted, the needle is too far posterior and there is a risk that the needle tip is located within the parotid gland. To correct, the dental hygienist should withdraw the needle almost completely out of the tissue, and redirect the barrel of the syringe more posteriorly over the molar teeth. Readvance the needle into the tissue until bone is gently contacted. Solution can then be deposited following a negative aspiration (see Figure 13-16).

4. Avoid larger gauge needles as they are more flexible and may deflect away from the bone.

Shortly following the inadvertent deposition of solution into the parotid gland, the patient will experience a

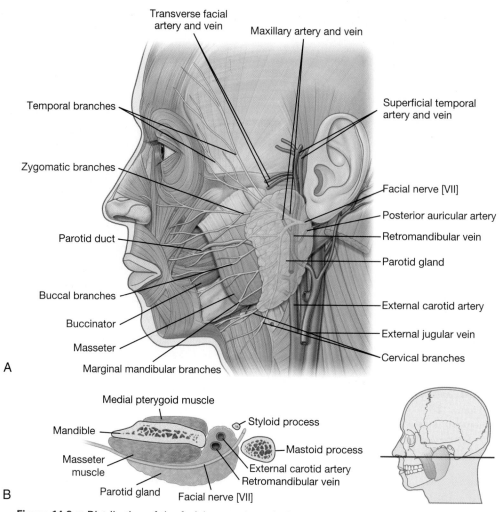

Figure 14-3 ■ Distribution of the facial nerve through the parotid salivary gland. (From Drake RL, Vogl AW, Mitchell AWM: *Gray's anatomy for students*, ed 2, Philadelphia, Churchill Livingstone, 2010, Elsevier.)

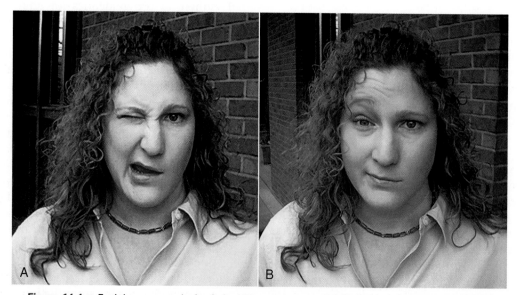

Figure 14-4 ■ Facial nerve paralysis. **A,** Inability to close eyelid. **B,** Drooping of lip on affected side (patient's left). (From Malamed S: *Handbook of local anesthesia*, ed 5, St Louis, 2004, Mosby.)

weakening of the facial expression muscles on the injection side, and no anesthesia of the inferior alveolar nerve. Management includes the following:

1. Reassure the patient. At the point of muscle weakening, the patient will be alarmed and immediate reassurance is necessary to alleviate the patient's fears. Reassure the patient that the paralysis is only temporary and will last only a few hours. Explain that weakness in the muscles will resolve as soon as the anesthetic action fades.

2. Ask the patient to remove contact lenses if applicable and to manually close his or her eye. Although the corneal reflex remains functional, this will assist in keeping the cornea lubricated.

3. There are no contraindications to completing the scheduled treatment. However, it may be advisable to reschedule treatment for a different time. This should be determined on an individual basis and predominantly depends on the patient's reaction to the situation. If treatment is to be continued, the IA block must be completed/reinjected because the target site was missed during the first injection.

4. Document the incident and the patient's reaction in the patient's chart.

5. Follow-up as indicated.

PARESTHESIA

Paresthesia is persistent anesthesia beyond the expected duration or altered sensation such as tingling or itching beyond a normal level. Paresthesia or prolonged anesthesia occurs occasionally causing the patient to feel numbness for many hours or days following the injection. Paresthesia can also be associated with a burning sensation, and patients can experience drooling, speech impediment, loss of taste, and tongue biting.[6] The risk for serious complications from paresthesia occurs when the anesthesia persists for days, weeks, or months. This condition is rare and occasionally may be unpreventable; however, it is one of the most frequent causes of dental malpractice litigation.[3]

Paresthesia most commonly occurs with the lingual and inferior alveolar nerve. During the administration of local anesthesia before treatment of mandibular teeth or their associated structures, the lingual or inferior alveolar neurovascular bundle can be traumatized by the sharp needle tip, the movement of the needle in the tissue, extraneural or intraneural hemorrhage from trauma to the blood vessels, or neurotoxic effects of the local anesthetic.[6-9] The primary factor in neurotoxicity of local anesthetics appears to be the concentration of the solution, with injuries increasing as concentration increases, particularly with articaine.[6,10] However, this hypothesis is controversial.[11,12] The original source of controversy surrounding articaine seems to have stemmed from an article published by Haas and Lennon[6] who analized cases of paresthesia reported to major dental malpractice carriers in Ontario, Canada. Analysis of the data indicates that articaine has a 4% higher occurrence of paresthesia than 2% or 3% local anesthetics. A more recent study of nonsurgical paresthesia in Ontario analogous to the Haas and Lennon study from the period of 1999 through 2008 yielded similar results.[13] The most recent study by Garisto et al,[14] analyzed reports of paresthesia from single agents of local anesthetics following dental procedures from November 1997 through August 2008 obtained from the U.S. Food and Drug Administration Adverse Event Reporting System. Paresthesia in, 94.5% of these cases involved the inferior alveolar (IA) block, and specifically the lingual nerve in 89% of these cases. Articaine 4% was involved in 51.3% of the cases, prilocaine 4% in 42.9% of the cases, and lidocaine 2% in 4.9% of the cases. Other studies have demonstrated no additionl risk. Pogrel,[15] studied a total of 57 patients who demonstrated nerve damage to the inferior alveolar or lingual nerve that could only have resulted from an IA block. Results on the basis of their estimated use indicated that paresthesia reports for articaine 4% were proportional to prilocaine 4% and lidocaine 2%. Because of the controversy and conflicting information surrounding this issue, more scientific-based evidence is needed to answer this difficult question. It is essential that the dental hygienist remain abreast of the current research of all anesthetics, and only administer a drug if the benefits outweigh the risks.

Paresthesia may be a result of irritation to the nerve following the administration of a contaminated local anesthetic solution with alcohol or other disinfectants. Edema caused by the irritation places pressure on the nerve, resulting in prolonged anesthesia. Hemorrhage around the nerve sheath may also contribute to paresthesia by creating excessive pressure on the nerve. Finally, paresthesia may also be caused by trauma to the nerve sheath resulting from the needle contacting the nerve during its insertion or removal from the tissues. This occurs most commonly with the lingual nerve producing a sensation of an electrical shock when it occurs.[2,3,5-9]

To prevent paresthesia, local anesthetic cartridges should be stored properly in their original containers. Cartridges should never be placed in disinfecting solution, basic injection protocol should be followed as described in Chapter 11, and injection techniques should be used as described in Chapters 12 and 13.

Most paresthesia is not serious and will typically resolve within 8 weeks. It most commonly occurs with the lingual and inferior alveolar nerve and produces only minimal sensory deficit. Fortunately, permanent nerve damage rarely occurs. The dental hygienist should following these recommendations for the management of paresthesia[3]:

1. Reassure the patient. The patient will typically call the dental office the day after the procedure concerned about the prolonged numbness. Reassure the patient that paresthesia is not uncommon following the administration of local anesthetics.

2. Arrange for the patient to be examined by the dentist to determine the extent of paresthesia. Instruct the patient that paresthesia may last up to 2 months and perhaps longer.

3. The patient should be examined by the dentist every 2 months until normal sensation returns. Consultation with an oral maxillofacial surgeon is advisable if the sensation deficit persists or deteriorates.

4. Thoroughly document the incident in the patient's chart, including a summary of all conversations with the patient. Inform your insurance carrier of the incident.

5. Dental and dental hygiene care may continue, avoiding injections to the traumatized nerve. Alternative pain control measures should be taken.

TRISMUS

Trismus occurs from spasms of the muscles of mastication resulting in soreness and difficulty opening the mouth. Trismus is a relatively common complication associated with the administration of local anesthesia. Trismus is most frequently a result of muscle trauma in the infratemporal space following intraoral injections. Multiple needle insertions, administration of contaminated solutions, deposition of large amounts of anesthetic solution in restricted areas causing distention of the tissues, hemorrhage leading to muscle dysfunction, and infection are all causes of trismus.

The following guidelines will help the dental hygienist prevent trismus:

1. Store anesthetic cartridges in a dark room in their original containers, and never place them in disinfecting solution.

2. Use sharp disposable needles and minimize the number of needle insertions.

3. Avoid contaminating the needle when not in use. Protective shields should be used to protect the needle, and the dental hygienist should know the location of an uncapped needle to avoid accidental contamination of the needle (Figure 14-5). Contaminated needles should not be used and should be discarded in appropriate sharps container.

4. Inject anesthetic solution slowly.

5. Use minimal amounts of solution in restricted tissue areas.

6. Adhere to recommended anesthetic techniques as described in Chapters 11, 12, and 13. Strive to improve your injection techniques to administer the most atraumatic injection possible and to decrease the necessary number of needle insertions.

Trismus is most commonly felt by the patient the day following the treatment and is typically associated with the inferior alveolar (IA) or posterior superior alveolar (PSA) blocks. Recommendations to reduce the soreness are as follows:

1. Arrange for the dentist to examine the patient.

2. Immediately instruct the patient to begin heat therapy: apply warm moist towels to the affected area for 20 minutes every hour. Analgesics can be used to manage muscle soreness. If the patient experiences severe discomfort, the dentist may prescribe codeine or muscle relaxants.

3. Instruct the patient to exercise the jaw by opening and closing the mouth, and by moving the mandible lateral from left to right for 5 minutes every 3 to 4 hours. Chewing gum is also a method to exercise the jaw.

4. Symptoms gradually diminish over time, typically within 48 hours after injection. Heat therapy, exercises, and analgesics should be continued until the condition resolves.

5. If pain and dysfunction persist despite the recommended therapy, refer the patient to an oral and maxillofacial surgeon for consultation.

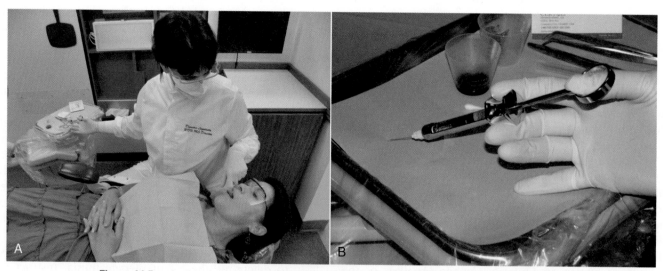

Figure 14-5 ■ Accidental contamination of an uncovered needle. **A,** Dental hygienist looking at patient. **B,** Close-up view of needle touching the instrument tray and contaminating the needle.

6. In the patient's chart, record the incident and a summary of all conversations and recommendations addressed with the patient.
7. Dental hygiene treatment should be avoided until all symptoms have resolved.

INFECTION

Infections caused by administration of local anesthetics are rare when sterile disposable needles and single-use glass cartridges are used. The most common cause of infection is the contamination of the anesthetic needle before the injection. Needle-track contamination can introduce pathogens into deeper tissues and can spread through the blood system. In addition, dental infections can spread to deeper tissues when local anesthetics are administered through areas of dental infection.[16] Infections may also result from improper handling of the local anesthetic before injection, using contaminated solutions, and/or improper tissue preparation.

The dental hygienist should follow these guidelines to prevent infection:

1. Use sterile disposable needles.
2. Carefully sheath and unsheath the needle before and after the injection. The dental hygienist should be aware of the location of the uncovered needle at all times to prevent the accidental contamination of the needle from a nonsterile surface (see Figure 14-5).
3. Store the anesthetic cartridges in their original container. If necessary, wipe the diaphragm of the anesthetic cartridge with a disinfectant before syringe assembly.
4. Prepare the tissues with a topical antiseptic or wipe the injection site with a piece of gauze to reduce the surface bacteria before needle insertion.
5. Do not administer local anesthetics through areas of dental infection.

Low-grade infections are very rare and often not easily recognized. The patient will express pain and discomfort to the region, and initially these symptoms should be treated as trismus. If the patient does not respond to the recommended treatment, antibiotics should be prescribed by the dentist or the physician.

EDEMA

Edema is an abnormal accumulation of fluid beneath the skin causing swelling of the tissues, and describes a clinical complication[17,18] (Figure 14-6). Edema following the administration of a local anesthetic agent may be caused by trauma during the injection, infection, administration of contaminated solutions, or an allergic response. Typically edema is manifested as localized pain and dysfunction. Edema associated with an allergic response is more serious and may produce airway obstruction, causing a life-threatening emergency.

To prevent edema, the dental hygienist should follow these guidelines:

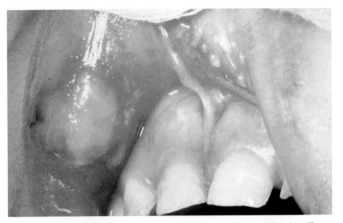

Figure 14-6 ■ Local edema in response to local anesthesia. (From Daniel S, Harfst S, Wilder R, Francis B, Mitchell S: *Dental hygiene concepts, cases and competencies*, ed 2, St Louis, 2008, Mosby.)

1. Conduct a thorough preanesthetic assessment.
2. Follow all recommended infection control procedures when storing or handling the local anesthetic armamentarium.
3. Follow all recommended guidelines for injection technique described in Chapters 11, 12, and 13.

The cause of edema will determine its course of treatment.[3] The following management procedures are recommended.

1. *Edema produced by an allergic response:* depends on the degree and location of swelling. If there is no airway obstruction, oral antihistamines should be administered. The patient should be referred to an allergist. If the airway is compromised, the guidelines described later in this chapter should be followed.
2. *Edema produced by contaminated solution or trauma:* no treatment is required, the symptoms usually subside after approximately 1–3 days. Recommend analgesics for discomfort.
3. *Edema produced by hemorrhage:* the tissue may be discolored and resemble a hematoma, and therefore should be managed as a hematoma.
4. *Edema produced by infection:* if the edema does not resolve within 3 days and the pain and discomfort continue, antibiotics should be prescribed by the dentist or physician.

SOFT TISSUE TRAUMA

Soft tissue trauma is due to the patient inadvertently self-inflicting damage to the tissues such as the lips, tongue, or cheek while anesthetized. This is most often observed in children and special needs patients. This type of trauma can lead to swelling and significant discomfort when the anesthetic effect fades (Figure 14-7).

To prevent soft tissue trauma, the dental hygienist should follow these guidelines:

1. Select an anesthetic duration that is appropriate for the length of the procedure.

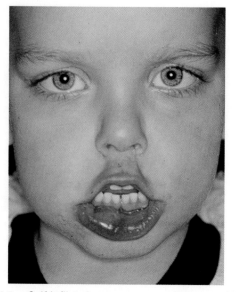

Figure 14-7 ■ Self-inflicted trauma caused by a child while anesthetized. (From Malamed S: *Handbook of local anesthesia*, ed 5, St Louis, 2004, Mosby.)

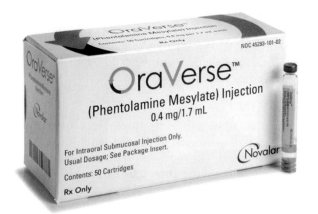

Figure 14-8 ■ OraVerse agent used for local anesthetic reversal is easily distinguished from local anesthetic cartridges by its translucent green label and blue aluminum cap. (Image courtesy of Novalar Pharmaceuticals.)

2. Warn the patient to not eat, drink hot fluids, or test the anesthesia area by biting until the anesthetic wears off and normal sensations have returned. The parent or guardian should also be warned about the dangers and be instructed to carefully watch young children and disabled individuals.

3. Cotton rolls can be placed between the teeth and soft tissues to protect the lips. They can be secured with dental floss wrapped around the teeth.

4. Consider the administration of phentolamine mesylate to patients who are particularly susceptible to self-mutilation. (Discussed later.)

5. Warning stickers are available to be placed on the patient's forehead to serve as a reminder to the parent and guardian that care should be taken while anesthetized.

Management of soft tissue injuries includes the following:

1. Analgesics may be taken as necessary for discomfort.

2. Infection due to soft tissue injuries are rare; however, if they occur, antibiotics can be prescribed by the dentist.

3. Recommend warm saline rinses to decrease swelling and discomfort.

4. Petrolatum can be used to coat the lips to minimize discomfort.

Phentolamine Mesylate

Phentolamine mesylate (Table 14-3) is an alpha-adrenergic receptor antagonist used in dentistry to reverse the effects of local anesthetics containing vasoconstrictors. Phentolamine mesylate, competes for the receptor sites of the vasoconstrictor, thus encouraging faster metabolic reuptake of the local anesthetic by way of increased vasodilation.[19] OraVerse (Novalar, 2008) is currently the only local anesthesia reversal agent available for use in dentistry. It is packaged in an anesthetic cartridge with a translucent green label and blue aluminum cap to distinguish it from local anesthetic cartridges (Figure 14-8).

Suggested clinical uses: OraVerse may be used when faster anesthetic recovery time is beneficial, such as when treating pediatric and special needs populations when the risk of self-inflicted oral trauma is increased due to lack of oral awareness, or when patients prefer not to feel numb for long durations. The manufacturer claims that, when used properly, OraVerse will reduce the length of prolonged anesthesia by almost half the original duration of action when an anesthetic with epinephrine is used.[20]

Dosage and administration technique: OraVerse is administered by submucosal injection at a 1:1 ratio (cartridge to cartridge ratio) of the previously administered local anesthetic containing a vasoconstrictor. The same techniques used for the local anesthetic injection should be used when administering OraVerse.[20] For example, if an inferior alveolar block was administered using 1 cartridge of local anesthetic with a vasoconstrictor, then a second inferior alveolar block should be administered following treatment using 1 cartridge of OraVerse. (See Table 14-3 for dosing guidelines.)

Contraindications: OraVerse is contraindicated in:

- Patients younger than age 6 years
- Patients weighing less than 15 kg or 33 lb
- Patients who are sensitive to phentolamine mesylate
- Patients with history of myocardial infarction
- Patients with angina
- Patients with coronary artery disease

Side effects: side effects are rare but may include the following:

- Nausea
- Vomiting
- Diarrhea
- Weakness
- Dizziness
- Orthostatic hypotension

TABLE 14-3	Phentolamine Mesylate (OraVerse)

Chemical Formula
phenol,3-[[(4,5-dihydro-1 H-imidazol-2-yl)methyl](4-methyl-phenyl)amino]-, methanesulfonate

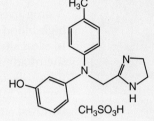

Proprietary names	OraVerse
Formulations in dentistry	0.4 mg phetolamine meslate in 1.7 mL of solution
Vasoactivity	Vasodilator
Duration of action	30–45 minutes
Toxicity	No known toxic levels
Metabolism	Liver
Excretion	Kidneys with 10% as unchanged drug
pKa	Not available
Onset of action	Rapid
Half-life	Approximately 2–3 hours
Dosage	1:1 ratio of OraVerse cartridge to local anesthetic cartridge containing epinephrine Children weighing 33–66 lb: 0.2 mg (1/2 cartridge) Children weighing more than 66 lb and up to 12 years old: 0.4 mg (1 cartridge) Not recommended for children younger than 6 years old or weighing less than 15 kg (33 lb)
Maximum recommended dose	The same MRD as calculated for the the local anesthetic drug administered
Pregnancy category C	To be used only when risks outweigh the benefits during pregnancy. Nursing mothers should use caution because excretion in breast milk is not known.
Contraindications	Age younger than 6 years
	Weight less than 15 kg or 33 lb
	Sensitivity to phentolamine mesylate
	History of myocardial infarction
	Angina
	Coronary artery disease
Product warning	Myocardial infarction, cerebrovascular spasm, and cerebrovascular occlusion have been reported to occur following the intravenous or intramuscular administration of phentolamine, usually in association with marked hypotensive episodes or shock-like states. Tachycardia and cardiac arrhythmias may occur with the use of phentolamine or other alpha-adrenergic blocking agents. Such effects are uncommon with OraVerse (phentolamine mesylate). However, the clinician should be cognizant of the signs and symptoms, particularly in patients with a history of cardiovascular disease.

Sources: Phentolamine. (2009). *Merck manuals: online medical library.* Retrieved (September 5, 2010) from Phentolamine Drug Information Provided by Lexi-Comp Merck Manual Professional.mht; OraVerse (2009). *Highlights of prescribing information.* Retrieved (September 5, 2010) from http://www.fda.gov/downloads/AdvisoryCommittees/CommitteesMeetingMaterials/PediatricAdvisoryCommittee/UCM214420.pdf.

- Flushing
- Tachycardia
- Cardiac arrhythmias

TISSUE SLOUGHING

Soft tissue sloughing is the loss of surface layers of epithelium that occurs after topical anesthetics are administered for extended periods. In addition, sloughing can occur from anesthetic sterile abscesses developed by prolonged ischemia due to the inclusion of a vasoconstrictor in the anesthetic solution. Sterile abscesses are most commonly observed on the hard palate (see Figure 4-5).

To prevent tissue sloughing, the dental hygienist should follow these guidelines:

1. Topical anesthetics should be minimally applied to the surface for a maximum of 1–2 minutes.
2. Avoid solutions with high concentrations of vasoconstrictors unless hemostasis is required. Epinephrine 1:50,000 is the dilutión most likely to cause prolonged ischemia increasing the likelihood of a sterile abscess.

Tissue sloughing usually requires no treatment and resolves on its own within a few days. Soft tissue sloughing associated with sterile abscesses typically take 7–10 days to

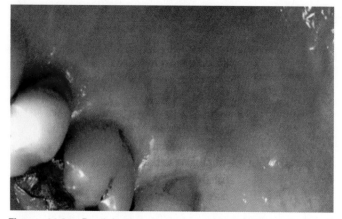

Figure 14-9 ■ Postinjection herpetic outbreak. (From Daniel S, Harfst S, Wilder R, Francis B, Mitchell S: *Dental hygiene concepts, cases and competencies*, ed 2, St Louis, 2008, Mosby.)

resolve. Topical ointments can be used to minimize discomfort.

POSTANESTHETIC INTRAORAL LESIONS

Intraoral lesions are occasionally reported a couple of days following intraoral injections. These lesions typically consist of recurrent aphthous stomatitis or herpes simplex, and may develop from trauma during the injection, or after the administration of the anesthetic solution (Figure 14-9). Lesions last approximately 7–10 days. Prevention of such lesions is difficult in susceptible patients. Using the appropriate technique during local anesthetic administration to minimize trauma reduces the occurrence. Topical anesthetic solutions and pastes, such as triamcinolone (Kenalog in Orabase), help alleviate the discomfort associated with these lesions.

▌SYSTEMIC COMPLICATIONS

Systemic complications associated with the administration of local anesthetics occur less frequently than local complications and are usually caused by high plasma concentrations of local anesthetic drugs after inadvertent intravascular injection, excessive dose or rate of injection, delayed drug clearance, or administration into vascular tissue. The dental hygienist can prevent 90% of potential life-threatening reactions due to the administration of local anesthetics by conducting a thorough preanesthetic patient assessment and by strictly following all local anesthetic administration guidelines.[17]

Systemic toxicity of anesthetics involves the central nervous system (CNS), the cardiovascular system (CVS), and the immune system. In relatively rare instances (<1%), the effects on the immune system can produce immunoglobulin E (IgE)-mediated allergic reaction. Most documented cases are associated with the use of amino esters, which are no longer available in dentistry. Some anesthetics, particularly prilocaine and benzocaine, are associated with hematologic effects, namely methemoglobinemia (see Chapter 7).

Cardiovascular effects are primarily those of direct myocardial depression and bradycardia, which may lead to cardiovascular collapse.

LOCAL ANESTHETIC OVERDOSE

A drug overdose reaction is the body's response to overly high blood levels of a drug in various organs and tissues.[3] In ideal situations, local anesthetics are absorbed from the site of administration into the circulation slowly and continuously until all the anesthetic is completely removed from the injection site. Concurrently, the local anesthetic is removed from the circulation as it undergoes biotransformation by the appropriate organs. If this steady sequence of events occurs, the risk of high plasma concentrations of the drug is rare. Toxicity of anesthetics is potentiated in patients when this sequence is disrupted causing plasma concentrations to increase. Table 14-4 summarizes the predisposing factors related to local anesthetic overdose reactions.

Causes and Prevention of Local Anesthetic Overdose

Biotransformation of anesthetic is unusually slow

A thorough review of the patient's medical history is important to determine the biotransformation capability of the local anesthetic agent by the patient.

1. Ester local anesthetics and the amide articaine are biotransformed in the blood by enzyme pseudocholinesterase. Ninety percent to 95% of articaine is metabolized in the blood and only 5%–10% is metabolized in the liver. The ester local anesthetic drugs undergo hydrolysis to para-aminobenzoic acid. Articaine's major metabolite is articainic acid. Patients with familial history of atypical pseudocholinesterase may be unable to detoxify the drug at the normal rate.
2. Biotransformation of amides occurs in the liver with prilocaine being metabolized in the liver and the lungs. Toxicity of these anesthetics may be potentiated in patients with hepatic and lung compromise.

Elimination of anesthetic through the kidneys is unusually slow

Only a small percentage of both esters and amides are excreted unmetabolized through the urine. Patients who have significant renal dysfunction could possibly develop a toxic level of anesthetic in their blood. However, in clinical situations this occurrence is rare and does not pose any additional risk to the administration of local anesthetics. It is recommended to use the minimal effective dose.

Total dose administered is too large

1. If excessive total dose of local anesthetic is administered to a patient, toxic effects may develop.
2. Calculation of maximum recommended dose (MRD) is very important. Guidelines exist for the dental hygienist to determine the patient's individual MRD based upon the patient's weight (see Chapter 8).

TABLE 14-4	Predisposing Factors to Local Anesthetic Overdose Reaction
PATIENT FACTORS	**CONTRIBUTORY FACTORS**
Age	Organs involved in the biotransformation of anesthetic drugs may not be fully developed in younger patients and may be diminished in older patients
Body weight	Lower body weight increases risk
Genetics	Genetic deficiencies may affect the biotransformation of certain drugs (e.g., atypical plasma cholinesterase)
Disease	Presence of disease may affect the ability of the body to biotransform the drug into an inactive metabolite (e.g., hepatic or renal dysfunction, cardiovascular disease)
Gender	Toxicity may be potentiated during pregnancy
DRUG FACTORS	**CONTRIBUTORY FACTORS**
Vasoactivity	Vasodilation increases risk
Drug dosage	Higher dose increases risk
Route of administration	Intravascular route increases risk
Rate of injection	Rapid injection increases risk
Addition of vasoconstrictors	Addition of vasoconstrictor decreases risk
Vascularity of injection site	Increased vascularity increases risk

Modified from Darby M, Walsh M: *Dental hygiene theory and practice*, ed 3, St Louis, 2010, Saunders, Elsevier.

3. Age of the patient and physical status affect the anesthetic dose, which should be adjusted accordingly due to immature or diminished organ function.

Absorption of anesthetic from the site of injection is unusually rapid

1. The addition of a vasoconstricting drug in the local anesthetic solution reduces the systemic toxicity of the anesthetic agent by slowing absorption into the circulatory system. Local anesthetic vasoconstrictor formulations should be used unless contraindicated by the patient's health status.
2. Limit area of use of topical anesthetics. Topical anesthetics are administered in high concentrations and are rapidly absorbed into the circulatory system. Applying topical anesthetic to large areas increases the possibility of an overdose.[3]

Anesthetic is administered intravascularly

Inadvertent intravascular injection is the most common cause of local anesthetic toxicity even when the anesthetic was administered within the recommended dose range.[2] Depositing the anesthetic solution directly into the bloodstream prevents the slow process of absorption of the drug into circulation and significantly increases systemic toxicity. Although all local anesthetic injections may be administered intravascularly, they are most common during nerve blocks such as the PSA, IA, and mental/incisive blocks. Overdose reactions can be avoided by following these guidelines:
1. *Know your anatomy:* the dental hygienist must be aware of all anatomic features in the area of the anesthetic deposition.
2. *Aspirate in two planes:* although the dental hygienist may properly aspirate, it is not always possible to avoid intravascular injection. The bevel of the needle may rest against the blood vessel during the negative

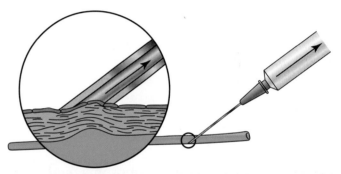

Figure 14-10 ■ Negative pressure during aspiration pulls the vessel wall against the bevel of the needle, giving a false-negative result. (Modified from Jastak T, Yagiela J, Donaldson D: *Local anesthesia of the oral cavity*, St Louis, 1995, Saunders.)

pressure produced by the aspiration. This simply draws the lining of the blood vessel over the lumen of the needle, preventing access of blood into the cartridge (Figure 14-10). Therefore it is important to aspirate on two planes, meaning to rotate the barrel of the syringe about 45 degrees and aspirate a second time. When injecting near highly vascular areas, such as near the pterygoid venous plexus with the PSA block, the dental hygienist should aspirate several times during the injection in case needle movement places the needle within the blood vessel.
3. *Use 25- or 27-gauge needle:* larger gauge needles provide easier access for blood to enter the cartridge during the aspiration.
4. *Administer drug slowly:* according to Malamed,[3] an excessively rapid injection (entire anesthetic cartridge [1.8 mL] deposited in 30 seconds or less) of a local anesthetic drug into a vein or artery produces blood levels in excess of that needed for an overdose to occur. The same volume of anesthetic administered within the recommended guidelines (a minimum of

60 seconds) produces blood levels lower than the blood levels needed to produce an overdose.[3] Injecting the anesthetic slowly is the most important factor in preventing an overdose. Therefore the dental hygienist should slowly inject a cartridge of anesthetic in approximately 2 minutes.

Clinical Manifestations of Overdose

After the administration of local anesthetic agents, consider new signs or symptoms as a possible sign of toxicity when evaluating patients. (see Table 14-5) The manifestation of toxicity depends on the organ system or systems that are affected. The following is a list of toxicity manifestations organized by the affected system.

Central nervous system signs

Initial symptoms
- Light-headedness
- Dizziness
- Visual and auditory disturbances (difficulty focusing and tinnitus)
- Disorientation
- Drowsiness

Higher-dose symptoms
- Often occur after an initial CNS excitation followed by a rapid CNS depression
- Muscle twitching
- Convulsions
- Unconsciousness
- Coma
- Respiratory depression and arrest
- Cardiovascular depression and collapse

Cardiovascular signs

Direct cardiac effects
- Toxic doses of local anesthetic agents can cause myocardial depression (tetracaine, bupivacaine), cardiac dysrhythmias (bupivacaine), and cardiotoxicity in pregnancy.
- Several anesthetics also have negative inotropic effects on cardiac muscle that lead to hypotension. Bupivacaine is especially cardiotoxic.

Peripheral effects
- Vasoconstriction at low doses
- Vasodilatation at higher doses (hypotension)

The range of signs and symptoms of cardiovascular toxicity includes the following:
- Chest pain
- Shortness of breath
- Palpitations
- Light-headedness
- Diaphoresis
- Hypotension
- Syncope

TABLE 14-5 Signs, Symptoms, and Management of a Local Anesthetic Overdose on CNS

SIGNS (OBSERVABLE-OBJECTIVE)	SYMPTOMS (SUBJECTIVELY FELT)	MANAGEMENT
Low to moderate blood levels		
Excitatory-nervousness-talkativeness	Disorientation	Terminate procedure
Slurred speech, general stutter	Nervousness	Reassure patient
Involuntary muscular twitching or shivering	Flushed skin color	Position patient in comfortable position
General light-headedness, dizziness	Apprehension	Administer oxygen
Tremor or twitching in muscles	Twitching tremors	Provide basic life support
Confusion, apprehension	Shivering	Monitor vital signs
Sweating	Dizziness	Summon medical assistance if needed
Vomiting	Light-headedness	Allow patient to recover and discharge
Elevated respiration	Visual disturbances	
Elevated heart rate	Auditory disturbances	
Increased blood pressure	Headache	
	Tinnitus	
	Metallic taste	
Moderate to high blood levels		
Convulsions, generally tonic-clonic	Muscle twitching	Terminate procedure
Respiratory depression (at high blood levels)	Seizures	Position patient supine, legs elevated
Depressed blood pressure and heart rate	Coma	Summon medical assistance
Unconsciousness		Manage seizure: protect patient from injury
CNS depression—coma—death		Provide basic life support
Respiratory depression and arrest		Administer oxygen
Cardiovascular depression and collapse		Monitor vital signs
		Administer an anticonvulsant (prolonged seizure)
		Stabilize patient's condition and transport to hospital

Sources: Malamed SF: *Medical emergencies in the dental office,* ed 6, St Louis, 2007, Mosby; Darby M, Walsh M: *Dental hygiene theory and practice,* ed 3, St Louis, 2010, Saunders, Elsevier.

Management of Local Anesthetic Overdose

The onset, intensity, and severity of the local anesthetic overdose will determine how to manage the emergency. In most cases the patient's symptoms will be mild, requiring little or no treatment. For moderate to severe reactions, specific, prompt management is necessary.[17]

In patients with suspected local anesthetic toxicity, the initial step is stabilization of potential life threats. Impending airway compromise, significant hypotension, and treatment of dysrhythmias and seizures take precedence. Once other possible etiologies of the patient's new symptoms have been excluded, management of the specific symptoms can begin. Table 14-5 describes the clinical signs, symptoms and management of mild, moderate, and severe overdose reactions.

EPINEPHRINE OVERDOSE

Epinephrine and levonordefrin are the two vasopressor drugs currently combined with local anesthetic agents for use in dentistry in the United States. Epinephrine is the most potent of the two and the most widely used.

Causes and Prevention of Epinephrine Overdose

An epinephrine overdose is more likely to occur when higher concentrations are administered. The use of a 1 : 50,000 concentration is twice as potent as the 1 : 100,000 concentration and is more likely to cause a toxic overdose with no added benefit to pain control. It has been stated that a dilution of 1 : 250,000 provides adequate duration of pain control for dental procedures with minimal risk of toxicity.[3] The only benefit to administering the 1 : 50,000 concentration is to increase hemostasis, which can be accomplished by infiltrating small volumes of solution to the site of excess bleeding. An overdose in this type of administration technique is rare.

Intravascular injection may also produce an epinephrine overdose reaction. As discussed previously, it is recommended for the dental hygienist to properly aspirate on several planes and to inject the solution slowly.

Patients with cardiovascular disease are much more susceptible to an epinephrine overdose, causing more strain to an already compromised cardiovascular system. The lowest possible effective dose should always be used when administering local anesthetics with epinephrine to all patients, whether healthy or medically compromised. The maximum recommended dose per visit of epinephrine for a healthy patient is 0.2 mg. The maximum recommended dose per visit of epinephrine for a cardiovascularly involved patient is 0.04 mg. The dental hygienist should use the lowest possible concentration to achieve the desired result and follow dosage guidelines as describe in Chapter 8.

Clinical Manifestations and Management of Epinephrine Overdose

Epinephrine overdose produces overstimulation of adrenergic receptors that can produce signs and symptoms normally observed from CNS stimulation and resemble the fight or flight response. Table 14-6 describes the signs, symptoms and management of an epinephrine overdose. Because the body is very efficient at removing vasoconstrictors, these adverse effects only last about 5–10 minutes and typically need little or no definitive treatment. In patients who are cardiovascularly compromised, or if prolonged reactions occur, a more serious response to the overdose may be observed, and the dental hygienist must be prepared to respond to the emergency situation.

■ ALLERGIC MANIFESTATIONS

Allergic reactions are derived by an immunologic reaction to a noninfectious foreign substance (antigen). They comprise a series of repeat reactions to a foreign substance. These foreign substances that trigger hypersensitivity reactions are called allergens or antigens.[18]

Amino esters are derivatives of *para-aminobenzoic acid* (PABA) and are associated with acute allergic reactions. Previous studies indicate a 30% rate of allergic reactions to procaine, tetracaine, and chloroprocaine. Amino amides are

TABLE 14-6	Clinical Manifestations and Management of a Patient with an Epinephrine Overdose Reaction

SIGNS AND SYMPTOMS	MANAGEMENT
Tension	Terminate procedure
Anxiety	Position patient upright
Apprehension	Reassure patient
Nervousness	Provide basic life support
Tremors	Monitor vital signs
Tension	Summon medical assistance if needed
Increased heart rate	Administer oxygen
Increased blood pressure	Allow patient to recover and discharge
Throbbing headache	
Hyperventilation	

Sources: Malamed SF: *Medical emergencies in the dental office*, ed 6, St Louis, 2007, Mosby; Darby M, Walsh M: *Dental hygiene theory and practice*, ed 3, St Louis, 2010, Saunders, Elsevier.

---

not associated with PABA and do not produce allergic reactions with the same frequency. Allergic reactions associated with amides in the past were associated with the preservative methylparaben, which has since been taken out of anesthetic solutions.

Allergic reactions associated with sodium bisulfite or metabisulfite are reported frequently.[21,22] Bisulfites are antioxidants added to local anesthetic solutions to prevent the oxidation of epinephrine. They are commonly used commercially in restaurants where they are sprayed on fruits and vegetables to prevent discoloration. They are also used to prevent bacterial contamination of wines, beers, and other distilled beverages.[17,23] Box 14-1 lists the common sulfite-containing agents. It is unknown whether bisulfites can trigger an anaphylactic reaction. Bisulfite allergies typically manifest as a severe respiratory allergy, commonly bronchospasm. It has been reported that up to 10% of people with asthma are allergic to bisulfites.[17,23]

Topical anesthetics are also possible allergens.[17] Benzocaine and tetracaine are commonly used ester topical anesthetics that can contribute to an allergic response. Lidocaine is the only amide anesthetic available topically and may contain preservatives such as parabens (methyl, ethyl, propyl), which could induce an allergic response. Careful consideration of the patient's potential for an allergic reaction should be determined before administering these agents.

PREVENTION OF ALLERGIC REACTIONS

The preanesthetic patient assessment is the most important measure that the dental hygienist can complete to prevent an allergic reaction. Patients who respond to questions related to asthma, hay fever, and allergies to foods have an increased potential for developing an allergic response to medications.[17] The dental hygienist should proceed with

further dialogue to determine whether a true allergy exists (Box 14-2). The dental hygienist should not use the anesthetic agent in question until the allergy is disproved. If questions remain following the dialogue history, the dental hygienist should consult the dentist and the patient's physician; referral to an allergist should be considered (Box 14-3).

CLINICAL MANIFESTATIONS AND MANAGEMENT OF ALLERGIC REACTIONS

Allergic responses are either delayed or immediate. Delayed signs and symptoms of an allergic reaction are less serious, and rapid signs and symptoms of an allergic reaction are more intense and serious. The amount of time between the administration of the anesthetic agent and the signs and symptoms of the allergic response determines how the dental hygienist will manage the reaction.

Allergic manifestations of local anesthetics include rash and urticaria. If these skin reactions appear alone after considerable time following the injection (more than 60 minutes), this is most likely a delayed allergic response and is usually not life-threatening. If the skin reaction develops immediately following the injection, a more serious and

TABLE 14-7	Clinical Manifestations and Management of an Allergic Reaction	
DELAYED ALLERGIC RESPONSE	**SIGNS AND SYMPTOMS**	**MANAGEMENT**
Skin	Erythema Urticaria (hives) Pruritus (itching) Angioedema (localized swelling of extremities, lips, tongue, pharynx, larynx)	Administer antihistamine Obtain medical consultation
Respiration	Bronchospasm Distress Dyspnea Wheezing Perspiration Flushing Cyanosis Tachycardia Anxiety	Terminate procedure Position patient semi-erect Reassure patient Provide basic life support as needed Summon medical assistance if needed Administer epinephrine Monitor vital signs Administer antihistamine Allow patient to recover and discharge
Laryngeal edema	Swelling of vocal apparatus and subsequent obstruction of airway Respiratory distress Exaggerated chest movements High-pitched sound to no sound Cyanosis Loss of consciousness	Terminate procedure Position patient supine Summon medical assistance Administer epinephrine Maintain airway Administer oxygen Additional drug management: antihistamine, corticosteroid Cricothyrotomy if needed Transfer patient to hospital
IMMEDIATE ANAPHYLAXIS	**SIGNS AND SYMPTOMS**	**MANAGEMENT**
Skin	Pruritus (itching) Flushing Urticaria (face and upper chest) Feeling of hair standing on end Conjunctivitis, vasomotor rhinitis	Terminate procedure Position the patient supine, legs elevated Provide basic life support as indicated Summon medical assistance Administer epinephrine Administer oxygen Monitor vital signs Additional drug management: antihistamine, corticosteroid Transport patient to hospital
Gastrointestinal or genitourinary	Abdominal cramps Nausea, vomiting diarrhea	Same as management of anaphylaxis related to skin
Respiratory	Substernal tightness or chest pain Cough, wheeze Dyspnea Cyanosis of mucous membranes, nail beds Laryngeal edema	Same as management of anaphylaxis related to skin
Cardiovascular	Pallor Light-headedness Palpitations, tachycardia Hypotension Cardiac dysrhythmias Unconsciousness Cardiac arrest	Same as management of anaphylaxis related to skin

Modified from Darby M, Walsh M: *Dental hygiene theory and practice*, ed 3, St Louis, 2010, Saunders, Elsevier.

generalized reaction, known as anaphylaxis, may occur and can be life-threatening. Anaphylaxis due to local anesthetics is very rare, but should be considered when a patient demonstrates intense itching and urticaria as well as wheezing or respiratory distress seconds following the administration of the local anesthetic agent.

Although allergic reactions to local anesthetics are extremely rare, these are treated by the dentist according to severity. Mild cutaneous reactions may be treated with diphenhydramine (Benadryl 25–50 mg for adult doses, 1 mg/kg for pediatric doses); treat patients with more serious reactions with 0.3 mL of epinephrine subcutaneously (1 : 1000), and closely monitor for further decompensation. Corticosteroids (125 mg methylprednisolone or 60 mg prednisone) should be given to the patient with severe allergic reactions (eg, respiratory distress, hypotension). Table 14-7 describes the signs, symptoms, and management of delayed allergic responses, as well as immediate anaphylactic reactions. The dental hygienist should be familiar with the use of a preloaded EpiPen (Figure 14-11).

MANAGEMENT OF MEDICAL EMERGENCIES

Life-threatening emergencies can occur during dental hygiene treatment with or without the administration of local anesthetics. Although these types of emergencies occur infrequently, the increasing number of older patients seeking dental treatment, medically compromised adults, patients taking multiple drugs, and longer dental appointments increase the likelihood of an emergency. These situations are compounded when the administration of local anesthetics is incorporated into the treatment. The dental hygienist should become familiar with the most common emergency situations, their management (including office procedures), and drugs used to treat such complications. The following guidelines are general measures to ensure emergency preparedness:

1. *Training:* all office personnel should be trained and retrained annually in emergency procedures. Office emergency simulations should be conducted every 6 months. Basic cardiac life support, that is, cardiopulmonary resuscitation is required. Advanced cardiac life support training is optional unless performing conscious sedation; however, it is recommended for dental hygienists practicing local anesthesia in states allowing its use without the physical presence of a dentist.

2. *Phone number:* telephone numbers of the closest physician, emergency department, and ambulance service (911) should be posted and programmed for "speed dial."

3. *Emergency equipment:* emergency equipment should include an oxygen tank, pocket mask, and automated external defibrillator (AED). All office personnel should know the location of the items, and all trained dental personnel who would use the oxygen and AED should be retrained on these devices annually.

4. *Drug kit:* drug therapy is always secondary to basic life support. Table 14-8 describes the common dental emergency drug kit.

5. *Recognition and management of an emergency:* the dental hygienist must maintain up-to-date education on

recognition and management of emergency situations. Table 14-9 describes the common medical emergencies and their management. Figure 14-12 illustrates actions that should be taken by the dental hygienist in an emergency situation when the patient loses consciousness.

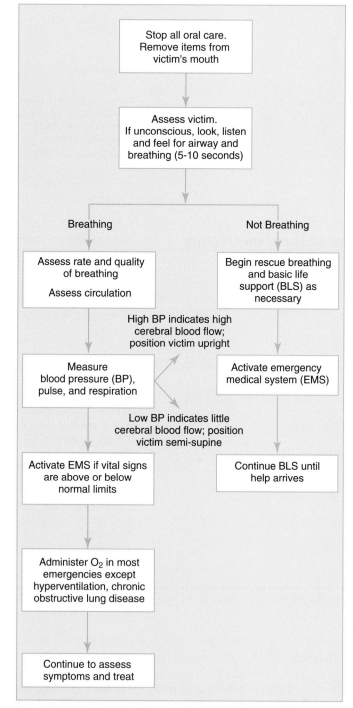

Figure 14-12 ■ Dental hygiene actions taken in an emergency situation when the patient loses consciousness. (From Darby M, Walsh M: *Dental hygiene theory and practice,* ed 3, St Louis, 2010, Saunders, Elsevier.)

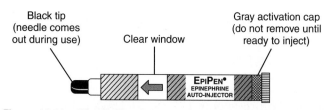

Figure 14-11 ■ The EpiPen is an emergency preloaded supply of epinephrine. (From Lehne R: *Pharmacology for nursing care,* ed 6, Philadelphia, 2007, Saunders. In Haveles E: *Applied pharmacology for the dental hygienist,* ed 6, St Louis, 2011, Mosby.)

TABLE 14-8 — Common Drugs in a Dental Emergency Kit

DRUG	ACTION AND USES
Nitroglycerin Amyl-nitrite	Coronary vessel dilator in angina pectoris
Ammonia	Irritant: increases respiratory rate
Wyamine sulfate	Vasopressors: to combat falling blood pressure
Atropine	Parasympathetic depressant to prevent vagal syncopes
Tigan	To combat nausea
Medihaler Ventolin (albuterol)	Bronchodilator
Glucola	Insulin shock
Valium	Depressant to combat convulsions
Talwin	To combat severe pain
Adrenalin	Antiallergic drug: to combat undue reactions to drugs such as penicillin or to combat severe asthmatic attack
Benadryl	Antiallergic drug: to combat undue reactions to drugs such as penicillin or to combat severe asthmatic attack
Aminophyllin	Antiallergic drug: to combat undue reactions to drugs such as penicillin or to combat severe asthmatic attack
Solu-Cortef	Antiallergic drug: to combat undue reactions to drugs such as penicillin or to combat severe asthmatic attack

TABLE 14-9 — Management of Specific Medical Emergencies

CONDITION	SIGNS AND SYMPTOMS	MANAGEMENT
Syncope (fainting)	Feeling of warmth, flushed skin, nausea, rapid heart rate, perspiration, pallor, diaphoresis. Sudden, transient loss of consciousness	Place in Trendelenburg's position (patient's head lower than legs). Loosen any binding clothes, maintain airway. Administer oxygen. Pass crushed ammonia capsule under patient's nose. Place cool, damp cloth on forehead, reassure. Monitor and record vital signs
Hyperventilation	Abnormally prolonged rapid and deep respirations, light-headedness, dizziness, tingling in extremities, tightness in the chest, rapid heartbeat, lump in throat, panic-stricken appearance. Impairment of problem-solving abilities, motor coordination, balance, and perceptual tasks	Terminate procedure, place patient in position of choice, usually upright. Use quiet tone of voice to calm and reassure patient; encourage slow, deep breaths. Loosen tight clothing in neck region. Work with patient to control rate of respirations. Have patient count to 10 in one breath, breathe through pursed lips or nose or in cupped hands
Asthma	Coughing, shortness of breath, periodic wheezing, dyspnea, anxiety, chest tightness, increased pulse rate	Assist patient to a position that facilitates breathing (upright is usually best). Have patient self-medicate with inhaler. Administer oxygen. Monitor vital signs. If necessary activate emergency medical services (EMS) and initiate basic life support (BLS)
Angina pectoris	Crushing, burning, or squeezing chest pain, radiating to left shoulder, arms, neck, or mandible and lasting 2–15 minutes; shortness of breath; diaphoresis (sweating)	Terminate procedure. Position patient upright. Monitor and record vital signs. Administer oxygen. Administer nitroglycerin (0.4 mg every 5 minutes for three doses). Activate EMS if patient's pain is not relived, and treat as a myocardial infarction
Myocardial infarction (heart attack)	Mild to severe chest pain; pain in the left arm, jaw, and possibly teeth, not relieved by rest and nitroglycerin; cold, clammy skin; nausea; anxiety; shortness of breath; weakness; perspiration; burning feeling of indigestion	Terminate procedure. Activate EMS. Place patient supine. Initiate BLS as needed. Prepare nitroglycerin from the emergency kit. Administer oxygen. Monitor and record vital signs

continued next page

TABLE 14-9   **Management of Specific Medical Emergencies—cont'd**

CONDITION	SIGNS AND SYMPTOMS	MANAGEMENT
Stroke	Sudden weakness of one side, difficulty of speech, temporary loss of vision, dizziness, change in mental status, nausea, severe headache, and/or seizures	Terminate procedure Monitor vital signs Monitor airway Administer oxygen Initiate BLS as needed Activate EMS
Seizures	Aura (change in taste, smell, or sight preceding seizure), loss of consciousness, sudden cry, involuntary tonic-clonic muscle contractions, altered breathing	Terminate procedure, lower dental chair and clear area of all sharp and dangerous objects Make no attempt to restrain patient Protect the patient's head Assess and establish an airway Monitor vital signs Initiate BLS and activate EMS if needed If the patient's condition is stable, allow patient to rest Arrange for medical follow-up Arrange for assistance in leaving the dental facility
Hypoglycemia (hyperinsulinism)	Mood changes, hunger, headache, perspiration, nausea, confusion irritation, dizziness and weakness, increased anxiety, possible unconsciousness	Terminate procedure Administer oral sugar; give concentrated form of oral sugar (e.g., sugar packet, cake icing, concentrated orange juice, apple juice, sugar-containing sodas) If patient is unconscious, activate EMS and place sugar on the oral mucosa of lower lip Initiate BLS
Hyperglycemia (ketoacidosis)	Excessive thirst, urination, and hunger; labored respirations; nausea; dry, flushed skin; low blood pressure; weak, rapid pulse; acetone breath ("fruity" smell), blurred vision, headache, unconsciousness	Terminate procedure, activate EMS, and provide BLS if needed If patient is conscious, ask when he or she ate last, whether insulin was taken, and whether patient brought insulin to the appointment If able, patient should self-administer the insulin Monitor and record vital signs
Mild allergic reaction	Itching, skin redness, hives	Call for assistance Prepare an antihistamine for administration; Be prepared to administer BLS if needed
Anaphylaxis	Urticaria (itchy wheals, also known as hives); angioedema of lips, tongue, larynx, pharynx; respiratory distress, wheezing, laryngeal edema, weak pulse, low blood pressure; may progress to unconsciousness and cardiovascular collapse	Terminate procedure, immediately activate EMS Establish and maintain airway Place in supine position Monitor vital signs Administer oxygen Initiate BLS as needed If qualified, administer epinephrine
Mild local anesthetic overdose	Disorientation, nervousness, flushed skin color, apprehension, twitching tremors, shivering, dizziness, light-headedness, visual disturbances, auditory disturbances, headache, tinnitus	Terminate procedure Reassure patient Position patient in comfortable position Administer oxygen Provide BLS if needed Monitor vital signs Summon medical assistance if needed Allow patient to recover and discharge
Severe local anesthetic overdose	Muscle twitching, convulsions	Terminate procedure Position patient supine, legs elevated Summon medical assistance Manage seizure: protect patient from injury Provide BLS if needed Administer oxygen Monitor vital signs Administer an anticonvulsant (prolonged seizure) Transport patient to hospital after condition is stabilized
Vasoconstrictor overdose	Tension Anxiety Apprehension Nervousness Tremors Increased heart rate Increased blood pressure Throbbing headache Hyperventilation	Terminate procedure Position patient upright Reassure patient Provide BLS if needed Monitor vital signs Summon medical assistance if needed Administer oxygen Allow patient to recover and discharge

Modified from Darby M, Walsh M: *Dental hygiene theory and practice*, ed 3, St Louis, 2010, Saunders, Elsevier.

DENTAL HYGIENE CONSIDERATIONS

- Most local and systemic reactions associated with the administration of local anesthetics can be avoided with thorough preanesthetic assessment, proper communication, careful choice of local anesthetic agent, and careful injection techniques. Conditions that place the patient at risk for an emergency should be recorded in red as a medical alert on the patient's medical history.
- Hematomas can occur even when the dental hygienist uses proper technique.
- Appropriate consultations or referrals must be completed before administering local anesthetics.
- Use stress reduction strategies to prevent stress-related emergencies. (See Chapters 1 and 7.)
- Baseline vital signs must be obtained before the administration of a local anesthetic. If an emergency occurs, the emergency rescue team will want to know preanesthetic vital signs.

- Always use the lowest effective dose and never exceed the maximum recommended dose (see Chapter 8).
- Record type of drug and doses administered in milligrams in the patient's chart. If an emergency occurs, the emergency rescue team will want to know what drug was administered and how much (in milligrams). (Medical personnel are unfamiliar with dental cartridge dosages, and all dosages must be converted to milligrams for appropriate documentation in the patient's chart.) (See Chapter 8.)
- Office staff must be competent in the use of emergency equipment, emergency drug kit, and office emergency procedures. Emergency drills should be conducted often.
- Thorough documentation is essential, including instructions to patient and patient responses.

CASE STUDY 14-1

Thanasi the athlete

Thanasi, a 23-year-old professional baseball player, comes in the dental office for a restorative procedure on tooth number 2. The dental hygienist, Stacey, is responsible for administration of all local anesthetics for the office. She thoroughly reviews Thanasi's medical history and determines that he is a healthy patient with no contraindications to the use of local anesthetics and vasoconstrictors. During the dialogue history when Stacey discusses his dental history, Thanasi responds by saying "I am pretty tough and can handle any dental procedure." A few minutes following Stacey's initial injection, Thanasi seems nervous and complains of dizziness, lightheadedness, and a racing heart. His color is ashen and his extremities feel cold and clammy.

Critical Thinking Questions
- According to the clinical symptoms described, what reaction is Thanasi experiencing?
- How should Stacey respond?

Thanasi has recovered from this condition when Stacey notices a faint bluish discoloration on his cheek. She checks intraorally and finds the same discoloration near the injection site along with swelling.

Critical Thinking Questions
- According to the clinical symptoms described, what reaction is Thanasi experiencing?
- What is the most probable cause of this mark?
- How should Stacey respond?

CHAPTER REVIEW QUESTIONS

1. What best describes a localized complication?
   A. A complication that occurs in a region of the injection and is attributed to the needle or the administered anesthetic
   B. A complication that is attributed only to the drug administered
   C. A complication that will resolve on its own and requires no treatment
   D. A complication that requires a definite plan of treatment.

2. What best describes a secondary complication?
   A. A complication that occurs in a region of the injection and is attributed to the needle
   B. A complication that is experienced by the patient after the injection
   C. A complication that will resolve on its own and requires no treatment
   D. A complication that requires a definite plan of treatment

3. If needle breakage occurs and the clinician can easily retrieve the needle, what is the next step?
   A. Inform the patient
   B. Call in the dentist
   C. Keep hand in the patient's mouth and ask him or her to open widely
   D. Take panoramic radiograph and refer to oral surgeon

4. Anaphylaxis is considered to be what type of complication?
   A. Localized and severe
   B. Systemic and mild
   C. Systemic and severe
   D. Localized and mild

5. When a blood vessel is punctured or lacerated by the anesthetic needle, an asymmetrical swelling and discoloration may occur. This is possibly a sign of:
   A. Hematoma
   B. Hemangioma
   C. Edema
   D. Trismus

6. What is the first step in managing a hematoma?
   A. Apply heat
   B. Apply cold compress
   C. Massage tissues
   D. Apply pressure

7. Soreness in the muscles caused by muscles spasms is called what?
   A. Trismus
   B. Nerve paralysis
   C. Hematoma
   D. Paresthesia

8. Edema can be caused by which of the following?
   A. Trauma during injections
   B. Infection
   C. Contaminated solutions
   D. Allergic reaction
   E. All of the above

9. Paresthesia occurs most commonly during which intraoral injection?
   A. MSA block
   B. PSA block
   C. IA block
   D. GG mandibular block

10. How can the dental hygienist decrease the risk of infection during an injection?
   A. Use sterile needles
   B. Store cartridges in original containers
   C. Use topical antiseptic
   D. Carefully sheath and unsheathe the needle before and after injections
   E. All of the above

11. Why should topical anesthetics only be applied for 1–2 minutes?
   A. To prevent tissue sloughing
   B. To prevent sterile abscesses
   C. To prevent soft tissues trauma
   D. B and C only
   E. All of the above

12. Systemic complications usually occur more frequently than local complications and are usually caused by high plasma concentration of the local anesthetic drug.
   A. Both statements are true
   B. Both statements are false
   C. First statement is true, second statement is false
   D. First statement is false, second state is true

13. All of the following can increase the risk of local anesthetic overdose EXCEPT:
   A. Fast biotransformation.
   B. Rapid deposit of solution
   C. Intravascular injection
   D. Atypical pseudocholinesterase

14. What are signs of central nervous system overdose?
   A. Dizziness
   B. Hypotension
   C. Chest pains
   D. Diaphoresis
   E. All of the above

15. Convulsions, respiratory distress, cardiovascular depression, and coma are all signs of what?
   A. Heart attack
   B. Cardiovascular toxicity
   C. Epinephrine overdose
   D. Local anesthetic overdose

16. Which of the following has the lowest concentration of epinephrine?
   A. 1:100,000 epinephrine
   B. 1:200,000 epinephrine
   C. 1:50,000 epinephrine
   D. 1:250,000 epinephrine

17. Which of the following is the appropriate treatment for a mild cutaneous reaction?
   A. Corticosteroids
   B. Diphenhydramine
   C. Nitroglycerin
   D. Aspirin

18. All are signs of angina pectoris EXCEPT:
   A. Crushing chest pain
   B. Pain in left arm
   C. Shortness of breath
   D. Dizziness

19. If the clinician strongly suspects the patient is having a myocardial infarction, he or she should terminate the procedure and then:

CHAPTER REVIEW QUESTIONS

A. Position the patient upright
B. Administer nitroglycerin
C. Activate EMS
D. Initiate BLS

20. If a patient starts to experience involuntary muscle contractions and altered breathing, what should the clinician suspect?

A. Respiratory distress
B. Hypoglycemia
C. Seizures
D. Asthma attack

REFERENCES

1. Bennett CR: *Monheim's local anesthesia and pain control in dental practice*, ed 7, St Louis, 1984, Mosby.

2. Jastak T, Yagiela J, Donaldson D: *Local anesthesia of the oral cavity*, St Louis, 1995, Saunders.

3. Malamed S: *Handbook of local anesthesia*, ed 5, St Louis, 2004, Mosby.

4. Darby M, Walsh M: *Dental Hygiene Theory and Practice*, ed 3, St Louis, 2010, Saunders.

5. Haas DA: Localized complications from local anesthesia, *J Calif Dent* 26: 677-682, 1998.

6. Haas DA, Lennon D: A 21-year retrospective study of reports of paresthesia following local anesthetic administration, *J Can Dent Assoc* 61: 319-330, 1995.

7. Pogrel MA, Bryan J, Regezi J: Nerve damage associated with inferior alveolar nerve blocks, *J Am Dent Assoc* 126: 1150-1155, 1995.

8. Pogrel MA, Thamby S: Permanent nerve involvement resulting from inferior alveolar nerve blocks, *J Am Dent Assoc* 131: 901-907, 2000.

9. Harn SD, Durham TM: Incidence of lingual nerve trauma and postinjection complications in conventional mandibular block anesthesia, *J Am Dent Assoc* 121: 519-523, 1990.

10. Kalichman MW, Moorhouse DF, Powell HC, Myers RR: Relative neural toxicity of local anesthetics, *J Neuropathol Exp Neurol* 52: 234-240, 1993.

11. Malamed SF: Local anesthetics: dentistry's most important drugs-clinical update 2006, *J Calif Dent Assoc* 34(12): 971-976, 2006.

12. Malamed SF: Articaine versus lidocaine: the author responds (comment on Dower JS Jr. Articaine vs lidocaine, *J Calif Dent Assoc* 2007;35(4): 240, 242, 244), *J Calif Dent Assoc* 35(6): 383-385, 2007.

13. Gaffen AS, Haas DA: Retrospective review of voluntary reports of nonsurgical paresthesia in dentistry, *J Can Dent Assoc* 75(8): 579, 2009.

14. Garisto GA, Gaffen AS, Lawrence HP, Tenenbaum HC, Haas DA: Occurrence of paresthesia after dental local anesthetic administration in the United States, *J Am Dent Assoc* 141(7): 836-844, 2010.

15. Pogrel MA: Permanent nerve damage from inferior alveolar nerve blocks-an update to include articaine, *CDA Journal* 35(4): 271-273, 2007.

16. Fehrenbach M, Herring S: Spread of dental infection, *Practical Hygiene* 13-19, September/October 1997.

17. Malamed SF: *Medical emergencies in the dental office*, ed 6, St Louis, 2007, Mosby.

18. Little JW, Falace DA, Miller CS, Rhodus NL: *Dental management of the medically compromised patient*, St Louis, 2008, Mosby.

19. Phentolamine: (2009). *Merck manuals: online medical library*. Retrieved (September 5, 2010) from Phentolamine Drug Information Provided by Lexi-Comp Merck Manual Professional. mht

20. OraVerse (2009): *Highlights of prescribing information*. Retrieved (September 5, 2010) from http://www.fda.gov/downloads/AdvisoryCommittees/CommitteesMeetingMaterials/PediatricAdvisoryCommittee/UCM214420.pdf.

21. Stevenson DD, Simon RA: Sensitivity to ingested metabisulfites in asthmatic subjects, *J Allergy Clin Immunol* 68: 26-32, 1981.

22. Sher TH, Schwartz HJ: Bisulfite sensitivity manifesting an allergic reaction to aerosol therapy, *Ann Allergy* 54: 224-226, 1985.

23. Borghesan F, Basso D, Chieco Bianchi F, et al: Allergy to wine, *Allergy* 59: 1135-1136, 2004.

ADDITIONAL RESOURCES

Haas DA: An update on local anesthetics in dentistry, *J Can Dent Assoc* 68: 546-551, 2002.

Goldfrank LR, Flomenbaum NE, Lewin NA, et al: *Goldfrank's toxicologic emergencies*, ed 6, New York, 1998, McGraw-Hill, 897-903.

Wang Q, Liu Y, Lei Y, et al: Shenfu injection reduces toxicity of bupivacaine in rats, *Chin Med J (Engl)* 116: 1382-1385, 2003.

Weinberg GL, Ripper R, Feinstein DL, Hoffman W: Lipid emulsion infusion rescues dogs from bupivacaine-induced cardiac toxicity, *Reg Anesth Pain Med* 28: 198-202, 2003.

Weinberg GL, Di Gregorio G, Ripper R, et al: Resuscitation with lipid versus epinephrine in a rat model of bupivacaine overdose, *Anesthesiology* 108: 907-913, 2008.

Chen AH: Toxicity and allergy to local anesthesia, *J Calif Dent Assoc* 26: 683-692, 1998.

Hogan Q: Local anesthetic toxicity: an update, *Reg Anesth* 21(6 Suppl): 43-50, 1996.

Katzung BG: *Basic and clinical pharmacology*, ed 6, New York, 1995, McGraw-Hill, 395-403.

McGee D: Local and topical anesthesia. In: Roberts JR, Hedges J, eds. *Clinical procedures in emergency medicine*, ed 4, Philadelphia, 2004, WB Saunders, 533-551.

CHAPTER 15

Legal Considerations and Risk Management

Demetra Daskalos Logothetis RDH, MS

CHAPTER OUTLINE

LEARNING OBJECTIVES

1. Discuss the importance of effective dental hygienist–to-patient communication before treatment.
2. Discuss the importance of effective dental hygienist–to-employer communication.
3. Discuss the legal issues related to dental hygiene treatment and prevention strategies to reduce the risk of litigation.
4. Define indirect and general supervision.
5. Describe the type of information that should be documented in a patient's chart for the administration of local anesthetics.
6. Describe the procedures to reduce the risk of accidental needle exposure.
7. Describe postexposure protocol.
8. Successfully complete review questions and activities for this chapter.

KEY TERMS

Occupational exposure A percutaneous injury (e.g., needlestick or cut with a sharp object) or contact of mucous membrane on nonintact skin (e.g., exposed skin that is chapped, abraded, or with dermatitis) with blood, saliva, tissue, or other body fluids that are potentially infectious.

Primary prevention Strive to use all protocols to prevent the injury from occurring.

Qualified health care professional Designated qualified health care professional responsible for care and follow-up of occupational exposures.

Secondary prevention Strive to contain the injury.

Tertiary prevention Strive to return to a functional state and prevent future injuries.

RISK MANAGEMENT

Every great mistake has a halfway moment when it can be recalled and perhaps remedied.

—Pearl S. Buck

The primary objective of providing dental hygiene care is to assist patients in preventing disease and maintaining oral health. With the delivery of these services, the dental hygienist may experience unanticipated and problematic outcomes. For example, local anesthetics administered for pain management to effectively maximize patient comfort and treatment may bring with it undesirable adverse reactions. Risk management identifies preventive methods to minimize or eliminate the risk of legal action associated with the delivery of oral care. Due to the scope of practice for dentists, they are more at risk for litigation. However, the dental hygienist is also exposed to legal risks, and there is a greater degree of accountability when a dental hygienist is licensed to administer local anesthetics. To reduce the risk of litigation, the dental hygienist should follow these important principles for risk management.

COMMUNICATION

Dental hygienist-patient communication: open and effective communication between the dental hygienist and the patient is an important risk management tool. Minimizing misunderstandings and resolving problems as they arise during the dental hygiene treatment reduces the likelihood of lawsuits. It is important to develop a one-on-one relationship with the patient to build confidence and trust.[1,2]

Before the administration of a local anesthetic, it is essential for the dental hygienist to clearly present the benefits and risks associated with the procedure. For this type of communication to be successful, the dental

hygienist should simplify technical terms to the appropriate level of the patient. Dental jargon can sound like "Greek" to most patients and should only be used with other health professionals. It is ultimately the patient's decision whether he or she wishes to accept the local anesthetic procedure. Usually, the patient does not fully understand the benefits of nonsurgical periodontal therapy with anesthesia, and he or she is more likely to decline the procedure. The dental hygienist must use effective communication skills to explain the procedure and the benefits for patient comfort, as well as explain the risks associated with no treatment or treatment that is difficult to effectively accomplish because the procedure is too painful. Box 15-1 is a sample conversation between the dental hygienist and the patient.

Dental hygienist–employer communication: the dental hygienist should have an open discussion with his or her employer regarding the potential liabilities for dental hygienists and prevention strategies. Office protocols should be written and reviewed periodically by all office employees. Dental hygienists should discuss with their employer the scope of dental hygiene practice and always practice within the regulations of their license, regardless of their employer's request.

BOX 15-1	**Sample Dialogue Regarding Nonsurgical Periodontal Therapy between the Patient and the Dental Hygienist**

Hygienist: Seated in a position that allows direct eye contact, and showing empathy and respect, the dental hygienist should begin the conversation outlining the treatment for the day:

Today, I will be treating the upper right quadrant (point to the upper right quadrant).

Utilizing the periodontal chart, or computerized program, discuss the periodontal involvement.

As you can see from this chart, in several areas you have "periodontal pockets," which have occurred in the past from the destruction of the supporting bone around these teeth. I will be debriding and root planing these areas with my instruments.

Patient: *Will this hurt?*

Hygienist: *As I recall from our previous visit when I was assessing the status of your teeth with my periodontal probe (show probe), it seems as if you were sensitive when I was walking the probe around your gums to determine the depth of the pocket. Is this a correct assumption?*

Patient: *Yes, it did feel uncomfortable.*

Hygienist: *Well, fortunately I can numb up the area to provide you with the maximum comfort for the procedure. What are your thoughts to receiving a local anesthetic?*

Patient: *Well gosh, I have had my teeth cleaned before at other dental offices and never had to get a shot. I don't think that is necessary.*

Hygienist: *I completely understand. Since I do not have the records from your other dental office, it is hard for me to comment on the procedures that you had in the past, or the condition of your mouth at that particular time. The type of treatment we provide is dependent upon the condition of your mouth at the time of treatment. Today your condition requires me to use my instruments a little deeper under your gums than you may have*

experienced in the past. I want you to be as comfortable as possible, and your comfort will allow me to successfully complete the procedure for your maximum benefit.

Patient: *Well, I do want the comfort, but I am scared of getting shots.*

Hygienist: *I understand your fear of shots; many individuals feel the same way you do. Let me explain the procedure, and then you can let me know what concerns or questions you may have.*

First, I will apply some topical anesthetic with a Q-tip to the area to numb the area where the injection will take place. I will then deposit the solution slowly. Once I start depositing the solution, it will only take a couple of seconds until the area begins to become numb.

Patient: *Wow, it only takes a couple of seconds.*

Hygienist: *Let me explain myself better, the injection will take longer because I will be injecting the solution slowly for better comfort to you, and to increase the safety of the injection. The tissue will begin to numb even before the injection is completed, and you will only feel a pinch for a couple of seconds.*

Patient: *OK, go ahead with this procedure, and I will tell you if I am uncomfortable during the shot.*

Hygienist: *It is fine if you want me to stop during the procedure, but it is best if you do not try to talk. Instead you can raise your hand, which will signal me that you want me to stop. (This is a strategy to let the patient know that you will stop if there is a concern, and it gives them the confidence to know that they are in control of the situation). OK, before we begin I will go over the benefits and risks associated with the treatment today, and any questions you may have. If you are OK with the procedures, we will then begin treatment.*

Patient: *OK, that sounds good.*

LEGAL ISSUES RELATED TO THE DENTAL HYGIENIST

A licensed dental hygienist has a contractual obligation (whether written or oral) to the patient to provide safe and thorough dental hygiene services. As a licensed practitioner, the dental hygienist is dependent upon the rules and regulation laws of the state in which he or she has obtained a license. The dental hygienist must assume the legal responsibilities of his or her own actions and should never assume that the employer should be held accountable for the dental hygienist's actions. A dental hygienist may be charged with malpractice if he or she induces harm to the patient or if a breech of duty exists. (See Box 15-2.) A dental hygienist may commit a negligent act during the administration of local anesthetics by causing paresthesia or if a needle breaks in the patient's tissue. Moreover, if a dental hygienist is unable to provide thorough nonsurgical periodontal therapy because the patient refuses anesthesia, he or she may be held accountable if the patient's periodontal status declines. Whatever the situation may be, malpractice may be determined if the contractual obligations are not met by the dental hygienist. The dental hygienist should do the following to prevent litigation:[2]

1. *Maintain proper licensure:* Be properly licensed in all dental hygiene functions required to engage in the practice of dental hygiene. Most states require the dental hygienist to apply for an additional local anesthesia license or certificate in lieu of a regular dental hygiene license to legally administer local anesthetics. Each state has different educational and examination requirements that need to be completed by the dental hygienist prior to the application process for licensure. The dental hygienist can easily obtain that information from the website of the dental board for each individual state.

2. *Take responsibility for lifelong learning:* The dental hygienist is responsible for maintaining his or her own professional competency and credentials as determined by the licensing board. Continuing education courses are critical to maintaining dental hygiene competence.

An investment in knowledge always pays the best interest.
—Benjamin Franklin

3. *Never exceed the scope of dental hygiene practice.* In some states, the scope of dental hygiene practice for all dental hygiene treatment, including local anesthesia requires the physical presence of a dentist. This means that the dentist must diagnose the patient's condition, authorize the procedures, and be physically on the premises where the dental hygienist is providing care. In other states, supervision laws do not require the physical presence of the dentist for dental hygiene treatment, but do require it during the administration of local anesthesia. Because of the confusion presented by two supervision laws and the scope of dental hygiene practice, the dentist may assume that the dental hygienist can legally administer local anesthetics without the physical presence of a dentist in this situation. It is the responsibility of the dental hygienist to know the supervision laws of the state as they pertain to the practice of dental hygiene and discuss them with the dentist. The dental hygienist should never administer local anesthetics without the physical presence of a dentist, even if requested by the supervising dentist, unless the laws of the state allow for this procedure. The dental hygienist should never administer local anesthetics unless properly licensed and should report any illegal activities by a health care provider to the responsible authorities.

In any moment of decision, the best thing you can do is the right thing. The worst thing you can do is nothing.
—Theodore Roosevelt

4. Obtain informed consent from the individual or parent/guardian before treatment. Individuals who incur a health care injury and allege that the dental hygienist did not fully inform them of the procedure to which they consented may file legal action. See Figure 11-3 for a sample consent form.

5. Before administration of local anesthetics, make appropriate referrals and consultations regarding the patient's medical status.

BOX 15-2	Dental Hygienist Legal Case: Dental Hygienist's Unlawful Administration Of Nitrous Oxide

This case[4] arises from a complaint by a dental hygienist against a former employer, Lowenberg and Lowenberg Corporation. The dental hygienist alleged that the defendant allowed dental hygienists working in their office to administer nitrous oxide to patients. Under state law, dental hygienists may not administer nitrous oxide. The Department of Education's Office of Professional Discipline investigated the complaint by using an undercover investigator. The investigator made an appointment for teeth cleaning. At the time of her appointment, she requested that nitrous oxide be administered. Agreeing to the investigator's request, the dental hygienist administered the nitrous oxide. There were no notations in the patient's chart indicating that she had been administered nitrous oxide.

A hearing panel found the involved dental hygienist guilty of administering nitrous oxide without being properly licensed. In addition, the hearing panel found that the dental hygienist had failed to record accurately in the patient's chart that she had administered nitrous oxide.

The New York Supreme Court, Appellate Division, held that the investigator's report provided sufficient evidence to support the hearing panel's determination. There is adequate evidence in the record to support a finding that the dentist's conduct was such that it could reasonably be said that he permitted the dental hygienist to perform acts that she was not licensed to perform.

6. Maintain patient privacy and confidentiality of information according to Health Insurance Portability and Accountability Act guidelines.
7. Always administer local anesthetic according to acceptable standards set by other practitioners with similar training.
8. Do not experiment on a patient with new local anesthetic techniques or drugs. Dental hygienists should frequently attend continuing education courses specifically on local anesthetics. New techniques, procedures, and local anesthetic drugs will be presented in an education environment conducive to safe and effective learning.
9. Administer the appropriate volume of anesthetic for the area that can reasonably be completed during one appointment. For nonsurgical periodontal therapy for patients with advanced periodontitis, care should be taken in developing the dental hygiene care plan as to not be overly aggressive in the care. If the dental hygienist is unsure of the difficulty of the case, it is best to administer local anesthetics for just one quadrant, or even a sextant, and to complete the area in its entirety before administering more anesthetic for the next quadrant or sextant. Once one quadrant or sextant is completed, the dental hygienist can administer more anesthetic (assuming the maximum recommended dose has not been administered), if time is available.
10. Never abruptly stop treatment or abandon the patient.
11. Keep the patient informed regarding the progression of treatment and results obtained.
12. Keep the patient informed of any unanticipated occurrences during and after the administration of the local anesthetic.
13. Document and keep accurate records.
14. Always practice in a manner consistent with the dental hygiene code of ethics.
15. Obtain professional liability insurance. The dental hygienist as a licensed professional should maintain adequate professional liability insurance and be familiar with the policy coverage. In the event of malpractice litigation, the dental hygienist cannot rely on being covered against malpractice under the employer's insurance policy.

DOCUMENTATION

Documentation in the patient's permanent record can be the dental hygienists' best defense, or worst enemy, in the event of a malpractice lawsuit.[1] In addition to the information necessary for all dental procedures, the patient record should include the following information specifically for the administration of local anesthetics:

1. Medical status of the patient including any pharmacologic history. Documentation regarding any contraindications to local anesthetics or vasoconstrictors should be included.

2. Vital signs taken before administration of the local anesthetic drug.
3. Dental history regarding the patient's psychological state as related to injections and nervousness.
4. Referrals or consultations obtained before the administration of the local anesthetic drug.
5. Any refusal of treatment by the patient and a brief statement documenting the discussion of risks associated with treatment refusal.
6. Comprehensive and chronologic documentation of treatment, including the patient's maximum recommended dose, the drug used and concentration, vasoconstrictor used if any, the amount administered in milligrams, the gauge and type of needle, the injections given, the time of anesthetic administration, and any patient reactions or complications.
7. Any unexpected occurrences or reactions.
8. Continued care intervals or maintenance schedule.
9. Any specific postcare instructions given to the patient.

EXPOSURE PREVENTION AND MANAGEMENT

An occupational exposure in dentistry is defined by the Centers for Disease Control and Prevention as a percutaneous injury (e.g., needlestick or cut with a sharp object) or contact of mucous membrane or nonintact skin (e.g., exposed skin that is chapped, abraded, or with dermatitis) with blood, saliva, tissue, or other body fluids that are potentially infectious.[3] Exposure incidents might place dental health care personnel at risk for hepatitis B virus (HBV), hepatitis C virus (HCV), or human immunodeficiency virus (HIV) infection, and therefore should be evaluated immediately following treatment of the exposure site by a qualified health care professional.[2]

All dental facilities must have a post exposure management protocol for occupational exposures. This protocol should contain written guidelines, according to the most current guidelines from the U.S. Public Health Service (USPHS), addressing the steps for post exposure, training and education requirements for dental personnel, types of exposures that put dental personnel at risk, and procedures for prompt reporting and evaluation. Guidelines must follow the Occupational Health and Safety Administration blood-borne pathogen standards and any state or local laws or regulations.

The three categories of prevention and management of injury should be followed:

Primary prevention: The dental hygienist should strive to use all protocols to prevent the injury from occurring.

Secondary prevention: If an injury occurs, the dental hygienist should strive to contain the injury.

Tertiary prevention: The dental hygienist should strive to return the patient to a functional state and prevent future injuries.

RISK REDUCTION PROTOCOL

Avoiding occupational exposure to blood is the primary way to prevent transmission of HBV, HCV, and HIV in health care settings. Methods used to reduce such exposures in dental settings include engineering and work practice controls and the use of personal protective equipment (PPE).

Primary prevention involves the dental hygienist striving to make every effort to avoid injury during the administration of local anesthetics and throughout the dental hygiene treatment. However, in a moment of distraction during or after treatment, a needlestick injury can occur. To minimize the risk, the dental hygienist should follow these guidelines:

- Use the most currently developed medical devices with safety features designed to prevent injuries and use the safest technique.
- Never recap the needle by hand; always use the scoop technique for capping needles. Needle-capping devices aid in effectively accomplishing this technique.
- Use disposable needle systems.
- Know the position of the uncapped needle at all times.
- Immediately after the injection, safely cap the needle before continuing with any procedure.
- Dispose of needle in appropriate sharps container. Caution should be taken when removing the needle from the syringe. Remember that the needle penetrating end that is embedded in the cartridge is contaminated after the injection, and care should be taken when removing it from the syringe.
- Create a neutral zone for the sharps. The needle should not be passed between health care workers.

POSTEXPOSURE MANAGEMENT

Postexposure management involves secondary and tertiary prevention strategies. The goal is to contain the injury to reduce the possibility of disease transmission. The exposed worker should review the most recent USPHS guidelines for postexposure. A qualified health care professional (QHCP) should be selected by the dental practice *before* the dental health care professionals are placed at risk for exposure. This QHCP should be experienced in conducting testing and providing antiretroviral therapy, and should be familiar with the unique nature of dental injuries so they can provide appropriate guidance on the need for antiretroviral prophylaxis. The QHCP determines the source patient's disease status through testing if consent is obtained. The following steps should be conducted following the exposure:

1. Wounds and skin sites that have been in contact with blood or body fluids should be cleansed with soap and water. Flush mucous membranes with water. Bleach or other caustic agents should not be used to cleanse the wound.
2. The QHCP should communicate to the source patient the incident and his or her role in the postexposure protocol. Excellent communication skills are critical at this point in the process.
3. Obtain consent for testing from the source patient if known.
4. Immediately set up testing for dental worker and source patient with the QHCP.
5. The incident report form (Figure 15-1) should be completed and recorded in the exposed person's confidential medical record. The following information should be recorded:
   - Date and time of exposure.
   - Details of the procedure performed, including where and how the exposure occurred, and whether the exposure involved a sharp device, the type of device, whether there was visible blood on the device, and how and when the exposure occurred.
   - Details of the exposure, including the type and amount of fluid or material and the severity of the exposure. For a percutaneous injury, details should include the depth of the wound, the gauge of the needle, and whether fluid was injected; for a skin or mucous membrane exposure, the estimated volume of material, the duration of contact, and the condition of the skin (e.g., chapped, abraded, or intact) would be included.
   - Details about the exposure source: (1) whether the patient was infected with HCV or HBV and the patient's hepatitis B e antigen (HBeAg) status and (2) whether the source was infected with HIV, the stage of disease, history of antiretroviral therapy, and viral load, if known.
   - Details about the exposed person (e.g., hepatitis B vaccination and vaccine-response status).
   - Details about counseling, postexposure management, and follow-up.
6. The qualified health care professionals must consider the following factors when assessing the need for follow-up of occupational exposures:
   Type of exposure
   - Percutaneous injury (e.g., depth, extent)
   - Mucous membrane exposure
   - Nonintact skin exposure
   - Bites resulting in blood exposure to either person involved
   Type and amount of fluid/tissue
   - Blood
   - Fluids containing blood
   Infectious status of source
   - Presence of hepatitis B surface antigen (HBsAg) and HBeAg
   - Presence of HCV antibody
   - Presence of HIV antibody
   Susceptibility of exposed person
   - Hepatitis B vaccine and vaccine response status
   - HBV, HCV, or HIV immune status
   - After conducting this initial evaluation of the occupational exposure, a qualified health care professional must decide whether to conduct further

---

BLOODBORNE EXPOSURE REPORT FORM

Exposed Employee Information:

Name_____ SS#_____ Job Title_____

Employer name _____ Address_____

Time of Occurrence_____Time Reported_____Date_____

Hepatitis B vaccination Yes_____   No_____

If yes, dates of vaccination: 1._____   2._____   3._____

Post-vaccination status, if known: Positive_____Titer_____ Negative_____

Last tetanus vaccination date:_____

Review of *Exposure Incident Follow-Up Procedures:* Yes_____

Exposure Incident Information:

If sharps-related injury:
Type of sharp: _____ Brand _____

Work area where exposure occurred:_____

Procedure in progress:_____

How incident occurred:_____

Location of exposure (e.g., right index finger):_____

Did sharps involved have engineered injury protection? yes:_____   no:_____

If yes:
Was the protective mechanism activated?   yes_____   no:_____

    If yes, did the injury occur: before activation of protective mechanism_____
                                    during activation of protective mechanism_____
                                      after activation of protective mechanism_____

If no:
Employee's opinion:

Could a mechanism have prevented the injury: yes_____   no_____

How could a mechanism have prevented the injury:_____
1 of 2

Figure 15-1 ◼ Exposure reporting form. (From Darby M, Walsh M: *Dental hygiene theory and practice*, ed 3, St Louis, 2010, Saunders, Elsevier.)

follow-up on an individual basis using all of the information obtained.

7. Written report/opinion of health care provider: Within 15 days of evaluation, the qualified health care provider sends a written opinion to the employer. The report documents that the employee was informed of evaluation results and the need for further follow-up treatment, and whether the HBV vaccine was indicated and if the employee received the vaccine. All other findings are confidential and not included. The employer keeps a copy of the report in a confidential medical record and provides a copy to the exposed employee.

The most important human endeavor is the striving for morality in our actions. Our inner balance, and even our very existence depends on it. Only morality in our actions can give beauty and dignity to our lives.

—Albert Einstein

BLOODBORNE EXPOSURE REPORT FORM

Employee's opinion:

Could any engineering, administrative, or work practice control have prevented the injury?
yes___   no___

Explain: _____

_____

Source Patient Information:

Name_____Chart No._____ Telephone No._____

	Yes	No
Release of information to evaluating healthcare professional?	___	___

Patient's signature_____

	Yes	No
Review of source patient medical history: Verbally questioned regarding:		
• History of hepatitis B, hepatitis C or HIV infection	___	___
• High risk history associated with these diseases	___	___
• Patient consents to be tested for HIV, HCV and HBV	___	___

If HIV-positive source patient:

List all current medications patient is taking for HIV infection:

1._____ 2._____ 3._____ 4._____

List all medication previously taken by patient to which he or she was resistant or medications that were ineffective:

1._____ 2._____ 3._____ 4._____

Provide most recent viral load: _____ date:_____

CD4 count if known:_____ date:_____

Healthcare worker referred to: _____

Questionnaire completed by_____

Bill for fees to:_____

Retain one copy in employee's confidential medical record; send one copy to evaluating healthcare professional. Retain copy with employee's and source patient's name removed as sharp's injury log.

2 of 2

Figure 15-1, cont'd

DENTAL HYGIENE CONSIDERATIONS

- Ethical principles guide the conduct of the health care professions regarding moral duties and obligations to the profession, to one's self, to the employers, and to the patients.
- Dental hygienists are accountable to their patients and employers, and must take responsibility for their actions.

- Obtain and maintain appropriate licensure before services are provided.
- A licensed dental hygienist has a contractual responsibility (whether written or oral) to the patient to provide safe and thorough dental hygiene services.
- A dental hygienist must meet the standard of care set by other practitioners with similar training.

DENTAL HYGIENE CONSIDERATIONS—cont'd

- Always obtain informed consent to allow the patient to formally accept or deny services.
- Communication between the dental hygienist and the patient is an important risk management tool. Always keep the patient informed of treatment and progress.
- Confidentiality of patient records is an important responsibility of the dental hygienist.
- The dental hygienist should always identify preventable methods to minimize or eliminate risk.

- Never recap the needle by hand; always use the scoop technique for capping needles.
- Always dispose of contaminated needles in approved containers.
- The dental hygienist should know the position of the uncapped needle at all times.
- Thorough documentation of treatment and reactions to treatment are essential.
- The dental hygienist must follow the most current postexposure guidelines set by the USPHS.

CASE STUDY 15-1

The anxious dental hygienist

Joan B., RDH, BSDH, graduated from a university dental hygiene program that did not teach the administration of local anesthetics. Joan was not concerned about not practicing this expanded function because she worked in a state where this function was not allowed for dental hygienists.

Her husband was offered a job transfer to a state where local anesthesia administration was legal for dental hygienists. Joan was thrilled to finally work in a state where she could perform that function. Joan was an experienced dental hygienist of 7 years and easily obtained a licensure by credentials in the state where she would soon be working. Joan took the necessary education required by the state to administer local anesthetic, passed the written and clinical examinations, and applied for her anesthesia licensure.

Joan received a job before her anesthesia license was sent by the board, but she was not concerned because she already had her dental hygiene license for that state. On her first day of the job, Joan was scheduled for several nonsurgical periodontal debridements requiring local anesthetics. She immediately became concerned because the dentist was scheduled to be in a continuing education class that day and would not be in the office. The dental hygienist approached the receptionist about the dentist not being in the building for the dental hygiene care. The receptionist informed the dental hygienist that the administration of local anesthesia by a dental hygienist without the physical presence of the dentist is allowed in the state, and the dentist already examined the patients and authorized the procedures.

Joan was embarrassed to reveal that she had not yet received her anesthesia license and was concerned about having to cancel the patients on her first day at work. She decided to go ahead and administer the anesthetic, because, after all, she took the appropriate education and passed all the clinical and written examinations. She convinced herself that the license was just a formality and not to be concerned with not having it in hand.

Ethical and Legal Issues

- Discuss how ethical values were violated in this case.
- Describe how both ethical and legal issues are intertwined in this case.

CHAPTER REVIEW QUESTIONS

1. Before administering local anesthetics, the dental hygienist should describe the risks and benefits to the patient. What type of terms should be used?
   A. Specific technical terms
   B. Phrases like "pokey thing" and "feels like an ouchie"
   C. Terms appropriate for the patient's education level
   D. Do not tell the patient anything. If you do not talk about it, then the patient will not be nervous.
2. Practicing within the legal scope of practice means?
   A. Practicing only within the limits set forth by your license and state's rules and regulations

   B. Practicing within the limits of your license, unless the dentist gives you permission to do expanded procedures
   C. Practicing any procedure as long the doctor is present in the office
   D. Performing procedures that the doctor has approved in the treatment plan
3. Which of the following statements is false regarding the administration of local anesthetics?
   A. Never abruptly stop treatment, or abandon the patient
   B. Keep the patient informed regarding the progression of treatment and results obtained

CHAPTER REVIEW QUESTIONS

C. Never inform the patient of any unanticipated occurrences during and after the administration of the local anesthetic

D. Document and keep accurate records

4. In most states the dental hygienist is not required to have malpractice insurance, because the dental hygienist will be covered under the dentist's insurance.
   A. Both the statement and the reason are true
   B. Both the statement and the reason are false
   C. The statement is false, but the reason is true
   D. The statement is true, but the reason is false

5. Dental hygienists are accountable for their own actions and practice; however, the dentist is always liable for any legal actions taken against the hygienist.
   A. Both statements are true
   B. Both statements are false
   C. The first statement is true, and the second statement is false
   D. The first statement is false, and the second statement is true

6. Dental hygienists who hold a current anesthesia license are always able to administer local anesthetics without the physical presence of a dentist, but only if the dentist authorizes the procedure.
   A. Both statements are true
   B. Both statements are false
   C. The first statement is true, and the second statement is false
   D. The first statement is false, and the second statement is true

7. What is the appropriate amount of anesthetic to be administered during a procedure?
   A. The amount necessary to complete the area that will be treated and finished in a single appointment
   B. The amount that covers most of the area, so that you do not have to give a second injection
   C. Enough for one tooth at a time; that way you can avoid the risk of toxicity
   D. Always give at least half the maximum recommended dose

8. Which of the following diseases is contractible if a needlestick occurs to the dental hygienist?
   A. HBV
   B. HCV
   C. HIV
   D. All of the above

9. Postexposure management protocol for occupational exposures should contain?
   A. Steps for postexposure
   B. Training and education requirements for dental personnel

C. Types of exposures that put dental personnel at risk
D. Procedures for prompt reporting and evaluation
E. All of the above
F. None of the above

10. Which statement is true regarding the handling of sharps?
    A. It is acceptable to throw unused needles in the regular trash
    B. It is acceptable to hand an uncapped needle to an assistant if you are unable to reach the cap
    C. It is acceptable to recap a needle with your hands as long as the needle has not been contaminated
    D. It is acceptable to recap a needle only using the scoop method

11. If a needlestick injury occurs, it is not necessary to report the details of what happened, only that you were possibly exposed.
    A. Both statements are true
    B. Both statements are false
    C. The first statement is true; the second is false
    D. The first statement is false; the second is true

12. Secondary prevention is when there is containment of an injury after it occurs. Tertiary prevention involves the return of the patient to a functional state and the prevention of further injuries.
    A. Both statements are true
    B. Both statements are false
    C. The first statement is true; the second is false
    D. The first statement is false; the second is true

13. What does *PPE* stand for?
    A. Patient protective equipment
    B. Personal protective equipment
    C. Person protective equipment
    D. Procedure protection equipment

14. When it comes to occupational exposure risks, a QHCP should be experienced in which of the following?
    A. Conducting testing
    B. Providing antiretroviral therapy
    C. Being familiar with the unique nature of dental injuries
    D. All of the above

15. Risk management occurs when:
    A. You refuse to treat any patient with foreseeable risks
    B. You identify preventive methods to reduce or eliminate the risk of legal actions
    C. You sue the patient back if the patients sues you
    D. You make notes in the chart as general as possible so as to give the same treatment to every patient

16. Following exposure, if there is not enough time to get tested right away it is okay to use bleach to cleanse

CHAPTER REVIEW QUESTIONS

the exposure site. However, if you are able to get tested immediately then you should just use soap and water.

A. Both statements are true
B. Both statements are false
C. The first statement is true; the second is false
D. The first statement is false; the second is true

17. Communication, documentation, and risk reduction protocols are all necessary elements when administering a local anesthetic. This is because they help to reduce the chance of possible litigation.

A. Both the statement and the reason are true
B. Both the statement and the reason are false
C. The statement is true, but the reason is false
D. The statement is false, but the reason is true

18. The QHCP must take into consideration which of the following factors when determining the need for follow-up of occupational exposures?

A. Infectious state of source
B. Type and amount of tissue/fluid
C. Type of exposure
D. Susceptibility of exposed person
E. All of the above
F. None of the above.

19. When handling a contaminated needle it is only important to avoid being exposed to the end that penetrated the tissues or fluids. The cartridge-penetrating end of the needle is not a risk for contamination.

A. Both statements are true
B. Both statements are false
C. The first statement is true; the second is false
D. The first statement is false; the second is true

20. It is the responsibility of the dental hygienist to report any illegal activities regarding the administration of local anesthesia to the proper authorities as well as to educate the dentist about current regulations regarding the hygienist's scope of practice.

A. Both statements are true
B. Both statements are false
C. The first statement is true; the second is false
D. The first statement is false; the second is true

REFERENCES

1. Darby M, Walsh M: *Dental hygiene theory and practice*, ed 3, St Louis, 2010, Saunders.
2. Beemsterboer PL: *Ethics and law in dental hygiene*, ed 2, St Louis, 2010, Saunders.
3. Centers for Disease Control: www.cdc.org.
4. Pozgar GP: Legal and ethical issues for health professionals, ed 2, Sudbury, 2010, Jones and Bartlett.

GLOSSARY

A Fibers The largest nerve fibers; can be either motor or sensory.

Absolute contraindication The administration of the offending drug should not be administered to the individual under any circumstances.

Absolute refractory period The interval during which a second action potential absolutely cannot be initiated to restimulate the membrane, no matter how large a stimulus is applied.

Action potential Nerve impulse that generates an electronic signal to and from the central nervous system (CNS).

Adrenergic drugs Drugs that stimulate the adrenergic nerves directly by mimicking the action of norepinephrine or indirectly by stimulating the release of norepinephrine.

Afferent nerves Nerves that conduct signals from sensory neurons to the spinal cord or brain *(carry toward)*.

Allergens or antigens Noninfectious foreign substances that trigger hypersensitivity.

All or none principle The minimal threshold stimulus sends an impulse along the axon that travels the full length of the fiber without additional stimulus.

Amide A local anesthetic agent made from a specific class of chemical compounds that are generally broken down by the liver and are more effective and longer-lasting than esters. This type of anesthetic rarely causes allergic reactions.

Anastomosis/anastomoses Connecting channel(s) among the blood vessels.

Analgesic A drug that relieves pain.

Anesthetic A drug that produces loss of feeling or sensation generally or locally.

Anesthetic allergy Hypersensitivity to a local agent, which is fairly common with esters but rarely occurs with amides. Allergy to bisulfites in vasoconstrictors is common.

Anesthetic cartridge A capsule-like vessel containing the local anesthetic solution that is inserted into the syringe in preparation for an injection; older term is *carpule*.

Anion The base form of the local anesthetic (lipid soluble and penetrates the nerve).

Anterior middle superior alveolar (AMSA) block A type of injection that anesthetizes most of the maxillary teeth and their associated periodontium, as well as most of the facial and lingual gingival tissue in one quadrant.

Anterior superior alveolar block (ASA) A type of injection that anesthetizes the maxillary anterior teeth and associated structures when the local anesthetic agent is deposited superior to the apex of the maxillary canine.

Anesthesiologist A physician trained in the administration of anesthesia.

Armamentarium Local anesthetic supplies, materials, and devices needed to successfully administer a local anesthetic. More generally, the equipment, pharmaceuticals, and methods used in medicine.

Arteriole Smaller vessels of the artery.

Artery A component of the vascular system that arises from the heart, carrying blood away from it.

Articaine An intermediate amide local anesthetic metabolized in the blood, noted for its highly lipid characteristics.

ASA physical status classification American Society of Anesthesiologists' rating system is a uniform system to assess the patients physical state prior to selecting an anesthetic before surgery, and a mean to communicate between colleagues regarding a patients physical status.

Aspirate on two planes The procedure of rotating the barrel of the syringe 45 degrees and aspirating following the initial aspiration test to ensure that the bevel of the needle is not abutting a blood vessel and producing a false-negative aspiration.

Aspiration test Negative pressure placed on the anesthetic syringe before depositing the anesthetic to determine whether the tip of the needle rests within a blood vessel; observed by absence or entry of blood into the cartridge.

Atypical pseudocholinesterase A hereditary trait in which individuals are unable to hydrolyze ester local anesthetics and other chemically related drugs.

Autonomic nervous system (ANS) A control system (part of the peripheral nervous system) that helps people adapt to change in their environment, adjusting some functions in response to stress.

Axon Cable-like structure of neuron.

Axon Hillock Specialized part of the neuron that emerges from the soma and connects to the axon where membrane potentials are summated before being transmitted to the axon.

B Fibers Lightly myelinated motor nerve fibers with medium diameters.of < 3 μm.

Benzocaine A common ester topical anesthetic.

Bevel The angled surface of the needle tip.

Blanching A temporary whitening of the tissue due to the diffusion of anesthetic solution that decreases the bloodflow in the area.

Biotransformation The process by which the local anesthetic is altered within the body by the action of enzymes to produce a less toxic metabolite.

Biphasic A process that occurs in two phases.

Bradycardia Decreased heart rate.

Bradykinin A pain mediator produced during cellular injury.

Breech-loading The process of inserting the glass anesthetic cartridge into the syringe through the side of the barrel.

Buccal block Type of injection that anesthetizes the buccal soft tissue of the mandibular molars.

Bupivacaine A long-acting amide local anesthetic that is metabolized in the liver.

Butamben An ester topical anesthetic; often combined with other topicals for use.

C fibers Unmyelinated nerve fibers primarily responsible for dull, aching pain.

Cartridge Contains the sterile local anesthetic drug and other contents.

Catecholamine Sympathomimetic "fight-or-flight" hormones released by the adrenal glands.

Cation Ionized ion in local anesthetic solution.

Canal Opening in bone that is long, narrow, and tubelike.

Cell Body The nucleus-containing central part of a neuron exclusive of its axons and dendrites that is the major structural element of the gray matter of the brain and spinal cord, the ganglia, and the retina. Rresponsible for protein synthesis; provides metabolic support for the neuron.

Computer-controlled local anesthetic delivery device (CCLAD) A machine that controls the amount and rate of administered anesthetic.

Condyle Oval bony prominence, usually part of a joint.

Concomitant Drugs Having two or more drugs in the systemic circulation at the same time.

Capillary Smaller vessels of the arterioles that form a network.

Cation A positively charged ion, specifically the ionized portion of the anesthetic molecule that is acidic and water soluble. The active form of the molecule that binds to the receptor sites in the sodium channel.

Connective tissue A form of fibrous tissue.

Central fibers Nerve fibers that extend from the cell body toward the CNS.

Central nervous system (CNS) The structural and functional center of the nervous system that includes the brain and the spinal cord.

Cocaine An ester local anesthetic drug with addictive properties.

Complication An adverse reaction or event.

Concentration gradient A ratio of different substances (ions): extracellular versus intracellular in relation to nerve conduction.

Core bundles Fasciculi located in the core region (inner core).

Coronoid notch Concavity in the anterior border of the ramus; the landmark for the inferior alveolar injection.

Crossover innervation Overlap of terminal nerve fibers from the contralateral side.

Deflection The deviation in direction of the anesthetic needle from its intended path.

Demyelination Disease of nervous system in which the myelin sheath encompassing a neuron is damaged (e.g., multiple sclerosis).

Dental plexus A network of vessels or nerves.

Dental phobia Unfounded fear or morbid dread of dental treatment.

Dendriticzone The most distal section of the neuron that includes an arborization of nerve endings.

Depolarization The process whereby the action potential causes sodium channels to open, allowing an influx of sodium ions to change the electrochemical gradient, which in turn produces a further rise in the membrane potential.

Depth of needle penetration Needle depth covered in tissue when target area is reached.

Deposit location The target area where local anesthetic will be deposited.

Dialogue history Orally communicating with the patient to gain more information regarding the patient's medical status.

Diaphragm Semipermeable material located at the top of the cartridge where the needle is inserted into the center of the rubber.

Diaphoresis Excessive sweating

Dilution ratio The strength of vasoconstrictor drug per volume of solution expressed as milligrams per milliliter (mg/mL).

Dissociation constant (pK$_a$) The pH at which 50% of molecules exist in the lipid-soluble tertiary form and 50% in the quaternary, water-soluble form.

Drug concentration The strength of the local anesthetic agent in the cartridge expressed as a percentage.

Dyclonine hydrochloride A ketone topical anesthetic

Edema Abnormal accumulation of fluid beneath the skin causing swelling of the tissues, and describes a clinical complication.

Efferent nerves Nerves that conduct signals away from the brain or spinal cord (*carry away*).

Electrical potential The electrical charge across the nerve membrane.

Elimination The process by which the kidney removes the local anesthetic drug, primarily its metabolites, from the body.

Endogenous Originating or produced within an organism, tissue, or cell.

Endoneurium Connective tissue that surrounds each axon by a layer of connective tissue.

Engineering controls Devices or controls developed to provide safer administration of local anesthetics such as safety syringes, sharps disposal containers, recapping devices.

Esters Short-acting local anesthetic agents made from a specific class of chemical compounds that are broken down by blood enzymes. They are less effective than amide anesthetics and more likely to cause allergic reactions. These are no longer used as an injection in the United States but are still used as a topical agent.

Epinephrine Naturally occurring catecholamine secreted by the adrenal medulla.

Epineurium Connective tissue that wraps the entire nerve.

Eutectic mixtures A mixture of two elements that have a lower melting point than any of the individual components.

Exogenous Coming from outside the body.

Extracellular Outside the nerve membrane.

Fasciculi Nerve fibers bundled together into groups.

False-negative aspiration A perceived negative aspiration where the needle tip lies within a blood vessel and is butting up against the wall of the vessel, preventing the entrance of blood into the cartridge.

Felypressin A synthetic hormone analogue of vasopressin.

Field block A form of regional anesthesia that is deposited near large terminal nerve branches.

Fight or flight response The body's primitive, automatic, inborn response that prepares the body to "fight" or "flee" from perceived attack, harm, or threat to survival.

Finger grip Winged or wingless component of the syringe that allows the clinician to hold and control the syringe.

Foramen/foramina Short, window-like opening in bone.

Fossa/fossae Depression on a bony surface.

Gauge The diameter of the tubular lumen (channel) of the needle.

General supervision Refers to the idea that a dentist has authorized the procedures to be performed for a patient but a dentist need not be present when the procedures are performed.

Generic Drug A nonproprietary agent.

Glial cells Nonneuronal cells that maintain homeostasis, form myelin, and provide support and protection for the brain's neurons.

Gow Gates mandibular block A type of injection that anesthetizes most of the mandibular nerve.

Greater palatine nerve block A type of injection that anesthetizes the lingual soft tissue distal to the maxillary canine in one quadrant.

H₂ receptor antagonists A class of drugs used to block the action of histamine on parietal cells in the stomach, decreasing the production of acid by these cells.

Half-life of drug The period of time required to eliminate the amount of drug in the body by one-half of its strength.

Harpoon A sharp tip attached to the internal end of the piston of an aspirating syringe that embeds into the silicone rubber stopper, allowing retraction for an aspiration test.

Hematoma Swelling that develops when a blood vessel, particularly an artery, is punctured or lacerated by the needle.

Hemostat An instrument used in dentistry to retrieve small items, such as broken needles.

Hemostasis A complex process that changes blood from a fluid to a solid state.

Henderson-Hasselbach equation A formula that calculates the pH of a buffer solution or the concentration of acid versus base molecules in an anesthetic solution.

Hub A plastic or metal adaptor that provides a means to attach the needle to the syringe.

Human needs paradigm The relationship between human need fulfillment and human behavior.

Hyperresponders Individuals who overly respond to local anesthetics.

Hyporesponders Individuals who underrespond to local anesthetics.

Hydrophilic group A portion of a local anesthetic agent's chemical structure, with strong water-attracting properties that enable the diffusion of the agent through the water portions of the tissues to the final destination in the nerves. Typically described in opposition to the lipophilic portion of a local anesthetic agent.

Impulse A wave of physical and chemical excitation along a nerve fiber in response to a stimulus, accompanied by a change in electric potential in the membrane.

Incisive block A type of injection that anesthetizes the teeth and associated periodontium as well as facial soft tissue anterior to the mental foramen.

Indirect supervision A dentist must be physically on the premises where the dental hygienist is administering the local anesthetic.

Inferior alveolar block A type of injection that anesthetizes the mandibular teeth and their associated periodontium and lingual soft tissue to the midline.

Infiltration injection A type of injection that provides soft tissue anesthesia of the smaller terminal nerve endings only in the area of anesthetic deposition.

Informed consent Written agreement from the patient consenting to treatment following a discussion of the benefits and risks associated with the treatment.

Infraorbital nerve (IO) A type of injection that anesthetizes the maxillary anterior and premolar teeth and associated structures when the local anesthetic agent is deposited at the infraorbital foramen.

Intracellular A term meaning "within the nerve membrane."

Interpapillary injection An infiltration injection depositing a small volume of local anesthetic into the buccal or lingual papilla.

Intermediate chain linkage The connector between the lipophilic and hydrophilic portions of a local anesthetic agent's chemical structure. Local anesthetic agent's classification is performed on the basis of whether the intermediate chain is made up of an ester or an amide.

Ion channels Membrane protein complexes and that facilitate the diffusion of ions across nerve membranes.

Ionized Cationic form of molecule.

Jet injector Needleless syringe that delivers anesthesia to mucous membranes at high pressure.

Kilogram The base unit of mass in the International System used to calculate and record maximum recommended doses, 1 pound equals 2.2 kilograms.

Levonordefrin A synthetic catecholamine manufactured in the United States as a 2% mepivacaine, 1:20,000 levonordefrin solution.

Lidocaine An amide local anesthetic metabolized in the liver.

Limiting factor The drug that limits the total amount of volume of anesthetic delivered based upon the patient's medical status.

Line Straight, small ridge of bone.

Lipophilic group A portion of a local anesthetic agent's chemical structure, with its fat-attracting properties that enable the agent to pass through the lipid membrane of the tissues to reach the nerve destination. Typically described in opposition to the hydrophilic portion of the local anesthetic agent.

Localized complication A complication that occurs in the region of the injection.

Lumen The inner tubular (channel) area of an anesthetic needle.

Malignant hyperthermia An inherited syndrome triggered by exposure to certain drugs used for general anesthesia and the neuromuscular blocking agent succinylcholine.

Mantle bundles Fasciculi located in the mantle region (outer core).

Maximum recommended dose The highest amount of an anesthetic agent that can safely be administered without complication to a patient while maintaining efficacy.

Maxillary nerve Second division (V_2) from the sensory root of the trigeminal nerve.

Mandibular nerve Third division (V_3) of the trigeminal nerve.

Membrane expansion theory Theory that suggests that the local anesthetic agents that are highly lipid insert themselves into the lipid bilayer of the cell membrane affecting the nerve membrane.

Membrane potential The difference in voltage or electrical potential between the interior and exterior of a cell.

Mental block A type of injection that anesthetizes the facial soft tissue anterior to the mental foramen.

Mepivacaine An amide local anesthetic that provides short to intermediate duration and is metabolized in the liver.

Methemoglobinemia A rare hereditary condition characterized by the inability of the blood to bind to oxygen that deprives oxygen to be carried effectively to body tissues.

Methylparaben A bacteriostatic agent and preservative that was added to local anesthetics agents without vasoconstrictors before 1984 to prevent bacterial growth.

Middle superior alveolar block (MSA) A type of injection that anesthetizes the maxillary premolars, and the mesial buccal root of the maxillary first molar and associated structures when the local anesthetic agent is deposited superior to the apex of the maxillary second premolar.

Mild complication A minor problem that will resolve without requiring treatment.

Milligram A unit of mass equal to one one-thousandth (1/1000th) a gram. It is used to calculate and record the maximum recommended dose.

Milliliter A measure of volume equal to one one-thousandth (1/1000th) of a liter.

Myelinated nerve Lipoprotein sheath that almost completely insulates the axon from the outside.

Mucobuccal fold The fold located in the vestibule where the labial or buccal mucosa meets the alveolar mucosa.

Nasopalatine nerve block A type of injection that anesthetizes the lingual soft tissue between the maxillary right and left canines.

Needle adapter A threaded tip of the syringe that allows the attachment of the needle to the barrel of the syringe.

Needle insertion point The injection site where the bevel of the needle is covered with tissue.

Needle shields A cover that protects the needle that is inserted in the tissue, as well as the cartridge-penetrating end of the needle.

Needle track infection An infection that can be spread into deeper tissues along a needle pathway.

Negative aspiration A clear air bubble entering the cartridge, or no return, after negative pressure is applied to the cartridge.

Negative pressure Pressure produced when the thumb ring of a syringe is pulled back, causing retraction of the rubber stopper to produce an aspiration test.

Nerve The sensitive pulp of the tooth that contains many bundles of peripheral axons.

Nerve block An injection of local anesthetic in the vicinity of a major nerve trunk to anesthetize the nerve's area of innervations, usually at a distance from the area of treatment.

Nerve fiber Any of the processes (as an axon or a dendrite) of a neuron that is comprised of axon and myelin sheath.

Neuron Basic functional unit of the nervous system that manipulates information and responds to either excitation or inhibition.

Neurotransmitters Endogenous chemicals that transmit signals from a neuron to a target cell across a synapse.

Nociception The neural processes of encoding and processing noxious stimuli.

Nodes of Ranvier Uninsulated gaps formed between myelin sheaths covering axons, allowing for the generation of electrical activity.

Nonselective beta blockers A class of drugs used to treat hypertension and cardiac arrhythmias.

Norepinephrine Naturally occurring catecholamine affecting primarily α receptors.

Normal responder An individual who responds typically to the duration of local anesthesia.

Notch An indentation at the edge of a bone.

Noxious stimulus A mechanical, chemical, or thermal stimulus that can actually or potentially damage tissue.

Nurse anesthetist A nurse who specializes in the administration of anesthesia.

Occupational exposure A percutaneous injury (e.g., needlestick or cut with a sharp object) or contact of mucous membrane or nonintact skin (e.g., exposed skin that is chapped, abraded, or with dermatitis) with blood, saliva, tissue, or other body fluids that are potentially infectious.

Oligodendrocytes A brain cell responsible for insulating axons.

Ophthalmic nerve First (V_1) division of the sensory root of the trigeminal nerve.

Overdose An administration of local anesthetic that results in signs and symptoms of CNS and CVS depression.

Pain An unpleasant sensory and emotional experience

Pain control The mechanism to alleviate pain.

Pain threshold The point at which a sensation starts to be painful and discomfort results.

Pain perception Neurologic experience of pain that differs little between individuals.

Pain reaction Personal interpretation and response to pain message; highly variable among individuals.

Parasympathetic nervous system Coordinates the body's normal resting activities and is known as the "rest or digest" response.

Paresthesia Persistent anesthesia (anesthesia well beyond the expected duration) or altered sensation (tingling or itching) well beyond the expected duration of anesthesia.

Penetrating end The part of the needle shaft that passes through the hub and penetrates the rubber diaphragm of the cartridge.

Perineurium Connective tissue that wraps each fascicle.

Periodontal ligament injection A supplemental injection used when pulpal anesthesia is indicated on a single tooth mainly in the mandibular arch.

Peripheral fibers Nerve fibers that extend from the cell body away from the CNS.

Peripheral nervous system (PNS) Nerve tissues that lie in the periphery.

Permanent complication A problem that leaves a residual effect.

Piston A solid metallic cylinder of the anesthetic syringe attached to the thumb ring that displaces anesthetic solution when positive pressure is exerted on the thumb ring.

Pharmacodynamics The study of the physiologic effects of drugs on the body and the mechanisms of drug action and its relationship between drug concentration and effect.

Pharmacokinetics The study of the action of drugs within the body.

Phenylephrine A synthetic sympathomimetic amine that exerts its action predominately on α receptors.

Positive aspiration Blood entering the cartridge following an aspiration test, indicating the needle tip is within a blood vessel.

Posterior superior alveolar nerve (PSA) A type of injection that anesthetizes the maxillary molars and associated structures when the local anesthetic solution is deposited superior to the apex of the maxillary second molar and posterior and superior to posterior border of maxilla at posterior superior alveolar foramina.

Pressor An exaggerated increase in blood pressure.

Prilocaine An intermediate amide local anesthetic that is metabolized in the lungs and the liver.

Primary complication Experienced by the patient at the time of the injection.

Primary prevention Utilizing all standard protocols to prevent injury. g.

Procaine An ester local anesthetic that is no longer available for use in dentistry due to its allergic potential (more commonly known as Novacaine).

Process General term for any prominence on a bony surface.

Propagation The process by which an action potential leaps along myelinated axons.

Proprietary Drug A drug that has brand name that is protected by a patent.

Pterygomandibular raphe The fibrous structure that extends from the hamulus to the posterior end of the mylohyoid line and is used as a landmark for the inferior alveolar injection.

Qualified health care professional Designated qualified health care professional responsible for care and follow up of occupational exposures.

Relative contraindication A contraindication to a local anesthetic that allow the administration of the offending drug to be used judiciously (i.e., administration of a minimal effective dose).

Relative refractory period The interval immediately following the absolute refractory period and before complete reestablishment to the resting state, during which initiation of a second action potential is possible if a larger stimulus is achieved to produce successful firing.

Repolarization Occurs once the peak of the action potential is reached and the membrane potential begins to move back toward the resting potential (-70 mV). Results from efflux of K+ ions.

Resting state A neurologic term to describe the polarized nerve membrane receiving little or no stimulation.

Safety syringe A plastic disposable syringe that decreases the risk of accidental exposure to the clinician from contaminated needles.

Saltatory conduction The propagation of action potentials along myelinated axons from one node of Ranvier to the next node, increasing the conduction velocity of action potentials without needing to increase the diameter of an axon.

Schwann cells Glia cells of the peripheral nervous system (PNS).

Scoop technique A method to safely recap contaminated needles using one hand to scoop the needle into the needle shield.

Secondary complication Apparent after the injection is completed. The problem arises separately from and after an earlier complication.

Secondary prevention A prevention strategy following an injury to minimize its complications.

Severe complication A problem that requires a definite plan of treatment to resolve the issue.

Shaft The length of the needle comprised of long tubular metal.

Shank Shaft.

Silicone rubber stopper A piece of equipment located at the bottom of the anesthetic cartridge, where the harpoon is embedded.

Sodium bisulfite A preservative added by the manufacturer to a local anesthetic cartridge containing a vasoconstrictor to delay the oxidation of the vasoconstrictor. Metabisulfite and sodium bisulfite are the most commonly used antioxidants.

Soft tissue sloughing The loss of surface layers of epithelium due to the administration of topical anesthetics for extended periods, or anesthetic sterile abscesses developed by prolonged ischemia due to the inclusion of a vasoconstrictor in the anesthetic solution.

Somatic nervous system (SNS) Subdivision of the efferent division of the PNS and controls the body's voluntary and reflex activities through somatic sensory and somatic motor components.

Specific receptor theory The theory that explains the binding of local anesthetics to specific receptor sites on the sodium channel to prevent the depolarization phase of the nerve impulse generation.

Stress Physical and emotional responses to particular situations.

Sulfonamides Synthetic antimicrobial agents.

Supraperiosteal injection A form of regional anesthesia deposited near large terminal nerve branches providing pulpal and soft tissue anesthesia of a single tooth.

Surface anesthesia Anesthesia achieved by application of topical anesthetics to the mucosal surface by gels, creams, or sprays to block the free nerve endings.

Sympathetic nervous system Division of ANS that prepares the body to deal with an emergency situation; involved in the fight or flight response.

Sympathomimetic drugs Drugs that mimic the effects of the sympathetic nervous system.

Synapses The junctions of nerve cells.

Syncope Fainting; loss of consciousness resulting from insufficient bloodflow to the brain.

Syringe Metal devices used to administer local anesthetic drugs.

Syringe barrel The part of the local anesthetic syringe that holds the glass cartridge.

Systemic complications Complications that affect the entire body; attributed to the drug administered.

Topical anesthetic A drug applied to the surface of the skin or mucosal tissues that produces local insensibility to pain.

Topical anesthetic spray Application of an aerosol spray directly on the surface of a mucous membrane, resulting in loss of nerve conduction.

Topical antiseptic An antimicrobial substance applied to tissue to reduce the risk of infection.

Tachycardia Increased heart rate.

Tachyphylaxis Increased tolerance to a drug that is administered repeatedly.

Tertiary prevention Prevention strategy that strives to prevent disease progression, and to return patient to a functional state.

Tetracaine hydrochloride An ester anesthetic that is considered most potent and used only as a topical anesthetic.

Thumb ring A portion of the syringe that is attached to the external end of the piston, allowing the clinician to advance or retract the piston.

Topical anesthetic An anesthetic that is applied to the body surface such as the skin or mucous membrane.

Transdermal A route of administration, delivered across the skin.

Transient complication May appear severe at the time of its observance, but eventually resolves without any residual effect.

Transoral A route of administration, delivered via oral mucosa.

Tricyclic antidepressant Drugs used primarily to treat depression.

Trigeminal nerve Fifth cranial nerve.

Trismus Spasms of the muscles of mastication resulting in soreness and difficulty opening the mouth.

Tonic-clonic seizure A type of generalized seizure that affects the entire brain.

Tuberosity Large, often rough prominence on the surface of bone.

Unionized Anionic form of molecule.

Unmyelinated A nerve that contains no myelin sheath for protection.

Vasoconstrictor An agent added to local anesthetic solutions to delay the absorption of local anesthetics.

Vasopressor Synonym for vasoconstrictor.

Vein Component of the vascular system that carries blood to the heart.

Venous sinuses Blood-filled spaces between the two layers of tissue.

Visual Analog Scale (VAS) A measurement instrument to measure pain.

INDEX

Page numbers followed by "f" indicate figures, "t" indicate tables, and "b" indicate boxes.